First Aid and Emergency Care Workbook

First Aid and Emergency Care Workbook

Alton L. Thygerson
Brigham Young University

Produced in cooperation with the

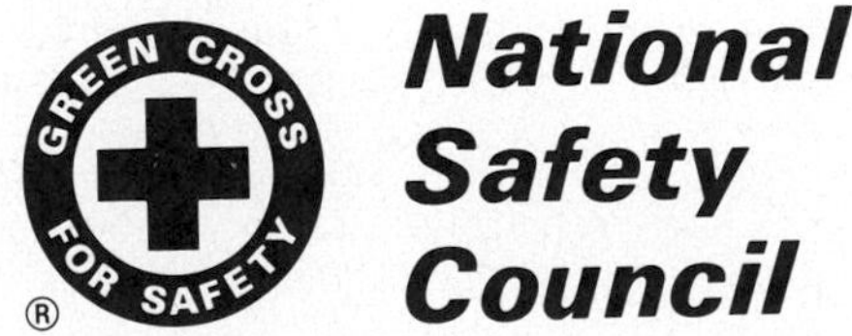

JONES AND BARTLETT PUBLISHERS, INC.
BOSTON PORTOLA VALLEY

Editorial offices: Jones and Bartlett Publishers, Inc.
30 Granada Court, Portola Valley, CA 94025

Sales and customer service offices:
Jones and Bartlett Publishers, Inc.
20 Park Plaza, Boston, MA 02116

Library of Congress Cataloging-in-Publication Data

Thygerson, Alton L.
First aid and emergency care workbook.

Includes index.
1. First aid in illness and injury. 2. Medical emergencies. I. Title. [DNLM: 1. Emergencies. 2. First aid. WA 292 T549fa]
RC86.7.T468 1987 616'.025 86-27771

ISBN 0-86720-071-5

Typing and Word Processing: Sherry I. Littler
Copy Editor: Margaret E. Hill
Illustrator: Chris Young
Illustrator of Flow Charts: Greg Kyle
Text Design: Rafael Millán
Front Cover Art and Cover Design: Vanessa Piñeiro
Typesetting: Delmas Typesetting

Printed in the United States of America

10 9 8 7 6 5 4 3 2

The first aid and emergency care procedures in this book are based on the most current recommendations of responsible medical sources. The author, the publisher, and the National Safety Council, however, make no guaranty as to, and assume no responsibility for, the correctness, sufficiency or completeness of such information or recommendations. Other or additional safety measures may be required under particular circumstances.

Preface

Everyone will be faced with situations involving injury and sudden illness. Therefore, everyone should be prepared to give first aid and emergency care. *First Aid and Emergency Care Workbook* is a unique book that has been produced in cooperation with the National Safety Council to help in such preparation.

Special features include:

• CONTENT: Up-to-date, accurate, concise first aid information backed by medical literature.

- 1986 Standards and Guidelines for Cardiopulmonary Resuscitation (CPR) and Emergency Cardiac Care (ECC) from the American Heart Association. Performance Sheets are also included.
- Hypothermia and Cold Water Near Drowning Guidelines from the State of Alaska
- Regional Poison Control Centers meeting the certification criteria of the American Association of Poison Control Centers
- First Aid for Epilepsy from the Epilepsy Foundation of America
- Dental Emergency Procedures from the American Dental Association
- Eye Injuries First Aid from the American Academy of Ophthalmology
- Diabetic Emergency Information from the American Diabetes Association

• FLOW CHARTS: Depict decision-making and appropriate first aid procedures. They also serve as a quick review.

• FULL COLOR ILLUSTRATIONS: Dramatic illustrations of many of the injuries discussed and likely to be seen by a first aider.

• LINE DRAWINGS: Show appropriate first aid techniques for bandaging, splinting, rescues, and more.

• TABLES: Important information in table form serves as a reference.

• LEARNING ACTIVITIES: Self-tests to evaluate one's understanding of key first aid concepts. Case situations offer opportunity to apply one's knowledge.

• PATIENT EDUCATION AIDS: Reprints of doctor-to-patient instructions for self-care from the popular physician journal, *Patient Care.*

• GLOSSARY: A collection of first aid terms with their meanings.

• QUICK REFERENCE INDEX: Aids the reader in finding what is wanted.

The National Safety Council's contribution to this Workbook has been invaluable, as the Council is recognized around the world as one of the most reliable sources of information pertaining to accidental injury.

TO THE INSTRUCTOR

First Aid and Emergency Care Workbook is the cornerstone of a comprehensive first aid teaching package. This seven-part package is designed to aid the instructor and to challenge, motivate and reinforce first aid and emergency care procedures and concepts for the student. The perforated pages and workbook format ensure active student involvement and enhanced learning in this very important course. In addition to the text, the package includes:

• *Instructor's Resource Manual* - containing answers to all end-of-chapter tests and cases, as well as a variety of teaching aids and suggestions.

• *Instructor's Test Bank* - containing over 700 multiple choice test questions of varying difficulty that correspond to the text chapter-by-chapter.

• *Trauma Slide Series* - containing over 100 color slides of various injuries.

• *Workbook Slide Series* - containing 54 color slides corresponding to the color photographs in the text.

• *Instructor's Acetate Transparency Set* - containing 54 acetate transparencies corresponding to the flow charts in the text.

• *First Aid and Emergency Care Film Series* - a collection of educational films on the subject.

Further information on this teaching package is available by contacting the publisher.

Alton Thygerson

Acknowledgments

The author gratefully acknowledges the following for permission to use some of their material in this text:

American Academy of Ophthalmology
American Association of Poison Control Centers
American Dental Association
American Diabetes Association
American Heart Association
Epilepsy Foundation of America
Patient Care Communications, Inc., 16 Thorndal Circle, Darien, CT 06820
RN, the full-service nursing journal (Medical Economics Company, Inc.)
State of Alaska, Department of Health and Social Services

Full Color Illustrations:

Bruce Argyle, M.D.
H.B. Bectal, M.D.
Michael D. Ellis, ed., *Dangerous Plants, Snakes, Arthropods and Marine Life—Toxicity and Treatment* (Hamilton, IL: Drug Intelligence Publications, Inc.)
Fitnus® for Life (© Algra, Inc.), 3125 19th Street, Suite 305, Bakersfield, CA 93301
Murray P. Hamlet, D.V.M.
Axel W. Hoke, M.D.
Sherman A. Minton, M.D.
Eugene Robertson, M.D.
Richard C. Ruffalo, D.M.D.
Jeffrey Saffle, M.D.
Clifford C. Snyder, M.D.
U.S. Department of Transportation

The author also wishes to acknowledge Jems Publishing Company, Inc., with special thanks to Jim Page and Gary R. Williams for their contribution of *Emergency First Aid Videotape*.

Jems Publishing Company, Inc.
P.O. Box 1026
215 South Highway 101, Suite 100
Solana Beach, CA 92075
(619) 481-1128

CONTENTS

1. **INTRODUCTION**
   Injury: Magnitude of the Problem **1**
   Need for First Aid Training **2**
   Legal Aspects of First Aid **2**
   Learning Activities **5**

2. **VICTIM ASSESSMENT**
   Physical Examination **8**
   History-Taking **8**
   Vital Signs **9**
   Head-to-Toe Examination **10**
   Triage **13**
   Learning Activities **15**

3. **BASIC LIFE SUPPORT**
   The 1986 Cardiopulmonary Resuscitation (CPR) Guidelines from the American Heart Association **18**
   Adult **18**
   Pediatric **32**
   Learning Activities **41**
   CPR and ECC Performance Sheets:
   - One-Rescuer CPR: Adult **47**
   - One-Rescuer CPR: Child **49**
   - One-Rescuer CPR: Infant **51**
   - Obstructed Airway: Conscious Adult **53**
   - Obstructed Airway: Conscious Child **55**
   - Obstructed Airway: Conscious Infant **57**
   - Obstructed Airway: Unconscious Adult **59**
   - Obstructed Airway: Unconscious Child **61**
   - Obstructed Airway: Unconscious Infant **63**

4. **SHOCK**
   Shock Due to Injury (Hypovolemic) **65**
   Anaphylactic Shock (Allergic Reaction) **66**
   Fainting **67**
   Flow Chart: Allergic Reaction **69**
   Flow Chart: Shock (Traumatic) **70**
   Flow Chart: Fainting **71**
   Learning Activities **73**

5. **BLEEDING**
   Types of External Bleeding **77**
   Types of Wounds **79**
   Wounds Requiring Medical Attention **81**
   Infection **83**
   Tetanus **84**
   Amputation **84**
   Animal Bites **85**
   Flow Chart: Bleeding Control **87**
   Flow Chart: Amputation **88**
   Flow Chart: Animal Bites **89**
   Learning Activities **91**

6. **SPECIFIC BODY AREA INJURIES**
   Head Injuries **95**
   Eye Injuries **97**
   Nosebleeds **98**
   Dental Emergencies **100**
   Larynx Injuries **100**
   Chest Injuries **101**
   Abdominal Injuries **102**
   Foreign Objects **103**
   Hand and Finger Injuries **106**
   Blisters **108**
   Flow Chart: Head Injury **111**
   Flow Chart: Eye Injuries **112**
   Flow Chart: Nosebleeds **113**
   Flow Chart: Tooth Injury **114**
   Flow Chart: Larynx Injuries **115**
   Flow Chart: Chest Injuries **116**
   Flow Chart: Abdominal Injuries **117**
   Flow Chart: Object in Nose **118**
   Flow Chart: Object in Ear **119**
   Flow Chart: Fishhook Removal **120**
   Flow Chart: Blisters **121**
   Learning Activities **123**

7. **POISONING**
   Poisoning by Ingestion **127**
   Insect Stings **134**
   Snakebites **136**
   Spider Bites **138**
   Scorpion Stings **139**
   Tick Removal **139**
   Poison Ivy, Sumac, and Oak **140**
   Carbon Monoxide **142**
   Marine Animal Injuries **143**
   Alcohol **143**
   Drugs **143**
   Flow Chart: Poisoning (Ingestion) **145**
   Flow Chart: Poisoning (Inhaled) **146**

Flow Chart: Insect Stings (Flying Insects) 147
Flow Chart: Snakebite 148
Flow Chart: Spider Bites and Scorpion Stings 149
Flow Chart: Tick Removal 150
Flow Chart: Poison Ivy, Oak, and Sumac 151
Learning Activities 153

8. BURNS
Thermal Burns 163
Sunburn 166
Chemical Burns 167
Electrical Burns 167
Flow Chart: Thermal Burns 169
Flow Chart: Chemical Burns 170
Flow Chart: Electrical Burns 171
Learning Activities 173

9. EXPOSURE TO COLD AND HEAT
Frostbite 177
Hypothermia 180
Heat-Related Emergencies 181
Flow Chart: Frostbite 184
Flow Chart: Hypothermia 185
Flow Chart: Cold Water Drowning 186
Flow Chart: Heat-Related Injuries 187
Learning Activities 189

10. BONE, JOINT, AND MUSCLE INJURIES
Fractures 194
Spinal Injuries 196
Joint Injuries 197
Muscle Injuries 201
Flow Chart: Fractures 203
Flow Chart: Spinal Injury 204
Flow Chart: Shoulder Injuries 205
Flow Chart: Knee Injuries 206
Flow Chart: Ankle Injuries 207
Flow Chart: Muscle Injuries 208
Flow Chart: Sprains, Strains, Contusions, Dislocations 209
Learning Activities 211

11. MEDICAL EMERGENCIES
Heart Attack 217
Stroke 219
Diabetic Emergencies 220
Epilepsy 222
Asthma 224
Abdomen Pain 225
Constipation 226
Cough 227
Diarrhea 228
Earache 228
Fever 229
Headache 231
Sore Throat 231
Vomiting 232
Hyperventilation 233
Bleeding (Respiratory and Digestive Tracts) 233
Flow Chart: Heart Attack 236
Flow Chart: Stroke 237
Flow Chart: Diabetic Emergencies 238
Flow Chart: Seizures 239
Flow Chart: Asthma 240
Flow Chart: Abdominal Pain 241
Flow Chart: Constipation 242
Flow Chart: Coughing 243
Flow Chart: Diarrhea 244
Flow Chart: Earache 245
Flow Chart: Fever 246
Flow Chart: Headache 247
Flow Chart: Sore Throat 248
Flow Chart: Vomiting 249
Flow Chart: Hyperventilation 250
Learning Activities 251

12. EMERGENCY CHILDBIRTH
Emergency Childbirth Procedures from the nursing journal *RN* 263
Flow Chart: Emergency Childbirth 269
Learning Activities 271

13. FIRST AID SKILLS
Bandaging 275
Splinting 282

14. MOVING AND RESCUING VICTIMS
Emergency Moves 289
Nonemergency Moves 290
Water Rescue 295

15. MEDICINE CHEST AND FIRST AID SUPPLIES
Medicine Chest 299
First Aid Supplies 300

16. PATIENT EDUCATION AIDS
Reprints from the physician journal, *Patient Care:*
"Helping your wound heal" 303
"Head injury instructions" 304
"Protecting yourself against bee stings" 305
"Tips for protecting yourself against ticks" 306
"How to identify poison ivy, poison oak, and poison sumac" 307
"Tips for safeguarding your family from plant poisoning"308
"Questions and answers about carbon monoxide poisoning" 310

"Tips for protecting yourself against sunburn" **312**
'First aid for burns" **313**
"Caring for a burn injury at home" **315**
"How to avoid frostbite" **316**
"What you should know about hypothermia" **318**
"Understanding and treating heat disorders" **319**
"Recognizing heart attack" **321**
"Understanding stroke" **322**
"Understanding diabetic emergencies" **324**
"Questions and answers about epilepsy" **326**
"First aid for epileptic seizures" **328**
"Questions and answers about asthma" **329**
"Helpful hints for controlling asthma" **331**
"Constipation" **332**
"Home care for diarrhea" **333**
"Tips for managing diarrhea while traveling" **334**
"How to take your child's temperature" **336**
"When your child has a fever" **340**
"Questions and answers about sore throat" **341**
"Facts about the common cold" **343**

GLOSSARY 345

CROSS REFERENCE TABLE FOR THE AMERICAN RED CROSS HANDBOOKS

Thygerson, *First Aid and Emergency Care Workbook* © '87	**ARC,** *Standard First Aid And Personal Safety* © '79	**ARC,** *Advanced First Aid and Emergency Care* © '79
Chapter 1	Chapter 1, pp. 11-13	Chapter 1, pp. 17-20
Chapter 2	Chapter 1, pp. 13-17	Chapter 1, pp. 20-23
Chapter 3	Chapter 5, pp. 66-94	Chapter 5, pp. 65-83 Chapter 6, pp. 84-94
Chapter 4	Chapter 4, pp. 60-65	Chapter 4, pp. 59-64
Chapter 5	Chapter 2, pp. 18-44	Chapter 2, pp. 24-45
Chapter 6	Chapter 3, pp. 45-59	Chapter 3, pp. 46-58
Chapter 7	Chapter 7, pp. 99-125 Chapter 8, pp. 126-143	Chapter 7, pp. 99-117 Chapter 8, pp. 118-133
Chapter 8	Chapter 9, pp. 144-159	Chapter 9, pp. 134-144
Chapter 9	Chapter 10, pp. 160-165 Chapter 11, pp. 166-169	Chapter 11, pp. 147-150 Chapter 12, pp. 151-154
Chapter 10	Chapter 14, pp. 195-224	Chapter 13, pp. 155-201
Chapter 11	Chapter 12, pp. 170-176	Chapter 15, pp. 225-246
Chapter 12		Chapter 16, pp. 147-253
Chapter 13	Chapter 13, pp. 177-194 Chapter 14, pp. 200-218	Chapter 14, pp. 202-223 Chapter 13, pp. 161-201
Chapter 14	Chapter 15, pp. 225-253	Chapter 17, pp. 254-284 Chapter 18, pp. 285-301 Chapter 6, pp. 91-94
Chapter 15	Chapter 13, pp. 192-194	Chapter 14, pp. 223-224
Chapter 16		

1 Introduction

- Injury: Magnitude of the Problem
- Need for First Aid Training
- Legal Aspects of First Aid

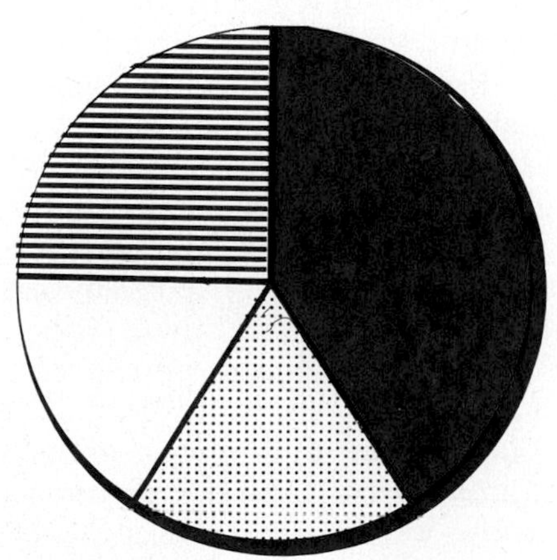

Heart Disease, 16.4%

Cancers, 18.0%

Injury, 40.8%

All other diseases, 24.8%

1-1. Percentages of years of potential life lost to injury, cancer, heart disease, and other diseases before age 65. Modified from Centers for Disease Control.

INJURY: MAGNITUDE OF THE PROBLEM*

Injuries are the most serious public health problem. Injuries are the leading cause of death and disability in children and young adults. They destroy the health, lives, and livelihoods of millions of people, yet they receive scant attention, compared with diseases and other hazards.

- Each year, more than 140,000 Americans die from injuries, and one person in three suffers a nonfatal injury.
- Injury is the last major plague of the young. Injuries kill more Americans aged 1–34 than all diseases combined, and they are the leading cause of death up to the age of 44.
- Preceded by heart disease, cancer, and stroke, injury is the fourth leading cause of death among all Americans.
- Injuries cause the loss of more working years of life than all forms of cancer and heart disease combined. See Figure 1-1.
- One of every eight hospital beds is occupied by an injured patient.
- Every year, more than 80,000 Americans join the ranks of those with unnecessary, but permanently disabling, injury of the brain or spinal cord.
- Injuries constitute one of our most expensive health problems, costing $75-$100 billion a year directly and indirectly.
- Injury is the leading cause of physician contacts. And more than 25% of hospital emergency room visits are for the treatment of injuries.

---

*Committee on Trauma Research of the National Research Council and the Institute of Medicine, *Injury in America: A Continuing Public Health Problem* (Washington, D.C.: National Academy Press, 1985).

NEED FOR FIRST AID TRAINING

The medical treatment of injury has a long history. Descriptions of treatments of 48 cases of head and foot injuries appear on papyrus dating to approximately 1600 B.C. In approximately 400 B.C., Hippocrates studied wounds and fractures and suggested causes of injury and methods of treatment. Most early physicians spent much time managing wounds that occurred in civilian life and in warfare.

With the size and magnitude of the injury problem, everyone must expect sooner or later to be on hand when an injury or sudden illness strikes. The outcome of such misfortune frequently depends not only on the severity of the injury or illness, but on the first aid rendered. Therefore, first aid knowledge and skills are essential in our society. Every person should be trained in first aid.

First aid is the immediate care given to an injured or suddenly ill person. First aid does not take the place of proper medical treatment. It consists only of furnishing temporary assistance until competent medical care, if needed, is obtained, or until the prognosis for recovery without medical care is assured. Remember that most injuries and illness are corrected with only first aid care.

A knowledge of first aid, when properly applied, may mean the difference between life and death, rapid recovery and long hospitalization, or temporary disability and permanent injury.

LEGAL ASPECTS OF FIRST AID

Duty to Act

No one is required to render aid when no legal duty to do so exists. For example, even a physician could ignore a stranger suffering a heart attack or a fractured bone. There may be moral obligations, but this is not always the same as a legal obligation to render aid.

Duty to act may occur in the following situations:

1. When under a contractual duty. In other words, if a preexisting relationship exists between two people (e.g., teacher-student, physician-patient, parent-child, lifeguard-swimmer, driver-passenger), there is a duty to render first aid.
2. When beginning first aid. Once you start first aid, you cannot stop. Duty to give first aid is usually questioned only when a person fails to act.

Obtain Consent

First aiders should obtain the victim's consent to receive first aid or they may risk incurring charges of technical assault and battery.

- Consent should be an informed consent. Oral consent is valid. The victim must understand that you are a first aider.
- Consent should be obtained from every conscious, mentally competent adult.
- Consent is implied for emergency lifesaving first aid to the unconscious victim.
- Consent should be obtained from the parent or guardian of a victim who is a child, or of one who is an adult but is mentally incompetent. If a parent or guardian is not available, emergency first aid to maintain life may be given without consent.
- Psychiatric emergencies present difficult problems of consent. Under most conditions, a police officer is the only person with the authority to restrain and transport a person against that individual's will. However, if the victim is not violent, the situation is similar to that for minors.

Abandonment

First aiders must remain with the victim until the victim is under the supervision of others of equal or greater competence, or until the victim refuses treatment and transportation. This may seem like an obvious requirement, but there have been cases where critically ill or injured victims were left.

The Right to Refuse Care

A perplexing problem is that of the conscious, rational, adult victim who is suffering from an actual or potential life-threatening injury or illness, but who refuses treatment or transportation. In such a situation, you should make every reasonable effort to convince the victim, or anyone who can influence the victim, to accept first aid and/or transportation. When a victim refuses to consent, you may not give first aid or transport the victim.

Should consent be refused, you should document this refusal on paper. Attempt to obtain the victim's signature and that of an impartial witness. It is hazardous to attempt to force the victim to submit to first aid; those who do may be subject to suits for assault.

Parent Refusing Permission to Help a Child

Very rarely will a first aider encounter a parent who refuses permission—usually on moral, ethical, or religious grounds—to care for a seriously injured or ill child. When a parent refuses permission to treat a child, every effort must be made to convince the parent of the seriousness of the problem and the necessity of the first aid. If you do not succeed, you should summon the police.

The Intoxicated or Belligerent Victim

As a first aider, you may encounter people who are in some stage of drug or alcohol intoxication and are injured. If an intoxicated victim refuses treatment, make every effort to persuade the individual to consent to first aid care. If refused, make sure to document the situation and attempt to have it signed by the victim and by an impartial witness.

If the intoxicated person consents to first aid, take the greatest possible care. Alcohol or drugs may mask vital symptoms, so that the seriously injured may also have a higher-than-average risk of death or disability.

Many first aiders may be repulsed by the intoxicated victim's appearance or attitude. If such is the case, you may overlook important symptoms that could be vital.

Good Samaritan Laws

Starting in the early 1960s, a number of states enacted statutes that were designed to provide freedom from liability to individuals who stopped and helped at the scene of an emergency. There are notable differences in the range of these laws among different states. First aiders are covered by a Good Samaritan law in some states, but this is not the situation in most cases. Some state laws cover only physicians and nurses, or only automobile accidents. It is recommended that you look carefully at your state law. Volunteer first aid personnel are usually given protection because there is no profit or expectation of payment involved.

The intention behind the Good Samaritan laws is good, but the results have not been. In fact, these laws are subject to serious constitutional questions that (in the judgment of some experts) may result in their being declared unconstitutional.

The Good Samaritan legislation only protects those acting in good faith and without gross negligence or willful misconduct. Accordingly, it is easy to sidestep any Good Samaritan legislation—all one has to do is allege that the first aider was negligent or malicious or did not act in good faith.

Many legal experts believe that the main effect of the Good Samaritan legislation has been to create a false sense of security in the minds of first aiders and health care professionals.

Statistics

LEARNING ACTIVITIES

Directions: In the left column list your estimate of the appropriate information. Your estimate should be for the entire United States for a period of one year. After you have completed your estimate, fill in the right column with information from your instructor or the National Safety Council's annual publication, *Accident Facts.*

	Estimate	*The Facts*
1. Annual number of deaths from all causes	________	________
2. Annual number of accidental deaths	________	________
3. Annual number of disabling injuries	________	________
4. The 4 leading causes of death	a ________	a ________
	b ________	b ________
	c ________	c ________
	d ________	d ________
5. The 6 leading causes of accidental death	a ________	a ________
	b ________	b ________
	c ________	c ________
	d ________	d ________
	e ________	e ________
	f ________	f ________
6. The two most dangerous regions for accidents in the United States	1 ________	1 ________
	2 ________	2 ________
7. Sex of most accident victims	________	________
8. Age group of most accident victims	________	________
9. Most accidental deaths occur in motor vehicles. Where do most injuries occur?	________	________
10. Day of the week on which accidental deaths and injuries occur most frequently	________	________
11. Months of the year in which accidental deaths and injuries occur most frequently	________	________

HOW TO GET QUICK EMERGENCY HELP*

To receive the best emergency medical help fast, you should keep a list of the following phone numbers near your telephone. If you have no such list, clip this section from the book and write in the appropriate phone numbers.

In many communities, to receive emergency assistance of every kind you just dial 911. Check to see if this is true in your community.

1. The Rescue Squad ____________________
Often part of the local fire department, these specially trained paramedics are likely to respond swiftly and competently.

2. The Police ____________________
They may or may not be able to respond with medically trained personnel, however, they can get someone to the hospital quickly.

3. Ambulance Service ____________________
Some services have trained paramedics; others do not.

4. Your Doctor ____________________
Your own doctor may not be available, but he or she should be alerted if an emergency has occurred.

5. Poison Control Center ____________________
In some communities, this service will give information to doctors only. Call before an emergency occurs to find out.

*Adapted from Consumer's Union, *Consumer's Reports.*

Give the following information over the phone:

1. *The victim's location.* Give city or town, street name, and street number. If calling at night, describe the building. This is probably the single most important piece of information.

2. *What has happened?* Tell the nature of the emergency—woman is bleeding badly, child has fallen and is unconscious, man has had a heart attack, and so on.

3. *Identify yourself.* Give your name. If it is different from the name of the homeowner or the apartment dweller, give that person's name as well.

4. *Give your phone number.* This information is required not only to help prevent false calls but, more important, to allow the center to call back for additional information.

5. *Tell them if they will need extra help.* Tell them if the victim is overweight, if there are several flights of stairs and no elevator, number of people involved, and so on.

6. *Ask for questions and advice.* Let the person on the other end of the line ask you questions and tell you what to do until help arrives.

7. *Always be the last to hang up the phone.* The police, ambulance, or fire department may need to ask more questions about how to find you. They may also tell you what to do until help arrives.

8. *Speak slowly and clearly.* Shouting is difficult to understand.

2 Victim Assessment

- Physical Examination
- History-Taking
- Vital Signs
- Head-to-Toe Examination
- Triage

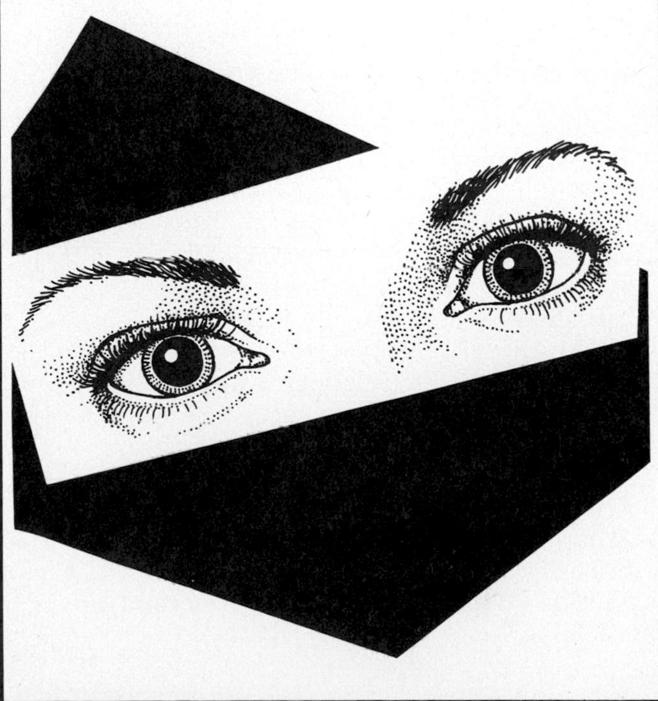

Examining a victim is essential to determine the extent of a victim's injury and/or illness in order to provide adequate emergency care. Such exams are, however, subject to error; and treatment, whether by a first aider or a physician, should not be founded upon the results of a single examination. Any examination that could affect someone must be repeated at least twice before it can be considered valid. Exception to this "two-time test rule" naturally occurs when a life threatening situation exists and time is crucial.

Injury victims, conscious or unconscious, should always be surveyed. Injury victims may have obvious as well as not-so-obvious injuries. Every unconscious person should also be examined, regardless of whether coma has been produced by injury or illness.

To find out the needs of an injured or suddenly ill person, first you must ask important questions and then examine the person carefully. You should look for signs and symptoms that help you tell how the person is and what kind of problem he or she may have.

There are certain basic things to ask and to look for in anyone who is sick or injured. Certainly, those with extensive experience in the field of emergency care may have their preferences as to what to ask and what to look for. However, the intent is to focus on the basics which are pertinent to the first aider level. The things the victim feels or reports (symptoms), as well as things you notice on examining him (signs), are the basics of a victim examination. Signs can be especially important in victims unable to talk.

A victim assessment has the following purposes:

- Gain the victim's confidence and thereby relieve some of the victim's anxiety due to discomfort and pain.
- Identify the victim's problem(s) and establish which problem(s) require immediate first aid.

• Obtain information about the victim that may not be readily available later in the hospital but could be useful to the attending medical personnel.

The information a first aider gains through a victim assessment depends largely on the way in which these procedures are performed. Victim assessment must be unhurried and systematic; a hasty approach always leads to omissions.

Urgent first aid may be required before you can stop to ask questions or perform a thorough examination, as in the case of a victim with an obstructed airway.

PHYSICAL EXAMINATION

The physical examination of either an injured victim or a medically ill victim is divided into two steps:

- Primary survey
- Secondary survey

Physical assessment begins with the primary survey, which covers the following areas:

A—Airway
B—Breathing
C—Circulation
H—Hemorrhage

The primary survey is the first step in the first aider's assessment of the victim and always takes precedence over all other aspects of the physical examination. Many times the primary survey will be completed in short order: when, for example, you encounter the alert victim with medical problems. Other times, however, close examination will be required to accomplish the primary survey: when the victim, for example, is unconscious or suffering from a major injury. If the primary survey uncovers any findings, such as an obstructed airway or massive bleeding, you must attend immediately to those injuries before proceeding with the victim assessment.

Having completed the primary survey and attended to any problems it uncovers, take a closer look at the victim and make a systematic examination from head to toe. This examination is called the secondary survey.

The secondary survey is done to discover problems that do not pose an immediate threat to life but may do so if they remain uncorrected. The secondary survey has three parts:

- History-taking
- Vital signs
- Head-to-toe examination

HISTORY-TAKING

History-taking begins as soon as you see the victim; before asking a single question, evaluate the victim's environment. History-taking may involve the victim, the victim's family, and bystanders. In general, if the victim is able to communicate, it is best to question him or her rather than the others. The victim is thus reassured that he or she is the center of interest. If you need to question others, do so one at a time.

When taking a history, obtain the victim's chief complaint—the problem that prompted the need for help. Often, it will be obvious; for example, the man who lies bleeding in the street after being struck by an automobile. However, there may be unexpected findings. The victim may have an obvious fracture of the left leg, and yet his chief complaint may be, "I can't breathe." Most chief complaints are characterized by pain, abnormal function, some change from a normal state, or an observation made by the victim.

After finding out about the chief complaint, obtain any pertinent information about the victim's past medical history that relates to the current problem. It is, for example, not especially relevant to learn whether the victim underwent a hernia operation five years earlier or had measles as a child ,when the problem is a second-degree burn over the back of the victim's body. In general, you will want to determine the following:

• Does the victim have any major underlying medical problems (for example, diabetes or serious condition that has required a doctor's care)?

• Does the victim take any medication regularly? If so, what are they? Medications may give important clues to a victim's underlying condition.

• Does the victim have known allergies?

Two mnemonic devices might help you identify the victim's problem: taking a S-A-M-P-L-E history and P-A-I-N.

*S*ymptoms (chief complaint)
*A*llergies
*M*edications
*P*revious illnesses (relating to the problem)
*L*ast meal (in case of surgery)
*E*vents prior to emergency

*P*eriod of pain (How long? What started it?)
*A*rea (Where?)
*I*ntensity
*N*ullify (What stops it? Rest, a certain position, medication?)

VITAL SIGNS

Pulse

A fingertip held over an artery where it either crosses a bone or lies close to the skin surface can easily feel characteristic pulsations as the pressure wave of blood causes the vessel wall to expand; hence the term pulse. Do not use your thumb to feel for the pulse—it has its own pulse.

The pulse rate can be determined at a number of points throughout the body, but the usual method is to palpate the radial point at the wrist (*see* Figure 2-1) or use the carotid point (*see* Figure 2-2) at the neck if you cannot feel the radial pulse. Do not palpate both carotid arteries at the same time. Pulsations are usually visible at the carotid artery in a victim lying down; pulsations disappear as the victim is elevated to a sitting position (usually a 45°angle). Never put too much pressure or massage the carotid, especially in victims who have had a heart attack—the heart's electrical conduction system may be disturbed.

Normal pulse at rest for adults is from 60 to 80 beats per minute. (Refer to Table 2-1.) For children, it is 80 to 100; and for babies, it is 100 to 140 beats per minute. As a general rule, the pulse increases 20 beats per minute for each degree rise in fever.

Respiration

The only concern for respiration during a primary survey is that the victim is breathing through an unobstructed airway. In the secondary survey, you should be concerned with the rate of respirations.

Count the number of breaths per minute. Between 12 and 20 breaths per minute is normal for adults and older children. Up to 30 breaths per minute is normal for children, and 40 is normal for babies.

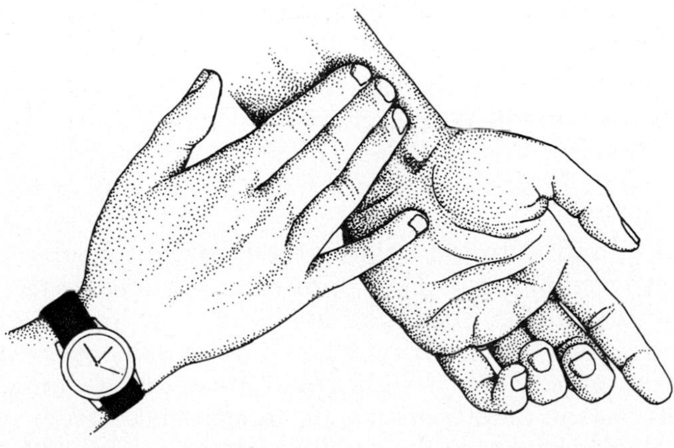

2-1. Palpating the radial pulse

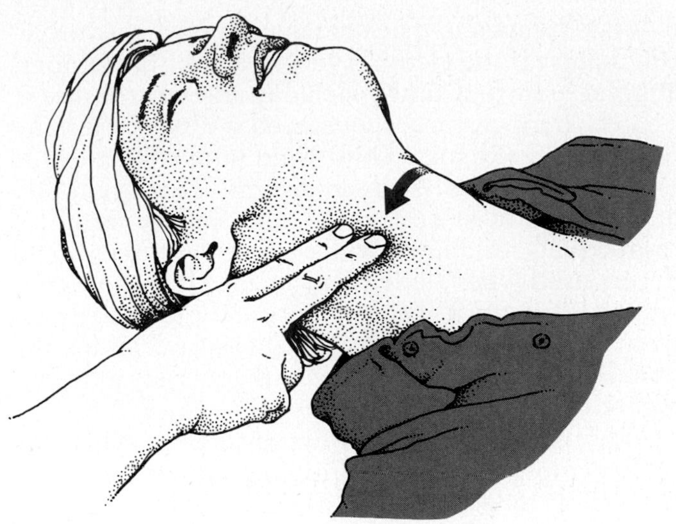

2-2. Palpating the carotid pulse

As you determine the rate of respirations, also listen for sounds, for example,

- A whistle or wheeze and difficulty breathing out can mean asthma.
- A gurgling or snoring noise and difficult breathing in an unconscious person may mean the tongue, mucus, or something else is stuck in the throat and does not let enough air get through.

Temperature

Body temperature measurement is important, as in cases of heat stroke or high fever. It is often wise to take a victim's temperature, even if he or she does not seem to have a fever.

Body temperature is often recorded when a person cannot receive medical care for some time, as in a rural area when snow or high water prevents the im-

TABLE 2-1. Normal Pulse Rates

60–70	Men
70–80	Women
80–90	Children over seven years
80–120	Children from one to seven years
110–130	Infants
Pulse Classified in Adults	
60 and below	Slow or subnormal
60–80	Normal (men, women)
80–100	Moderate increase
100–120	Quick
120–140	Rapid
140 and above	Running (hard to count)

Source: U.S. Public Health Service, *The Ship's Medicine Chest and Medical Aid at Sea.*

mediate transfer of a sick or injured person to a medical facility. If the victim is very sick, take the temperature at least four times each day and write it down.

Body temperature is measured with a thermometer that is held for a short time under the tongue, within the rectum, or in an armpit. The techniques are referred to as oral, rectal, and axillary (armpit), respectively. A standard glass thermometer should not be used when there is any chance that the victim will bite through it. Temperature at the axilla is usually a degree lower than that measured under the tongue, and rectal temperature is generally a degree higher.

Although 98.6°F is considered to be normal, the body temperature of healthy individuals may vary from 97°F to 99°F. (Refer to Table 2–2.)

TABLE 2-2. What Body Temperatures Mean

Fahrenheit (F)		Centigrade (C)
108°	Usually Fatal	42.2°
107 106 105	Critical Condition	41.7 41.1 40.6
104 102 103	High Fever	40.0 39.4 38.9
101 100 99	Moderate Fever	38.3 37.8 37.2
98.6	Healthy (Normal) Temperature in Mouth	37.0
98 97 96 95	Subnormal Temperature	36.7 36.1 35.6 35.0

Source: U.S. Public Health Service, *The Ship's Medicine Chest and Medical Aid at Sea.*

If there is no thermometer, you can get an idea of the temperature by putting the back of one hand on the victim's forehead and the other on your own or that of another healthy person. If the victim has a fever, you should feel the difference. Fingertips may be somewhat insensitive because of calluses.

Skin Color

The color of the skin, especially in Caucasian victims, reflects the circulation immediately underlying the skin as well as the oxygen saturation of the blood. In darkly pigmented individuals, these changes may not be apparent in the skin, but may be assessed by examining the mucous membranes (mouth, inner eyelids, and nailbeds). If the skin vessels constrict or heart output drops, the skin becomes pale, mottled, or cyanotic (a bluish discoloration). If the blood vessels of the skin dilate or blood flow increases, the skin becomes warm and pink.

Table 2–3 identifies possible medical conditions related to pulse, respirations, temperature, skin color, and pupil signs.

HEAD-TO-TOE EXAMINATION

Once as much pertinent information as possible has been obtained, the first aider should move to a head-to-toe examination of the victim, looking for other signs of injury or disease. Be careful not to aggravate injuries or contaminate wounds. Take great care not to move the victim because there could be undetected neck and spinal injuries.

Removal of clothing from the victim during the head-to-toe examination is not usually necessary.

Head and Neck

Check the scalp for lacerations and contusion. Is there blood in the hair? Where is it coming from? Do not move the head during this procedure. Pay particular attention to the area over the mastoid bone, just behind the ear. Bluish discoloration of this area is called Battle's sign and indicates a probable basal skull fracture.

Check the ears and nose for discharge of clear fluid or blood. Blood draining from the ears may be a sign of skull fracture; clear fluid draining from the nose or ears may be cerebrospinal fluid (CSF), again indicating a skull fracture. Do not attempt to stop the flow.

Inspect the mouth for blood or foreign materials such as broken dentures. The lips should be observed for cyanosis in victims with trauma or suspected cardiorespiratory problems.

Eyes

Pay attention to the size of the pupils (*see* Figure 2–3). Very large pupils can mean a state of shock; very small pupils can mean poison or the effect of certain drugs.

A difference in the size of the two pupils is almost always a medical emergency. Unequal pupils may be due to a stroke or a head injury. However, this unequal condition occurs normally in 2% to 4% of the population.

Use a small bright light source (beam from a flashlight) to determine if the pupils are reactive. If there is no flashlight, cover the eye with your hand and notice the pupil reaction when the eye is uncovered. No pupil reaction to light could mean death, coma, cataracts in older persons, or an artificial eye.

While inspecting the pupils of the eye, look at the inner surface of the eyelids. They are pink in all normal, healthy people regardless of skin color. If the

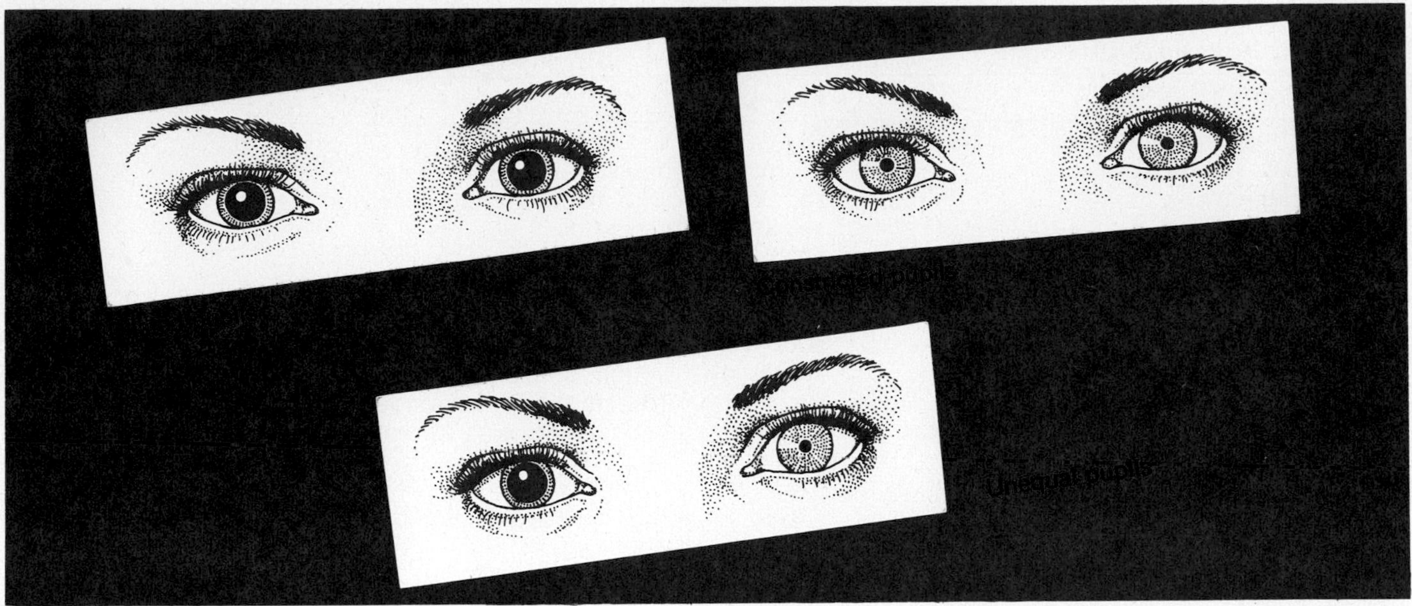

2-3. Changes in pupil size can have medical significance.

eyelids are pale in color, it may indicate anemia or blood loss. Remember that eyelids should be pink in color.

Chest

Check the chest for cuts, bruises, penetrations, and impaled objects. Warn the victim that you are going to apply pressure to the sides of the chest. Pain from squeezing or compressing the ribs may indicate possible rib fractures(s). Check to see if both sides of the chest expand normally when the victim breathes.

Abdomen

If something is protruding from the abdomen, it will be obvious. Less obvious and perhaps even difficult to see will be a wound produced by a small caliber bullet or a long thin weapon such as an ice pick.

If a person has pain in the abdomen, try to find out exactly where it hurts. When you examine the abdomen, first look at it for any unusual swelling or lumps.

The location of the pain often gives a clue to the cause (for example, pain in the upper right quadrant may be from a gallbladder). First, ask the person to point with one finger where it hurts. Then, beginning on the opposite side from the spot the victim has pointed to, press gently on different parts of the abdomen to see where it hurts the most. Feel for any abnormal lumps and hardened areas in the abdomen, but be extremely careful about pushing too deeply—lightly palpate the victim's abdomen. The victim who has tenderness may guard the painful area by tightening abdominal muscles. Palpate the four abdominal quadrants.

If a person has a constant pain in the abdomen, with nausea and has not been able to move his bowels, put an ear on the abdomen and listen for gurgles in the intestines. If you hear nothing after about two minutes, this is a danger sign of an abdominal emergency.

Other procedures could be performed, but the ones discussed here form a basis to help first aiders determine what a particular victim's problem is.

Extremity Assessment

In the trauma victim, the first aider should inspect the extremities for bruises and deformities, always checking for the presence of a pulse, sensation, and motion. Circulation to the extremities may also be gauged by the warmth of the limb and the degree of capillary refill in the nailbed. To assess capillary refill, you should exert gentle pressure on the nailbed sufficient to whiten the underlying tissue. Then, release the pressure and observe the rate at which the nailbed become pink again. If there is good circulation of the extremity, the capillaries should refill almost instantly, with prompt return of a pink coloring beneath the nail. Refill time greater than two seconds is definitely abnormal.

The first aider should check the victim's pulses. A normal pulse is full, easily felt, and equal to the corresponding pulse on the opposite side. The first aider should use the radial and pedal pulses to check circulation of the extremities. The sudden disappearance of a pulse in one extremity, together with sharp, sudden, severe pain in the limb may indicate occlusion of an artery in that extremity.

TABLE 2-3. Diagnostic Signs

Observation	Examples
1. **Pulse**	
a. **Rapid, strong:**	fright, apprehension, heat stroke
b. **Rapid, weak:**	shock, bleeding, diabetic coma, heat exhaustion
c. **Slow, strong:**	stroke, skull fracture
d. **None:**	cardiac arrest, death
2. **Respirations**	
a. **Shallow:**	shock, bleeding, heat exhaustion, insulin shock
b. **Deep, gasping, labored:**	airway obstruction, chest injury, diabetic coma, heart disease
c. **None:**	respiratory arrest due to any number of illnesses/injuries
d. **Bright, frothy blood coughed up:**	lung damage possibly due to fractured ribs or penetrating objects
3. **Skin temperature**	
a. **Cool, moist:**	shock, bleeding, heat exhaustion
b. **Cool, dry:**	exposure to cold
c. **Hot, dry:**	heat stroke, high fever
4. **Face color**	
a. **Red:**	high blood pressure, heat stroke, diabetic coma
b. **Pale/white/ashen:**	shock, bleeding, heat exhaustion, insulin shock
c. **Blue:**	heart failure, airway obstruction, some poisonings
Note: Blue results from poor oxygenation of circulating blood. For people with dark skin pigmentation, blue may be noted around the finger nails, palms of hands and mouth.	
5. **Pupils of the eyes**	
a. **Dilated:**	shock, bleeding, heat stroke, cardiac arrest
b. **Constricted:**	opiate addiction
c. **Unequal:**	head injury, stroke
6. **State of consciousness**	
a. **Confusion:**	most any illness/injury, fright, apprehension, alcohol, drugs
b. **Coma:**	stroke, head injury, severe poisoning, diabetic coma
7. **Inability to move upon command**—an indicator of paralysis.	
a. **One side of body:**	stroke, head injury
b. **Arms and legs:**	damage to spinal cord in neck
c. **Legs:**	damage to spinal cord below neck
8. **Reaction to physical stimulation**—an indicator of paralysis.	
a. **No sensation in arms and/or legs**	damage to spinal cord as indicated above
b. **Numbness in arms and/or legs:**	damage to spinal cord as indicated above
Note: No sensation or indication of pain when there is an obvious injury can also be due to hysteria, violent shock, or excessive alcohol or drug use.	

Source: National Highway Traffic Safety Administration, *Emergency Medical Services: First Responder Training Course* (Washington, D.C.: U.S. Superintendent of Documents).

In injured victims, the first aider should look for abnormal positioning of the legs. For example, a leg that is externally rotated suggests a hip fracture.

Assessment of the Back

When examining the back, remember to avoid excessive movement of the victim. In all victims with possible spinal injury as well as those with suspected stroke, the first aider should check strength and sensation in all extremities. The victim with a spinal injury may show paraplegia (paralysis of both legs) or quadriplegia (paralysis of all four extremities); the stroke victim is more likely to have hemiplegia (paralysis of an arm or leg on the same side of the body). The loss of movement in the extremities is usually accompanied by a loss of sensation in those extremities. It is very important that the first aider recognize this finding and appropriately immobilize the victim.

Putting It All Together

The physical exam will be influenced by whether the victim is suffering from a medical problem or is injured, whether the victim is conscious or unconscious, and whether life-threatening conditions are present. Table 2-4 shows the suggested sequence for conducting a victim assessment. Remember to first conduct the primary survey and correct any problems it uncovers before continuing on to the secondary survey.

TRIAGE

Triage is the sorting of victims into highest, second, and lowest priority based on injuries and medical emergencies. If triage is not performed, a victim with a minor wound could receive care while someone in cardiac arrest goes unnoticed, or a victim may not be thought to be serious when, in fact, he or she is.

You cannot begin to treat victims at random. Treat those victims who have the highest priority based on need of care.

As a first aider, use the following classification for triage:

Highest Priority (must be treated at the scene and immediately transported)

1. Airway and breathing difficulties
2. Cardiac arrest
3. Severe bleeding
4. Open chest or abdominal wounds
5. Severe head injuries
6. Burns:
   a. All that are complicated by other major injuries or involve respiratory tract.
   b. Third degree, > 10% BSA (involving face, hands, or feet)
   c. Second degree, > 30% BSA
7. Coma (unconscious)
8. Hypovolemic and anaphylactic shock

Second Priority (transportation and medical care at hospital can be delayed)

1. Burns:
   a. Third degree, 2%–10% BSA (not including face, hands, or feet)
   b. Second degree, 15%–30% BSA
   c. First degree, 50%–75% BSA
2. Major or multiple fractures (open)
3. Back injuries with or without spinal damage
4. Moderate bleeding
5. Severe eye injuries

TABLE 2-4. Victim Assessment

Primary Survey

A—Airway?
B—Breathing?
C—Circulation: pulse?
H—Hemorrhage?

Secondary Survey

History-Taking

S— Symptoms (chief complaint)
A— Allergies
M—Medications
P— Previous illnesses (relating to the problem)
L— Last meal (in case of surgery)
E— Events prior to emergency

P— Period of pain (how long? what started it?)
A— Area (where?)
I— Intensity
N—Nullify (what stops it? rest, a certain position, medication?)

Vital Signs

Pulse rate
Respiration rate
Temperature
Skin color

Head-to-Toe Examination

Head and neck—Bleeding? Deformity? CSF? Cyanosis?
Eyes—Pupils equal? Pupils react? Eyelid color?
Chest—Pain? Wounds?
Abdomen—Pain? Wounds?
Extremities—Deformity? Pulses? Sensation?
Back—Extremities checked for sensation and movement
Medical Alert Symbols—check for tags, bracelets, etc.

Lowest Priority (to be treated or transported last)

1. Obviously dead
2. Obvious mortal wounds where first aid is not practical
3. Burns:
   a. Third degree, < 2% BSA
   b. Second degree, < 15% BSA
   c. First degree, < 20% BSA
4. Minor fractures (closed fractures)
5. Minor soft tissue injuries and minor bleeding

Not everyone agrees completely with the preceding classifications. Variations do occur, but they tend to be minor.

Victim Assessment LEARNING ACTIVITIES

T F 1. There are two major parts to a good victim examination: primary and secondary.
T F 2. Use your thumb to feel for a victim's pulse.
T F 3. A pulse can be felt usually at either the radial point at the wrist or the carotid point at the neck.
T F 4. Feeling both carotid arteries at the same time is permissible.
T F 5. Normal pulse rate for adults is 60–80 beats per minute.
T F 6. Normal respiration rate for adults is between 12 and 20 breaths per minute.
T F 7. Normal body temperature of healthy individuals may vary below and above 98.6°F.
T F 8. Large pupils of the eyes can mean a state of shock.
T F 9. A difference in the size of the two pupils of the eyes may indicate a stroke or head injury.
T F 10. Inner surfaces of the eyelids in all people, regardless of skin color, is pink.
T F 11. A clear, water-like fluid called cerebrospinal fluid coming from an ear may indicate a skull fracture.
T F 12. If you hear nothing for two minutes after placing your ear on a victim's abdomen and the person has had constant pain with nausea, the victim is all right.

Signs and Symptoms
Designate which of the following are signs (with an A) and which are symptoms (with a B).

_________ 1. Sherry states that she feels dizzy.
_________ 2. Matt says he feels like throwing up.
_________ 3. Steve's skin is red and blistered.
_________ 4. Jim says that he has no feeling in his right arm.
_________ 5. Scott's pulse rate is 88 beats per minute.
_________ 6. Joni's oral temperature is 104°F.
_________ 7. Justin's pupils are unequal.
_________ 8. Mike begins to vomit.
_________ 9. Blood is spurting from Tom's leg.
_________ 10. Carla has a fruity odor on her breath.
_________ 11. Glen has an impaled object in his eye.
_________ 12. Cerebrospinal fluid is coming from Joann's ear.
_________ 13. Wes has a deformity in his wrist after falling on it.
_________ 14. Lisa is wheezing while breathing.
_________ 15. After falling, Whitney's ankle becomes swollen.

Triage
For each of these injuries, indicate whether it is:

A. Highest priority
B. Second priority
C. Lowest priority

_________ 1. Second degree burns completely covering both arms and hands
_________ 2. Severe head injury
_________ 3. Severe bleeding of the right forearm
_________ 4. Fracture of the ulna
_________ 5. Difficult breathing with gasping respirations
_________ 6. Back injury with suspected spinal damage
_________ 7. Chest wound with breathing problems
_________ 8. Abrasions on both knees
_________ 9. Minor bleeding from a lacerated toe
_________ 10. Sprained ankle
_________ 11. Sunburn over all of an individual's legs

3 Basic Life Support

- The 1986 Cardiopulmonary Resuscitation (CPR) Guidelines from the American Heart Association (Performance sheets are also included)
- Adult
- Pediatric

Sudden death from heart disease is the most prominent medical emergency today. It is possible that a large number of deaths can be prevented by prompt action to provide early entry into the emergency medical services (EMS) system, cardiopulmonary support using CPR, or both.

The only chance for survival for a substantial number of persons who experience cardiac arrest is successful resuscitation. Early bystander CPR remains the critical element in the prevention of sudden death. When coupled with an efficient emergency medical service system and advanced cardiac life support capability, the chances for survival are over 40%. Large numbers of laypeople trained in basic life support (BLS) and a rapid response system of well-trained paramedical personnel could save an estimated 100,000 to 200,000 lives each year in the United States. In addition, a number of victims who die of drowning, electrocution, suffocation, and drug intoxication could most likely be saved by the prompt and proper application of CPR.

The greatest risk of death from heart attack is in the first two hours after the onset of symptoms. Laypeople, both those recognized to be at high risk and their immediate family and friends, must first be educated to recognize the usual manifestations of heart attack. They then must know how to gain access to the EMS system. The fastest way for an emergency medical team to respond is through the use of a universal emergency telephone number, such as 911.

Usually the majority of lay individuals taking CPR courses are young adults who are not often exposed to high-risk individuals. An emphasis must be placed on the need to train families, neighbors, and coworkers of high-risk individuals.

One-rescuer CPR by the lay individual is emphasized in most CPR training. Two-rescuer CPR is seldom, if ever, used by lay rescuers because when help is summoned it most often comes in the form of EMS personnel who then relieve the lay rescuer. Learning the skills of two-rescuer CPR adds complexity, likely leading to decreased retention of the main techniques of one-rescuer CPR.

First aiders should initiate CPR to the best of their knowledge and capability in cases they recognize as cardiac arrest. First aiders who initiate BLS should continue resuscitation efforts until one of the following occurs:

1. Effective circulation and ventilation have been restored.
2. Resuscitation efforts have been transferred to another responsible person who continues BLS.
3. A physician or a physician-directed person or team assumes responsibility.
4. The victim is transferred to properly trained personnel charged with responsibilities for emergency medical services.
5. The rescuer is exhausted and unable to continue resuscitation.

There has been no instance known in which a layperson who has performed CPR reasonably has been sued successfully.

The following eleven pages contain the Standards and Guidelines for Cardiopulmonary Resuscitation (CPR) and Emergency Cardiac Care (ECC). (Reprinted with permission. © *JAMA*, June 6, 1986. American Heart Association.)

Adult Basic Life Support

Basic life support (BLS) is that particular phase of emergency cardiac care that either (1) prevents circulatory or respiratory arrest or insufficiency through prompt recognition and intervention or (2) externally supports the circulation and ventilation of a victim of cardiac or respiratory arrest through cardiopulmonary resuscitation (CPR).[1] The major objective of performing CPR is to provide oxygen to the brain, heart, and other vital organs until appropriate, definitive medical treatment (advanced cardiac life support) can restore normal heart and ventilatory action. Speed is critical—the key to success. The highest hospital discharge rate has been achieved in those patients for whom CPR was initiated within four minutes of the time of the arrest and who, in addition, were provided with advanced cardiac life support measures within eight minutes of their arrest.[2] Early bystander CPR intervention and fast emergency medical system (EMS) response are therefore essential in improving survival rates[3-5] and good neurological recovery rates.[6,7]

Basic life support includes the teaching of primary and secondary prevention. The basic concept, put forward by the American Heart Association during the last 20 years, that "it is possible to prevent and control coronary heart disease,"[8] should be reinforced during the teaching of BLS, with an emphasis on "prudent heart living" and the role of risk factor modification. The earlier this information is transmitted to the community, the stronger the impact on mortality and morbidity; therefore, efforts must be made to include BLS in the curricula of schools. Cardiopulmonary resuscitation training should include information on danger signals, actions for survival, and entry into the EMS system in order to help prevent sudden death in individuals who have sustained myocardial infarctions.

INDICATIONS FOR BLS

Respiratory Arrest

When there is primary respiratory arrest, the heart can continue to pump blood for several minutes, and existing stores of oxygen in the lungs and blood will continue to circulate to the brain and other vital organs.[9] Early intervention for victims in whom respirations have stopped or the airway is obstructed can prevent cardiac arrest. Respiratory arrest can result from drowning, stroke, foreign-body airway obstruction, smoke inhalation, drug overdose, electrocution, suffocation, injuries, myocardial infarction, injury by lightning, and coma of any cause leading to airway obstruction.

Cardiac Arrest

When there is primary cardiac arrest, oxygen is not circulated, and oxygen stored in the vital organs is depleted in a few seconds. Cardiac arrest can be accompanied by the following electrical phenomena: ventricular fibrillation, ventricular tachycardia, asystole, or electromechanical dissociation.

THE SEQUENCE OF BLS: ASSESSMENT AND THE *ABC*s OF CPR

The assessment phases of BLS are crucial. No victim should undergo any one of the more intrusive procedures of cardiopulmonary resuscitation (ie, positioning, opening the airway, rescue breathing, and external chest compression) until the need for it has been established by the appropriate assessment. The importance of the assessment phases should be stressed in the teaching of CPR.

Each of the *ABC*s of CPR, *A*irway, *B*reathing, and *C*irculation, begins with an assessment phase: "determine unresponsiveness," "determine breathlessness," and "determine pulselessness," respectively. Assessment also involves a more subtle, constant process of observing and interacting with the victim.

1. Assessment: Determine Unresponsiveness.—The rescuer arriving at the scene of the collapsed victim must quickly assess any injury and determine whether the individual is unconscious (Fig 1, top). If the victim has sustained trauma to the head and neck, the rescuer should move the victim only if absolutely necessary because improper movement may cause paralysis in the victim with a neck injury.

The rescuer should tap or gently shake the victim and shout, "Are you OK?" This precaution will prevent injury from attempted resuscitation of a person who is not truly unconscious.

2. Call for Help.—If the victim does not respond to attempts at arousal, call out for help (Fig 1, center). When someone responds, send that person to activate the EMS system.

3. Position the Victim.—For CPR to be effective, the victim must be supine and on a firm, flat surface (Fig 1, bottom); even flawlessly performed external chest compressions will produce inadequate blood flow to the brain if the head is positioned higher than the thorax. If the victim is lying face down, the rescuer must roll the victim as a unit so that the head, shoulders, and torso move simultaneously with no twisting. The head and neck should remain in the same plane as the torso, and the body should be moved as a unit. Once the body is supine, the victim's arms should be placed alongside the body. The victim is now appropriately positioned for the next step in CPR.

4. Rescuer Position.—By kneeling at the level of the victim's shoulders, the rescuer can perform, in turn, rescue breathing and chest compression without moving the knees.

5. Open Airway.—The most important action for successful resuscitation is immediate opening of the airway. In the absence of sufficient muscle tone, the tongue and/or the epiglottis will obstruct the pharynx and the larynx, respectively (Fig 2, top).[10-14] The tongue is the most common cause of airway obstruction in the unconscious victim. Since the tongue is attached to the lower jaw, moving the lower jaw forward will lift the tongue away from the back of the throat and open the airway. Either the tongue or the epiglottis,[13] or both, may produce obstruction also when negative pressure is created in the airway by inspiratory effort, causing a valve-type mechanism to occlude the entrance to the trachea.

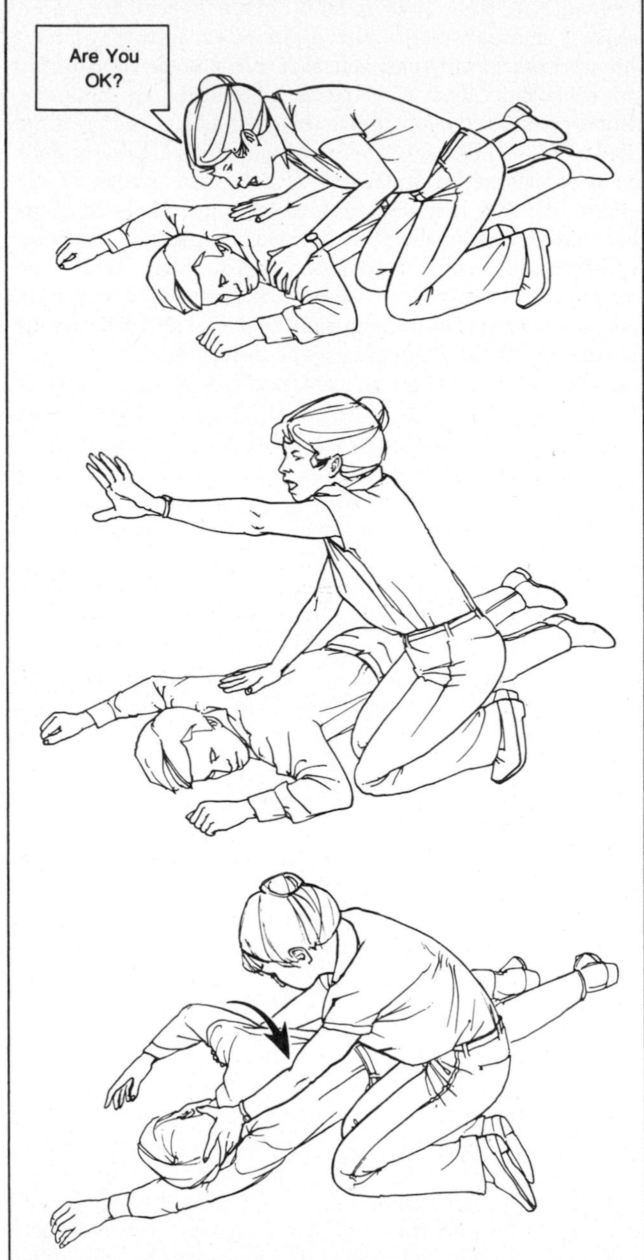

Fig 1.—Initial steps of cardiopulmonary resuscitation. Top, Determining unresponsiveness; center, calling for help; bottom, positioning the victim.

The rescuer should use the head-tilt/chin-lift maneuver, described below, to open the airway (Fig 2, bottom). If foreign material or vomitus is visible in the mouth, it should be removed. Excessive time must not be taken. Liquids or semiliquids should be wiped out with the index and middle fingers covered by a piece of cloth; solid material should be extracted with a hooked index finger. The mouth can be opened by the "crossed-finger" technique.[15]

Head-Tilt/Chin-Lift Maneuver.—Head-tilt/chin-lift is more effective in opening the airway than the previously recommended head-tilt/neck-lift.[16] Head-tilt is accomplished by placing one hand on the victim's forehead and applying firm, backward pressure with the palm to tilt the head back. To complete the head-tilt/chin-lift maneuver, place the fingers of the other hand under the bony part of the lower jaw near the chin and lift to bring the chin forward and the teeth almost to occlusion, thus supporting the jaw and helping to tilt the head back. The fingers must not press deeply into the soft tissue under the chin, which might obstruct the airway. The thumb should not be used for lifting the chin. The mouth should not be completely closed (unless mouth-to-nose breathing is the technique of choice for that particular victim). When mouth-to-nose ventilation is indicated, the hand that is already on the chin can close the mouth by applying increased force and in this way provide effective mouth-to-nose ventilation.[13] If the victim has loose dentures, head-tilt/chin-lift maintains their position and makes a mouth-to-mouth seal easier.[16] Dentures should be removed if they cannot be managed in place.

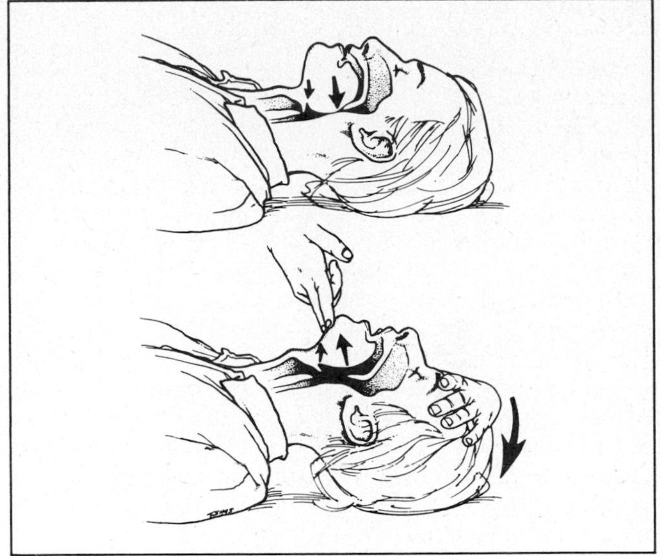

Fig 2.—Opening the airway. Top, Airway obstruction produced by tongue and epiglottis; bottom, relief by head-tilt/chin-lift.

Jaw-Thrust Maneuver.—Forward displacement of the mandible can be accomplished by grasping the angles of the victim's lower jaw and lifting with both hands, one on each side, displacing the mandible forward while tilting the head backward.[15,17] The rescuer's elbows should rest on the surface on which the victim is lying. If the lips close, the lower lip can be retracted with the thumb. If mouth-to-mouth breathing is necessary, the nostrils may be closed by placing the rescuer's cheek tightly against them.[15] This technique is very effective in opening the airway[18,19] but is very fatiguing and technically difficult.[16]

The jaw-thrust technique without head-tilt is the safest first approach to opening the airway of the victim with suspected neck injury because it usually can be accomplished without extending the neck. The head should be carefully supported without tilting it backward or turning it from side to side. If jaw-thrust alone is unsuccessful, the head should be tilted backward very slightly.

Recommendations for Opening the Airway.—A layperson should learn only one maneuver for opening the airway. The recommended technique must be simple, safe, easily learned, and effective. Since head-tilt/chin-lift meets these criteria, it should be the method of choice.

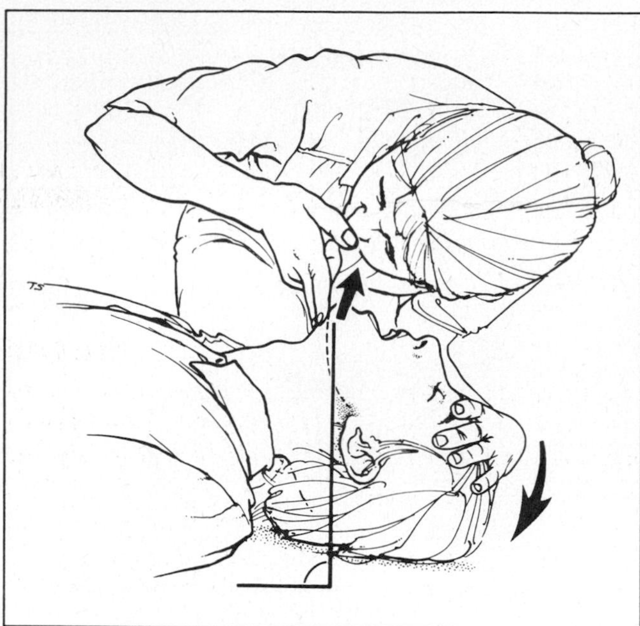

Fig 3.—Determining breathlessness.

Professional rescuers (emergency medical technicians and other medical and health care providers) should be trained in both head-tilt/chin-lift and jaw-thrust.

Breathing

6. Assessment: Determine Breathlessness.—To assess the presence or absence of spontaneous breathing, the rescuer should place his or her ear over the victim's mouth and nose while maintaining an open airway (Fig 3). Then, while observing the victim's chest, the rescuer should (1) *look* for the chest to rise and fall; (2) *listen* for air escaping during exhalation; (3) *feel* for the flow of air. If the chest does not rise and fall and no air is exhaled, the victim is breathless. This evaluation procedure should take only 3 to 5 seconds.

It should be stressed that, although the rescuer may notice that the victim is making respiratory efforts, the airway may still be obstructed and opening the airway may be all that is needed. If the victim resumes breathing, the rescuer should continue to help maintain an open airway.

7. Perform Rescue Breathing.—*Mouth-to-Mouth.*—Rescue breathing using the mouth-to-mouth technique is a quick and effective way of providing the necessary oxygen to the victim's lungs (Fig 4, top).[20] The rescuer's exhaled air contains sufficient oxygen to supply the victim's needs. Rescue breathing requires that the rescuer inflate the victim's lungs adequately with each breath. Keeping the airway open by the head-tilt/chin-lift maneuver, the rescuer gently pinches the nose closed using the thumb and index finger of the hand on the forehead, thereby preventing air from escaping through the victim's nose. The rescuer takes a deep breath and seals his or her lips around the outside of the victim's mouth, creating an airtight seal; then the rescuer gives two full breaths.

Adequate time for the two breaths (1 to 1½ seconds per breath) should be allowed to provide good chest expansion and decrease the possibility of gastric distention. (Measurements of time "per breath" given herein are, more precisely, measurements of the victim's inspiratory time.) The rescuer should take a breath after each ventilation, and each individual ventilation should be of sufficient volume to make the chest rise. In most adults, this volume will be 800 mL (0.8 L). Adequate ventilation usually does not need to exceed 1,200 mL (1.2 L). An excess of air volume and fast inspiratory flow rates are likely to cause pharyngeal pressures that exceed esophageal opening pressures, allowing air to enter the stomach and, thus, resulting in gastric distention.[21-23] Indicators of adequate ventilation are (1) observing the chest rise and fall and (2) hearing and feeling the air escape during exhalation.

If the initial attempt to ventilate the victim is unsuccessful, reposition the victim's head and repeat rescue breathing. Improper chin and head positioning is the most common cause of difficulty with ventilation. If the victim cannot be ventilated after repositioning the head, proceed with foreign-body airway obstruction maneuvers (see "Foreign-Body Airway Obstruction," below).

Mouth-to-Nose.—This technique is more effective in some cases than mouth-to-mouth (Fig 4, center).[24] The technique is recommended when it is impossible to ventilate through the victim's mouth, the mouth cannot be opened (trismus), the mouth is seriously injured, or a tight mouth-to-mouth seal is difficult to achieve. The rescuer keeps the victim's head tilted back with one hand on the forehead and uses the other hand to lift the victim's lower jaw (as in head-tilt/chin-lift) and close the mouth. The rescuer then takes a deep breath, seals the lips around the victim's nose, and blows into the nose. The rescuer's mouth is then removed, and the victim exhales passively. It may be necessary to open the victim's mouth intermittently or separate the lips (with the thumb) to allow air to be exhaled since nasal obstruction may be present during exhalation.[25]

Mouth-to-Stoma.—Persons who have undergone a laryngectomy (surgical removal of the larynx) have a permanent stoma (opening) that connects the trachea directly to the skin.[26] The stoma can be recognized as an opening at the front base of the neck. When such an individual requires rescue breathing, direct mouth-to-stoma ventilation should be performed (Fig 4, bottom). The rescuer's mouth is sealed around the stoma and air is blown into the victim's stoma until the chest rises. When the rescuer's mouth is removed from the stoma, the victim is permitted to exhale passively.

Other persons may have a temporary tracheostomy tube in the trachea. To ventilate these persons, the victim's mouth and nose usually must be sealed by the rescuer's hand or by a tightly fitting face mask to prevent leakage of air when the rescuer blows into the tracheostomy tube. This problem is alleviated when the tracheostomy tube has a cuff that can be inflated.

Recommendations for Rescue Breathing.—(1) The "four quick" initial ventilations formerly recommended in one-rescuer CPR have been changed to two initial breaths of 1 to 1½ seconds each. Those ventilations should no longer be given to create a "staircase" effect. By giving the ventilations with a slower inspiratory flow rate and by avoiding trapping air in the lungs between breaths, the possibility of exceeding the esophageal opening pressure will be less.

FIRST-AID FOR CHOKING

OBSTRUCTED AIRWAY TECHNIQUES FOR ADULTS (AGES 9 AND OVER)

Fitnus For Life

Conscious Victim Standing

1 Recognize choking signs.

Choking victim will have severe difficulty speaking, breathing, coughing and may be clutching throat between thumb and fingers (Universal Distress Signal). Ask if he or she is choking. **If able to speak or cough effectively, do not interfere.**

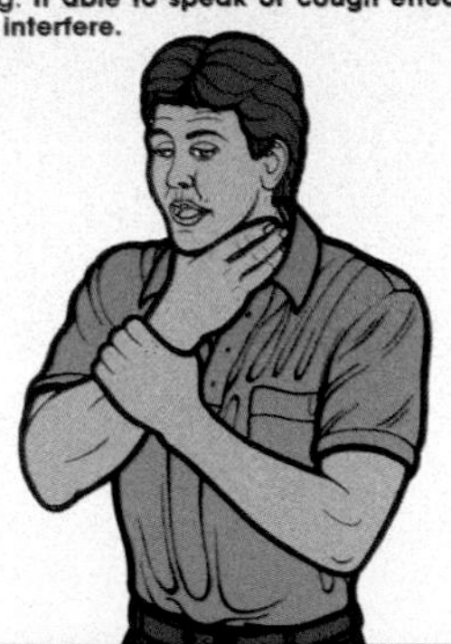

2 If choking— Give 6-10 abdominal thrusts.

Stand behind victim and wrap arms around his or her waist. Make a fist with one hand. Place thumb side of fist into abdomen above navel and below rib cage. Grasp fist with other hand and press inward and upward with 6-10 quick thrusts.

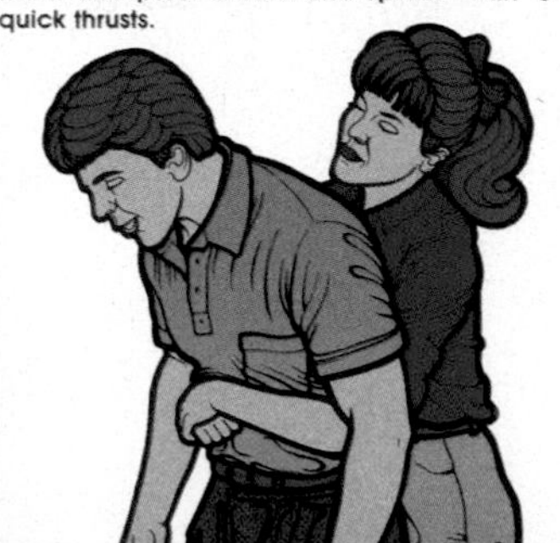

3 If pregnant or obese— Give 6-10 chest thrusts.

Stand behind victim, placing your arms under victims armpits, and encircle chests. Place thumb side of fist on the middle of the breastbone. Grasp fist with other hand and press backward with 6-10 quick thrusts.

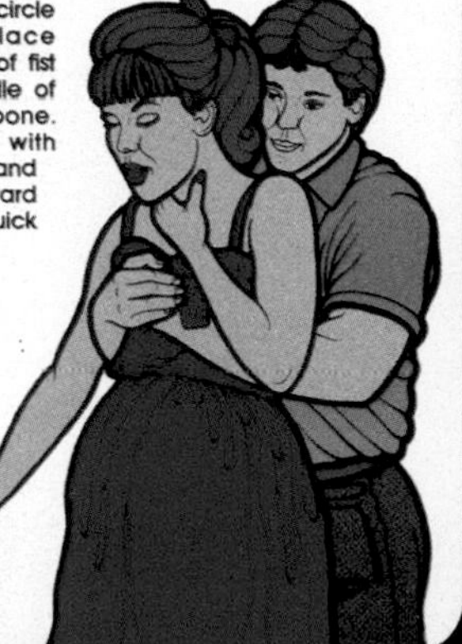

Victim Lying Conscious or Unconscious

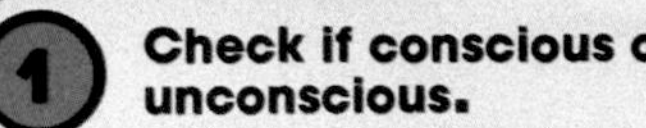

1 Check if conscious or unconscious.

Gently tap and shake shoulders to determine if victim is ok. If unresponsive call out for "Help!"

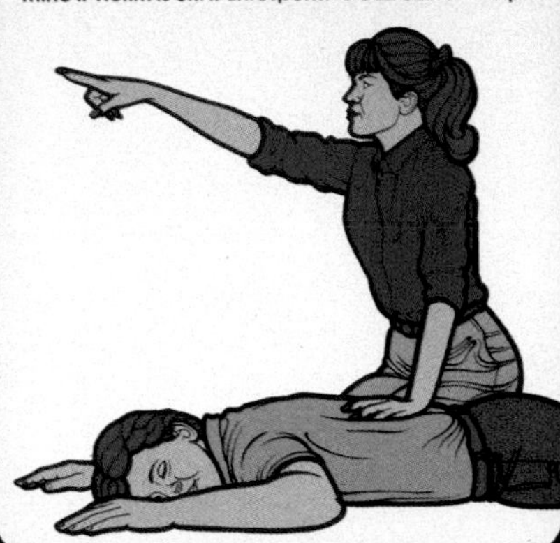

2 Position victim carefully on back.

If lying face down, roll victim flat onto back. Supporting head, neck, and torso carefully turn victim as a unit without twisting.

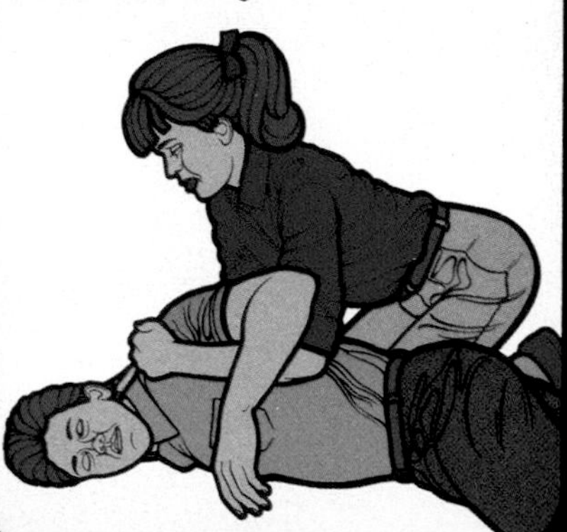

3 Open airway. Check for breathing.

Apply downward pressure with hand on forehead and gently lift with other hand just under chin. Place ear close to victim's mouth and nose. **LOOK** for rise and fall of chest. **LISTEN** and **FEEL** for breathing.

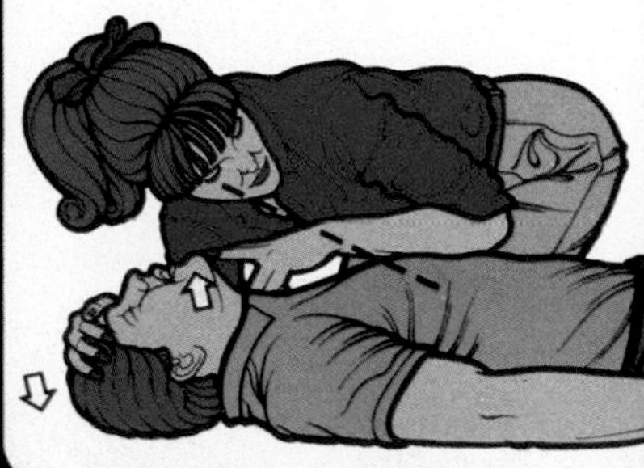

4 Attempt to ventilate.

Keeping head tilted and airway open, pinch victim's nose with thumb and index finger. Cover victim's mouth and attempt to get air into the lungs.

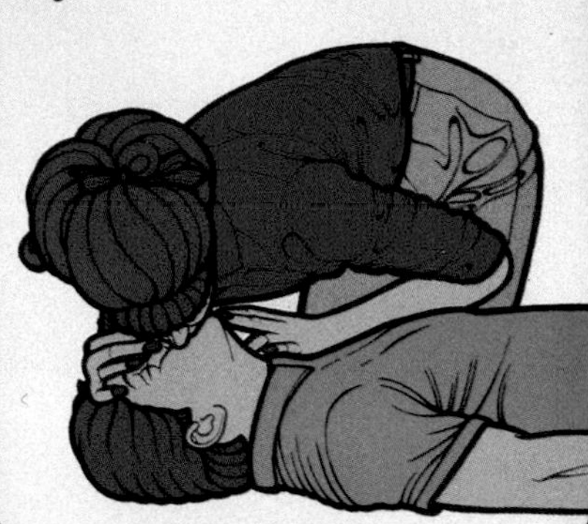

5 If unsuccessful— Give 6-10 abdominal thrusts.

Kneeling close to victim's hips, place heel of hand on victim's abdomen above navel and below rib cage. Put other hand on top of first, and press into abdomen with 6-10 quick inward and upward thrusts.

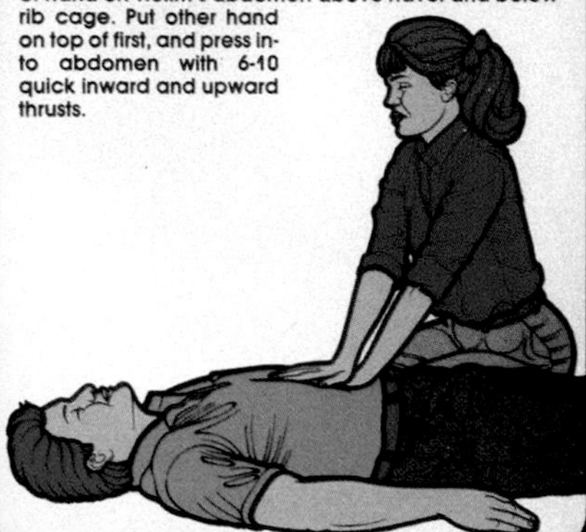

6 Finger sweep for foreign object.

Open victim's mouth by grasping tongue and lower jaw, and lift. Insert index finger of other hand deep into mouth along the cheek. Using hooked finger try to dislodge object.

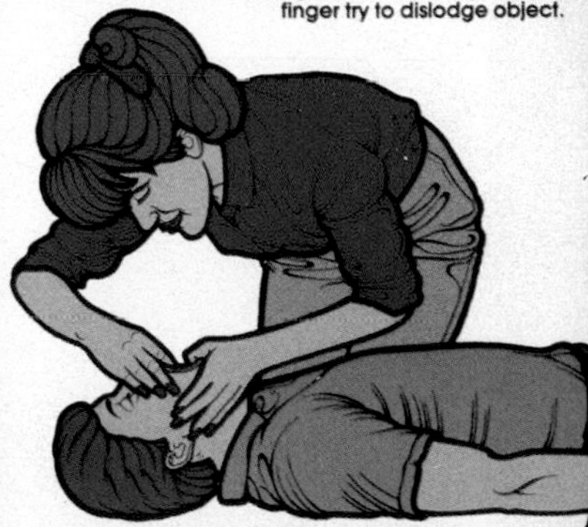

• If unsuccessful reattempt to ventilate •

Fitnus® For Life 3125 19th Street, Suite 305 • Bakersfield, CA 93301 • (805) 861-1100 Algra, Inc. 1986

18x24" posters available from Fitnus® for Life, 3125 19th Street, Suite 305, Bakersfield, CA 93301

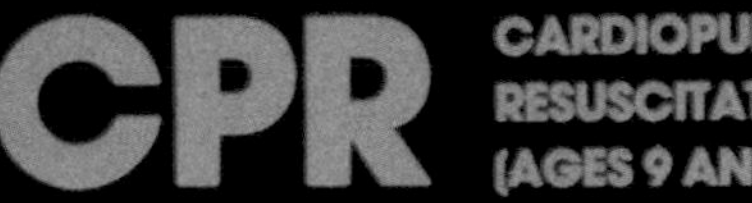

CPR

CARDIOPULMONARY RESUSCITATION FOR ADULTS (AGES 9 AND OVER)

Fitnus For Life

1 Check if conscious or unconscious.

Gently shake shoulders and shout: "Are you OK?" Call out for "Help!" If positioning is necessary support head and neck and roll victim as a unit onto back.

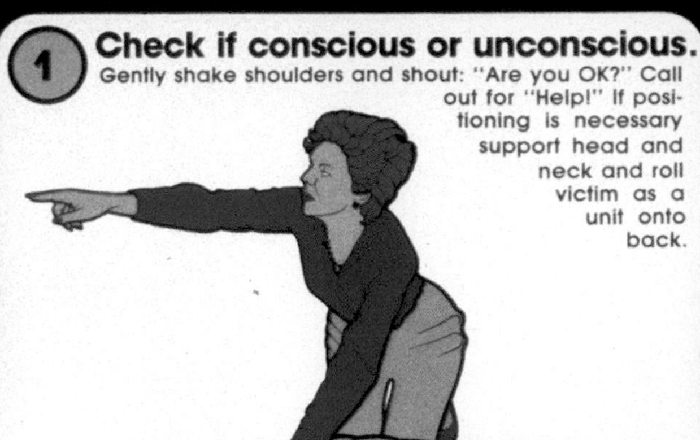

2 Open airway. Check for breathing.

Place palm of one hand on forehead and apply firm pressure backward. Place fingers of other hand just under chin and gently lift. Do not close victim's mouth completely. Put ear close to victim's mouth and nose. **LOOK** for rise and fall of the chest. **LISTEN** and **FEEL** for breathing.

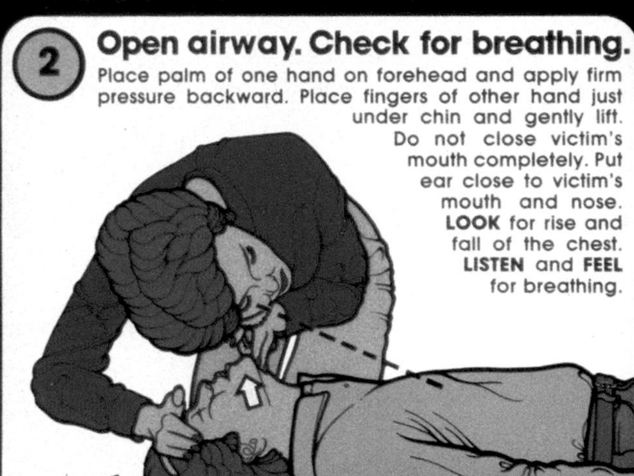

3 If not breathing - Give 2 full breaths.

Keeping airway open, pinch nose using thumb and index finger. Open your mouth wide and take a deep breath. Place your mouth over victim's mouth making a tight seal. Give 2 full breaths with a pause between to take a breath.

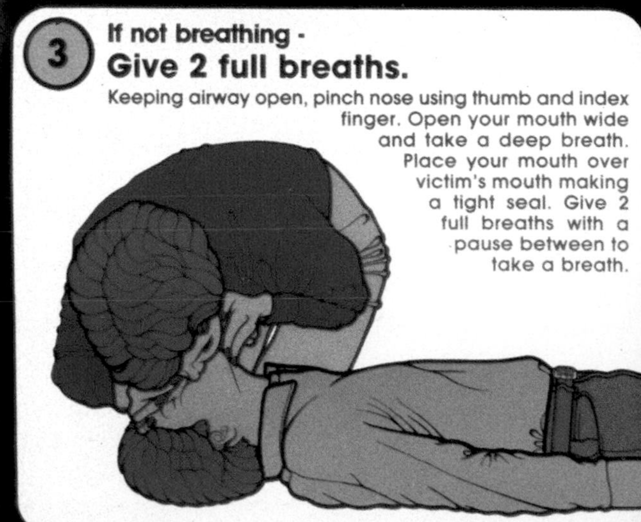

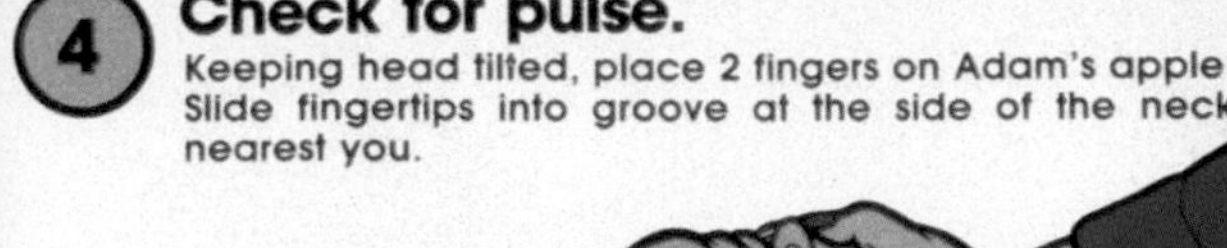

4 Check for pulse.

Keeping head tilted, place 2 fingers on Adam's apple. Slide fingertips into groove at the side of the neck nearest you.

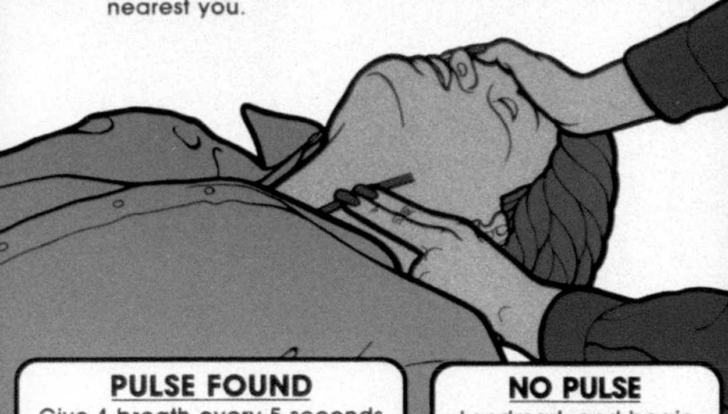

PULSE FOUND
Give 1 breath every 5 seconds until breathing resumes
(DO NOT GO TO STEPS 5 AND 6)

NO PULSE
Landmark and begin chest compressions
(GO TO STEPS 5 AND 6)

5 Landmark for hand position.

Run fingers up lower edge of rib cage to notch where ribs meet breastbone. Place middle finger on notch, index finger next to it. Put heel of other hand next to fingers. Place hand you located notch with on top or interlace fingers. Keep fingers up off chest.

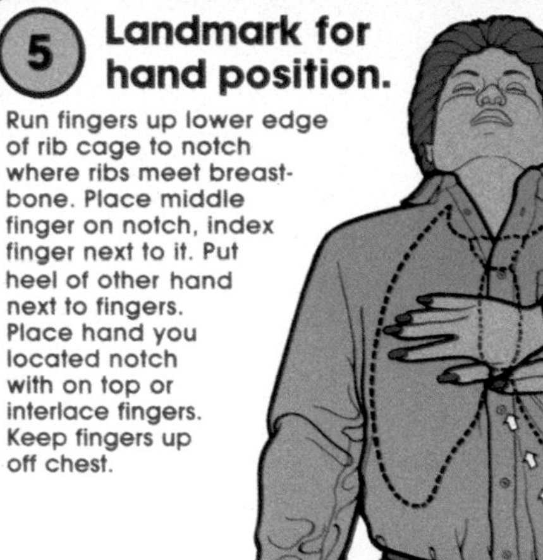

6 Chest compressions.

Place shoulders and weight directly over hands, keeping elbows straight. Pushing straight down with smooth and even movements, compress chest cavity 1½ - 2 inches at a rate of 80 - 100 compressions per minute. Give 15 compressions counting: "one and two and three and . . ." Follow 15 compressions with 2 breaths and repeat.

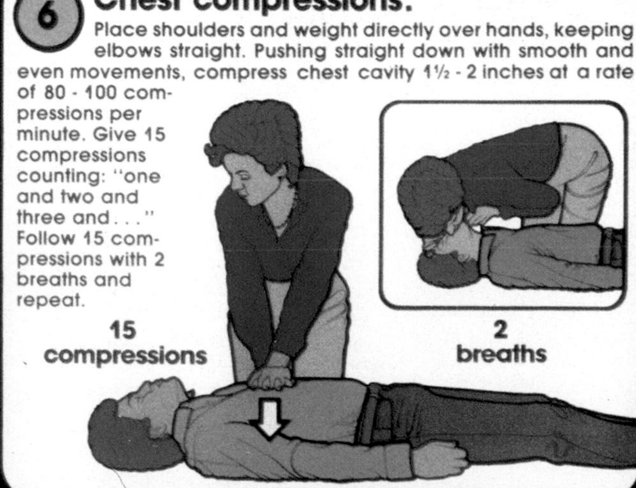

18x24" posters available from Fitnus® for Life, 3125 19th Street, Suite 305, Bakersfield, CA 93301

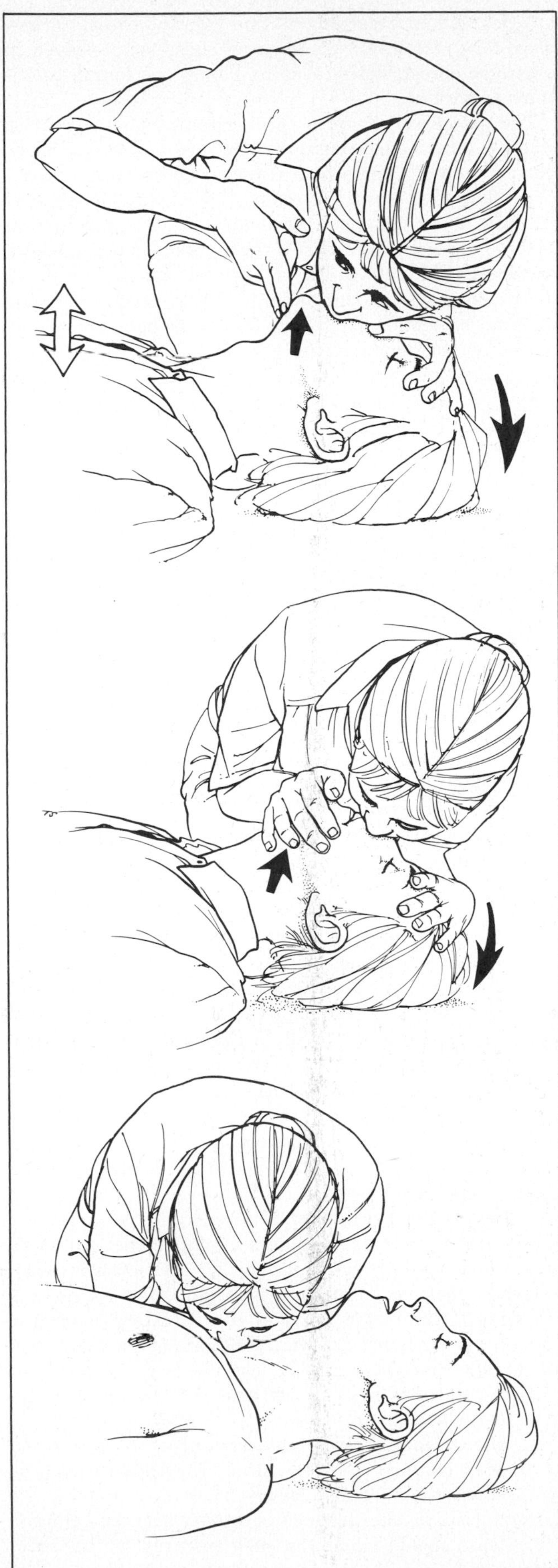

Fig 4.—Rescue breathing. Top, Mouth-to-mouth; center, mouth-to-nose; bottom, mouth-to-stoma. (Adapted from *Cardiopulmonary Resuscitation*. Washington, DC, American National Red Cross, 1981, pp 16-17. Used by permission.)

This technique should result in less gastric distention, regurgitation, and aspiration. Also, an equal number of initial and subsequent ventilations should enhance retention by trainees. (2) In two-rescuer CPR, a pause for ventilations should be allowed after every five external chest compressions. However, such pauses for ventilations (1 to 1½ seconds) decrease the total number of compressions per minute, affecting the blood flow to vital organs; therefore, a faster compression rate than was previously recommended is necessary for adequate blood flow (see "Recommendations for External Chest Compressions").

Circulation

8. Assessment: Determine Pulselessness.—Cardiac arrest is recognized by pulselessness in the large arteries of the unconscious victim (Fig 3). The pulse check should take 5 to 10 seconds, and the carotid artery should be used. It lies in a groove created by the trachea and the large strap muscles of the neck. While maintaining head-tilt with one hand on the forehead, the rescuer locates the victim's larynx with two or three fingers of the other hand. The rescuer then slides these fingers into the groove between the trachea and the muscles at the side of the neck where the carotid pulse can be felt. The pulse area must be pressed gently—to avoid compressing the artery. This technique is usually more easily performed on the side nearest the rescuer. Adequate time should be allowed since the pulse may be slow, irregular, or very weak and rapid. This is the most accessible, reliable, and easily learned technique for locating the pulse in adults and children. The pulse in the carotid artery will persist when more peripheral pulses (eg, radial) are no longer palpable. For health care professionals, or in the hospital setting, determining pulselessness using the femoral pulse is also acceptable; however, this pulse is difficult to locate in a fully clothed patient.

Proper assessment of the victim's condition must be made since performing external chest compressions on a patient who has a pulse may result in serious medical complications. If a pulse is present but there is no breathing, rescue breathing should be initiated at a rate of 12 times per minute (once every 5 seconds) after initial two breaths of 1 to 1½ seconds each.

If no pulse is palpated, the diagnosis of cardiac arrest is confirmed. If not yet done, the EMS system should be activated and external chest compression begun after the initial two breaths.

9. Activate the EMS System.—The EMS system is activated by calling the local emergency telephone number (911, if available). This number should be widely publicized in each community. The person who calls the EMS system should be prepared to give the following information as calmly as possible[27]: (1) where the emergency is (with names of cross streets or roads, if possible); (2) the telephone number from which the call is made; (3) what happened—heart attack, auto accident, etc; (4) how many persons need help; (5) condition of the victim(s); (6) what aid is being given to the victim(s); (7) any other informa-

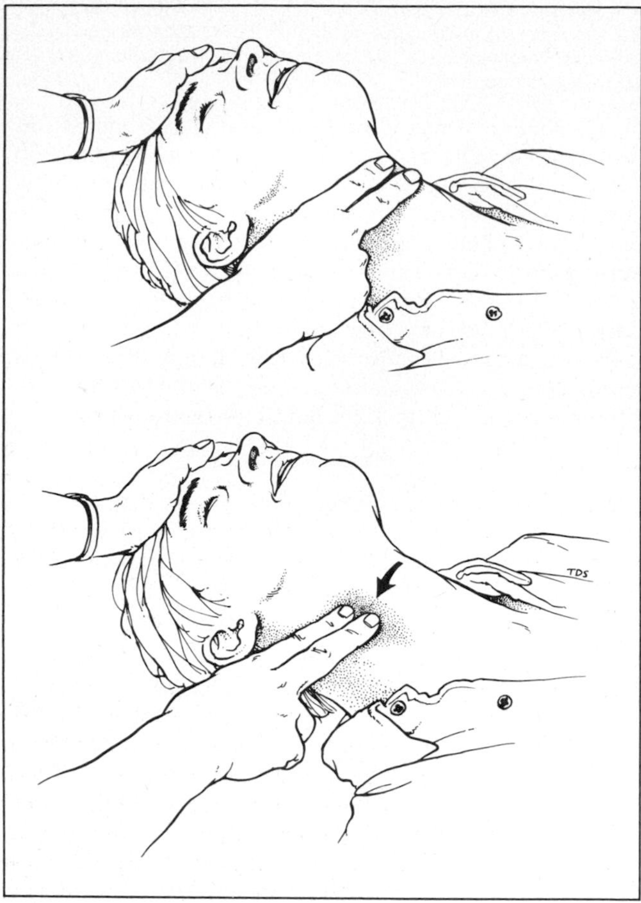

Fig 5.—Determining pulselessness.

tion requested. To ensure that EMS personnel have no more questions, the caller should hang up last.

If no one responds to the call for help and the rescuer is alone, CPR should be performed for about one minute and then help should be summoned. The decision when to leave the victim to telephone for help is affected by a number of variables, including the possibility of someone else arriving on the scene. If the rescuer is unable to activate the EMS system, the only option is to continue with CPR.

10. External Chest Compressions.—Cardiac arrest is recognized by pulselessness in the large arteries of the unconscious, breathless victim. All the *ABC*s of CPR are required in rapid succession to optimize the chances for survival.

The external chest compression technique consists of serial, rhythmic applications of pressure over the lower half of the sternum (Fig 5).[28] These compressions provide circulation to the heart, lungs, brain, and other organs as a result of a generalized increase in intrathoracic pressure and/or direct compression of the heart. Blood circulated to the lungs by external chest compressions will receive sufficient oxygen to maintain life when the compressions are accompanied by properly performed rescue breathing.[29]

During cardiac arrest, properly performed external chest compressions can produce systolic blood pressure peaks of more than 100 mm Hg, but the diastolic blood pressure is low, the mean blood pressure in the carotid arteries seldom exceeding 40 mm Hg. The carotid artery blood flow resulting from external chest compressions on a cardiac arrest victim usually is only one fourth to one third of normal.

The patient must be in the horizontal supine position when external chest compressions are performed. Even during properly performed external chest compressions, blood flow to the brain is reduced. With any elevation of the head above the heart, blood flow to the brain is further reduced or even eliminated. If the victim is in bed, a board, preferably the full width of the bed, should be placed under the back of the patient. Elevation of the lower extremities, while keeping the rest of the body horizontal, may promote venous return and augment artificial circulation during external chest compressions.

Proper Hand Position.—Proper hand placement is established by the following guidelines (Fig 6, left):

1. With the middle and index finger of the hand nearest the victim's legs, the rescuer locates the lower margin of the victim's rib cage on the side next to the rescuer.
2. The fingers are then moved up the rib cage to the notch where the ribs meet the sternum in the center of the lower part of the chest.
3. With the middle finger on this notch, the index finger is placed next to it on the lower end of the sternum.
4. The heel of the hand nearest the patient's head (which had been used on the forehead to maintain head position) is placed on the lower half of the sternum, close to the index finger that is next to the middle finger in the notch. The long axis of the heel of the rescuer's hand should be placed on the long axis of the sternum. This will keep the main force of compression on the sternum and decrease the chance of rib fracture.
5. The first hand is then removed from the notch and placed on top of the hand on the sternum so that both hands are parallel to each other.
6. The fingers may be either extended or interlaced but must be kept off the chest.
7. Because of the varying sizes and shapes of different persons' hands, an alternate acceptable hand position is to grasp the wrist of the hand on the chest with the hand that has been locating the lower end of the sternum. This technique is helpful for rescuers with arthritic problems of the hands and wrists.

Proper Compression Techniques.—Effective compression is accomplished by attention to the following guidelines (Fig 6, right):

1. The elbows are locked into position, the arms are straightened, and the shoulders of the rescuer are positioned directly over the hands so that the thrust for each external chest compression is straight down on the sternum. If the thrust is other than straight down, the torso has a tendency to roll, losing part of the force, and the chest compression may be less effective.
2. The sternum must be depressed 1.5 to 2 in (3.8 to 5.0 cm) for the normal-sized adult.
3. The external chest compression pressure is released to allow blood to flow into the heart. The pressure must be released completely and the chest allowed to return to its normal position after each compression. The time allowed for release should equal the time required for compression.

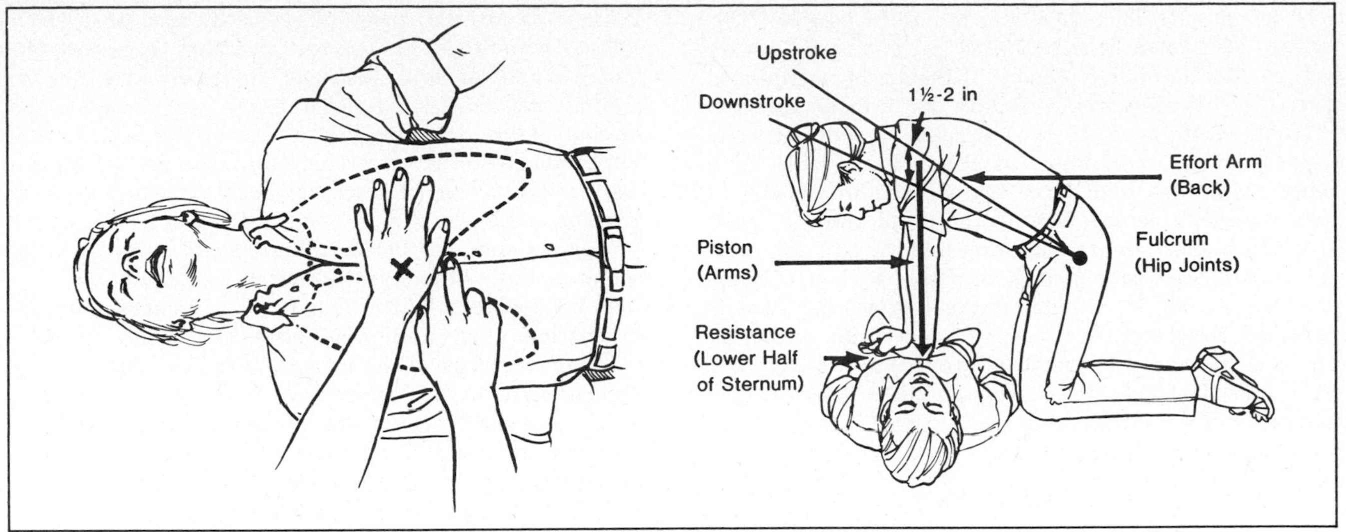

Fig 6.—External chest compression. Left, Locating the correct hand position on the lower half of the body; Right, Proper position of the rescuer, with shoulders directly over the victim's sternum and elbows locked (Adapted from *Cardiopulmonary Resuscitation*. Washington, DC, American National Red Cross, 1981, p 25. Used by permission.)

4. The hands should not be lifted from the chest or the position changed in any way, lest correct hand position be lost.

Rescue breathing and external chest compression must be combined for effective resuscitation of the cardiopulmonary arrest victim.

Physiology of Circulation.—"Closed-Chest Cardiac Massage" was published in 1960.[28] Soon after that this technique was well accepted by professional people and, later, laypersons. It became known as "standard" or "conventional" CPR.

It was believed that external chest compression resulted in the direct compression of the heart between the sternum and the spine, with an increase in pressure within the ventricles and a closure of the valves (mitral and tricuspid). This pressure was thought to cause blood to move into the pulmonary artery (lungs) and the aorta (blood flow to the organs).

In support of this "cardiac pump theory"[30] are the recent studies that demonstrated higher stroke volume and coronary blood flow with high-impulse (moderate force and brief duration) external chest compressions at high rates.[31] Preliminary studies reported that there is valve motion and cardiac chamber compression during the initial five minutes of external chest compression.[32]

This conventional theory of blood flow during CPR has been challenged by several workers who have advanced the "thoracic pump mechanism."[33,34] According to this latter theory, external chest compression produces a rise in the intrathoracic pressure that is transmitted equally to all intrathoracic vascular structures. Because arteries resist collapse, there is nearly full transmission of pressure from intrathoracic to extrathoracic arteries. Competent venous valves and venous collapse prevent full transmission of pressure to extrathoracic veins. An extrathoracic arteriovenous pressure gradient is produced, which causes blood to flow. This thoracic pump theory is supported by the following observations:

1. In patients with flail chests and who need CPR, the arterial pressure does not increase during chest compressions unless the chest is stabilized with a belt, which allows an increase in intrathoracic pressure.[34]

2. It has been observed that some patients who sustain a cardiac arrest and are asked to cough vigorously before loss of consciousness are able to remain conscious and that the systolic arterial pressure during coughing is higher than 100 mm Hg. This significant increase in intrathoracic pressure provides blood flow to the brain.[35] The increase in intrathoracic pressure during coughing results from the contraction of the diaphragm, intercostal, and abdominal muscles against a closed glottis.

3. Two-dimensional echocardiography shows that mitral and tricuspid valves remain open during CPR,[36] supporting the concept that the heart is a passive conduit, rather than a pump.

Recently, there has been important research in new techniques to improve blood flow during CPR: (1) simultaneous chest compression and ventilation (SCV-CPR),[37] (2) abdominal compression with synchronized ventilation,[38] (3) CPR augmented with military antishock trousers,[39] (4) interposed abdominal compression (IAC-CPR),[40] and (5) continuous abdominal binding.[41] Because many of the proposed techniques require the use of devices (eg, endotracheal intubation, binders, trousers, and mechanical compressors), they cannot be recommended as BLS techniques. Additionally, more information regarding survival rates, neurological outcome, and complications is needed before changes in the technique of external chest compressions are recommended.

It is possible that both mechanisms for blood flow play a role during external chest compression. Which one is predominant in a particular victim may depend on several factors, including the size of the heart, ventrodorsal chest diameter, compliance of the chest wall, the magnitude of chest compressions, and perhaps others that are unknown.

Recommendations for External Chest Compression.—The only change from past practice recommended at this time is an increase in the compression rate. The external chest compression rate should be increased to a minimum of 80 per minute, and to 100 per minute if possible. This change is consistent with both the "cardiac pump" theory and the "thoracic pump" theory. If the direct compression of the heart is operative, it is clear that a faster rate will increase blood flow. If the increase in intrathoracic pressure is the mechanism of blood flow during CPR, compression with high force and a duration of 50% of cycle time will increase flow to the brain and the heart. However, higher compression force and the 50% compression duration are very difficult to obtain with a compression rate of 60 per minute; if the compression rate is increased, the result is an optimal compression relaxation duration. A faster compression rate will also allow for a pause for ventilation (in two-rescuer CPR), which is now delivered at an inspiratory flow rate slower than previously recommended.

Cough CPR

Self-induced CPR is possible; however, its applications are limited to clinical situations in which the patient has a cardiac monitor, the arrest was recognized before loss of consciousness (usually within 10 to 15 seconds from the cardiac arrest), and the patient has the ability to cough forcefully. The increase in intrathoracic pressure will generate blood flow to the brain to maintain consciousness for a longer period of time.[42]

CPR PERFORMED BY ONE RESCUER AND BY TWO RESCUERS

CPR Performed by One Rescuer

A lay person should learn only one-rescuer CPR. The previously recommended two-rescuer technique is thought to cause too much confusion and to be infrequently used by laypersons in actual rescue situations. Teaching only one-rescuer CPR should result in better skill retention and possibly better performance. One-rescuer CPR is effective in maintaining adequate circulation and ventilation but is more exhausting than two-rescuer CPR. When trained professionals arrive at the scene of an emergency, they will proceed with two-rescuer CPR and advanced cardiac life support, as appropriate for the situation. The lay rescuer is relieved of responsibility at this point.

One-rescuer CPR should be performed as follows:

A. Airway.—(1) Assessment: determine unresponsiveness (tap or gently shake and shout), (2) call for help, (3) position the victim, and (4) open the airway by the head-tilt/chin-lift maneuver.

B. Breathing.—Assessment: determine breathlessness. *If the victim is breathing,* (1) monitor breathing, (2) maintain an open airway, and (3) activate the EMS system (if not done previously). *If the victim is not breathing,* perform rescue breathing by giving two initial breaths. If unable to give two breaths, (1) reposition the head and attempt to ventilate again, and (2) if still unsuccessful, perform the foreign-body airway obstruction sequence. If successful, continue to the next step.

C. Circulation.—(1) Assessment: determine pulselessness. If pulse is present, continue rescue breathing at 12 times per minute and activate the EMS system. (2) If pulse is absent, activate the EMS system (if not previously done) and continue to the next step. (3) Begin external chest compression: (a) Locate proper hand position. (b) Perform 15 external chest compressions at a rate of 80 to 100 per minute. Count "one and, two and, three and, four and, five and, six and, seven and, eight and, nine and, ten and, eleven and, twelve and, thirteen and, fourteen and, fifteen." (Any mnemonic that accomplishes the same compression rate is acceptable.) (c) Open the airway and deliver two rescue breaths. (d) Locate the proper hand position and begin 15 more compressions at a rate of 80 to 100 per minute. (e) Perform four complete cycles of 15 compressions and two ventilations.

D. Reassessment.—After four cycles of compressions and ventilations (15:2 ratio), reevaluate the patient.

Check for return of the carotid pulse (5 seconds). If it is absent, resume CPR with two ventilations followed by compressions. If it is present, continue to next step.

Check breathing (3 to 5 seconds). If present, monitor breathing and pulse closely. If absent, perform rescue breathing at 12 times per minute and monitor pulse closely.

If CPR is continued, stop and check for return of pulse and spontaneous breathing every few minutes. Do not interrupt CPR for more than 7 seconds except in special circumstances.

One-Rescuer CPR With Entry of a Second Rescuer

When another rescuer is available at the scene, it is recommended that this second rescuer should activate the EMS (if not done previously) and perform one-rescuer CPR when the first rescuer, who initiated CPR, becomes fatigued.

The following steps are recommended for entry of the second rescuer. The second person should identify himself or herself as a qualified rescuer who is willing to help. If the first rescuer is fatigued and has requested help, the logical sequence is as follows: (1) The first rescuer stops CPR after two ventilations. (2) The second rescuer kneels down and checks for pulse for 5 seconds. (3) If there is no pulse, the second rescuer gives two breaths. (4) The second rescuer commences external chest compressions at the recommended rate and ratio for one-person CPR. (5) The first rescuer assesses the adequacy of the second rescuer's ventilations and compressions. This can be done by watching the chest rise during rescue breathing and by checking the pulse during the chest compressions.

CPR Performed by Two Rescuers

All professional rescuers (emergency medicine technicians and medical and health care professionals) should learn both the one-rescuer technique and the two-rescuer coordinated technique, which is less fatiguing. Since this is a two-rescuer technique done by professionals, mouth-to-mask ventilation is an acceptable alternative for rescue breathing.

One person is positioned at the victim's side and performs external chest compression while the other remains at the victim's head, maintains an open airway, monitors the carotid pulse for adequacy of chest compressions, and provides rescue breathing. The compression rate for two-rescuer CPR is 80 to 100 per minute. The compression-ventilation ratio is 5:1, with a pause for ventilation (1 to 1½ seconds). When the compressor becomes fatigued, the rescuers should exchange positions as soon as possible.

Two rescuers should be able to coordinate and perform the following sequences, as appropriate:

1. If CPR is in progress by one rescuer, the logical time for entrance of the two-professionals rescuer team is immediately after the first rescuer has completed a cycle of 15 compressions and two breaths:

One rescuer moves to the head, opens the airway, and checks for a pulse, while the other member of the team locates the area for external chest compressions and finds the proper hand position. This should take 5 seconds.

If there is no pulse, the ventilator gives one breath and the compressor begins external chest compressions at the rate of 80 to 100 per minute, counting "one-and, two-and, three-and, four-and, five."

At the end of the fifth compression a pause should be allowed for the ventilation (1 to 1½ seconds per breath). The compression-ventilation ratio for two rescuers is 5:1. The pause for ventilation may be shorter or may be interposed if the victim is intubated, as faster inspiratory flow rates are possible without the problem of gastric distention, regurgitation, and aspiration. After the airway is protected by the placement of an esophageal obturator airway or endotracheal tube, ventilations may be given in an asynchronous mode at a rate of 12 to 15 per minute.

2. If no CPR is in progress and both rescuers arrive on the scene at the same time, both must determine what needs to be done and start immediately, without wasting time. One rescuer should ensure that the EMS system is activated. If this person leaves the area, the other person should institute one-person CPR.

If both persons are available, one rescuer should go to the head of the victim and proceed as follows: (1) determine unresponsiveness, (2) position the victim, (3) open the airway, (4) check for breathing, (5) if breathing is absent, say "No breathing" and give two ventilations, (6) check for pulse. If there is no pulse, say "No pulse."

The second rescuer should simultaneously (1) find the location for external chest compressions, (2) assume the proper hand position, and (3) initiate external chest compressions after the first rescuer states "No pulse."

Monitoring the Victim

The victim's condition must be monitored to assess the effectiveness of the rescue effort. The ventilator assumes this responsibility for monitoring the pulse and breathing, which serves to (1) evaluate the effectiveness of compressions and (2) determine if the victim resumes spontaneous circulation and breathing.

To assess the effectiveness of the partner's external chest compressions, the pulse should be checked during the compressions. To determine if the victim has resumed spontaneous breathing and circulation, chest compressions must be stopped for 5 seconds at about the end of the first minute and every few minutes thereafter. When the compressor is fatigued, the rescuers should exchange places.

FOREIGN-BODY AIRWAY OBSTRUCTION MANAGEMENT

Causes and Precautions

Upper airway obstruction can cause unconsciousness and cardiopulmonary arrest, but far more often upper airway obstruction is caused by unconsciousness and cardiopulmonary arrest.

An unconscious patient can develop airway obstruction when the tongue falls backward into the pharynx, obstructing the upper airway. The epiglottis could block the entrance of the airway in unconscious victims. Regurgitation of stomach contents into the pharynx, resulting in an obstructed airway, can occur during a cardiopulmonary arrest or during resuscitative attempts. Head and facial injuries may also result in blood clots obstructing the upper airway, particularly if the patient is unconscious.

The National Safety Council[43] reported that foreign-body obstruction of the airway accounted for approximately 3,100 deaths in 1984. Management of upper airway obstruction should be taught within the context of BLS because of the associated ventilatory and circulatory problems if the victim becomes unconscious. Any victim, especially in younger age groups, who suddenly stops breathing, becomes cyanotic, and falls unconscious for no apparent reason should have foreign-body airway obstruction considered in the differential diagnosis.

Foreign-body obstruction of the airway usually occurs during eating. In adults, meat is the most common cause of obstruction, although a variety of other foods and foreign bodies have been the cause of choking in children and some adults. Common factors associated with choking on food include (1) large, poorly chewed pieces of food, (2) elevated blood alcohol levels, and (3) upper and/or lower dentures. This emergency, when it occurs in restaurants, has been mistaken for a heart attack, giving rise to the name "cafe coronary."[44]

The following precautions may prevent foreign-body airway obstruction: (1) cutting food into small pieces and chewing slowly and thoroughly, especially if one is wearing dentures; (2) avoiding laughing and talking during chewing and swallowing; (3) avoiding excessive intake of alcohol before and during meals; (4) restricting children from walking, running, or playing with food or foreign objects in their mouths, and (5) keeping foreign objects, (eg, marbles, beads, and thumbtacks) away from infants and small children.

Recognition of Foreign-Body Airway Obstruction

Because early recognition of airway obstruction is the key to successful management, it is important to distinguish this emergency from fainting, stroke, heart attack, epilepsy, drug overdose, or other conditions that cause sudden respiratory failure but are managed differently.

Foreign bodies may cause either partial airway obstruction or complete airway obstruction. With partial airway obstruction, the victim may be capable of either "good air exchange" or "poor air exchange." With good air exchange, the victim can cough forcefully, although frequently there is wheezing between coughs. As long as good air exchange continues, the victim should be encouraged to persist with spontaneous coughing and breathing efforts. At this point, do not interfere with attempts to expel the foreign body; stay with the victim and monitor these attempts. If partial airway obstruction persists, activate the EMS system.

Poor air exchange may occur initially, or good air

exchange may progress to poor air exchange, as indicated by a weak, ineffective cough, high-pitched noise while inhaling, increased respiratory difficulty, and possibly, cyanosis. A partial obstruction with poor air exchange should be managed as if it were a complete airway obstruction.

With complete airway obstruction the victim is unable to speak, breathe, or cough and may clutch the neck between the thumb and fingers (Fig 7). (The public should be encouraged to use this sign, the universal distress signal.) Ask the victim if he or she is choking. Movement of air will be absent if complete airway obstruction is present. Oxygen saturation in blood will decrease rapidly because the obstructed airway prevents entry of air into the lungs. The brain will develop an oxygen deficit resulting in unconsciousness, and death will follow rapidly if prompt action is not taken.

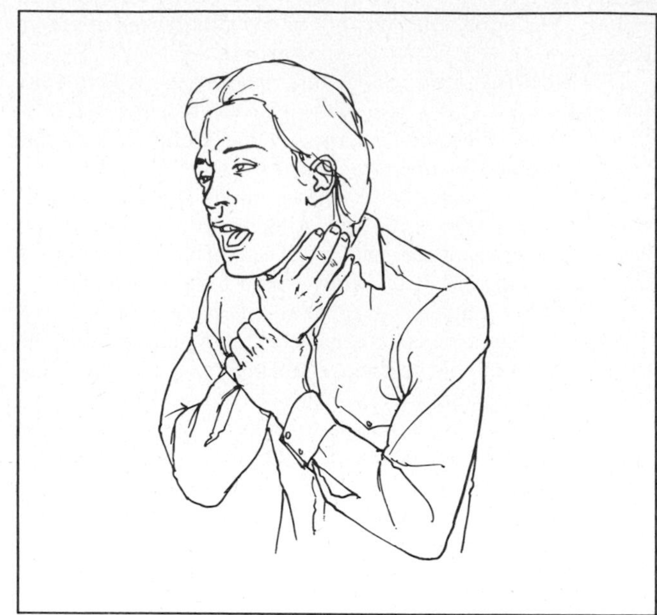

Fig 7.—Universal distress signal for foreign-body airway obstructions.

Management of the Obstructed Airway

The Heimlich maneuver (subdiaphragmatic abdominal thrusts) is recommended for relieving foreign-body airway obstruction.[45] (The term "abdominal thrust" has been used synonymously with the term "Heimlich maneuver" since 1976.[46] For the sake of uniformity, "Heimlich maneuver" should be employed, with the more descriptive "subdiaphragmatic abdominal thrusts" or "abdominal thrusts" used interchangeably, depending on the circumstance.)

A subdiaphragmatic abdominal thrust, by elevating the diaphragm, can force air from the lungs in sufficient quantity to create an artificial cough intended to move and expel an obstructing foreign body in an airway.[47-53] Each individual thrust should be administered with the intent of relieving the obstruction. It may be necessary to repeat the thrust six to ten times to clear the airway. An important consideration during application of the maneuver is possible damage to internal organs, such as rupture or laceration of abdominal or thoracic viscera.[54,55] The rescuer's hands should never be placed on the xiphoid process of the sternum or on the lower margins of rib cage. They should be below this area but above the navel and in the midline. Regurgitation may occur as a result of abdominal thrusts. Training and proper performance should minimize these problems.

Heimlich Maneuver With Victim Standing or Sitting (Conscious).—The rescuer should stand behind the victim, wrap his or her arms around the victim's waist, and proceed as follows (Fig 8): Make a fist with one hand. Place the thumb side of the fist against the victim's abdomen, in the midline slightly above the navel and well below the tip of the xiphoid process. Grasp the fist with the other hand. Press the fist into the victim's abdomen with a quick upward thrust. Each new thrust should be a separate and distinct movement.[45,51,52,56]

Heimlich Maneuver With Victim Lying (Unconscious).—The victim should be placed in the supine position with the face up (Fig 9). The rescuer kneels astride the victim's thighs. The rescuer places the heel of one hand against the victim's abdomen, in the midline slightly above the navel and well below the tip of the xiphoid, and the second hand directly on top of the first. The rescuer presses into the abdomen with a quick upward thrust. If the rescuer is in the correct position, he has a natural midabdominal position and is thus unlikely to direct the thrust to the right or left. A rescuer too short to reach around the victim's waist who is conscious can use this technique. The rescuer can use his or her body weight to perform the maneuver.

Finger Sweep.—This maneuver should be used only in the unconscious victim. With the face up, open the victim's mouth by grasping both the tongue and lower jaw between the thumb and fingers and lifting the mandible (tongue-jaw lift). This action draws the tongue away from the back of the throat and away from a foreign body that may be lodged there. This alone may partially relieve the obstruction. Insert the index finger of the other hand down along the inside of the cheek and deeply into the throat to the base of the tongue. Then use a hooking action to dislodge the foreign body and maneuver it into the mouth so that it can be removed. It is sometimes necessary to use the index finger to push the foreign body against the opposite side of the throat to dislodge and remove it. Be careful not to force the object deeper into the airway. If the foreign body comes within reach, grasp and remove it.

The Self-Administered Heimlich Maneuver.—Treatment of one's own complete foreign-body airway obstruction is as follows: Make a fist with one hand, place the thumb side on the abdomen above the navel and below the xiphoid process, grasp the fist with the other hand, and then press inward and upward toward the diaphragm with a quick motion. If this is unsuccessful, the victim should press the upper abdomen quickly over any firm surface such as the back of a chair, side of a table, or porch railing. Several thrusts may be needed to clear the airway.

Chest Thrusts With Victim Standing or Sitting (Conscious).—This technique is to be used only in the advanced stages of pregnancy or in the markedly obese victim. The rescuer should stand behind the victim, rescuer's arms directly under victim's armpits, and encircle the victim's

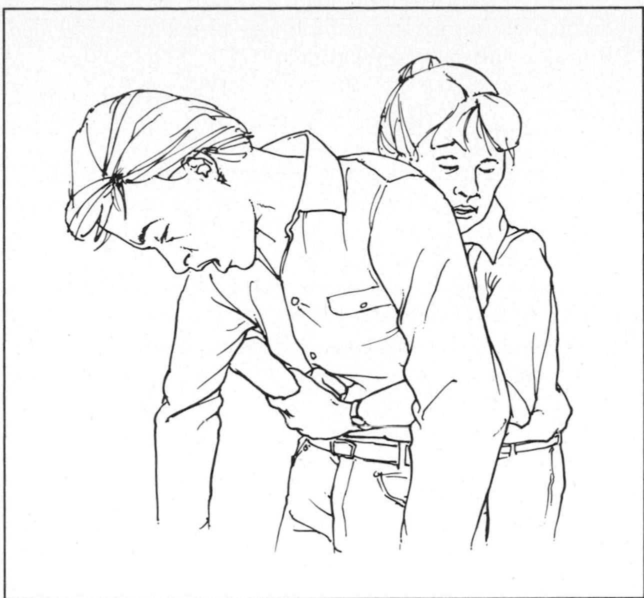

Fig 8.—Heimlich maneuver administered to conscious victim of foreign-body airway obstruction.

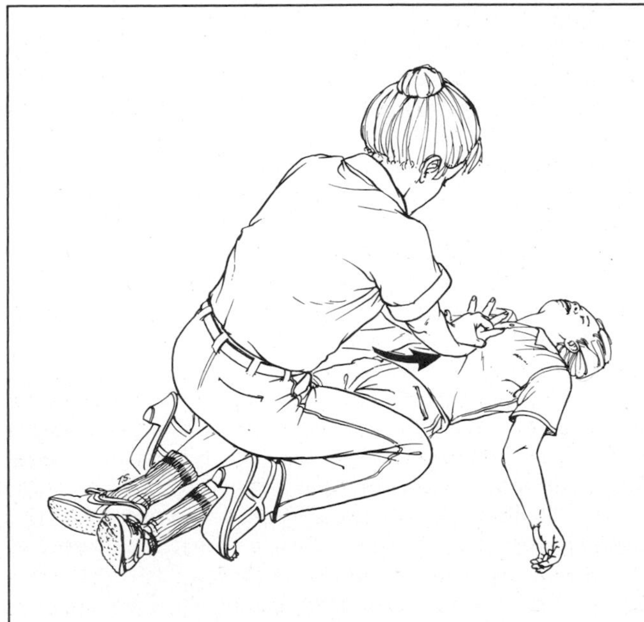

Fig 9.—Heimlich maneuver administered to unconscious victim of foreign-body airway obstruction.

chest. The rescuer should place the thumb side of his or her fist on the middle of the breastbone, taking care to avoid the xiphoid process and the margins of the rib cage. The rescuer should then grab his or her fist with the other hand and perform backward thrusts until the foreign body is expelled or the victim becomes unconscious. Each thrust should be administered with the intent of relieving the obstruction.

Chest Thrusts With Victim Lying (Unconscious).—This maneuver must be used only in the advanced stages of pregnancy and when the rescuer cannot apply the Heimlich maneuver effectively to the unconscious, markedly obese victim. The rescuer should place the victim on the victim's back and kneel close to the side of the victim's body. The hand position for the application of chest thrusts is the same as that for external heart compressions, eg, in the adult, the heel of the hand is on the lower half of the sternum. Each thrust should be delivered slowly, distinctly, and with the intent of relieving the obstruction.

Recommended Sequence for the Conscious Victim or the Victim Who Becomes Unconscious.—(1) Identify airway obstruction and ask the victim if he or she is choking. (2) Apply the Heimlich maneuver until the foreign body is expelled or the victim becomes unconscious. (3) Open the mouth of the now unconscious victim and perform the finger sweep. (4) Open the airway and attempt rescue breathing. (5) If unable to ventilate, perform additional (six to ten) subdiaphragmatic abdominal thrusts. (6) Open the mouth and perform finger sweep. (7) Attempt to ventilate. (8) Repeat the sequence of Heimlich maneuver, finger sweep, and attempt to ventilate. (9) Persist in these efforts as long as necessary. (10) A second person, if available, should activate the EMS as soon as possible.

Recommended Sequence for the Unconscious Victim.—If a rescuer has found an unconscious victim and is unable to ventilate, he or she should reposition the head and try again to ventilate. If this is unsuccessful, subdiaphragmatic abdominal thrusts, followed by the finger sweep, should be performed. If unsuccessful in removing the foreign body, repeat the sequence: thrusts, finger sweep, and attempt to ventilate.

General Recommendations.—(1) The Heimlich maneuver, or subdiaphragmatic abdominal thrusts, is the recommended technique for foreign-body airway obstruction removal in the adult. The use of only this method, which is at least as effective and as safe as any other single method, will simplify training programs and should result in better skills retention. (2) It has previously been recommended that the chest thrust be used in the markedly obese person and in the advanced stages of pregnancy when there is no room between the enlarging uterus and the rib cage in which to perform the thrusts.[52,57] There was no evidence reported at the national conference to suggest that this recommendation should not be continued. It is acknowledged that these incidents are rare. Further investigation is necessary to resolve this dilemma. Until such time the chest thrust should remain as an alternative for the victim of foreign-body airway obstruction in advanced pregnancy and in the markedly obese. (3) Data were presented at the conference that suggest that, as a single method, back blows may not be as effective as the Heimlich maneuver in adults.[47] Because of these data, and in an effort to simplify training, the Heimlich maneuver is the only method recommended at this time. More research and investigation are necessary. (4) Under no circumstances should students practice subdiaphragmatic abdominal thrusts (the Heimlich maneuver) on each other during CPR training. (5) The use of devices for relieving foreign-body airway obstruction is restricted to those properly trained in their use and application. The use of devices by persons who are not proficient in their use is unacceptable, and any efforts to support such activity, by legislation or other means, are seen by this conference as a distinct threat to the well-being of patients in need of emergency airway care. The two types of conventional forceps that are acceptable at the present time, but only in the hands of trained persons proficient in their use, are the Kelly clamp and the Magill forceps. Both should be used only with direct visualization of the foreign body. Either a laryngoscope or tongue blade and flashlight can be used to permit direct visualization.

WARNING SIGNS OF STROKE

Cerebrovascular disease (stroke) may precipitate conditions requiring rescue breathing, external chest compressions, or both. The lay public and health care professionals should know the early warning signs of stroke, and this information should be included in CPR classes so that prompt, early action can be taken.

Emergency care of the stroke victim should be initiated as soon as warning signs or symptoms are recognized. The warning signs or symptoms of stroke may include (1) paralysis on one or both sides of the body, (2) loss of speech or difficulty in speaking, (3) severe dizziness or stupor, (4) loss of vision, particularly in one eye, and (5) loss of consciousness.

The above warning signs of stroke may also be temporary. They may last less than 24 hours and, indeed, often last for only a few minutes. If any of these signs or symptoms occur, a physician should be sought immediately or the EMS system activated, depending on the severity of the symptoms. Similar signs may also be due to alcohol, drugs, insulin reactions, or other diseases; but they may also be warning signs of stroke, even when transient.

UNIQUE SITUATIONS

Changing Location.—A victim should not be moved from a cramped or busy location for convenience until effective CPR has been started and the victim has a spontaneous pulse, or until help arrives so that CPR can be performed without interruption.

Stairways.—In some instances a victim has to be transported up or down a flight of stairs. It is best to perform CPR effectively at the head or the foot of the stairs and, at a predetermined signal, to interrupt CPR and move as quickly as possible to the next level, where CPR should be resumed. Interruptions should not last longer than 30 seconds and should be avoided if possible.

Litters.—While transferring a victim into an ambulance or other mobile emergency care unit, CPR should not be interrupted. Even as the victim is being moved to an ambulance, CPR must continue. With a low-wheeled litter the rescuer can stand alongside, maintaining the locked-arm position for compression. With a high litter or bed, the rescuer may have to kneel beside the victim on the bed or litter to gain the needed height over the victim's sternum.

Cardiopulmonary resuscitation should not be interrupted for more than 7 seconds unless endotracheal intubation is being performed by trained individuals or there are problems with transportation.

PITFALLS AND COMPLICATIONS

If CPR is performed improperly or inadequately, external chest compression and rescue breathing may be ineffective in supporting life. Even properly performed CPR may result in complications.[58-61]

Rescue Breathing

Techniques for opening the airway should be carefully followed to avoid potential neck and spine complications. The most common reason for inability to ventilate a patient is improper head position.

The major problem associated with excess ventilation volume and fast ventilatory flow rates is gastric distention. Rescue breathing frequently causes distention of the stomach, especially in children. This usually occurs when excessive inflation pressures are used, or if the airway is partially or completely obstructed. Gastric distention can be minimized by maintaining an open airway and limiting ventilation volumes to the point at which the chest rises, and not exceeding esophageal opening pressures. Other techniques have been reported to prevent gastric distention:

1. Mouth-to-nose ventilation.[13] The rationale for this recommendation is that the nose, by providing greater resistance to the flow of ventilating gases, will decrease the pressure of the gases reaching the pharynx.
2. Slow inflation time during ventilation.[13,22] The slower inspiratory flow rates will produce less pressure in the pharynx and thereby minimize the risk of gastric distention.
3. Cricoid pressure. This technique consists of applying backward pressure on the cricoid cartilage against the cervical vertebra to prevent regurgitation.[62,63] Cricoid pressure has been found to be effective in preventing regurgitation against esophageal pressure of up to 100 cm of water.[64] This technique should be applied only by health care professionals in two-rescuer CPR situations; its application is simple but requires an assistant.

Marked distention of the stomach may promote regurgitation and reduce lung volume by elevation of the diaphragm. If the stomach becomes distended during rescue breathing, recheck and reposition the airway, observe the rise and fall of the chest, and avoid excessive airway pressure. Continue rescue breathing without attempting to expel the stomach contents. Experience has shown that attempting to relieve stomach distention by manual pressure over the victim's upper abdomen is almost certain to cause regurgitation if the stomach is full. If regurgitation does occur, turn the victim's entire body to the side, wipe out the mouth, return the body to the supine position, and continue CPR.

If severe gastric distention results in inadequate ventilation, apply pressure over the epigastrium after placing the victim on the side to expel the air from the stomach. This maneuver may be necessary despite the risk of inducing regurgitation and aspiration. The use of suction by trained individuals will minimize aspiration in this situation.

Continuous pressure should not be maintained on the abdomen to help prevent gastric distention because of the danger of trapping the liver, possibly causing liver rupture.[65,66] An additional reason to avoid such pressure is the possibility of regurgitation and aspiration of gastric contents.

External Chest Compression

Care should be taken to comply with the recommendations concerning external chest compression techniques. Pulselessness must be established prior to performing compressions. Proper CPR techniques lessen the possibilities of complications resulting from improperly performed compressions.

Even properly performed external chest compression can cause rib fractures in some patients. Other complications that may occur despite proper CPR techniques include fracture of the sternum, separation of the ribs from the sternum, pneumothorax, hemothorax, lung contusions, lacerations of the liver and spleen, and fat emboli. These complications may be minimized by careful attention to details of performance but cannot be entirely prevented. Accordingly, concern for injuries that may result even from properly performed CPR should not impede prompt and energetic application of the technique. The only alternative to timely initiation of effective CPR for the cardiac arrest victim is death.

Improper hand position for external chest compression should be avoided by careful identification of landmarks. Applying pressure too low on the chest may cause the tip of the sternum to cut into the liver and cause internal bleeding.

The rescuer's fingers should not rest on the victim's ribs during compression. Interlocking the fingers of the hands may help avoid this. Pressure with fingers on the ribs or lateral (sideways) pressure increases the possibility of rib fractures and costochondral separations. Between compressions, the heel of the hand must completely release its pressure but should remain in constant contact with the chest wall over the lower half of the sternum.

Compressions should be smooth, regular, and uninterrupted except for rescue breathing. There should be equal compression and relaxation cycles. Sudden or jerking movements should be avoided. Jabs can increase the possibility of injury to the ribs and internal organs and may decrease the amount of blood circulated by each compression. The lower half of the sternum of an adult must be depressed about 1.5 to 2 in (3.8 to 5 cm) during chest compression. Less depth of compression may be ineffective.

SPECIAL RESUSCITATION SITUATIONS

Near Drowning

The most important consequence of prolonged underwater submersion without ventilation is hypoxemia. There are four elements in the management of a near-drowning victim.

1. Rescue From the Water.—When attempting to rescue a near-drowning victim, the rescuer should get to the victim as quickly as possible, preferably with some conveyance (boat, raft, surfboard, or flotation device). The rescuer must always be aware of personal safety in attempting a rescue and should exercise caution to minimize the danger.

2. Rescue Breathing.—Initial treatment of the near-drowning victim consists of rescue breathing using the mouth-to-mouth or mouth-to-nose technique. Rescue breathing should be started as soon as possible, even before the victim is moved out of the water, into a boat, or onto a surfboard, provided it can be accomplished without undue risk to the rescuer.

Appliances (such as a snorkel using the mouth-to-snorkel technique) may permit specially trained rescuers to perform rescue breathing in deep water. However, rescue breathing should not be delayed for lack of such equipment if it can otherwise be provided safely; untrained rescuers should not attempt the use of such adjuncts.

If neck injury is suspected, however, the victim's neck should be supported in a neutral position (without flexion or extension), and the victim should be floated supine onto a horizontal back support before being removed from the water. If the victim must be turned, the head, neck, chest, and body should be aligned, supported, and turned as a unit to the horizontal supine position. If artificial respiration is required, maximal head-tilt should not be used. Rescue breathing should be provided with the head maintained in a neutral position, ie, jaw-thrust without head-tilt, or chin-lift without head-tilt, should be used.

3. Foreign Matter in the Airway.—The need for clearing the lower airway of aspirated water has not been proved scientifically, although there are anecdotal reports of clinical response to a subdiaphragmatic abdominal thrust.[83] At most, only a modest amount of water is aspirated by the majority of both freshwater and seawater drowning victims, and freshwater is rapidly absorbed from the lungs into the circulation.[84] Furthermore, 10% to 12% of victims do not aspirate at all due to laryngospasm or breath holding.[84,85] An attempt to remove water from the breathing passages by any means other than suction may be unnecessary and dangerous because it could eject gastric contents and cause aspiration.[85]

Since the risk-benefit ratio of a subdiaphragmatic abdominal thrust in this setting is unknown, the only time it definitely should be used is when the rescuer suspects that foreign matter is obstructing the airway or if the victim does not respond appropriately to mouth-to-mouth ventilation. Then, if necessary, CPR should be reinstituted after the Heimlich maneuver has been applied.[86-88] The Heimlich maneuver is performed on the near-drowning victim as described in the treatment of foreign-body airway obstruction (unconscious supine) except that in near drowning the victim's head should be turned sideways.

Further investigation is needed to define better the need for, the risk of, and the timing of a subdiaphragmatic abdominal thrust in this situation.

4. Chest Compressions.—External chest compression should not be attempted in the water unless the rescuer has had special training in techniques of in-water CPR because the brain is not perfused effectively unless the victim is maintained in the horizontal position and the back is supported. It is usually not possible to keep the victim's body horizontal and still keep the victim's head above water, in position for rescue breathing.

On removal from the water, the victim must be assessed immediately for adequacy of circulation. The pulse may be difficult to appreciate in a near-drowning victim because of peripheral vasoconstriction and a low cardiac output. If a pulse cannot be felt, CPR should be started at once.

5. Definitive Advanced Life Support Care.—There should be no delay in moving the victim to a life support unit where advanced life support is provided. Every submersion victim, even one who requires only minimal resuscitation and regains consciousness at the scene, should be transferred to a medical facility for follow-up care. It is imperative that life support measures be continued en route and that oxygen be administered if it is available in the transport vehicle.

Successful resuscitation with full neurological recovery has occurred in near-drowning victims with prolonged submersion in cold water.[89,90] An absolute time limit beyond which resuscitation is not indicated has not been established. Since it is often difficult for rescuers to obtain an accurate time of submersion, attempts at resuscitation should be initiated by rescuers at the scene unless there is obvious physical evidence of death (such as putrefaction). The victim should be transported with continued CPR to an advanced life support facility where a physician can decide whether to continue resuscitation. Aggressive continued attempts at resuscitation on hospital arrival should be encouraged.

Traumatic Injury

Survival from cardiac arrest due to traumatic injury is generally poor.[91-96] External chest compression may not provide adequate circulation in the severely hypovolemic trauma arrest victim.[92] Emphasis should be placed on rapid transport of such patients to a trauma center where circulating blood volume can be restored and the underlying vascular injury corrected.

1. Basic Life Support.—Lay rescuers coming onto the scene of an accident should request help as soon as possible. If an automobile accident victim is pinned, the untrained lay rescuer should not attempt to move the victim unless there is further imminent danger to life, such as fire. The unconscious trauma victim should be assessed and treated using the standard *ABC*s of CPR, taking care to protect the cervical spine and attempting to control any obvious severe bleeding with direct manual compression of the wound.

In trauma victims, it is imperative that caution be used to avoid inflicting further injury by backward tilt of the head when there is a possibility of cervical spine fracture. Cervical spine fracture should be suspected in any patient with the following: (1) an injury above the clavicle or a head injury resulting in an unconscious state or (2) a mechanism of injury that may have subjected the spine to sudden acceleration or deceleration (diving, fall, automobile crash, or airplane crash).

If cervical spine fracture is suspected, all forward, backward, lateral, or head-turning movement should be avoided. If turning is necessary, the head, neck, chest, and body should be supported and turned as a unit. The jaw-thrust maneuver without head-tilt or the chin-lift without head-tilt should be used to open the airway.

The different agencies involved in teaching rescue techniques to laypersons should have a coordinated effort for standardization and simplification of first aid techniques and should include basic CPR and special techniques for the trauma victim (eg, hemorrhage control, positioning of the unconscious victim, positioning of the victim in shock, and special techniques for airway control and ventilation).

Electric Shock

Complications that may follow an electric shock depend largely on the amplitude and duration of contact with the current. Electrical burns and injuries caused by falling may require prompt attention. Consequences likely to require CPR include the following:

1. Tetany of the breathing muscles. This is usually limited to the duration of current exposure. If current exposure is prolonged and tetany persists, cardiac arrest may occur because of hypoxia.
2. Prolonged paralysis of breathing muscles. This may result from massive convulsive phenomena, which last for minutes after the shock current has terminated, and result in hypoxic cardiac arrest.
3. Cardiac arrest. Ventricular fibrillation or ventricular asystole may occur as a direct result of electric shock and require CPR. Other serious cardiac arrhythmias, including ventricular tachycardia that may progress to ventricular fibrillation, may result from exposure to low- or high-voltage currents (110 to 220 V) sustained for several seconds and may require advanced cardiac life support monitoring and treatment or resuscitation.

The prognosis for victims of electric shock is not readily predictable, since the amplitude and duration of the charge usually are not known. Failure of either respiration or circulation is likely to result.

1. Basic Life Support.—It is critically important that the rescuer be certain that rescue efforts will not put him or her in danger of electrical shock. After safely clearing a victim from an energized object, the rescuer should determine the victim's cardiopulmonary status immediately. If spontaneous respiration or circulation is absent, the technique of CPR outlined in these standards and guidelines should be initiated.

In cases where electric shock occurs in a location that is not readily accessible, as on a public utility pole, rescue breathing should be started at once. The victim must therefore be lowered to the ground as quickly as possible. Cardiopulmonary resuscitation is effective only when performed on a victim who is in the horizontal position.

Lightning acts as a massive direct current countershock, depolarizing the entire myocardium at once, following which the heart's normal rhythm may resume. Patients most likely to die of lightning injury are those who suffer immediate cardiac arrest.[97] Patients who do not experience arrest immediately have an excellent chance of recovery. Therefore, when multiple victims are simultaneously struck by lightning, individuals who appear clinically dead immediately following the strike should be treated before other victims showing signs of life.

Hypothermia

Severe accidental hypothermia (below 30 °C) is associated with marked depression in cerebral blood flow and oxygen requirement, reduced cardiac output, and decreased arterial pressure. Victims can appear to be clinically dead due to marked depression of brain function. Peripheral pulses may be difficult to detect because of bradycardia and vasoconstriction.

1. Basic Life Support.—If the victim is not breathing, rescue breathing should be started. Chest compression is indicated in the pulseless, unmonitored, suspected hypothermia victim in the field, but a longer time to check for a pulse (up to one minute) may be necessary.[98]

The victim should be transported with continued CPR as quickly as possible to an advanced life support treatment facility. It is important to prevent further heat loss from the core by insulating the victim and adding heat (if possible) by applying external warm objects (eg, hot water bottles or warm packs) and/or warm, moist oxygen.[99]

References

1. *A Manual for Instructors in Basic Life Support.* Dallas, American Heart Association, 1977.

2. Eisenberg MS, Bergner L, Hallstrom A: Cardiac resuscitation in the community. Importance of rapid provision and implications for program planning. *JAMA* 1979;241:1905-1907.

3. Cobb LA, Werner JA, Trobaugh GB: Sudden cardiac death: Parts 1 and 2. *Med Concepts Cardiovasc Dis* 1980;49:31-36, 37-42.

4. Eisenberg MS, Copass MK, Hallstrom AP, et al: Treatment of out-of-hospital cardiac arrest with rapid defibrillation by emergency medical technicians. *N Engl J Med* 1980;302:1379-1383.

5. Myerburg RJ, Kessler KM, Zaman L, et al: Survivors of prehospital cardiac arrest. *JAMA* 1982;247:1485-1490.

6. Abramson N, Safar P, Detre K, et al: An international collaborative clinical study mechanism for resuscitation research. *Resuscitation* 1982; 10:141-147.

7. Longstreth WT, Diehr P, Inui TS: Prediction of awakening after out-of-hospital cardiac arrest. *N Engl J Med* 1983;308:1378-1382.

8. *Risk Factors and Coronary Disease: A Statement for Physicians.* Dallas, American Heart Association, 1980.

9. Safar P: The pathology of dying and reanimation, in Schwartz G, Safar P, Stone J, et al (eds): *Principles and Practice of Emergency Medicine,* ed 2. Philadelphia, WB Saunders Co, 1985.

10. Safar P: Ventilatory efficacy of mouth-to-mouth artificial respiration. Airway obstruction during manual and mouth-to-mouth artificial respiration. *JAMA* 1958;167:335-341.

11. Safar P, Escarraga L, Change F: A study of upper airway obstruction in the unconscious patient. *J Appl Physiol* 1959;14:760-764.

12. Morikawa S, Safar P, DeCarlo J: Influence of head position upon upper airway patency. *Anesthesiology* 1961;22:265.

13. Ruben H, Elam JO, Ruben AM, et al: Investigation of upper airway problems in resuscitation. *Anesthesiology* 1961;22:271-279.

14. Boidin MP: Airway patency in the unconscious patient. *Br J Anaesth* 1985;57:306-310.

15. Safar P: *Cardiopulmonary Cerebral Resuscitation.* Philadelphia, WB Saunders Co, 1981.

16. Guildner CW: Resuscitation—opening the airway: A comparative study of techniques for opening an airway obstructed by the tongue. *JACEP* 1976;5:588-590.

17. Esmarch F: *The Surgeon's Handbook.* London, Sampson Low Marston Searle & Rivington, 1878, pp 114-118.

18. Elam JO, Greene DG, Schneider MA, et al: Head tilt method of oral resuscitation. *JAMA* 1960;172:812-815.

19. Safar P, Lind B: Triple airway maneuver, artificial ventilation and oxygen inhalation by mouth-to-mask and bag-valve-mask techniques, in *Proceedings of the 1973 National Conference on CPR.* Dallas, American Heart Association, 1975.

20. Elam JO, Greene DG: Mission accomplished. Successful mouth-to-mouth resuscitation. *Anesth Analg Curr Res* 1961;40:440-442, 578-680, 672-676.

21. Ruben H, Knudsen EJ, Carugati G: Gastric inflation in relation to airway pressure. *Acta Anaesth Scand* 1961;5:107-114.

22. Melker R: Asynchronous and other alternative methods of ventilation during CPR. *Ann Emerg Med* 1984;13(pt 2):758-761.

23. Melker R: Recommendations for ventilation during cardiopulmonary resuscitation. Time for change? *Crit Care Med* 1985;13:882-883.

24. Ruben H: The immediate treatment of respiratory failure. *Br J Anaesth* 1964;36:542-549.

25. Safar P, Redding J: 'Tight jaw' in resuscitation. *Anesthesiology* 1959;20:701-702.

26. *First Aid for (Neck Breathers) Laryngectomees.* New York, American Cancer Society, 1971.

27. *Instructors Manual for Basic Life Support.* Dallas, American Heart Association, 1985.

28. Kouwenhoven WB, Jude JR, Knickerbocker GG: Closed-chest cardiac massage. *JAMA* 1960;173:1064-1067.

29. Safar P, Brown TC, Holtey WH, et al: Ventilation and circulation with closed-chest cardiac massage in man. *JAMA* 1961;176:574-580.

30. Babbs CF: New versus old theories of blood flow during CPR. *Crit Care Med* 1980;8:191-195.

31. Maier GW, Tyson GS, Olsen CO, et al: The physiology of external cardiac massage: High impulse cardiopulmonary resuscitation. *Circulation* 1984;70:86-101.

32. Deshmukh H, Weil MH, Swindall A, et al: Echocardiographic observations during cardiopulmonary resuscitation: A preliminary report. *Crit Care Med* 1985;13:904-906.

33. Niemann JT, Garner D, Rosborough J, et al: The mechanism of blood flow in closed chest cardiopulmonary resuscitation, abstracted. *Circulation* 1979;60(suppl 2):74.

34. Rudikoff MT, Maughan WL, Effron M, et al: Mechanism of blood flow during cardiopulmonary resuscitation. *Circulation* 1980;61:345-352.

35. Criley JM, Blaufuss AH, Kissel GL: Cough-induced cardiac compression. Self-induced form of cardiopulmonary resuscitation. *JAMA* 1976; 236:1246-1250.

36. Werner JA, Greene HL, Janko CL, et al: Visualization of cardiac valve motion during external chest compression using two-dimensional echocardiography. Implications regarding the mechanism of blood flow. *Circulation* 1981;63:1417.

37. Chandra N, Rudikoff M, Weisfelt M: Simultaneous chest compression and ventilation at high airway pressure during cardiopulmonary resuscitation. *Lancet* 1980;1:175-178.

38. Rosborough JP, Niemann JT, Criley JM, et al: Lower abdominal compression with synchronized ventilation: A CPR modality. *Circulation* 1981;64:303.

39. Bircher N, Safar P, Steward R: A comparison of standard 'MAST'-augmented, and open-chest CPR in dogs: A preliminary investigation. *Crit Care Med* 1980;8:147-152.

40. Ralston SH, Babbs CF, Niebauer MJ: Cardiopulmonary resuscitation with interposed abdominal compression in dogs. *Anesth Analg* 1982; 61:645-651.

41. Niemann JT, Rosborough JP, Ung S, et al: Hemodynamic effects of continuous abdominal binding during cardiac arrest and resuscitation. *Am J Cardiol* 1984;53:269-274.

42. Niemann JT, Rosborough J, Hausknecht M, et al: Cough CPR. Documentation of systemic perfusion in man and in an experimental model: A 'window' to the mechanism of blood flow in external CPR. *Crit Care Med* 1980;8:141-146.

43. *Accident Facts.* Chicago, National Safety Council, 1984, p 7.

44. Haugen RK: The cafe coronary. *JAMA* 1963;186:142-143.

45. Heimlich HJ: A life-saving maneuver to prevent food-choking. *JAMA* 1975;234:398-401.

46. Committee on Emergency Medical Services, Assembly of Life Sciences, National Research Council: *Report of Emergency Airway Management.* National Academy of Sciences, 1976.

47. Day RL, Crelin ES, DuBois AB: Choking: The Heimlich abdominal thrust vs back blows: An approach to measurement of inertial and aerodynamic forces. *Pediatrics* 1982;70:113-119.

48. Day RL, DuBois AB: Treatment of choking. *Pediatrics* 1983;71:300-301.

49. Day RL: Differing opinions on the emergency treatment of choking. *Pediatrics* 1983;71:976-977.

50. Patrick EA: *Decision Analysis in Medicine: Methods and Applications.* Boca Raton, Fla, CRC Press Inc, 1979, pp 90-93.

51. Heimlich HJ, Hoffman KA, Canestri FR: Food-choking and drowning deaths prevented by external subdiaphragmatic compression: Physiological basis. *Ann Thorac Surg* 1975;20:188-195.

52. Heimlich HJ, Uhtley MH: The Heimlich maneuver. *Clin Symp* 1979;31:22.

53. Patrick EA: Choking: A questionnaire to find the most effective treatment. *Emergency* 1980;12:59-63.

54. Visintine RE, Baick CH: Ruptured stomach after Heimlich maneuver. *JAMA* 1975;234:415.

55. Palmer E: The Heimlich maneuver misused. *Curr Prescribing* 1979;5:45-49.

56. Heimlich HJ: Pop goes the cafe coronary. *Emerg Med* 1974; 6:154-155.

57. Standards and Guidelines for Cardiopulmonary Resuscitation (CPR) and Emergency Cardiac Care (ECC). *JAMA* 1980;244:453-509.

58. Nagel EI, Fine EG, Krischer JP, et al: Complications of CPR. *Crit Care Med* 1983;9:424.
59. Bjork RJ, Snyder BD, Campion DC, et al: Medical complications of cardiopulmonary arrest. *Arch Intern Med* 1982;142:500-503.
60. Atcheson SG, Fred HL: Complications of cardiac resuscitation. *Am Heart J* 1975;89:263-264.
61. McGrath RB: Gastroesophageal lacerations: A fatal complication of closed chest cardiopulmonary resuscitation. *Chest* 1983;83:571-572.
62. Keith A: Mechanism underlying the various methods of artificial respiration. *Lancet*, March 1909, p 747.
63. Sellick BA: Cricoid pressure to control regurgitation of stomach contents during induction of anesthesia. *Lancet* 1961;2:404-406.
64. Salem MR, Wong AY, Mani M, et al: Efficacy of cricoid pressure in preventing gastric distention during bag-mask ventilation in pediatric patients. *Anesthesiology* 1974;40:96-98.
65. Wilder RJ, Weir D, Rush BE, et al: Methods of coordinating ventilation and closed-chest cardiac massage in the dog. *Surgery* 1963; 53:186-194.
66. Harris LC, Kirimli B, Safar P: Augmentation of artificial circulation during cardiopulmonary resuscitation. *Anesthesiology* 1967;28:730-734.
67. *Recommendations for Decontaminating Manikins Used in Cardiopulmonary Resuscitation: Hepatitis Surveillance*, report 42. Atlanta, Centers for Disease Control, 1978, pp 34-36.
68. Bond WW, Petersen NJ, Favero MS: Viral hepatitis B: Aspects of environmental control. *Health Lab Sci* 1977;14:235-252.
69. Bond WW, Favero MS, Petersen NJ, et al: Inactivation of hepatitis B virus by intermediate- to high-level disinfectant chemicals. *J Clin Microbiol* 1983;18:535-538.
70. Favero MS: Sterilization, disinfection and antisepsis in the hospital, in Lenette EH, Balows A, Hausler WJ Jr, et al (eds): *Manual of Clinical Microbiology*, ed 4. Washington, DC, American Society of Microbiology, 1985, pp 129-137.
71. Centers for Disease Control: Acquired immune deficiency syndrome (AIDS): Precautions for clinical and laboratory staffs. *MMWR* 1982; 31:577-580.
72. Centers for Disease Control: Prevention of acquired immune deficiency syndrome (AIDS): Report of inter-agency recommendations. *MMWR* 1983;32:101-103.
73. Task Force on the Acquired Immunodeficiency Syndrome: Infection control guidelines for patients with acquired immunodeficiency syndrome (AIDS). *N Engl J Med* 1983;309:740-744.
74. Bond WW: Inactivation of AIDS virus in clothing. *JAMA* 1985; 253:258.
75. Lettau LA, Bond WW, McDougal JS: Hepatitis and diaphragm fitting. *JAMA* 1985;254:752.
76. Martin LS, McDougal JS, Loskoski SL: Disinfection and inactivation of the human T lymphotrophic virus type III/lymphadenopathy-associated virus. *J Infect Dis* 1985;152:400-403.
77. McDougal JS, Cort SP, Kennedy MS, et al: Immunoassay for detection and quantitation of infectious viral particles of the human retrovirus lymphadenopathy-associated virus (LAV). *J Immunol Methods* 1985;76:171-183.
78. Spire B, Dormont D, Barré-Sinoussi F, et al: Inactivation of lymphadenopathy-associated virus by heat, gamma rays and ultraviolet light. *Lancet* 1985;1:188-189.
79. Recommendations for preventing transmission of infection with human T-lymphotropic virus type III/lymphadenopathy-associated virus in the workplace. *MMWR* 1985;34:681-696.
80. MacCauley C, Todd C: Physical disability among cardiopulmonary resuscitation students. *Occupational Health Nurse* 1978;3:17-19.
81. Greenberg M: CPR: A report of observed medical complications during training. *Ann Emerg Med* 1983;12:194-195.
82. Memon A, Salyer J, Hillman E, et al: Fatal myocardial infarction following CPR training: The question of risk. *Ann Emerg Med* 1982; 11:322-323.
83. Heimlich HJ: Subdiaphragmatic pressure to expel water from the lungs of drowning persons. *Ann Emerg Med* 1981;10:476-480.
84. Modell JH, Davis JH: Electrolyte changes in human drowning victims. *Anesthesiology* 1969;30:414-420.
85. Modell JH: Is the Heimlich maneuver appropriate as first treatment for drowning? *Emerg Med Serv* 1981;10:63-66.
86. Patrick EA: The Heimlich maneuver. *Emergency* 1981;13:45-47.
87. Heimlich HJ: The Heimlich maneuver: First treatment for drowning victims. *Emerg Med Serv* 1981;10:58-61.
88. Heimlich HJ: Editorial commentary. *Emerg Med Serv* 1982;11:93-96.
89. Siebke H, Rod T, Breivik H, et al: Survival after 40 minutes submersion without cerebral sequelae. *Lancet* 1975;1:1275-1277.
90. Southwick FS, Dalglish PH: Recovery after prolonged asystolic cardiac arrest in profound hypothermia. A case report and literature review. *JAMA* 1980;243:1250-1253.
91. Baker CC, Thomas AN, Trunkey DD: The role of emergency room thoracotomy in trauma. *J Trauma* 1980;20:848-855.
92. Mattox KL, Feliciano DV: Role of external cardiac compression in truncal trauma. *J Trauma* 1982;22:934-936.
93. Vij D, Simoni E, Smith RF, et al: Resuscitative thoracotomy for patients with traumatic injury. *Surgery* 1983;94:554-561.
94. Shimazu S, Shatney CH: Outcomes of trauma patients with no vital signs on hospital admission. *J Trauma* 1983;23:213-216.
95. Cogbill TH, Moore EE, Millikan JS, et al: Rationale for selective application of emergency department thoracotomy in trauma. *J Trauma* 1983;23:453-460.
96. Flynn TC, Ward RE, Miller PW: Emergency department thoracotomy. *Ann Emerg Med* 1982;11:413-416.
97. Cooper MA: Lightning injuries: Prognostic signs for death. *Ann Emerg Med* 1980;9:134-138.
98. Steinman AM: The hypothermic code: CPR controversy revisited. *J Emerg Med Serv* 1983;10:32-35.
99. Samuelson T, Doolittle W, Hayward J, et al: Hypothermia and cold water near drowning: Treatment guidelines. *Alaska Med* 1982;24:106-111.
100. Zell SC, Kurtz KJ: Severe exposure hypothermia: A resuscitation protocol. *Ann Emerg Med* 1985;14:339-345.
101. Reuler JB: Hypothermia: Pathophysiology, clinical settings, and management. *Ann Intern Med* 1978;89:519-527.
102. Elenbass RM, Mattson K, Cole H, et al: Bretylium in hypothermia-induced ventricular fibrillation in dogs. *Ann Emerg Med* 1984;13:994-999.
103. Althaus U, Aeberhard P, Schupbach P, et al: Management of profound accidental hypothermia with cardiorespiratory arrest. *Ann Surg* 1982;195:492-495.

Pediatric Basic Life Support

Cardiopulmonary resuscitation (CPR) in the pediatric age group should be part of a communitywide effort that smoothly integrates pediatric basic life support (BLS), pediatric advanced life support (ALS), and postresuscitation care. Basic life support is that phase of emergency care that (1) prevents respiratory and circulatory arrest through prompt recognition and intervention or (2) supports or provides ventilation and, if necessary, circulation to a victim, without the use of adjuncts. Except in the newborn period, the number of children who require resuscitation is small; for best results, therefore, each community must ensure that its emergency medical services (EMS) personnel are optimally trained and equipped to care for pediatric emergencies. There is evidence that this is not currently the case.[1] It is further recommended that (1) BLS for infants and children be the major focus of courses offered to certain audiences, ie, parents of young children, day care personnel, and parents of infants at high risk for sudden infant death; (2) personnel in ALS emergency facilities have demonstrated competence in pediatric BLS and pediatric ALS; and (3) each ALS facility have an ongoing agreement with an identified tertiary pediatric service where postresuscitation care for infants and children can be given in a pediatric intensive care unit under the supervision of trained personnel.

CAUSES OF CARDIOPULMONARY ARREST

Cardiac arrest in the pediatric age group is rarely primarily of cardiac origin; more commonly, it results from a low oxygen level secondary to respiratory difficulty or arrest. Since the cardiac arrest is the result of a long period of hypoxemia, it is not surprising that outcomes of CPR in children who have suffered a cardiac arrest have been poor.[2,3] On the other hand, the outcome of resuscitation from respiratory arrest, before the development of cardiac arrest, is considerably better.[2] It should be possible, theoretically, to improve the current poor results with an educational program—directed at parents, child care personnel, and members of the EMS system—that emphasizes prevention, early recognition of the child in distress, and rapid intervention before cardiac arrest occurs.

The major events that may necessitate resuscitation include (1) injuries, (2) suffocation caused by foreign bodies (ie, toys, foods, plastic covers, etc), (3) smoke inhalation, (4) sudden infant death syndrome, and (5) infections, especially of the respiratory tract. Injuries account for nearly 9,000 pediatric fatalities annually in the United States and represent approximately 44% of deaths in children between the ages of 1 and 14 years. Of these, 45% involve motor vehicles, 17% drowning, and 21% burns, firearms, and poisoning. In children younger than 1 year of age, 41% of accidental deaths involve poisons, suffocation, or motor vehicles.[4]

The vast majority of emergency situations requiring CPR are preventable, and special attention must therefore be paid to producing environments for children that are safe and protective without suppressing their need for exploration and discovery. Children should be taught respect for matches and fires, and young children should not be left unsupervised. Toys given to toddlers should be carefully examined for small parts that could be aspirated. Beads, small toys, marbles, and peanuts must be kept away from infants and preschool children. In automobiles, age-appropriate restraints, including infant car seats and seat belts, should be used. Children should be taught to swim, and water safety should be emphasized. It is important to remember that time spent mastering CPR is much less productive than time spent preventing the situation leading to its need.

THE SEQUENCE OF CPR

1. Determine Unresponsiveness or Respiratory Difficulty

The rescuer must quickly assess the extent of any injury and determine whether the child is unconscious. Special care must be taken if the victim has sustained head or neck trauma so as not to cause spinal cord injury. Unconsciousness is determined by gently shaking the victim to elicit a response. If the child is struggling to breathe but is conscious, the child should be transported as rapidly as possible to an ALS facility. Children will often find the best position in which to keep a partially obstructed airway open and should therefore be allowed to maintain the position affording them the greatest comfort.

2. Call for Help

After determining unresponsiveness or respiratory difficulty, the rescuer should call out for help. If the rescuer is alone and the child obviously is not breathing, CPR should be performed for one minute before calling for help.

3. Position the Victim

In order for CPR to be effective, the victim must be lying on his or her back on a firm, flat surface. Great care must be taken in moving a child into this position, especially if there is evidence of head and neck injury. The circumstances in which the child is found should influence the care that may be needed in positioning him or her. The likelihood of neck, spine, or bone injuries is greater if a child is found unconscious at the scene of an accident—for example, at the base of a tree—than if an infant is found in bed not breathing. The size of the child will also influence how she or he is positioned, but the principle to bear in mind is that the child must be turned as a unit, with firm support of the head and neck so that the head does not roll, twist, or tilt backward or forward.

4. Open the Airway

The small air passages of an infant or child can easily be obstructed by mucus, blood, vomitus, or, in an unconscious victim, the tongue. The tongue is attached to the lower jaw; with loss of consciousness the muscles relax and the tongue falls back, obstructing the airway.[5] The first maneuver, after determining unconsciousness and turning the victim into the supine position, is to open the airway. This is accomplished by the head-tilt/chin-lift maneuver.[5,6] If the child is having respiratory difficulty but is conscious, time should not be wasted on an attempt to open the airway; the child should be transported to an ALS facility as rapidly as possible.

Head-Tilt/Chin-Lift (Fig 1).—The rescuer places the hand closest to the child's head on the forehead and tilts the head gently back into a sniffing or neutral position in infants, and slightly further back in children. Some believe that overextension of the head closes the trachea in small babies; there are no data that this is so, but since

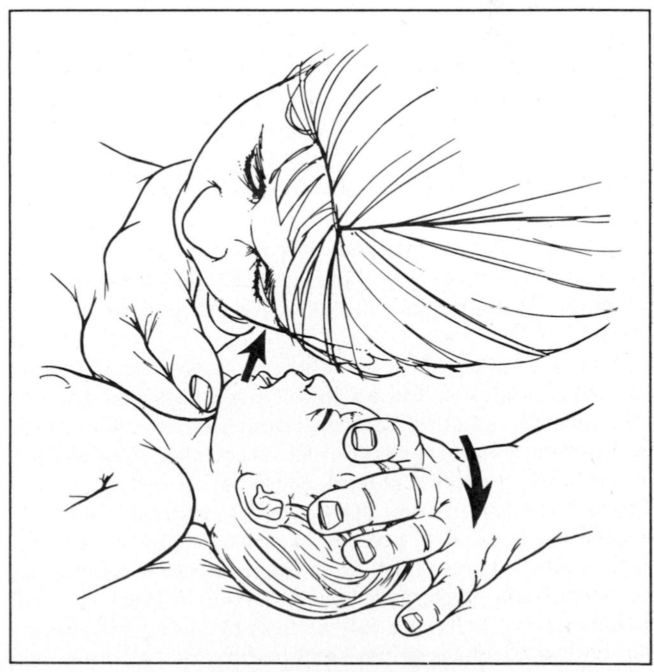

Fig 1.—Head-tilt/chin-lift.

it is unnecessary, overextension is best avoided. The head should not be tilted in suspected neck injury; jaw-thrust without head-tilt may be used instead.

To augment head-tilt, the rescuer lifts the chin, with its attached structures, including the tongue, from the airway. The fingers, but not the thumb, of the hand away from the victim's head are placed under the bony part of the lower jaw at the chin, and the chin is lifted upward. So as not to obstruct the airway, care must be exercised not to close the mouth completely or to push on the soft parts of the underchin. Except in cases of suspected neck injury, the rescuer's other hand continues to tilt the head backward.

Jaw-Thrust (Fig 2).—The rescuer places two or three fingers under each side of the lower jaw at its angle and lifts the jaw upward. The rescuer's elbows should rest on the surface on which the victim is lying. Jaw-thrust may be accompanied by slight head-tilt or can be used alone. Jaw-thrust, without head-tilt, is the safest technique for opening the airway when neck injury is suspected.

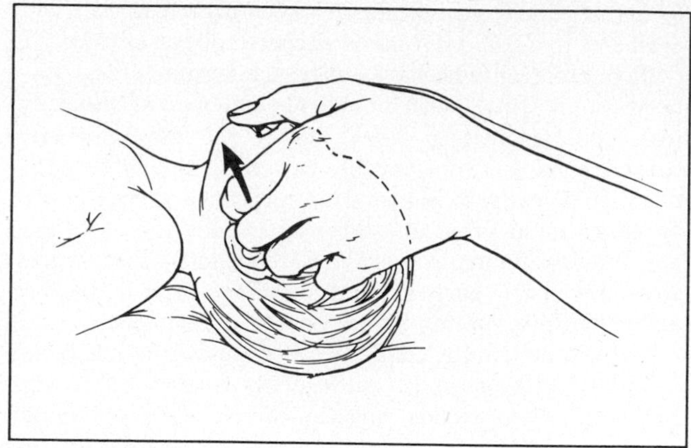

Fig 2.—Jaw-thrust.

5. Determine Whether the Victim Is Breathing

If it is unclear whether the victim is breathing, the airway is opened and, while patency is being maintained, the rescuer places his or her ear close to the victim's mouth and nose while *look*ing at the chest and abdomen for movement, *listen*ing for exhaled air, and *feel*ing for exhaled air flow (Fig 1). If the child is breathing, continued patency of the airway must be maintained. If no breathing is detected, the rescuer must breathe for the victim.

6. Breathe for the Victim

If after the airway is opened the victim does not breathe, rescue breathing must be applied to provide the victim's lungs with oxygen. While continuing to maintain patency of the airway, the rescuer takes a breath and makes a seal between his mouth and the mouth, or mouth and nose, of the victim. If the victim is an infant, the rescuer's mouth will make a tight seal with the mouth and nose (Fig 3). If the victim is larger, the nose is pinched tightly with the fingers of the hand that is maintaining head-tilt, and a mouth-to-mouth seal is made (Fig 4). Two slow breaths (1.0 to 1.5 seconds per breath) are given, with a pause between for the rescuer to take a breath. (Measurements of time "per breath" given herein are, more precisely, measurements of the victim's inspiratory time.)

The volume of air in an infant's lungs is smaller than that in an adult's, and an infant's air passages are also considerably smaller, with resistance to flow potentially quite high. Since these differences are also relative, it is impossible to make a recommendation about the force or volume of the rescue breaths. The critical things to remember are that (1) rescue breaths are the single most important maneuver in assisting a nonbreathing child victim; (2) an appropriate volume is that volume that will make the chest rise and fall; and (3) by giving the breaths slowly, an adequate volume will be provided at the lowest possible pressure, thereby avoiding gastric distention.[6,7]

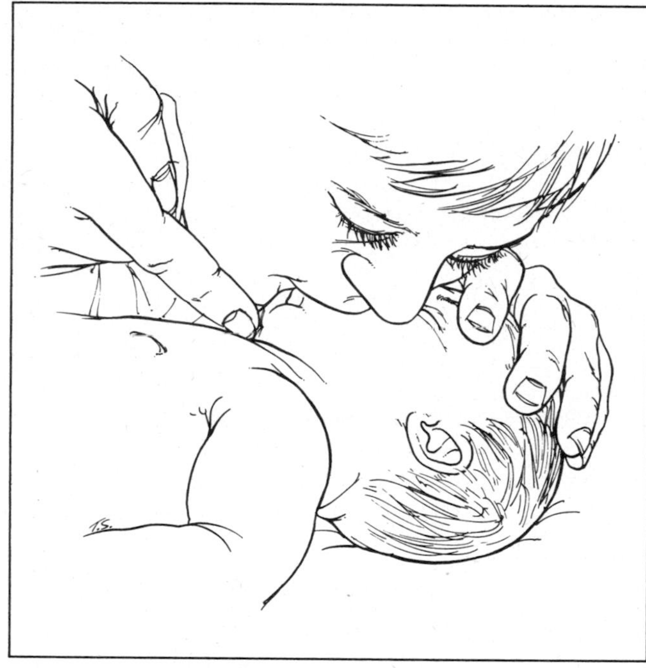

Fig 3.—Mouth-to-mouth and nose seal.

If air enters freely and the chest rises, the airway is clear. If air does not enter freely (ie, the chest does not rise), the airway is obstructed. Improper opening of the airway is the most common cause of obstruction, and head-tilt/chin-lift should be adjusted. If a repeated rescue breathing attempt does not allow air to enter freely as evidenced by lack of chest movement, a foreign-body obstruction should be suspected.

Gastric Distention.—Rescue breathing, especially if rapidly applied, can cause gastric distention,[6,7] which, if excessive, can interfere with rescue breathing by elevating the diaphragm, thus decreasing lung volume. The incidence of gastric distention can be minimized by limiting the rate of chest inflation and the ventilation volume to the point at which the chest rises, thereby not exceeding the esophageal opening pressure. Attempts at relieving gastric distention by pressure on the abdomen should be avoided because of the danger of aspiration of stomach contents into the lungs.

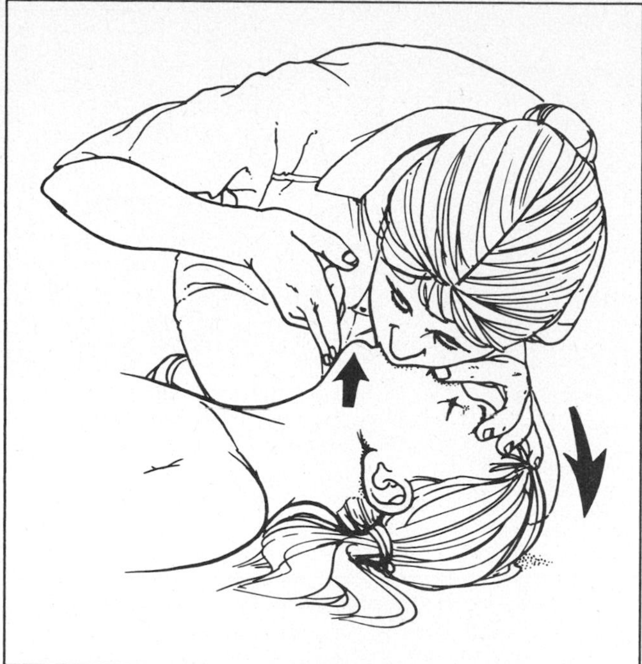

Fig 4.—Mouth-to-mouth seal.

Gastric decompression should be attempted only if the abdomen is so tense that ventilation is ineffective. In such a situation the victim's entire body is turned as a unit onto the side, with the head down if possible, before pressure is applied to the abdomen.

7. Circulation: Check the Pulse

Ineffective or absent cardiac contractions are recognized by the absence of a pulse in a large central artery. In a child older than 1 year of age the carotid is the most central and accessible artery; in an infant younger than 1 year of age, the short, chubby neck makes the carotid difficult to palpate and so the brachial artery is recommended instead.[8] The femoral pulse is often used by health professionals in a hospital setting; however, it is recommended that lay rescuers be instructed in locating the carotid and brachial arteries only.

The carotid artery lies on the side of the neck between the windpipe and the strap muscles. While maintaining head-tilt with one hand on the forehead, the rescuer locates the victim's Adam's apple with two or three fingers of the other hand. The fingers are then slid into the groove, on the side closest to the rescuer, between the trachea and the neck muscles, and the artery is gently palpated (Fig 5).

The brachial pulse is located on the inside of the upper arm, between elbow and shoulder. With the rescuer's thumb on the outside of the arm, the index and middle fingers are pressed gently until the pulse is felt (Fig 6).

When there is a pulse but no breathing, rescue breathing should be initiated and continued until spontaneous breathing resumes. For an infant the rescue breathing rate should be once every 3 seconds, or 20 times a minute; for a child, once every 4 seconds, or 15 times a minute. If a pulse is not present, a diagnosis of cardiac arrest is made and chest compressions must be initiated and coordinated with rescue breathing.

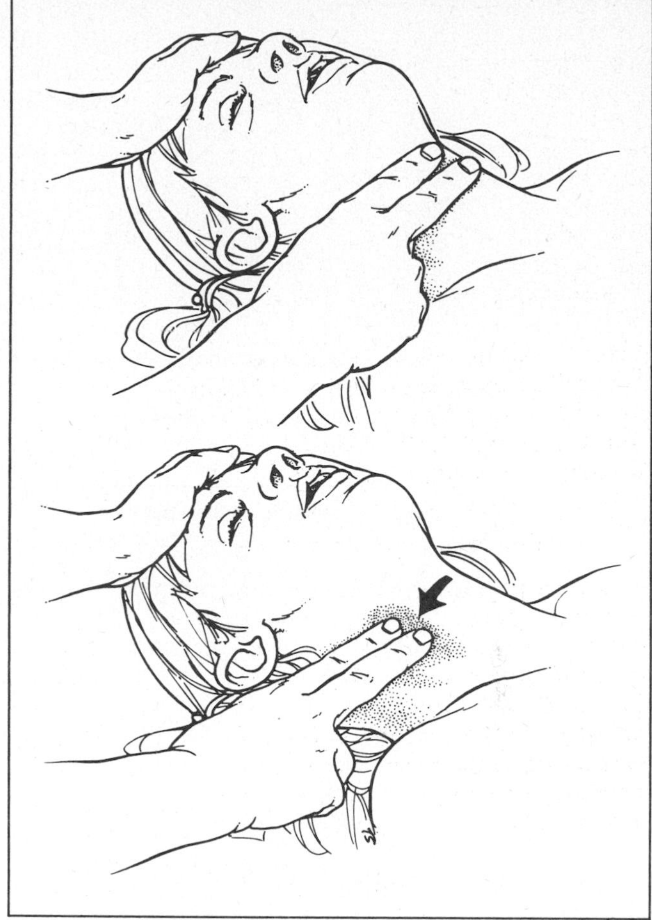

Fig 5.—Locating and palpating carotid artery pulse.

8. Activate the EMS System

If a second rescuer is present or arrives to help, one rescuer should activate the EMS system by calling the local emergency telephone number, in many communities 911. (The emergency number should be widely publicized.) If no help is forthcoming, the decision when to leave the victim in order to telephone is a difficult one and is affected by a number of variables, including the probability of someone else arriving on the scene. If the rescuer is unable to activate the EMS system, the only option is to continue CPR.

The rescuer calling the EMS system should give the following information: (1) the location of the emergency, including address and names of streets or landmarks; (2) the telephone number from which the call is being made; (3) what happened, ie, auto accident, drowning, etc; (4) the number of victims; (5) the condition of the victim(s); (6) the nature of the aid being given; (7) any other information requested. To ensure this last item, the caller should hang up last.

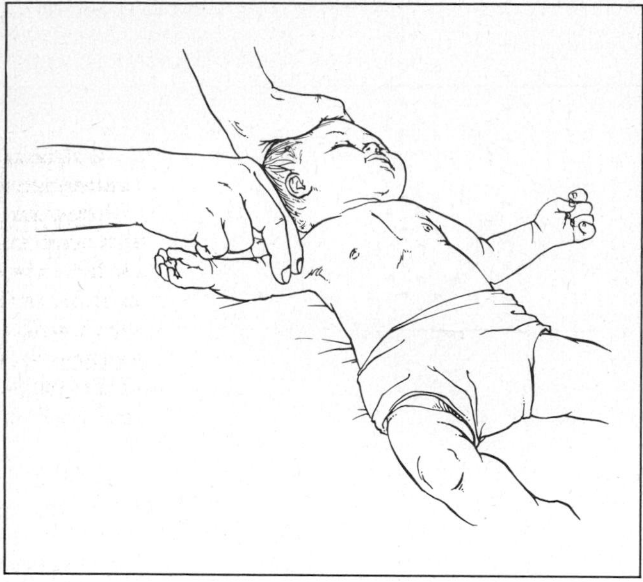

Fig 6.—Locating and palpating brachial pulse.

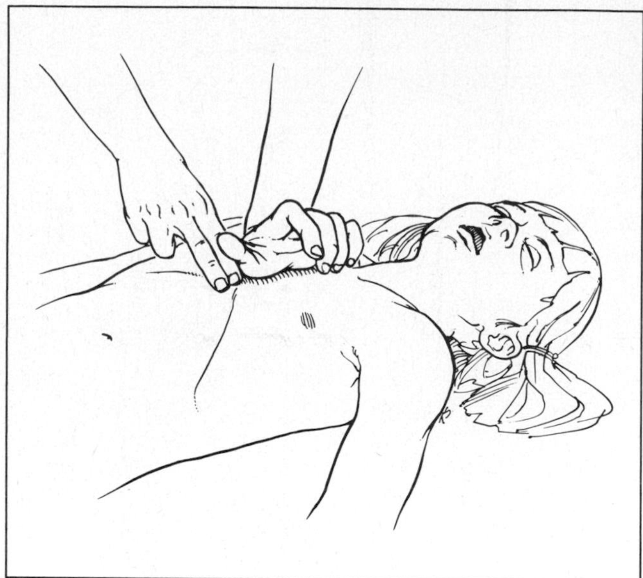

Fig 8.—Locating hand position for chest compressions in child.

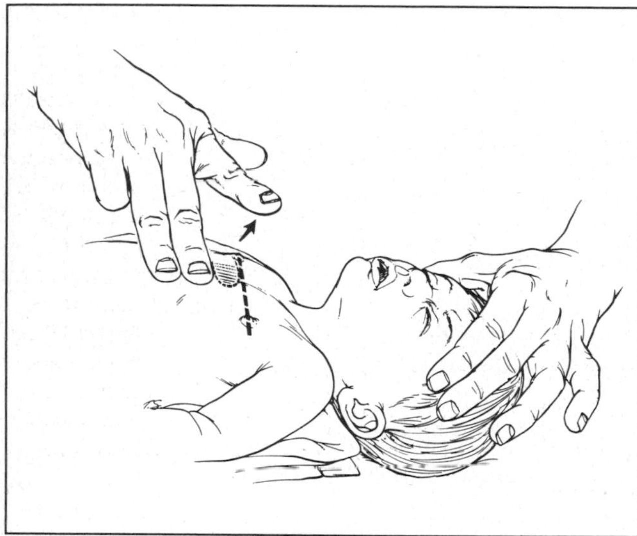

Fig 7.—Locating finger position for chest compressions in infant.

9. Perform Chest Compressions

External chest compression consists of serial, rhythmic compressions of the chest by which blood is circulated to the vital organs (heart, lungs, and brain) to keep them viable until ALS care can be given. Chest compressions must always be accompanied by rescue breathing. The mechanism by which blood is circulated by chest compressions is still a subject of controversy. It is not clear whether this takes place by a change in the thoracic pressures, by direct compression of the heart, or by a combination of both,[9-12] but direct heart compression may be the more important mechanism in the pediatric age group.[13]

For optimal compressions the child must be in a horizontal supine position on a hard surface. In an infant, the hard surface can be the palm of the hand not performing the compressions; head-tilt is then provided by the weight of the head and a slight lift of the shoulders.

Recent evidence[14] has shown that the heart of the infant is lower in relation to the external chest landmarks than was previously thought. In the following recommendations, therefore, the area of compression for infants is lower than in previous standards.

In the Infant (Fig 7).—(1) An imaginary line between the nipples is located over the breast bone. (2) The index finger of the hand farthest from the infant's head is placed just under the intermammary line where it intersects the sternum. The area of compression is one finger's width below this intersection, at the location of the middle and ring fingers. (3) Using two or three fingers, the breast bone is compressed to a depth of 0.5 to 1 in (1.3 to 2.5 cm) at a rate of at least 100 times per minute. (4) At the end of each compression, pressure is released and the sternum is allowed to come to its normal position, without removing the fingers from the sternum. A compression-relaxation rhythm should be developed that has equal time allotted to each and is smooth, ie, without jerky movements.

In the Child (Fig 8).—(1) The lower margin of the victim's rib cage is located on the side next to the rescuer, with the middle and index fingers. (2) The margin of the rib cage is followed with the middle finger to the notch where the ribs and breast bone meet. (3) With the middle finger on this notch, the index finger is placed next to the middle finger. (4) The heel of the hand is placed next to the index finger, with the long axis of the heel parallel to that of the sternum. (5) The chest is compressed with one hand to a depth of 1 to 1.5 in (2.5 to 3.8 cm) at a rate of 80 to 100 times per minute. The fingers should be kept off the ribs. (6) The compressions should be smooth, not jerky; the chest should be allowed to return to its resting position after each compression, but the hand should not be lifted off the chest. Each compression and relaxation phase should be equal in time. (7) If the child is large or older

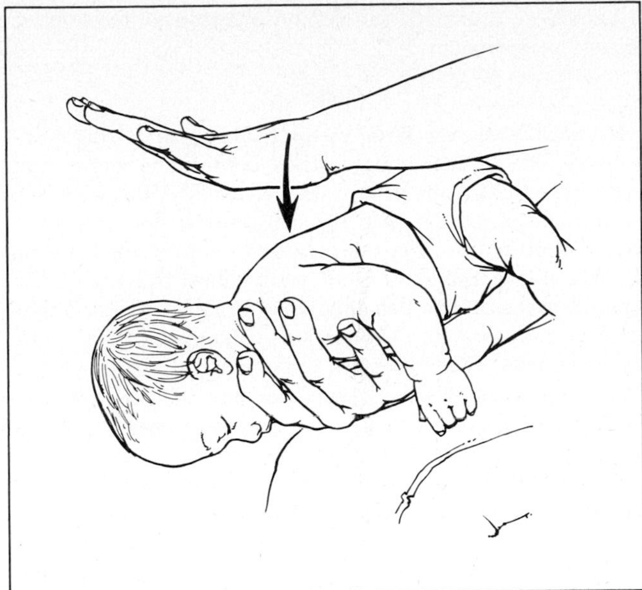

Fig 9.—Back blow in infant.

than approximately 8 years, the method described for adults in Part II should be used.

10. Coordinate Compressions and Rescue Breathing

External chest compressions must always be accompanied by rescue breathing. At the end of every fifth compression a pause should be allowed for a ventilation (1.0 to 1.5 seconds per breath). In the infant and child the 5:1 compression-ventilation ratio is maintained for both one and two rescuers. The two-rescuer technique should be used only by health care professionals. Since compressions must be briefly interrupted to allow for an adequate ventilation, a compression rate of 80 to 100 per minute is recommended. The infant and child should be reassessed after ten cycles of compressions and ventilations (approximately one minute) and every few minutes thereafter.

AIRWAY OBSTRUCTION MANAGEMENT

More than 90% of deaths from foreign-body aspiration in the pediatric age group occur in children younger than 5 years of age, and 65% are in infants. The 1985 National Conference noted the marked decline in pediatric deaths from foreign-body aspiration since the last conference. The reason for this decline is not clear. Aspirated materials include foods (ie, hot dogs, round candies, nuts, and grapes)[15] and other small objects. Foreign-body airway obstruction should be suspected in infants and children experiencing acute respiratory distress associated with coughing, gagging, or stridor (a high-pitched, noisy breathing).

Signs and symptoms of airway obstruction may also be due to infections that cause airway swelling, such as epiglottitis and croup. Children with an infectious cause of airway obstruction need prompt attention in an ALS facility, and time should not be wasted in a futile attempt to relieve their obstruction. Attempts at clearing the airway should be considered for (1) children whose

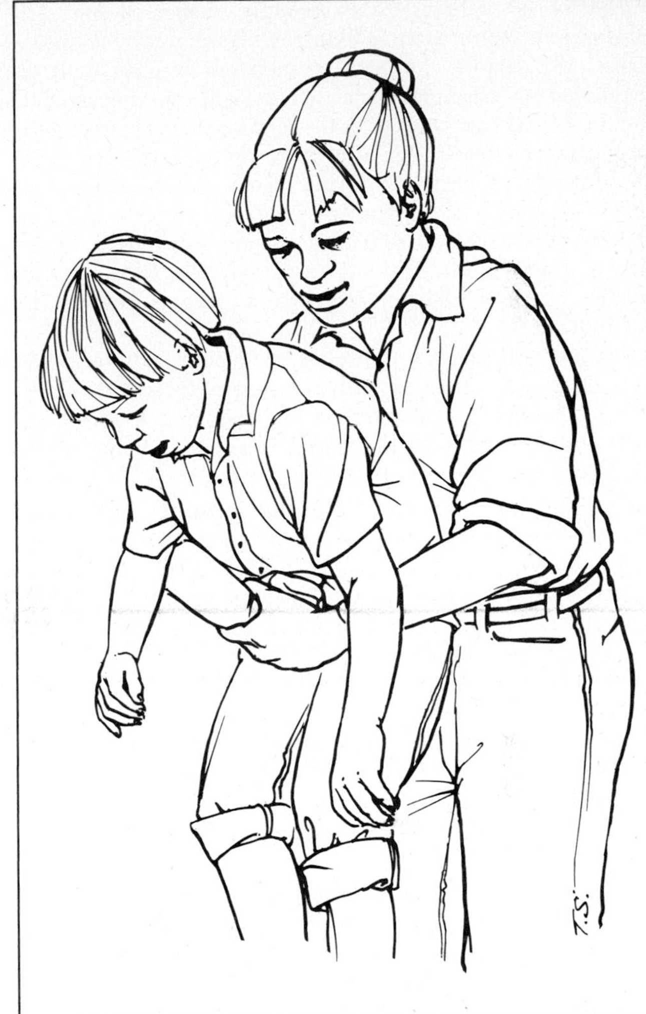

Fig 10.—Heimlich maneuver with child standing.

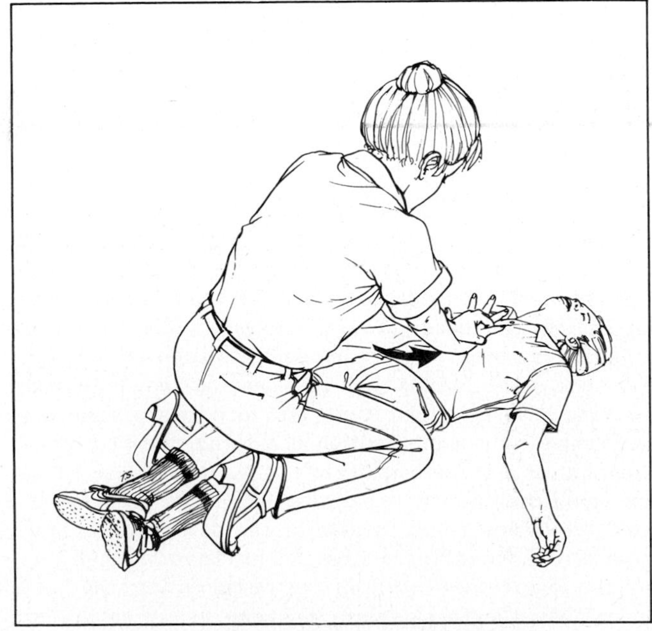

Fig 11.—Heimlich maneuver with child lying.

aspiration is witnessed or strongly suspected and (2) unconscious, nonbreathing children whose airways remain obstructed despite the usual maneuvers to open it. In a witnessed or strongly suspected aspiration, the rescuer should encourage the child to persist with spontaneous coughing and breathing efforts as long as the cough is forceful. Relief of the obstruction should be attempted only if the cough is, or becomes, ineffective and/or there is increased respiratory difficulty accompanied by a high-pitched noise while inhaling (stridor). The EMS system should be activated as soon as a second rescuer is available.

The optimal method for relief of foreign-body obstruction remains a matter of controversy, and further data are needed to distinguish opinions and personal experiences from objective facts. If the victim is a child, the Heimlich maneuver, a series of subdiaphragmatic abdominal thrusts, is recommended.[16-19] This maneuver, by increasing intrathoracic pressures, creates an artificial cough that forces air and, it is hoped, a foreign body out of the airway. Six to ten thrusts are repeated in rapid sequence until the foreign body is expelled. However, although the conference recognized the pedagogical value of uniformity, there was concern for potential intra-abdominal injury resulting from subdiaphragmatic abdominal thrusts in infants younger than 1 year of age. In this age group, therefore, the combination of back blows and chest thrusts continues to be recommended.[20] Some believe that in the infant this combination is an indirect application of the Heimlich maneuver.

Following maneuvers to remove an airway obstruction, the airway is opened using head-tilt/chin-lift and, if spontaneous breathing is absent, rescue breathing is performed. If the chest does not rise, the head is repositioned, the airway is opened, and rescue breathing is attempted again. If rescue breathing is still unsuccessful (the chest does not rise), maneuvers to relieve foreign-body obstruction should be repeated.

Infant

The infant is straddled over the rescuer's arm, with the head lower than the trunk, and the head is supported by firmly holding the jaw. The rescuer rests his or her forearm on his or her thigh and delivers four back blows forcefully with the heel of the hand between the infant's shoulder blades (Fig 9). After delivering the back blows, the rescuer places his free hand on the infant's back so that the victim is sandwiched between the two hands, one supporting the neck, jaw, and chest, while the other supports the back. While continuing to support the head and neck, the infant is turned, placed on the thigh with the head lower than the trunk, and four chest thrusts are performed in the same location as external chest compressions but at a slower rate (Fig 7). Rescuers whose hands are small may find it physically difficult to perform the back blows and chest thrusts in the described manner, especially if the infant is large. An alternate method is to lay the infant face down on the rescuer's lap, the head lower than the trunk, with the head firmly supported. After the four back blows have been performed, the infant is turned as a unit to the supine position and the chest thrusts performed.

Child

Heimlich Maneuver With Victim Standing or Sitting (Conscious).—The rescuer should stand behind the victim and wrap his or her arms around the victim's waist, with one hand made into a fist (Fig 10). The thumb side of the fist should rest against the victim's abdomen in the midline slightly above the navel and well below the tip of the xiphoid process. The fist should be grasped by the other hand and pressed into the victim's abdomen with a quick upward thrust. The rescuer's hands should not touch the xiphoid process or the lower margins of the rib cage because of possible damage to internal organs.[21,22] Each thrust should be a separate and distinct movement.

Heimlich Maneuver With Victim Lying (Conscious or Unconscious).—The rescuer should position the child face up on his or her back and kneel at the child's feet, if the child is on the floor, or stand at the child's feet, if the child is on a table[19] (Fig 11). (The astride position is not recommended for small children but may be used in the case of a large child.) The rescuer should place the heel of one hand on the child's abdomen in the midline slightly above the navel and well below the rib cage. The other hand should be placed on top of the first and pressed into the abdomen with a quick upward thrust. Care should be exercised to direct the thrusts upward in the midline and not to either side of the abdomen. Several thrusts may be necessary to expel the object. In small children the maneuver must be applied gently.

Finger Sweep

Blind finger sweeps are to be avoided in infants and children since the foreign body may be pushed back into the airway, causing further obstruction. In the unconscious, nonbreathing victim following the chest thrusts or subdiaphragmatic abdominal thrusts, the victim's mouth is opened by grasping both the tongue and the lower jaw between the thumb and finger and lifting (tongue-jaw lift). This action draws the tongue away from the back of the throat and may itself partially relieve the obstruction. If the foreign body is visualized, it should be removed.

References

1. Seidel JS, Hornbein M, Yoshiyama K, et al: Emergency medical services and the pediatric patient: Are the needs being met? *Pediatrics* 1984;73:769.

2. Ludwig S, Kettrick RG, Parker M: Pediatric cardiopulmonary resuscitation. *Clin Pediatr* 1984;23:71.

3. Torphy DE, Minter MG, Thompson BM: Cardiorespiratory arrest and resuscitation of children. *AJDC* 1984;138:1099.

4. Statistical Resources Branch, Division of Vital Statistics: *Final Mortality Statistics, 1981.* Hyattsville, Md, National Center for Health Statistics, 1984.

5. Ruben H, Elam JO, Ruben AM, et al: Investigation of upper airway problems in resuscitation. *Anesthesiology* 1961;22:271.

6. Melker R: Asynchronous and other alternative methods of ventilation during CPR. *Ann Emerg Med* 1984;13(pt 2):758.

7. Melker RJ, Banner MJ: Ventilation during CPR: Two rescuer standards reappraised. *Ann Emerg Med* 1985;14:397.

8. Cavallaro D, Melker R: Comparison of two techniques for determining cardiac activity in infants. *Crit Care Med* 1983;11:189.

9. Babbs CF: New versus old theories of blood flow during CPR. *Crit Care Med* 1980;8:191.

10. Rudikoff MT, Maughan WC, Effron M, et al: Mechanism of blood flow during cardiopulmonary resuscitation. *Circulation* 1980;61:345.

11. Werner JA, Greene H, Janko CL, et al: Visualization of cardiac valve motion during external chest compression using two-dimensional echocardiography: Implications regarding the mechanism of blood flow. *Circulation* 1981;63:1417.

12. Maier GW, Tyson GS, Olsen CO, et al: The physiology of external cardiac massage: High impulse cardiopulmonary resuscitation. *Circulation* 1984;70:86.

13. Koehler RC, Michael JR, Guerci AD, et al: Beneficial effects of epinephrine infusion on cerebral and myocardial blood flows during CPR. *Ann Emerg Med* 1985;14:744.

14. Orlowski JP: Optimal position for external cardiac massage in infants and children. *Crit Care Med* 1984;12:224.

15. Harris CS, Baker SP, Smith GA, et al: Childhood asphyxiation by food: A national analysis and overview. *JAMA* 1984;251:2231.

16. Day RL, Crelin ES, Dubois AB: Choking: The Heimlich abdominal thrust vs. back blows: An approach to measurement of inertial and aerodynamic forces. *Pediatrics* 1982;70:113.

17. Day RL, Dubois AB: Treatment of choking. *Pediatrics* 1983;71:300.

18. Day RL: Differing opinions on the emergency treatment of choking. *Pediatrics* 1983;71:976.

19. Heimlich HJ: A life-saving maneuver to prevent food choking. *JAMA* 1975;234:398.

20. Standards and guidelines for cardiopulmonary resuscitation (CPR) and emergency cardiac care (ECC). *JAMA* 1980;244:475.

21. Visintine RE, Baick CH: Ruptured stomach after Heimlich maneuver. *JAMA* 1975;234:415.

22. Palmer E: The Heimlich maneuver misused. *Curr Prescribing* 1979;5:45.

CPR Review

Item	Adult	Child	Infant
How to determine unresponsiveness	Tap shoulder Shout "Are you OK?"	Same	Same
How to open airway?	Head-tilt/chin-lift	Same	Same
How to check breathing?	Look, listen, feel (3-5 sec.)	Same	Same
What kind of breaths are given?	2X at 1-1 1/2 sec. observe chest rise	Same	Same
Where to check pulse?	Carotid (5-10 sec.)	Same	Brachial
Hand position for sternum compressions?	1 finger's width above sternum notch	Same	1 finger's width below imaginary line between nipples
How far are compressions?	1 1/2-2 inches	1 - 1 1/2 inches	1/2-1 inch
Compression rate?	80-100 per min.	Same	100+ per min.
Compression/ ventilation cycles	15:2	5:1	5:1
Pause to check pulse?	5 sec.	Same	Same
Pause to move victim?	<30 sec., avoid if possible	Same	Same
How often to reassess?	Every few minutes	Same	Same
After reassessment, continue CPR with	2 breaths	1 breath	1 breath

BLS Exam

LEARNING ACTIVITIES

Multiple Choice:

__B__ **1.** If the victim's mouth is injured or your mouth is too small to give mouth-to-mouth breathing:

A. Give mouth-to-nose breathing
B. Wait for an ambulance equipped with breathing equipment

__A__ **2.** You should push air out of the victim's stomach only when the stomach is bulging with air and you cannot inflate the lungs.

A. True
B. False

__A__ **3.** When you take a breath in mouth-to-mouth breathing, turn your head to look at the victim's:

A. Chest
B. Forehead

__B__ **4.** When you tip the head with the chin lift, where do you place your fingertips?

A. Under the soft part of the throat near the chin
B. Under the bony part of the jaw near the chin

__A__ **5.** Which is the safer way to open the airway of a person who may have neck or back injuries?

A. Push the jaw forward from the corners
B. Tip the head very gently, part way back

__B__ **6.** You find a victim who has just been hit by a car. You should probably:

A. Position the victim on the back immediately for mouth-to-mouth breathing or CPR
B. Check for breathing before you move the victim at all

__A__ **7.** How should you roll a victim onto the back for mouth-to-mouth breathing or CPR?

A. In one motion—keep the body from twisting
B. One part at a time—first the head, then the shoulders, then the legs

__A__ **8.** How should you check for stopped breathing?

A. Look at the chest; listen and feel for air coming out of the mouth
B. Look at the pupils of the eyes
C. Check the pulse

__B__ **9.** After you give two breaths, how often do you give breaths to an adult in mouth-to-mouth breathing?

A. Once every 3 seconds
B. Once every 5 seconds
C. Once every 10 seconds

__A__ **10.** When you give breaths to an adult, the breaths should be:

A. Large and full
B. Small and gentle

__B__ **11.** How do you find where to push on the chest for chest compressions?

A. Push on the xiphoid
B. Measure up one finger-width from the middle finger on the xiphoid notch

____ 12. In one-rescuer CPR, give chest compressions to an adult at the rate of:

A. 100 per minute
B. 80 per minute
C. 60 per minute
D. 40 per minute

____ 13. Before deciding whether to give CPR, check the victim's pulse for:

A. 1–3 seconds
B. 3–5 seconds
C. 5–10 seconds
D. 10–20 seconds

____ 14. Give chest compressions:

A. With a quick jerk
B. Smoothly and regularly

____ 15. Compress an adult's chest at least:

A. 1/4 to 1/2 inch
B. 1-1/2 to 2 inches

____ 16. What is the pattern of compressions and breaths in one-rescuer CPR for an adult victim?

A. 15 compressions, 2 breaths
B. 15 compressions, 1 breath
C. 5 compressions, 2 breaths
D. 5 compressions, 1 breath

____ 17. Pushing on the xiphoid increases the:

A. Amount of blood circulation
B. Chance of internal injuries

____ 18. Push on a victim's chest:

A. At an angle
B. Straight down

____ 19. Are chest compressions likely to work if the victim is on a soft surface?

A. Yes, a soft surface is OK.
B. No, the surface should be hard.

____ 20. You find a victim who needs CPR. An ambulance will arrive in a few minutes. You should:

A. Wait for the ambulance
B. Start CPR right away

____ 21. When should you stop giving CPR?

A. When other persons take over or the heart starts to beat
B. When you see an ambulance arrive at the scene

____ 22. Which position is better for CPR?

A. Victim's feet and legs elevated (raised)
B. Victim's head and shoulders elevated

____ 23. You are giving CPR and find that the pulse starts again but breathing does not. You should:

A. Keep giving CPR
B. Get the victim to a life-support unit

C. Give mouth-to-mouth breathing without chest compressions
D. Give chest compressions without mouth-to-mouth breathing

B **24.** A victim who seems to be choking CAN speak. Should you give abdominal thrusts?

A. Yes
B. No

B **25.** A victim is coughing forcefully. Should you give back blows and thrusts?

A. Yes
B. No

A **26.** Give abdominal thrusts quickly:

A. Inward and upward
B. Straight back

C **27.** When you give abdominal thrusts to a conscious victim, what part of your fist do you place against the victim?

A. The palm side
B. The little finger side
C. The thumb side

B **28.** Where do you place your fist to give abdominal thrusts?

A. Over the rib cage
B. Between the rib cage and the waist
C. Below the waist

B **29.** For a victim who is very fat or in advanced pregnancy, it is better to give:

A. Abdominal thrusts
B. Chest thrusts

A **30.** A person is coughing weakly and making wheezing noises. You should:

A. Give abdominal thrusts
B. Let the person alone and watch closely

A **31.** A conscious person is coughing forcefully trying to dislodge an object. Then the person stops coughing and cannot speak. You should:

A. Give abdominal thrusts
B. Let the person alone and watch closely

A **32.** To give abdominal thrusts to a victim who is lying down, place the heel of one hand:

A. Between the rib cage and the waist
B. Over the edge of the rib cage
C. Below the waist

B **33.** The tongue is more likely to block the airway if an unconscious person is lying:

A. On the side
B. On the back

B **34.** The first time you try to give breaths, you cannot inflate the lungs. You should:

A. Sweep in the mouth
B. Retip the head and try again

A **35.** Check a baby's pulse at the:

A. Middle of the upper arm
B. Wrist

B 36. After giving two breaths, give a baby one breath of air every ________ for mouth-to-mouth respiration.

A. 5 seconds
B. 3 seconds

D 37. You believe a baby has an object caught in its airway; it cannot cough or cry. What do you do?

A. Let it alone and watch closely
B. Give abdominal thrusts
C. Chest thrusts
D. Back Blows

A 38. When you give back blows to a baby, hold the baby with its head:

A. Lower than its chest
B. Higher than its chest

A 39. A baby's stomach can fill up with air if you:

A. Blow too hard or if the airway is partially blocked
B. Do not blow hard enough or tip the head too far

A 40. Give a baby chest compressions at the rate of:

A. 100 per minute
B. 80 per minute
C. 60 per minute

B 41. How far do you compress a baby's chest?

A. 1-1/2 to 2 inches
B. 1/2 to 3/4 inch

B 42. Push on the chest of a child or baby one finger-width:

A. Above nipple line
B. Below nipple line
C. Above xiphoid notch

B 43. When giving chest compressions to a *child,* use:

A. 2 or 3 fingers or heel of one hand
B. The heel of one hand and the other hand on top

A 44. When giving chest compressions to a *baby,* use:

A. 2 or 3 fingers
B. The heel of one hand

D 45. Give babies and children:

A. 15 compressions, 2 breaths
B. 5 compressions, 2 breaths
C. 15 compressions, 1 breath
D. 5 compressions, 1 breath

C 46. Your neighbor collapses while mowing his lawn. You determine that he is unresponsive. Next, you should:

A. Quickly run into your house and call an ambulance
B. Check for pulse and begin compressions, if necessary
C. Position the victim to open the airway and check breathing

A 47. The tongue is the most common cause of airway obstruction in the unconscious victim. The simplest technique to open the airway in most cases is:

A. Tilting the victim's head back
B. Opening the mouth with the cross finger technique
C. Delivering sharp blows to the back

__C__ **48.** Which of the following statements is FALSE?

A. Opening the airway may allow the victim to start breathing for himself
B. The airway must be open to assess breathing accurately
C. An open airway will increase the possibility of stomach distension from artificial ventilation
D. It is not possible to ventilate a victim properly unless the airway is open

__B__ **49.** After opening the airway, the most reliable way to assess breathing is to:

A. Check the pulse
B. Place your ear close to the victim's mouth, face the chest and look, listen, and feel for signs of air and chest movement
C. Place your hand on the chest to feel breathing movements

__C__ **50.** The victim's pulse should first be checked:

A. For 5 seconds immediately after opening the airway
B. For 5–10 seconds after determining unresponsiveness
C. For 5–10 seconds after the first two ventilations

__C__ **51.** To perform chest compressions on an adult, kneel beside the victim's chest, place one hand on top of the other with the heel of the lower hand on:

A. The lower half of the sternum
B. The xiphoid process
C. The middle sternum

__D__ **52.** When doing chest compressions, the rescuer's shoulders should be directly over the victim's sternum and elbows should be kept straight. This body position is important because:

A. Compressions should be straight down
B. You will achieve adequate pressure for effective compression depth
C. You will tire less quickly using your body weight rather than pushing with your arms
D. All of the above

__B__ **53.** The depth of compressions for the average adult is:

A. 1 to 1-1/2 inches
B. 1-1/2 to 2 inches
C. 2 to 2-1/2 inches

__A__ **54.** The compression rate for one-rescuer CPR is:

A. 60 times per minute
B. 40 times per minute
C. 80 times per minute

__C__ **55.** When one-rescuer is performing CPR on an adult victim, the ratio of compressions to ventilations is:

A. 10 compressions to 2 ventilations
B. 5 compressions to 1 ventilation
C. 15 compressions to 2 ventilations

__B__ **56.** Cardiac compressions are most effective when:

A. Done rhythmically, with compression time equal to release time
B. The chest is allowed to return to its normal position on release

C. There is no pause between compressions
D. All of the above

Case 1: You find a child (age about 6) cyanotic in the facial area. The child appears to be choking; he is violently gasping for air.

1. What is the immediate emergency care to alleviate the problem? What should be done?

____
____
____
____

2. Describe how the proper procedure for the immediate emergency care necessary in this situation is properly performed.

____
____
____
____

Case 2: A frantic mother calls to report that her infant suddenly has stopped breathing. Within minutes, you cross the street to the neighbor's and find that the mother has already begun mouth-to-mouth breathing. A check of the infant's pulse reveals no pulse.

1. What is the immediate emergency care in this situation?

____
____
____
____

2. For an infant, how many cardiac compressions per minute should you complete?

_____ A. 60–80
__X__ B. 80–100
_____ C. 100–120

3. For a small infant, how far down should you compress the chest wall?

_____ A. 1/4 inch
_____ B. 1/4 to 1/2 inch
_____ C. 1/2 to 3/4 inch
__X__ D. 3/4 to 1 inch
_____ E. 1 to 1-1/4 inches

4. When taking an infant's pulse, the best location to use is:

_____ A. carotid artery
_____ B. left nipple
__X__ C. brachial artery
_____ D. femoral artery

The following pages contain the CPR and ECC Performance Sheets. Reprinted with permission of the American Heart Association.

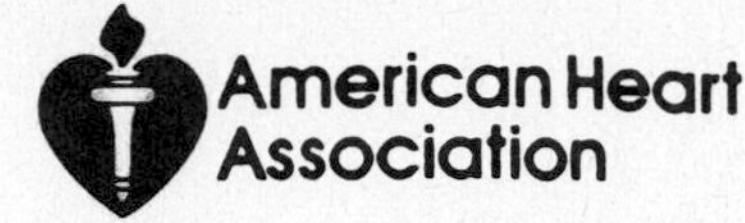

CPR and ECC Performance Sheet

One-Rescuer CPR: Adult

Name ______________________ Date ______________

Step	Activity	Critical Performance	S	U
1. Airway	Assessment: Determine unresponsiveness.	Tap or gently shake shoulder.		
		Shout "Are you OK?"		
	Call for help.	Call out "Help!"		
	Position the victim.	Turn on back as unit, if necessary, supporting head and neck (4–10 sec).		
	Open the airway.	Use head-tilt/chin-lift maneuver.		
2. Breathing	Assessment: Determine breathlessness.	Maintain open airway.		
		Ear over mouth, observe chest: look, listen, feel for breathing (3–5 sec).		
	Ventilate twice.	Maintain open airway.		
		Seal mouth and nose properly.		
		Ventilate 2 times at 1–1.5 sec/inspiration.		
		Observe chest rise (adequate ventilation volume.)		
		Allow deflation between breaths.		
3. Circulation	Assessment: Determine pulselessness.	Feel for carotid pulse on near side of victim (5–10 sec).		
		Maintain head-tilt with other hand.		
	Activate EMS system.	If someone responded to call for help, send him/her to activate EMS system.		
		Total time, Step 1—Activate EMS system: 15–35 sec.		
	Begin chest compressions.	Rescuer kneels by victim's shoulders.		
		Landmark check prior to hand placement.		
		Proper hand position throughout.		
		Rescuer's shoulders over victim's sternum.		
		Equal compression–relaxation.		
		Compress 1 1/2 to 2 inches.		
		Keep hands on sternum during upstroke.		
		Complete chest relaxation on upstroke.		
		Say any helpful mnemonic.		
		Compression rate: 80–100/min (15 per 9–11 sec).		
4. Compression/Ventilation Cycles	Do 4 cycles of 15 compressions and 2 ventilations.	Proper compression/ventilation ratio: 15 compressions to 2 ventilations per cycle.		
		Observe chest rise: 1–1.5 sec/inspiration; 4 cycles/52–73 sec.		
5. Reassessment*	Determine pulselessness. (If no pulse: Step 6.)†	Feel for carotid pulse (5 sec).		
6. Continue CPR	Ventilate twice.	Ventilate 2 times.		
		Observe chest rise; 1–1.5 sec/inspiration.		
	Resume compression/ventilation cycles.	Feel for carotid pulse every few minutes.		

* 2nd rescuer arrives to replace 1st rescuer: (a) 2nd rescuer identifies self by saying "I know CPR. Can I help?" (b) 2nd rescuer then does pulse check in Step 5 and continues with Step 6. (During practice and testing only one rescuer actually ventilates the manikin. The 2nd rescuer simulates ventilation.) (c) 1st rescuer assesses the adequacy of 2nd rescuer's CPR by observing chest rise during ventilations and by checking the pulse during chest compressions.

† If pulse is present, open airway and check for spontaneous breathing: (a) If breathing is present, maintain open airway and monitor pulse and breathing. (b) If breathing is absent, perform rescue breathing at 12 times/min and monitor pulse.

Instructor ______________________ Check: Satisfactory _____ Unsatisfactory _____

4/86

CPR and ECC Performance Sheet

One-Rescuer CPR: Child*

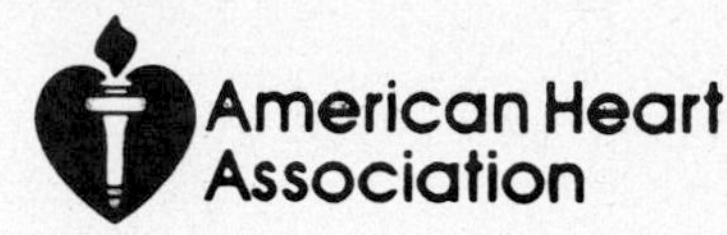

Name ______________________________ Date ______________

Step	Activity	Critical Performance	S	U
1. Airway	Assessment: Determine unresponsiveness.	Tap or gently shake shoulder.		
		Shout "Are you OK?"		
	Call for help.	Call out "Help!"		
	Position the victim.	Turn on back as unit, if necessary, supporting head and neck (4–10 sec).		
	Open the airway.	Use head-tilt/chin-lift maneuver.		
2. Breathing	Assessment: Determine breathlessness.	Maintain open airway.		
		Ear over mouth, observe chest: look, listen, feel for breathing (3–5 sec).		
	Ventilate twice.	Maintain open airway.		
		Seal mouth and nose properly.		
		Ventilate 2 times at 1–1.5 sec/inspiration.		
		Observe chest rise.		
		Allow deflation between breaths.		
3. Circulation	Assessment: Determine pulselessness.	Feel for carotid pulse on near side of victim (5–10 sec).		
		Maintain head-tilt with other hand.		
	Activate EMS system.	If someone responded to call for help, send him/her to activate EMS system.		
		Total time, Step 1—Activate EMS system: 15–35 sec.		
	Begin chest compressions.	Rescuer kneels by victim's shoulders.		
		Landmark check prior to initial hand placement.		
		Proper hand position throughout.		
		Rescuer's shoulders over victim's sternum.		
		Equal compression–relaxation.		
		Compress 1 to 1 1/2 inches.		
		Keep hands on sternum during upstroke.		
		Complete chest relaxation on upstroke.		
		Say any helpful mnemonic.		
		Compression rate: 80–100/min (5 per 3–4 sec).		
4. Compression/Ventilation Cycles	Do 10 cycles of 5 compressions and 1 ventilation.	Proper compression/ventilation ratio: 5 compressions to 1 slow ventilation per cycle.		
		Observe chest rise, 1–1.5 sec/inspiration (10 cycles/60–87 sec).		
5. Reassessment†	Determine pulselessness. (If no pulse: Step 6.)‡	Feel for carotid pulse (5 sec).		
6. Continue CPR	Ventilate once.	Ventilate one time.		
		Observe chest rise; 1–1.5 sec/inspiration.		
	Resume compression/ventilation cycles	Palpate carotid pulse every few minutes.		

* If child is above age of approximately 8 years, the method for adults should be used.

† 2nd rescuer arrives to replace 1st rescuer: (a) 2nd rescuer identifies self by saying "I know CPR. Can I help?" (b) 2nd rescuer then does pulse check in Step 5 and continues with Step 6. (During practice and testing only one rescuer actually ventilates the manikin. The 2nd rescuer simulates ventilation.) (c) 1st rescuer assesses the adequacy of 2nd rescuer's CPR by observing chest rise during ventilations and by checking the pulse during chest compressions.

‡ If pulse is present, open airway and check for spontaneous breathing. (a) If breathing is present, maintain open airway and monitor breathing and pulse. (b) If breathing is absent, perform rescue breathing at 15 times/min and monitor pulse.

Instructor ______________________________ Check: Satisfactory _____ Unsatisfactory _____

4/86

CPR and ECC Performance Sheet

One Rescuer CPR: Infant

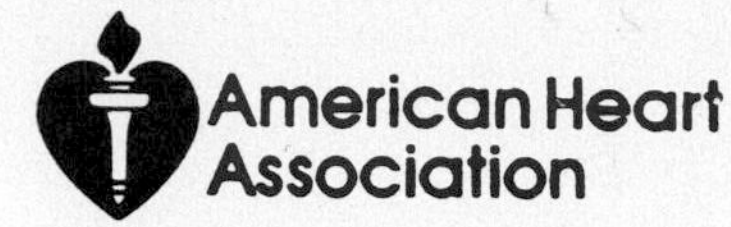

Name ______________________ Date ______________

Step	Activity	Critical Performance	S	U
1. Airway	Assessment: Determine unresponsiveness.	Tap or gently shake shoulder.		
	Call for help.	Call out "Help!"		
	Position the infant.	Turn on back as unit, supporting head and neck.		
		Place on firm, hard surface.		
	Open the airway.	Use head-tilt/chin-lift maneuver to sniffing or neutral position.		
		Do not overextend the head.		
2. Breathing	Assessment: Determine breathlessness.	Maintain open airway.		
		Ear over mouth, observe chest: look, listen, feel for breathing (3–5 sec).		
	Ventilate twice.	Maintain open airway.		
		Make tight seal on infant's mouth and nose with rescuer's mouth.		
		Ventilate 2 times, 1–1.5 sec/inspiration.		
		Observe chest rise.		
		Allow deflation between breaths.		
3. Circulation	Assessment: Determine pulselessness.	Feel for brachial pulse (5–10 sec).		
		Maintain head-tilt with other hand.		
	Activate EMS system.	If someone responded to call for help, send him/her to activate EMS system.		
		Total time, Step 1–Activate EMS system: 15–35 sec.		
	Begin chest compressions.	Draw imaginary line between nipples.		
		Place 2–3 fingers on sternum, 1 finger's width below imaginary line.		
		Equal compression-relaxation.		
		Compress vertically, 1/2 to 1 inches.		
		Keep fingers on sternum during upstroke.		
		Complete chest relaxation on upstroke.		
		Say any helpful mnemonic.		
		Compression rate: at least 100/min (5 in 3 sec or less).		
4. Compression/Ventilation Cycles	Do 10 cycles of 5 compressions and 1 ventilation.	Proper compression/ventilation ratio: 5 compressions to 1 slow ventilation per cycle.		
		Pause for ventilation.		
		Observe chest rise: 1–1.5 sec/inspiration; 10 cycles/45 sec or less.		
5. Reassessment	Determine pulselessness. (If no pulse: Step 6.)*	Feel for brachial pulse (5 sec).		
6. Continue CPR	Ventilate once.	Ventilate 1 time.		
		Observe chest rise; 1–1.5 sec/inspiration.		
	Resume compression/ventilation cycles.	Feel for brachial pulse every few minutes.		

* If pulse is present, open airway and check for spontaneous breathing. (a) If breathing is present, maintain open airway and monitor breathing and pulse. (b) If breathing is absent, perform rescue breathing at 20 times/min and monitor pulse.

Instructor ______________________ Check: Satisfactory ______ Unsatisfactory ______

4/86

CPR and ECC Performance Sheet

Obstructed Airway: Conscious Adult

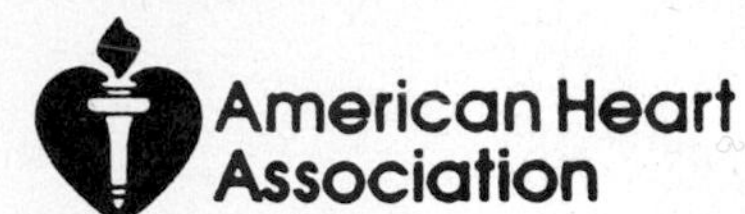

Name ______________________ Date ____________

Step	Activity	Critical Performance	S	U
1. Assessment	Determine airway obstruction.	Ask "Are you choking?"		
		Determine if victim can cough or speak.		
2. Heimlich Maneuver	Perform abdominal thrusts.	Stand behind the victim.		
		Wrap arms around victim's waist.		
		Make a fist with one hand and place the thumb side against victim's abdomen in the midline slightly above the navel and well below the tip of the xiphoid.		
		Grasp fist with the other hand.		
		Press into the victim's abdomen with quick upward thrusts.		
		Each thrust should be distinct and delivered with the intent of relieving the airway obstruction.		
		Repeat thrusts until either the foreign body is expelled or the victim becomes unconsious (see below).		

Victim with Obstructed Airway Becomes Unconscious (Optional Testing Sequence)

Step	Activity	Critical Performance	S	U
3. Additional Assessment	Position the victim.	Turn on back as unit.		
		Place face up, arms by side.		
	Call for help.	Call out "Help!" or, if others respond, activate EMS system.		
4. Foreign Body Check	Perform finger sweep.*	Keep victim's face up.		
		Use tongue-jaw lift to open mouth.		
		Sweep deeply into mouth to remove foreign body.		
5. Breathing Attempt	Attempt ventilation (airway is obstructed).	Open airway with head-tilt/chin-lift.		
		Seal mouth and nose properly.		
		Attempt to ventilate.		
6. Heimlich Maneuver	Perform abdominal thrusts.	Straddle victim's thighs.		
		Place heel of one hand against victim's abdomen, in the midline slightly above the navel and well below the tip of the xiphoid.		
		Place second hand directly on top of first hand.		
		Press into the abdomen with quick upward thrusts.		
		Perform 6–10 abdominal thrusts.		
7. Foreign Body Check	Perform finger sweep.*	Keep victim's face up.		
		Use tongue-jaw lift to open mouth.		
		Sweep deeply into mouth to remove foreign body.		
8. Breathing Attempt	Attempt ventilation.	Open airway with head-tilt/chin-lift.		
		Seal mouth and nose properly.		
		Attempt to ventilate.		
9. Sequencing	Repeat sequence.	Repeat Steps 6–8 until successful.†		

* During practice and testing, simulate finger sweeps.

† After airway obstruction is removed, check for pulse and breathing. (a) If pulse is absent, ventilate a second time and start cycles of compressions and ventilations. (b) If pulse is present, open airway and check for spontaneous breathing. (c) If breathing is present, monitor breathing and pulse closely, maintain open airway. (d) If breathing is absent, perform rescue breathing at 12 times/min and monitor pulse.

Instructor ______________________ Check: Satisfactory _____ Unsatisfactory _____

4/86

CPR and ECC Performance Sheet

Obstructed Airway: Conscious Child*

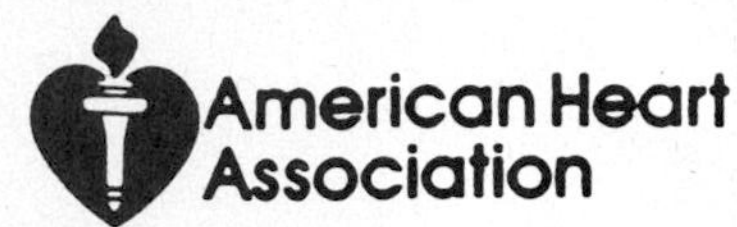

Name ______________________ Date ______________

Step	Activity	Critical Performance	S	U
1. Assessment	Determine airway obstruction.*	Ask "Are you choking?"		
		Determine if victim can cough or speak.		
2. Heimlich Maneuver	Perform abdominal thrusts (only if victim's cough is ineffective and there is increasing respiratory difficulty).	Stand behind the victim.		
		Wrap arms around victim's waist.		
		Make a fist with one hand and place the thumb side against victim's abdomen, in the midline slightly above the navel and well below the tip of the xiphoid.		
		Grasp fist with the other hand.		
		Press into the victim's abdomen with quick upward thrusts.		
		Each thrust should be distinct and delivered with the intent of relieving the airway obstruction.		
		Repeat thrusts until either the foreign body is expelled or the victim becomes unconsious (see below).		
Victim with Obstructed Airway Becomes Unconscious (Optional Testing Sequence)				
3. Additional Assessment	Position the victim.	Turn on back as unit.		
		Place face up, arms by side.		
	Call for help.	Call out "Help!" or if others respond, activate EMS system.		
4. Foreign Body Check	Perform tongue-jaw lift. Do not perform blind finger sweep; remove foreign body only IF VISUALIZED.	Keep victim's face up.		
		Use tongue-jaw lift to open mouth.		
		Look into mouth and remove foreign body IF VISUALIZED.		
5. Breathing Attempt	Attempt ventilation (airway is obstructed).	Open airway with head-tilt/chin-lift.		
		Seal mouth and nose properly.		
		Attempt to ventilate.		
6. Heimlich Maneuver	Perform abdominal thrusts.	Kneel at victim's feet if on the floor, or stand at victim's feet if on a table.		
		Place heel of one hand against victim's abdomen, in the midline slightly above navel and well below tip of xiphoid.		
		Place second hand directly on top of first hand.		
		Press into the abdomen with quick upward thrusts.		
		Perform 6–10 abdominal thrusts.		
7. Foreign Body Check	Perform tongue-jaw lift. Do not perform blind finger sweep; remove foreign body only IF VISUALIZED.	Keep victim's face up.		
		Use tongue-jaw lift to open mouth.		
		Look into mouth and remove foreign body IF VISUALIZED.		
8. Breathing Attempt	Attempt ventilation.	Open airway with head-tilt/chin-lift.		
		Seal mouth and nose properly.		
		Attempt to ventilate.		
9. Sequencing	Repeat sequence.	Repeat Steps 6–8 until successful.†		

* This procedure should be initiated in a conscious child only if the airway obstruction is due to a witnessed or strongly suspected aspiration and if respiratory difficulty is increasing and the cough is ineffective. If obstruction is caused by airway swelling due to infection such as epiglottitis or croup, these procedures may be harmful; the child should be rushed to the nearest ALS facility, allowing the child to maintain the position of maximum comfort.

† After airway obstruction is removed, check for pulse and breathing. (a) If pulse is absent, ventilate a second time and start cycles of compressions and ventilations. (b) If pulse is present, open airway and check for spontaneous breathing. (c) If breathing is present, monitor breathing and pulse closely and maintain an open airway. (d) If breathing is absent, perform rescue breathing at 15 times/min and monitor pulse.

Instructor ______________________ Check: Satisfactory _____ Unsatisfactory _____

4/86

CPR and ECC Performance Sheet

Obstructed Airway: Conscious Infant*

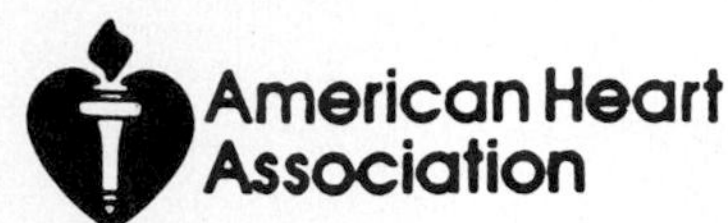

Name ______________________ Date ____________

Step	Activity	Critical Performance	S	U
1. Assessment	Determine airway obstruction.*	Observe breathing difficulties.*		
2. Back Blows	Deliver 4 back blows.	Supporting head and neck with one hand, straddle infant face down, head lower than trunk, over your forearm supported on your thigh.		
		Deliver 4 back blows, forcefully, between the shoulder blades with the heel of the hand (3–5 sec).		
3. Chest Thrusts	Deliver 4 chest thrusts.	While supporting the head, sandwich infant between your hands and turn on back, with head lower than trunk.		
		Deliver 4 thrusts in the midsternal region in the same manner as external chest compressions, but at a slower rate (3–5 sec).		
4. Sequencing	Repeat sequence.	Repeat Steps 2 and 3 until either the foreign body is expelled or the infant becomes unconscious (see below).		

Infant with Obstructed Airway Becomes Unconscious (Optional Testing Sequence)

Step	Activity	Critical Performance	S	U
5. Call for Help.	Call for help.	Call out "Help!" or, if others respond, activate EMS system.		
6. Foreign Body Check	Perform tongue-jaw lift. Do not perform blind finger sweep; remove foreign body only IF VISUALIZED.	Do tongue-jaw lift by placing thumb in infant's mouth over tongue. Lift tongue and jaw forward with fingers wrapped around lower jaw.		
		Remove foreign body IF VISUALIZED.		
7. Breathing Attempt	Attempt ventilation (airway is obstructed).	Open airway with head-tilt/chin-lift.		
		Seal mouth and nose properly.		
		Attempt to ventilate.		
8. Back Blows	Deliver 4 back blows.	Supporting head and neck with one hand, straddle infant face down, head lower than trunk, over your forearm supported on your thigh.		
		Deliver 4 back blows, forcefully, between the shoulder blades with the heel of the hand (3–5 sec).		
9. Chest Thrusts	Deliver 4 chest thrusts.	While supporting the head and neck, sandwich infant between your hands and turn on back, with head lower than trunk.		
		Deliver 4 thrusts in the midsternal region in the same manner as external chest compressions, but at a slower rate (3–5 sec).		
10. Foreign Body Check	Perform tongue-jaw lift, not blind finger sweep.	Do tongue-jaw lift.		
		Remove foreign body IF VISUALIZED.		
11. Breathing Attempt	Reattempt ventilation.	Open airway with head-tilt/chin-lift.		
		Seal mouth and nose properly.		
		Attempt to ventilate.		
12. Sequencing	Repeat sequence.	Repeat Steps 8–11 until successful.†		

* This procedure should be initiated in a conscious infant only if the airway obstruction is due to a witnessed or strongly suspected aspiration and if respiratory difficulty is increasing and the cough is ineffective. If the obstruction is caused by airway swelling due to infections, such as epiglottitis or croup, these procedures may be harmful; the infant should be rushed to the nearest ALS facility, allowing the infant to maintain the position of maximum comfort.

† After airway obstruction is removed, check for breathing and pulse. (a) If pulse is absent, ventilate a second time and start cycles of compressions and ventilations. (b) If pulse is present, open airway and check for spontaneous breathing. (c) If breathing is present, monitor breathing and pulse closely and maintain an open airway. (d) If breathing is absent, perform rescue breathing at 20 times/min and monitor pulse.

Instructor ______________________ Check: Satisfactory _____ Unsatisfactory _____

4/86

CPR and ECC Performance Sheet

Obstructed Airway: Unconscious Adult

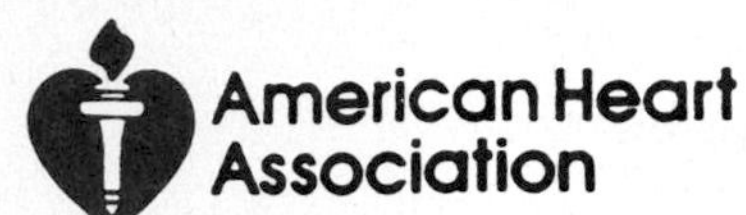

Name ______________________ Date ______________

Step	Activity	Critical Performance	S	U
1. Assessment/Airway	Determine unresponsiveness.	Tap or gently shake shoulder. Shout "Are you OK?"		
	Call for help.	Call out "Help!"		
	Position the victim.	Turn on back as unit, if necessary, supporting head and neck (4–10 sec).		
	Open the airway.	Use head-tilt/chin-lift maneuver.		
	Determine breathlessness.	Maintain open airway.		
		Ear over mouth, observe chest: look, listen, feel for breathing (3–5 sec).		
2. Breathing Attempt	Attempt ventilation (airway is obstructed).	Maintain open airway.		
		Seal mouth and nose properly.		
		Attempt to ventilate.		
	Reattempt ventilation (airway remains blocked).	Reposition victim's head.		
		Seal mouth and nose properly.		
		Reattempt to ventilate.		
	Activate EMS system.	If someone responded to call for help, send him/her to activate EMS system.		
		Total time, Steps 1 and 2: 15–35 sec.		
3. Heimlich Maneuver	Perform abdominal thrusts.	Straddle victim's thighs.		
		Place heel of one hand against victim's abdomen in the midline slightly above the navel and well below the tip of the xiphoid.		
		Place second hand directly on top of first hand.		
		Press into the abdomen with quick upward thrusts.		
		Each thrust should be distinct and delivered with the intent of relieving the airway obstruction.		
		Perform 6–10 abdominal thrusts.		
4. Foreign Body Check	Perform finger sweep.*	Keep victim's face up.		
		Use tongue-jaw lift to open mouth.		
		Sweep deeply into mouth to remove foreign body.		
5. Breathing Attempt	Attempt ventilation.	Open airway with head-tilt/chin-lift maneuver.		
		Seal mouth and nose properly.		
		Attempt to ventilate.		
6. Sequencing	Repeat sequence.	Repeat Steps 3–5 until successful.†		

* During practice and testing simulate finger sweeps.

† After airway obstruction is removed, check again for pulse and breathing. (a) If pulse is absent, ventilate a second time and start cycles of compressions and ventilations. (b) If pulse is present, open airway and check for spontaneous breathing. (c) If breathing is present, monitor breathing and pulse closely, maintain open airway. (d) If breathing is absent, perform rescue breathing at 12 times/min and monitor pulse.

Instructor ______________________ Check: Satisfactory _____ Unsatisfactory _____

4/86

CPR and ECC Performance Sheet

Obstructed Airway: Unconscious Child

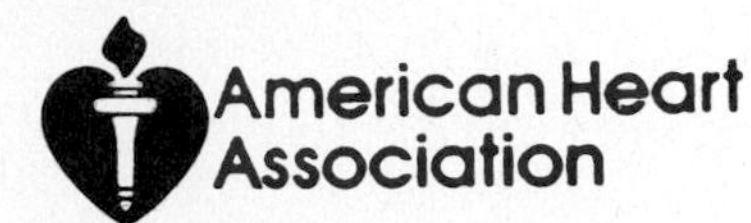

Name ______________________ Date ______________

Step	Activity	Critical Performance	S	U
1. Assessment/Airway	Determine unresponsiveness.	Tap or gently shake shoulder.		
		Shout "Are you OK?"		
	Call for help.	Call out "Help!"		
	Position the victim.	Turn on back as unit, if necessary, supporting head and neck (4–10 sec).		
	Open the airway.	Use head-tilt/chin-lift maneuver.		
	Determine breathlessness.	Maintain open airway.		
		Ear over mouth, observe chest: look, listen, feel for breathing (3–5 sec).		
2. Breathing Attempt	Attempt ventilation (airway is obstructed).	Maintain open airway.		
		Seal mouth and nose properly.		
		Attempt to ventilate.		
	Reattempt ventilation (airway remains blocked).	Reposition victim's head.		
		Seal mouth and nose properly.		
		Reattempt to ventilate.		
	Activate EMS system.	If someone responded to call for help, send him/her to activate EMS system.		
		Total time, Steps 1 and 2: 15–35 sec.		
3. Heimlich Maneuver	Perform abdominal thrusts.	Kneel at victim's feet if on the floor, or stand at victim's feet if on a table.		
		Place heel of one hand against victim's abdomen in the midline slightly above navel and well below tip of xiphoid.		
		Place second hand directly on top of first hand.		
		Press into the abdomen with quick upward thrusts.		
		Each thrust should be distinct and delivered with the intent of relieving the airway.		
		Perform 6–10 abdominal thrusts.		
4. Foreign Body Check	Perform tongue-jaw lift. Do not perform blind finger sweep; remove foreign body only IF VISUALIZED.	Keep victim's face up.		
		Use tongue-jaw lift to open mouth.		
		Look into mouth and remove foreign body IF VISUALIZED.		
5. Breathing Attempt	Reattempt ventilation.	Open airway with head-tilt/chin-lift maneuver.		
		Seal mouth and nose properly.		
		Attempt to ventilate.		
6. Sequencing	Repeat sequence.	Repeat Steps 3–5 until successful.*		

* After airway obstruction is removed, check for pulse and breathing. (a) If pulse is absent, ventilate a second time and start cycles of compressions and ventilations. (b) If pulse is present, open airway and check for spontaneous breathing. (c) If breathing is present, monitor breathing and pulse closely and maintain an open airway. (d) If breathing is absent, perform rescue breathing at 15 times/min and monitor pulse.

Instructor ______________________ Check: Satisfactory _____ Unsatisfactory _____

4/86

CPR and ECC Performance Sheet

Obstructed Airway: Unconscious Infant

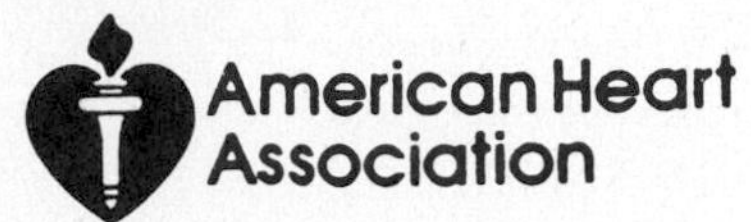

Name ______________________________ Date ________________

Step	Activity	Critical Performance	S	U
1. Assessment/Airway	Determine unresponsiveness.	Tap or gently shake shoulder.		
	Call for help.	Call out "Help!"		
	Position the infant.	Turn on back as unit, if necessary, supporting head and neck.		
		Place on firm, hard surface.		
	Open the airway.	Use head-tilt/chin-lift maneuver to sniffing or neutral position.		
		Do not overextend the head.		
	Determine breathlessness.	Maintain open airway.		
		Ear over mouth, observe chest: look, listen, feel for breathing (3–5 sec).		
2. Breathing Attempt	Attempt ventilation (airway is obstructed).	Maintain open airway.		
		Make tight seal on mouth and nose of infant with rescuer's mouth.		
		Attempt to ventilate.		
	Reattempt ventilation (airway remains blocked).	Reposition infant's head.		
		Seal mouth and nose properly.		
		Reattempt to ventilate.		
	Activate EMS system	If someone responded to call for help, send him/her to activate EMS system.		
		Total time, Steps 1 and 2: 10–25 sec.		
3. Back Blows	Deliver 4 back blows.	Supporting head and neck with one hand, straddle infant face down, head lower than trunk, over your forearm supported on your thigh.		
		Deliver 4 back blows, forecefully, between the shoulder blades with the heel of the hand (3–5 sec).		
4. Chest Thrusts	Deliver 4 chest thrusts.	While supporting the head and neck, sandwich infant between your hands and turn on back, with head lower than trunk.		
		Deliver 4 thrusts in the midsternal region in the same manner as external chest compressions, but at a slower rate (3–5 sec).		
5. Foreign Body Check	Perform tongue-jaw lift. Do not perform blind finger sweep; remove foreign body only IF VISUALIZED.	Do tongue-jaw lift by placing thumb in infant's mouth over tongue. Lift tongue and jaw forward with fingers wrapped around lower jaw.		
		Remove foreign body IF VISUALIZED.		
6. Breathing Attempt	Reattempt ventilation.	Open airway with head-tilt/chin-lift.		
		Seal mouth and nose properly.		
		Attempt to ventilate.		
7. Sequencing	Repeat sequence.	Repeat Steps 3–6 until successful.*		

* After airway obstruction is removed, check for breathing and pulse. (a) If pulse is absent, ventilate a second time and start cycles of compressions and ventilations. (b) If pulse is present, open airway and check for spontaneous breathing. (c) If breathing is present, monitor breathing and pulse closely and maintain an open airway. (d) If breathing is absent, perform rescue breathing at 20 times/min and monitor pulse.

Instructor ______________________________ Check: Satisfactory _____ Unsatisfactory _____

4/86

4 Shock

- Shock Due to Injury (Hypovolemic)
- Anaphylactic Shock (Allergic Reaction)
- Fainting

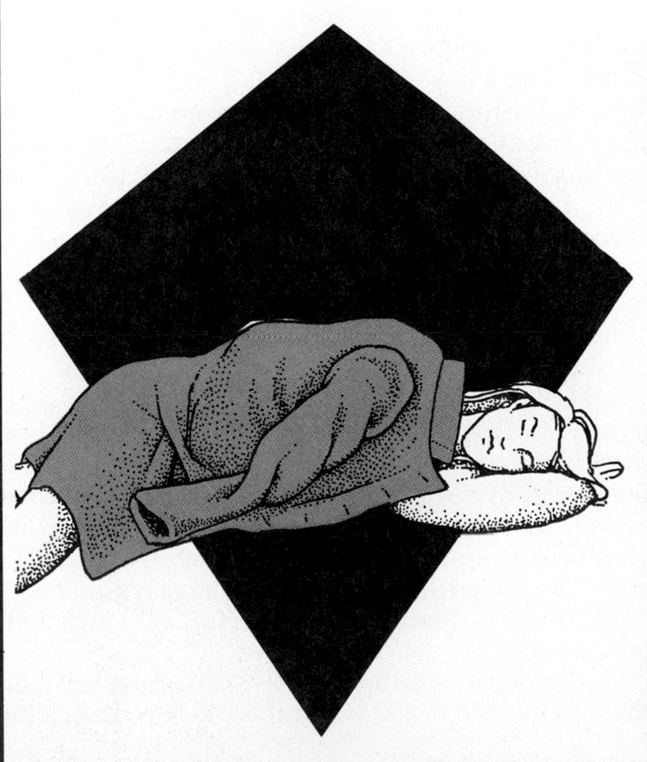

Shock occurs when the tissues or organs are inadequately supplied with oxygenated blood. Three factors are necessary to maintain normal perfusion: (1) a functioning heart, (2) adequate amount of blood, and (3) an intact circulatory system. Abnormalities in any one of these can produce shock.

Shock can be categorized into various types:

- Hypovolemic Shock (blood loss)—There is insufficient blood in the system to provide adequate circulation to all body organs. This causes hemorrhage and dehydration.
- Respiratory Shock (inadequate breathing There is insufficient oxygen in the blood.
- Neurogenic Shock—Enlargement of the vascular container so that there is insufficient blood to fill it.
- Psychogenic Shock (fainting)—Temporary dilation of the blood vessels results in decreased blood supply to the brain.
- Cardiogenic Shock (inadequate functioning of the heart)—The heart muscle no longer imparts sufficient pressure to the blood to drive it through the system.
- Septic Shock (severe infection)—Bacteria attack small blood vessel walls so they dilate.
- Anaphylactic Shock (allergic reaction)—This is a severe allergic reaction caused by foods, drugs, insect stings, and inhaled substances. It can occur in minutes or even seconds following contact with the substance to which the victim is allergic.
- Metabolic Shock (bodily loss of fluid)—A severe fluid loss occurs from a severe untreated illness.

SHOCK DUE TO INJURY (HYPOVOLEMIC)

Hypovolemic shock is a life threatening situation in which the body's vital functions are seriously threat-

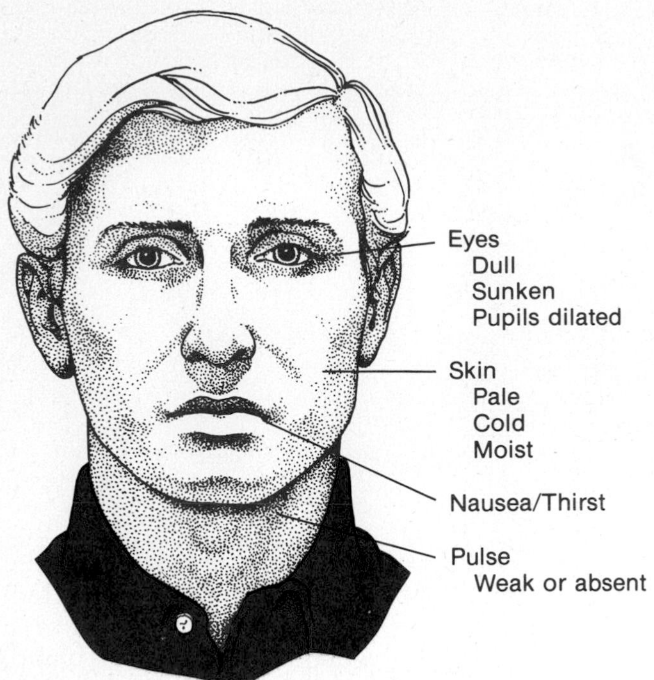

4-1. Signs and symptoms of shock

ened by insufficient blood, or oxygen in the blood, reaching the body tissues.

Some degree of shock can be attributed to every injury. Therefore, a first aider should treat for shock in all serious injuries. A first aider cannot reverse shock once it develops, but he or she can prevent it from worsening.

Signs and symptoms of shock include: pale or bluish and cool skin; moist and clammy skin; overall weakness; vomiting; dull, sunken look to the eyes; pupils widely dilated; and unusual thirst. (*See* Figure 4–1.)

Unfortunately there is little that a first aider can do. First aid for hypovolemic shock includes:

1. Maintain an open airway.
2. Control all obvious bleeding.
3. Elevate the lower extremities about twelve inches unless the injury makes this impossible or when it is not advisable, such as chest injuries, unconsciousness, etc. This allows the blood in the legs to be returned to the heart more readily.
4. Prevent the loss of body heat by putting blankets under and over the victim. Do not attempt to warm the victim.
5. Generally, keep the victim supine. However, some victims in shock may require another position. (*See* Figure 4–2.) For example, those with head or chest injury or stroke should have their heads and upper bodies elevated. This will reduce pressure on the brain. Those with lung disease or a heart attack should also have been in a semi-sitting position. These victims can breathe better. An unconscious or vomiting victim should lie on his or her side.
6. Do not give the victim anything to eat or drink. Eating or drinking may cause the victim to become nauseated and vomit.
7. Handle victims gently.

ANAPHYLACTIC SHOCK (ALLERGIC REACTION)

Although the incidence of severe allergic reactions to various substances is very low, when it happens, it can be a life-threatening emergency. Substances that most often cause allergic reactions may be grouped as follows:

1. *Insect stings.* Stings of the bee, wasp, yellow jacket, or hornet can cause very rapid and severe anaphylactic reactions.
2. *Injections.* The injections from various medications (e.g., tetanus antitoxin or drugs such as penicillin) may cause severe reactions.
3. *Ingestion.* Eating foods such as fish, shellfish, or berries or taking medications or drugs such as oral penicillin can cause slower but equally severe reactions to someone who is sensitive to any of them.
4. *Inhalation.* The inhalation of dusts, pollens, or materials to which an individual is especially sensitive may cause rapid and severe reactions.

If the sting is from a honeybee, carefully remove the stinger by gently scraping with a knife blade or fingernail. Removing the stinger reduces the amount of venom entering the body. Do not squeeze the stinger while removing it because you could be injecting more venom.

Quickly assess the victim's skin around the sting. If it is red and inflamed, an allergic reaction is occurring and there is danger of developing anaphylactic shock. Other signs of anaphylactic shock include: weakness, coughing and/or wheezing, breathing difficulty, severe itching or hives, nausea and vomiting, and dizziness.

Maintain an open airway and restore breathing if necessary.

Immediately ask the victim if he has an anaphylaxis kit (commonly known as an emergency bee sting kit). These are available only by prescription. If the individual does, inject the epinephrine, and then massage the injection site vigorously to speed the distribution of epinephrine throughout the victim's body. The injection should relieve the reaction; but if the kit is not available, the victim's anaphylaxis will worsen rapidly.

Continue to assess the victim's airway and ask if he is having trouble breathing or if he feels as though his

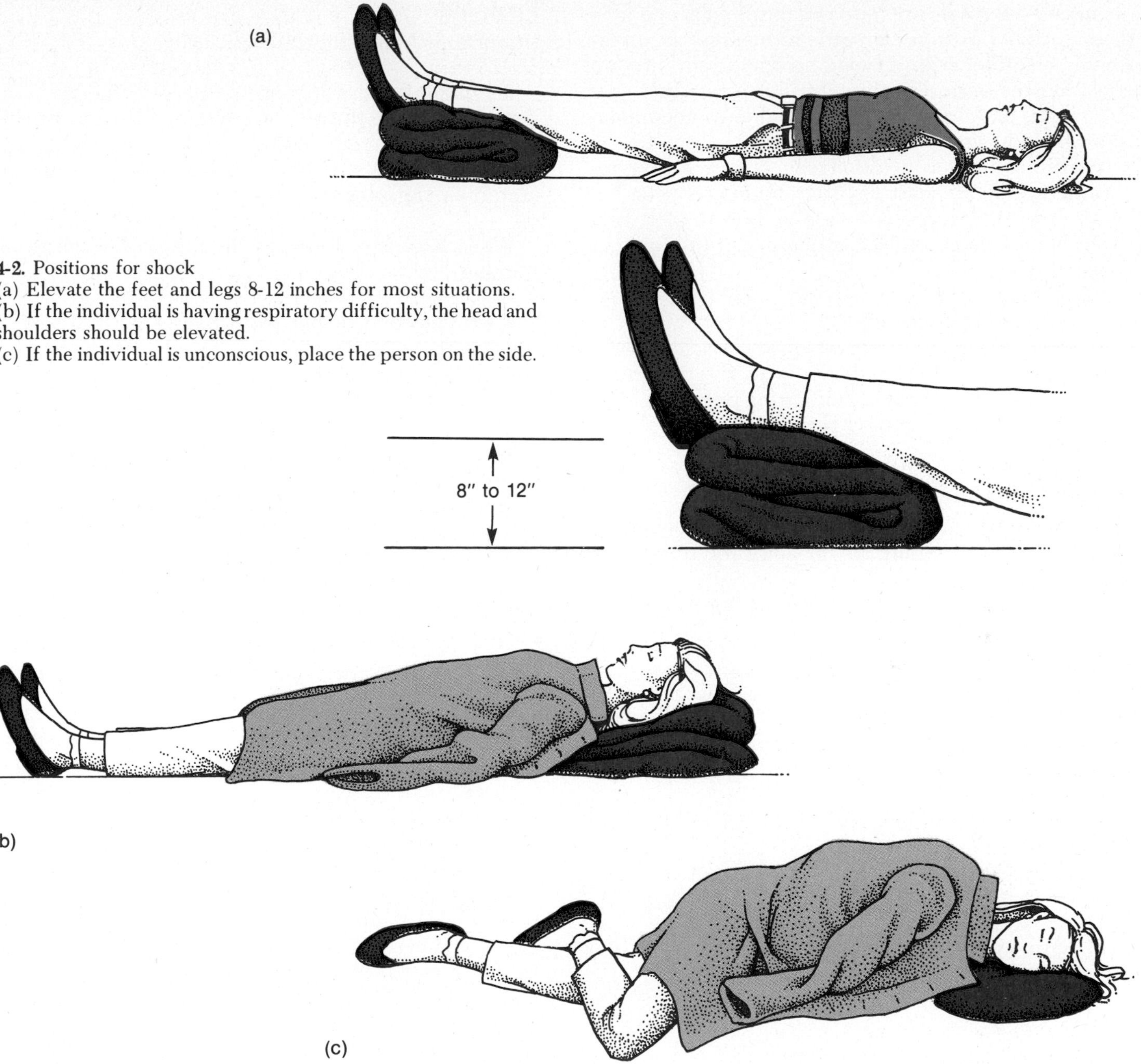

4-2. Positions for shock
(a) Elevate the feet and legs 8-12 inches for most situations.
(b) If the individual is having respiratory difficulty, the head and shoulders should be elevated.
(c) If the individual is unconscious, place the person on the side.

throat is closing up. Apply a constriction band just above the sting site, if on an arm or leg. Seek medical attention promptly, preferable at the nearest hospital emergency room.

The victim may have breathing difficulty as bronchospasm and swelling of the larynx develop. If the victim stops breathing, open the airway and begin resuscitation. Trained medical personnel could perform a cricothyrotomy or tracheotomy. First aiders should *not* perform these medical maneuvers. Remember, the only really effective treatment for severe allergic reactions is an immediate injection of epinephrine.

FAINTING

Fainting is a loss of consciousness. Staying conscious is dependent on normal brain function. To function normally, the brain needs a large supply of oxygen. When the oxygen supply to the brain is interrupted, fainting may occur.

Fainting may result from many different causes, the most common being a psychic disturbance of an unpleasant nature, which sets off a chain of effects not unlike those seen in shock. Some persons faint from merely seeing blood or from seeing or hearing unpleasant things. Also, there is a type of fainting that occurs in those who are required to spend a long time in an upright position with little movement as, for instance, a soldier who is being held at attention for a considerable period of time. In such a case there is a loss of circulating blood volume, due to accumulation of blood in the legs.

There are numerous other causes of fainting, including epilepsy, heart disorder, and cerebrovascular disease. Many are not serious, but an alert first aider should be especially concerned if the fainting victim:

- Is over forty years old.
- Has had repeated attacks of unconsciousness.
- Does not awaken within four to five minutes.
- Loses consciousness while sitting or lying down.
- Faints for no apparent reason.

Signs of Fainting

Fainting may occur suddenly or may be preceded by warning signs, including any or all of the following:

- Dizziness and the victim tells of "spots" before his eyes
- Nausea
- Paleness
- Sweating

First Aid

Important things not to do include:

- *Do not* pour water on the person's face.
- *Do not* give the person anything to drink until he or she has fully recovered.
- *Do not* use stimulants such as smelling salts or ammonia capsules.

When a person looks as though on the verge of fainting:

- Prevent him or her from falling.
- Lie the victim on his or her back and elevate the legs eight to twelve inches.

After fainting has occurred or if fainting is anticipated:

- Lie the victim down and elevate the legs eight to twelve inches.
- If vomiting begins, turn the person on his or her side to keep the airway open and clear.
- Loosen clothing around the person's neck (such as a tight necktie or collar).
- Wet a cloth with cool water and wipe the person's forehead and face.

Most cases of fainting are not serious and the victim regains consciousness quickly. However, seek medical attention if recovery is not complete within five minutes. If the victim has fallen, assess for injuries.

Allergic Reaction

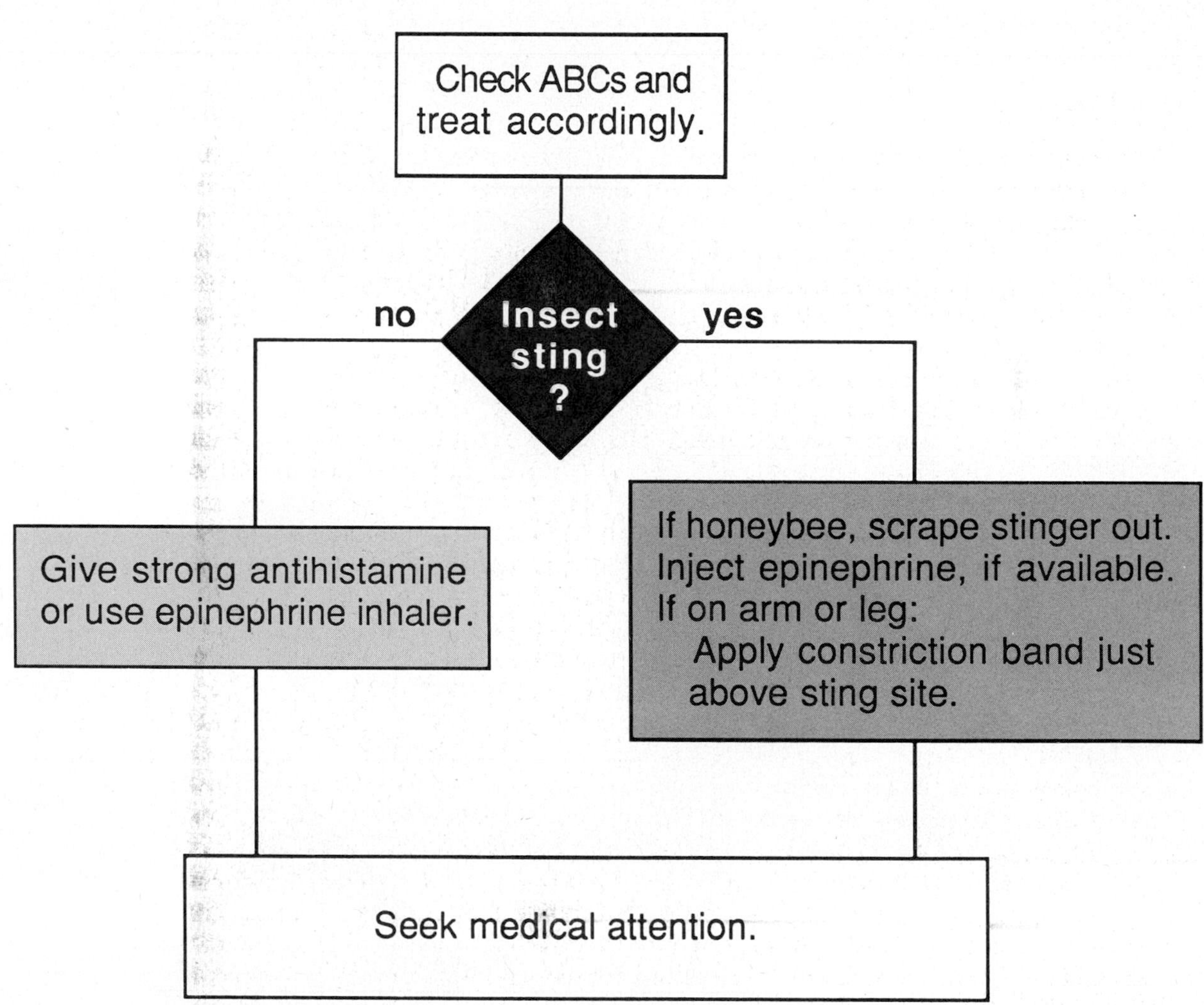

Shock (Traumatic)

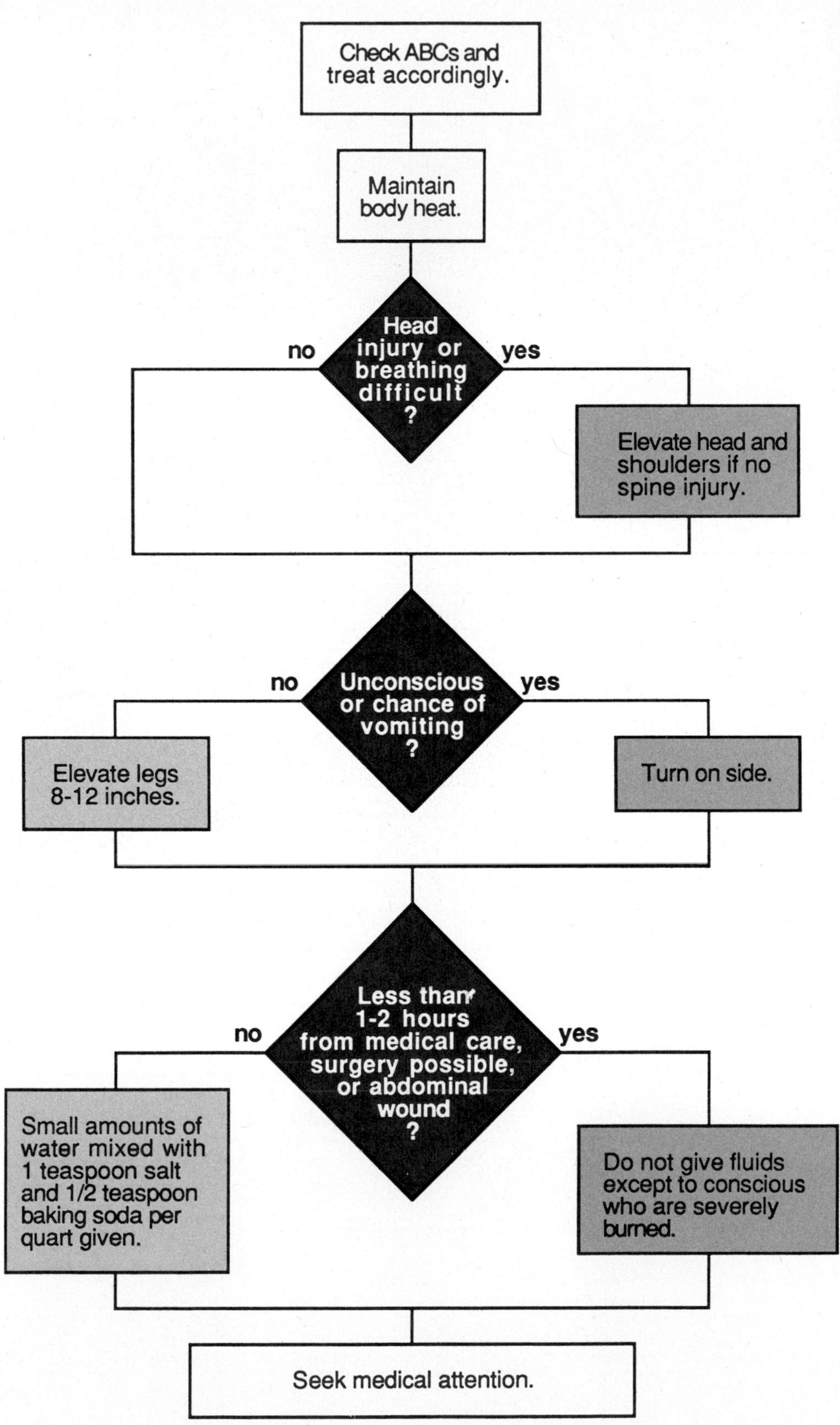

Fainting

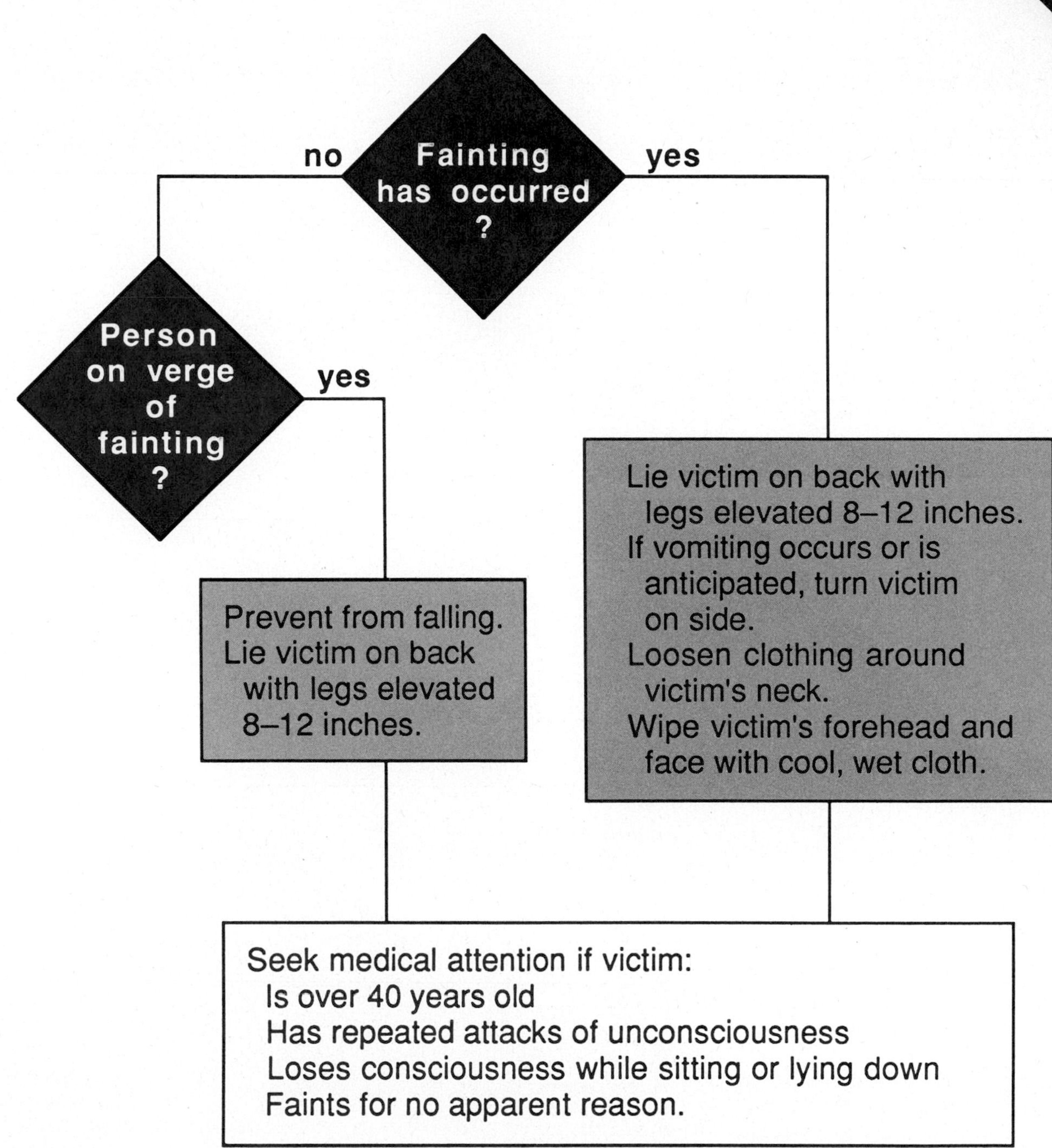

Fainting has occurred ?
no
yes
Person on verge of fainting ?
yes
Prevent from falling.
Lie victim on back with legs elevated 8–12 inches.
Lie victim on back with legs elevated 8–12 inches.
If vomiting occurs or is anticipated, turn victim on side.
Loosen clothing around victim's neck.
Wipe victim's forehead and face with cool, wet cloth.
Seek medical attention if victim:
Is over 40 years old
Has repeated attacks of unconsciousness
Loses consciousness while sitting or lying down
Faints for no apparent reason.

Shock

LEARNING ACTIVITIES

Case 1: A car carrying a young couple rounded a curve on a country road at an excessive speed. The 17-year-old girl slid across the front seat, hit the passenger door and rolled out of the car. She is lying face up on the grassy shoulder of the road. Her eyes are glassy with dilated pupils; a look of extreme fear is on her face. Her skin is pale and she does not respond to direct questioning. A quick physical examination does not evoke a pain response; her skin is pale, cool, and moist. Her face and hands are covered with minor abrasions and lacerations.

1. This victim is in what type of shock?

   ____

   ____

2. If internal injuries are suspected, what other type of shock should be considered?

   ____

   ____

3. In which of the following positions should the victim be placed?

   A. ______ elevate entire body
   B. ______ elevate legs only (12 inches)

4. What is a possible reason to place someone in a position other than the correct answer selected above?

   ____

   ____

5. What other care should be initiated for the victim at this time? ______________________________

   ____

6. When providing emergency medical care, what are two priority conditions that should be treated before shock?

   ____

   ____

7. A form of shock related to that in this case is simple fainting or ______________ shock?

Case 2: While chopping firewood for his evening campfire, a middle-aged man deeply lacerated his lower left leg. Fellow campers managed initial control of the profuse bleeding.

1. Upon arrival at the campground, the first aider would most likely find this man in

   A. ______ neurogenic shock
   B. ______ cardiogenic shock
   C. ______ hypovolemic shock
   D. ______ septic shock

2. This victim may be expected to exhibit which of the following signs and symptoms? Check *all* appropriate answers.

   A. ______ sunken eyes
   B. ______ ashen gray skin
   C. ______ high skin temperature
   D. ______ body covered with a clammy sweat
   E. ______ pulse rapid, weak
   F. ______ complaints of thirst

3. The most important action for the first aider to consider in this and most other emergency situations involving shock is to

   ____

   ____

Shock Positions

In shock, the proper position of the victim's body depends on the injuries received. Indicate the most desirable body position for the types of injuries listed below.

Type of Injury	*Shock Position*
1. Neck injury	1. ______
2. Unconscious	2. ______
3. Abdominal wound	3. ______
4. Head injury	4. ______
5. Sucking wound of chest	5. ______
6. Heart attack	6. ______
7. Fractured legs	7. ______
8. Avulsed fingers	8. ______

Anaphylactic Shock

Case: In an orchard, you see a man lying next to a pickup truck with several bystanders gathered around. A short distance away is a wooden out-building which appears to have an active beehive. The victim is in apparent respiratory distress; he is wheezing, and his eyelids appear swollen.

1. This victim is in what type of shock?

______

______

2. What are the four causes and four examples of this type of shock?

Cause	Example
A. ______	A. ______
B. ______	B. ______
C. ______	C. ______
D. ______	D. ______

3. The emergency care for the type of shock experienced by this victim would include which of the following? Check *all* appropriate answers.

A. ______ emergency transport to medical facility
B. ______ transport in a prone position to ease respiration
C. ______ determine if victim has an emergency bee sting kit
D. ______ give liquid to the victim if requested

Fainting

T F 1. Smelling salts should be used in cases of fainting.
T F 2. Splashing water on a person's face helps revive him.
T F 3. There are many causes for a person to faint.
T F 4. Fainting may be preceded by warning signs.
T F 5. Most cases of fainting are not serious.

Case: While donating blood, Scott reports to the nurse that he is not feeling well and may faint. After this warning, Scott collapses.

1. The most common cause of fainting is ______.

2. Soldiers faint when they are required to ______.

3. Name other examples of why people faint.

A. ______
B. ______

4. Cite things *not* to do for fainting.

A. ______________________________

B. ______________________________

C. ______________________________

5. What can be done in case of fainting?

A. ______________________________

B. ______________________________

C. ______________________________

5 Bleeding

- Types of External Bleeding
- Types of Wounds
- Wounds Requiring Medical Attention
- Infection
- Tetanus
- Amputation
- Animal Bites

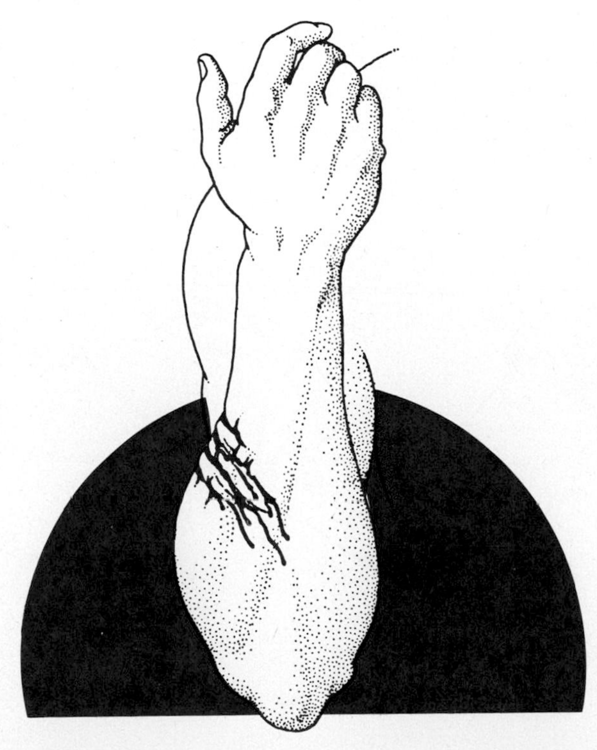

Of all the injuries seen by first aiders, bleeding may not only be the most visible but may also be the most often cared for.

The total blood volume in an average-sized individual is between five and six quarts. Although the average healthy adult can easily tolerate losses of a pint (the amount usually taken from blood donors), rapid loss of one quart or more of the total blood volume by bleeding often leads to irreversible shock and to death.

TYPES OF EXTERNAL BLEEDING

External bleeding classifications include:

Arterial: Blood from an artery spurts, and it is bright red in color because it is rich in oxygen. Arterial bleeding is less likely to clot than other types of bleeding. When completely severed, arteries often constrict and seal themselves off. However, if an artery is not completely severed but is torn or has a hole in its wall, it will probably continue to bleed. The blood loss from the wound is often rapid and profuse, as blood spurts from the wound. Unless a very large artery has been severed, it is unlikely that a person will bleed to death before control measures can be put into effect.

Unlike bleeding from other vessels, arterial bleeding, unless it is from only a small artery, will not clot because a blood clot can form only when there is a slow flow or no flow at all. Therefore, arterial bleeding is dangerous, and some external means of control must be used to stop the flow.

Some vessels are so large and carry such pressure that, even if a clot did form, it would be forced out. This might happen, too, if inept handling of a wound disturbed a clot or if pressure were released too soon. Therefore, once arterial bleeding is stopped, control must be maintained long enough for the injured person to be safely transported to an adequate medical facility.

Venous: Bleeding from a vein is steady and is dark bluish-red color. This type of bleeding may be profuse, but it is easier to control than arterial bleeding.

With venous bleeding, particularly from a large vein, do not overlook the danger of an air bubble or air embolism. This can happen because the blood in the larger veins is being sucked back toward the heart; hence, when a large vein is cut, air may actually be sucked into the opening in the vein. The air bubble can be large enough to interfere with the ability of the heart to pump the blood because of the air block that is formed. Therefore, venous bleeding must be controlled quickly.

Veins are usually located closer to the body surface than are arteries. Most veins collapse when they are cut;however, bleeding from deep veins can be as profuse and as hard to control as arterial bleeding.

Capillary: Blood oozes from a capillary and is similar in color to venous blood. Capillary bleeding is usually not serious and is easily controlled. It is characterized by a general ooze from the tissues, the blood dripping steadily from the wound or gradually forming a puddle in it. This type of bleeding is not immediately dangerous. Quite frequently, this type of bleeding will more or less control itself by clotting spontaneously.

In hemophilia, the tendency to bleed, as well as the inability of the blood to clot, may be so great as to threaten life. Bleeding in a person with this condition is especially difficult to control because the problem is in the failure of the blood clotting mechanism itself, and there is as yet no known specific cure. Hospitalization is required. As an emergency care measure, firm compression on the bleeding site should be applied.

Controlling External Bleeding

The first aider's major concern with open wounds is to control bleeding. This can be accomplished in almost all cases by:

Direct pressure: Direct pressure with the hand over the wound using a dressing or gauze pad stops most bleeding. If the bleeding does not stop, apply additional pressure with your hand. (*See* Figures 5-1 and 5-2.)

If sterile gauze is not available, use any clean fabric—handkerchief, bed sheet, sanitary napkin, and so on—never remove a dressing once it is in place because bleeding may start again. Apply another dressing on top of the blood-soaked one and hold them both in place.

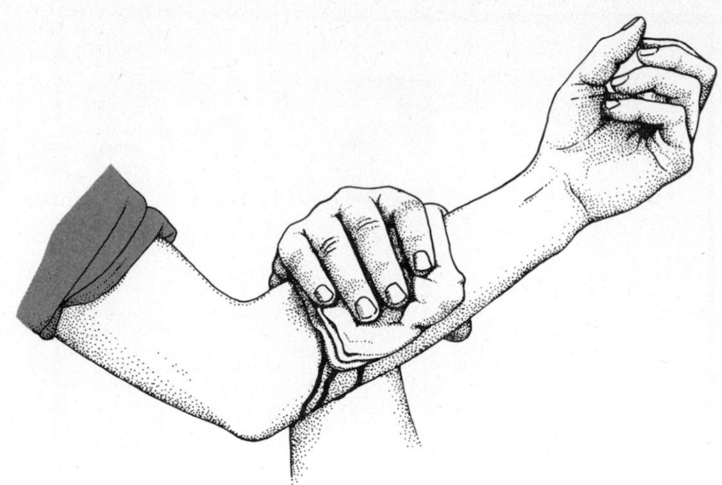

5-1. Applying direct pressure to a wound

If bleeding remains uncontrolled, try to grasp the blood vessel between your fingers or compress it between one finger and a bony part of the victim's body. However, do not waste valuable time attempting this. Direct pressure is usually the quickest and most efficient means of controlling external bleeding.

Elevation: Elevation may help control bleeding of an extremity. Application of direct pressure, however, on the wound site is still needed. When elevation of an extremity is used, gravity helps to reduce blood pressure and thus slows bleeding. (*See* Figure 5-3.)

Pressure points: If direct pressure is not controlling severe bleeding in the arm or leg, pressure points may be used. Such pressure can be applied most ef-

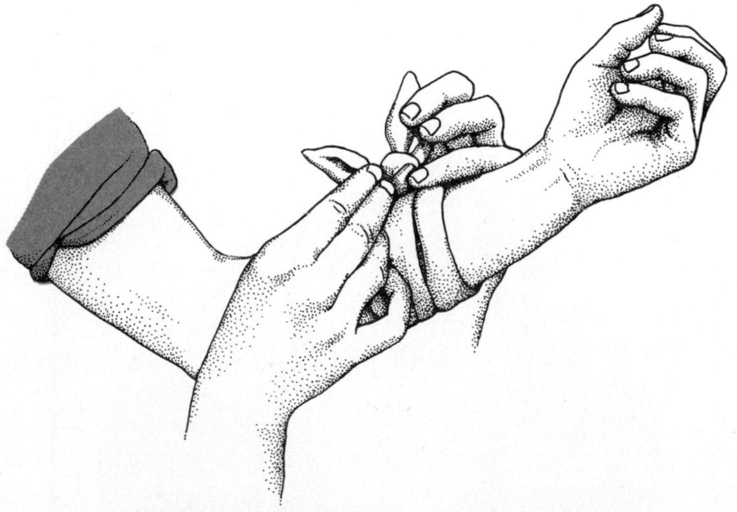

5-2. Applying a pressure bandage

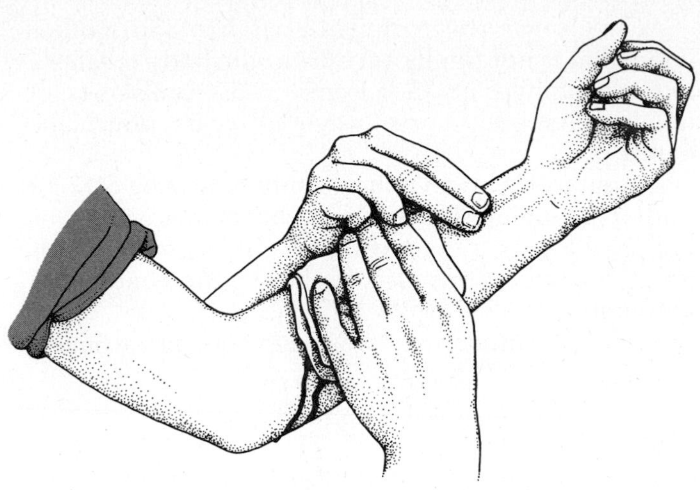

5-3. Applying direct pressure to a wound and elevating the wound above the victim's heart

fectively at the point where an artery is relatively near the surface and where it passes close to a bony structure against which it can be compressed. These points are known as pressure points. There are twenty-two such points, eleven on each side. Of these eleven, two are usually used to control most cases of external bleeding. The two easiest and most commonly used are the brachial point in the arm and the femoral point in the groin. (*See* Figure 5-4.)

Use pressure points only after direct pressure and elevation have failed to control the bleeding.

Tourniquet: A tourniquet is used only in a severe emergency when other means will not stop bleeding in an extremity. A tourniquet can damage nerves and blood vessels and can result in the loss of an arm or leg.

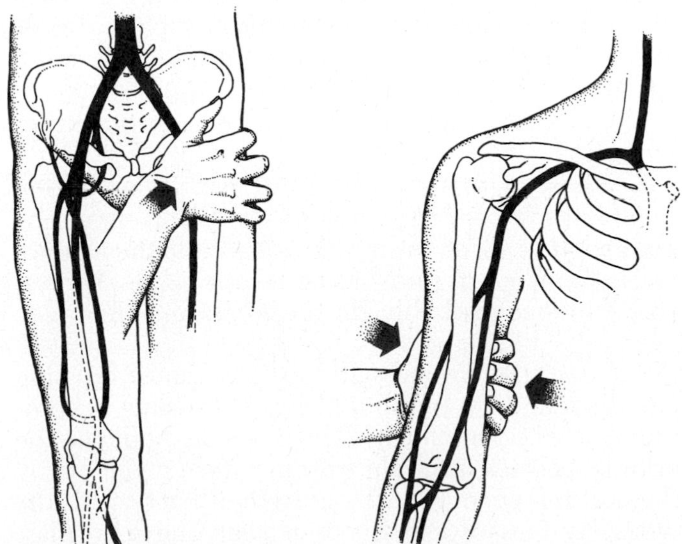

5-4. Proper hand positions for applying brachial and femoral pressure

Once you apply a tourniquet, do not loosen it. If a tourniquet is loosened, clots may be dislodged resulting in enough blood loss to cause severe shock and death. By leaving the tourniquet in place, more limbs may possibly be lost, but more lives will be saved.

Use a tourniquet only as a last resort to control a life-threatening bleeding that cannot be stopped by any other means. Besides, tourniquets are rarely, if ever, necessary.

TYPES OF WOUNDS

Soft-tissue injuries involve the skin and usually are classified as closed or open. In a closed injury, such as a bruise or contusion, there is damage to the soft tissue beneath the skin but no actual break in the skin. Contusions are marked by local pain and swelling. If small blood vessels beneath the skin have been broken, there will be a black and blue mark as well. If large vessels have been torn beneath the contused area, a hematoma, or collection of blood beneath the skin, will be evident as a lump with bluish discoloration. Closed wounds should be treated with pressure and cold applications to minimize swelling but otherwise require no specific treatment.

An open wound is one in which there is disruption in the continuity of the skin and, therefore, is susceptible to external bleeding and contamination. Open wounds may be of several types.

An abrasion, as shown in Figure 5–5, is a superficial wound caused by rubbing or scraping resulting in partial loss of the skin surface.

A laceration, as illustrated in Figure 5–5, is a cut made by a sharp instrument, such as a knife or razor blade, that produces a jagged incision through the skin surface and underlying structures. A laceration can be the source of significant bleeding if the sharp instrument also has disrupted the wall of a blood vessel, especially an artery. Thus, significant bleeding can result from lacerations in regions of the body where major arteries lie close to the surface, such as in the wrists.

A puncture wound, also shown in Figure 5–5, is a stab from a pointed object, such as a nail, ice pick, or knife. Special treatment of the puncture wound is required when the object causing the injury remains impaled in the wound. A discussion of this type of wound is provided in the section concerning impaled objects.

An incision is an open wound caused by sharp objects such as knives, razor blades, and sharp glass or metal edges. (*See* Figure 5–5.) The wound is smooth edged and bleeds freely. The amount of bleeding depends upon the depth, location, and size of the wound. There may be severe damage to muscles, nerves, and tendons if the wound is deep.

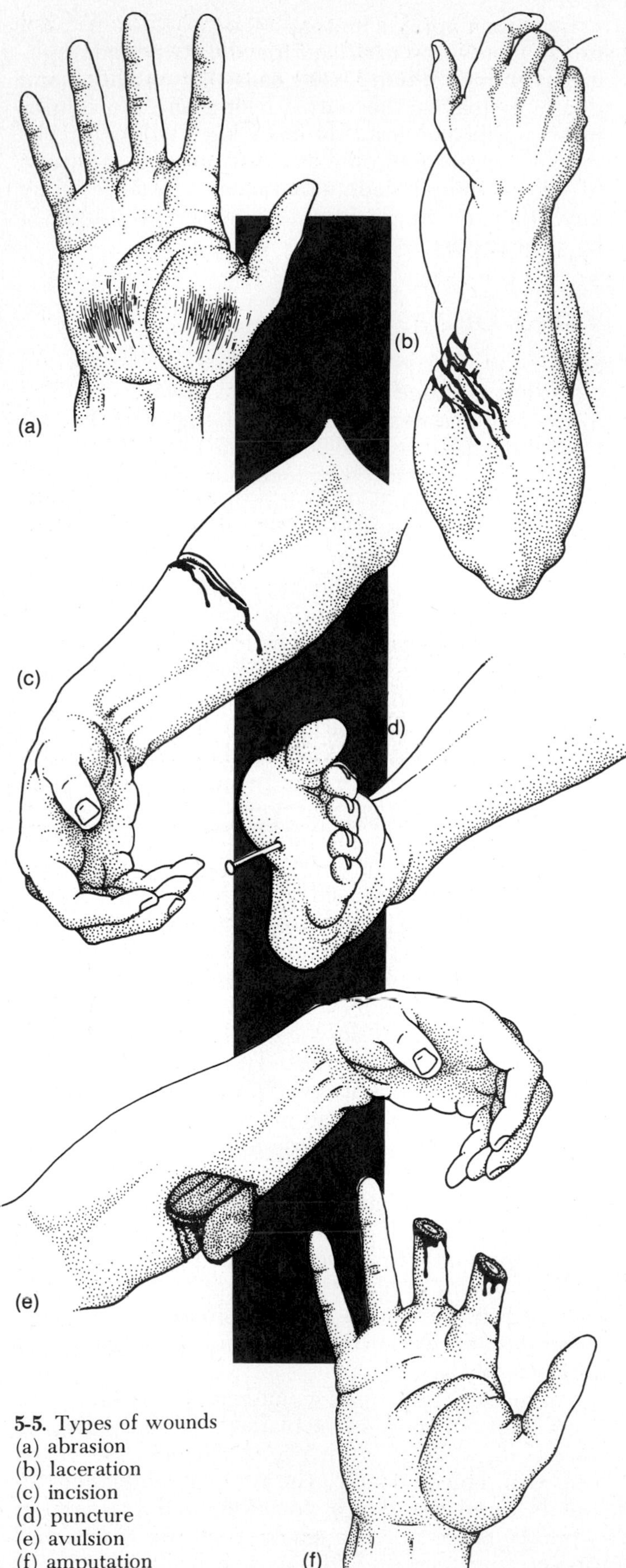

5-5. Types of wounds
(a) abrasion
(b) laceration
(c) incision
(d) puncture
(e) avulsion
(f) amputation

An avulsion is the tearing of a patch of skin or other tissue that if not totally torn from the body creates a loose, hanging flap. (*See* Figure 5-5.) Avulsions can involve such body parts as eyeballs, ears, fingers, or hands.

Amputations involve the cutting or tearing off of a body part such as fingers, toes, hands, feet, arms, or leg. (*See* Figure 5-5.) A discussion of severed or amputated parts is provided in the section concerning amputations.

Table 5-1 summarizes information on open wounds.

Minor Wounds

Cuts resulting in minor wounds are commonplace. In fact, the most frequently seen injury is a minor wound. During an average day, everyone can expect to see a bandage covering a minor wound. Every home, especially those with small children, should have an ample supply of bandages.

Minor wounds involve only the superficial layers of the skin and are not associated with severe bleeding. Most of these injuries can be handled safely without professional medical help. When caring for minor cuts and wounds, take the following steps:

1. When possible, wash hands in a vigorous scrubbing action using soap and water.

2. Allow the wound to bleed slightly. Apply direct pressure to the wound with a clean cloth. Continue pressure for three minutes. (Clotting may take six to seven minutes.)

3. Using a sterile gauze pad or a clean cloth saturated with soap and water, gently wash dirt away from the wound edges. Hydrogen peroxide (3% solution) helps to bubble away old blood and clots—not to disinfect the wound or destroy anaerobic bacteria as is often thought. Foreign bodies—such as dirt or gravel—must be removed to avoid infection and a tattoo look after the skin is healed.

4. Flush the wound liberally with large quantities of water.

5. Those who feel they must use an antiseptic should use isopropyl (rubbing) alcohol. It should be applied, if at all, on the intact skin around the wound, not in the wound. First aid antiseptic salves, sprays, and solutions probably do no good, and they may even retard healing.

6. Cover the wound with a sterile gauze dressing and bandage. A Band-aid™-type dressing is commonly used on small cuts. The dressing should not be airtight because it might trap moisture given off by the skin and encourage the growth of bacteria. If the wound is more of a scrape than a cut, one of the plastic "non-stickable" coverings may be helpful because they do not stick to the wound.

7. Small (less than one inch) lacerations heal faster and with less scarring if the wound edges are brought together by one or more pieces of tape. These are commonly known as "butterfly" bandages and can be made or purchased. (*See* Figure 5-6.)
8. If the wound bleeds after a bandage is applied and the bandage becomes stuck, it is best to leave it on as long as the wound is healing normally. Pulling the scab loose to change the dressing can only retard healing and increase the chances of infection. If a bandage must be removed, soak it in warm water or hydrogen peroxide to help soften the scab and make removal easier.

Dressings for a wound are most needed usually in the first twenty-four hours after an injury. During this time the scab has not yet formed and the wound is especially susceptible to infection.

Dressings serve a number of functions, including:

1. Protecting the wound from outside contamination.
2. Shielding the wound from further injury.
3. Preventing the spread of germs, blood, and other wound materials to surrounding areas.
4. Preventing the wound from getting either too wet or too dry.
5. Increasing the comfort of the victim while covering the wound site so the victim and others are not disturbed by its appearance.

WOUNDS REQUIRING MEDICAL ATTENTION

In today's world, many hazards cause a variety of wounds and bleeding. (Refer to Table 5-1.) These injuries generate a fair amount of anxiety and concern, especially regarding the question of whether or not to acquire professional medical care for the victim.

All of us will have the opportunity to decide about obtaining medical assistance for a wounded victim. To aid in this decision, consider the following types of wounds that require medical care:

1. Arterial bleeding.
2. Bleeding that cannot be controlled.

TABLE 5-1. Types of Open Wounds

Type	Cause(s)	Signs and Symptoms	First Aid
Abrasion (scrape)	Rubbing or scraping	Only skin surface affected Little bleeding	Remove all debris. Wash away from wound with soap and water.
Incision (cut)	Sharp objects	Smooth edges of wound Severe bleeding	Control bleeding. Wash wound.
Laceration (tearing)	Blunt object tearing skin	Veins and arteries can be affected Severe bleeding Danger of infection	Control bleeding. Wash wound.
Puncture (stab)	Sharp pointed object pierces skin	Wound is narrow and deep into veins and arteries Embedded objects Danger of infection	Do not remove impaled objects.
Avulsion (torn off)	Machinery, Explosives	Tissue torn off or left hanging Severe bleeding	Control bleeding. Take avulsed part to medical facility.

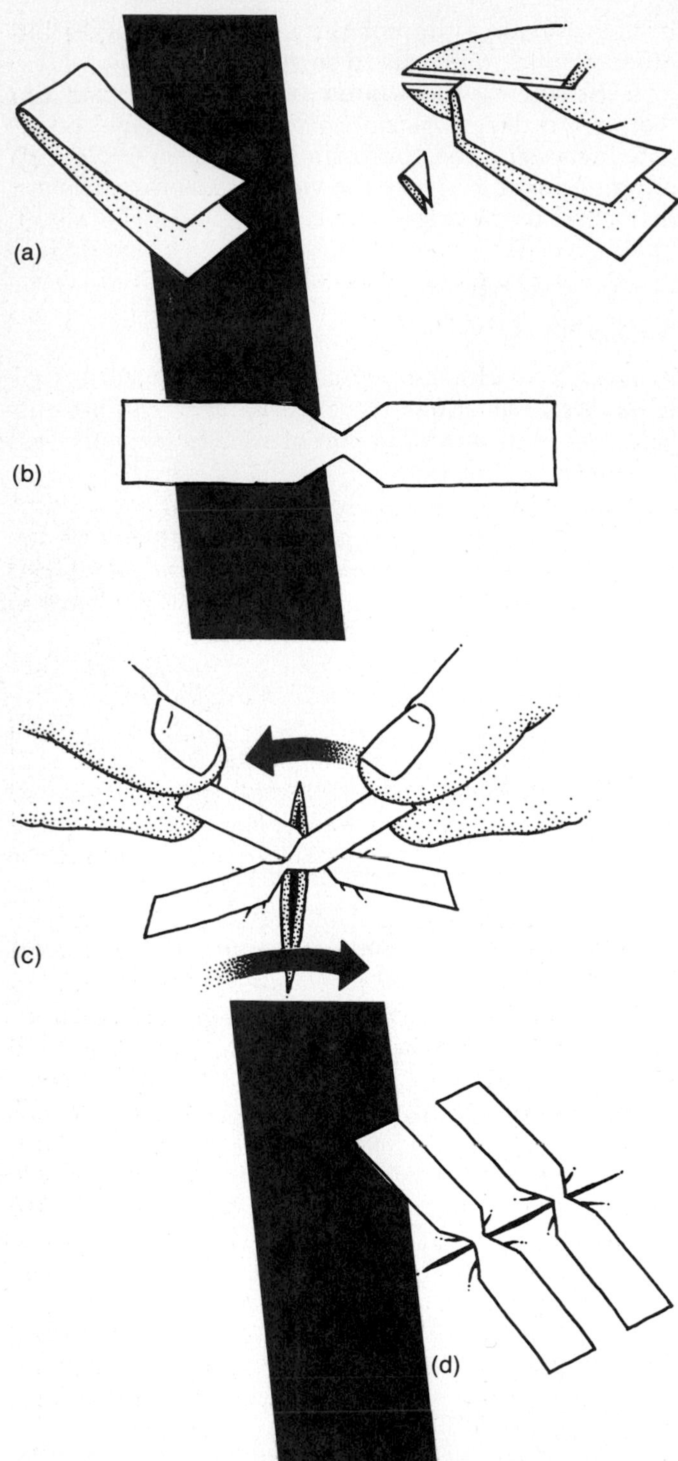

5-6. Butterfly bandage
(a) Fold a piece of tape and cut off both corners at the fold.
(b) The straightened tape reveals the "butterfly."
(c) Pull two butterfly bandages together to close and hold the wound edges together.
(d) Butterfly bandages holding edges together. Cover the butterflies and wound with a sterile dressing.

3. Any deep incision, laceration, or avulsion that:

a. Goes into the muscle or bone

b. Is located on a body part that ends and puts stress on the cut (elbows, knees, etc.)

c. Tends to gape widely

d. Is on the thumb or palm of hand (because nerves may be cut, later affecting the sense of touch).

4. Any puncture that is large or deep, is made by a dirty object, or does not bleed freely.

5. Large embedded objects.

6. Deeply embedded objects of any size.

7. Foreign matter left in a wound.

8. Human and animal bites.

9. Wounds where a scar would be noticeable. Stitched cuts usually heal with less scarring than unstitched ones.

10. Cuts to eyelids need sutures to prevent later drooping.

11. A slit lip needs stitches because it scars easily.

12. Any wound that a first aider is not certain how to care for.

Stitches

Stitches should be placed within six to eight hours of the injury. If the amount of contamination is small and the wound area is very vascular, the time may be extended to twelve hours.

It is good to stitch up cuts and wounds for several reasons:

1. Healing occurs more quickly.
2. Infection is less likely.
3. Scarring is lessened.

Most stitched wounds do well if the physician's advice is followed. The physician's instructions usually include:

- Keep the stitches clean and dry. Gently clean the wound area with a cotton-tipped applicator and hydrogen peroxide once or twice a day.
- Notify the physician promptly if the wound area becomes red or swollen or if pus begins to form because the wound has become infected.

Removal of most stitches follows these guidelines:

1. Face: three to five days
2. Scalp: six to eight days
3. Trunk: seven to ten days
4. Extremities: seven to ten days
5. Joints: twelve to sixteen days
6. Hands: seven to ten days
7. Feet: seven to ten days

Wounds not requiring stitches include:

1. Cut edges of the skin that tend to fall together.
2. Cuts less than one inch long that are not deep.

Gaping wounds may be closed by using the butterfly bandage only if all of the following are found:

1. The wound is less than eight to twelve hours old.
2. The wound is very clean; and
3. It is impossible to get to a physician to stitch it the same day the wound occurred.

INFECTION

All wounds, large or small, present one common danger—infection. Serious wounds also present the danger of severe bleeding. Most people are alert to these hazards.

Microorganisms grow in abundance on the skin and especially on the hands because our hands touch so many things. Once an infection begins, damage can be extensive, so prevention is the best way to avoid this problem.

Every cut, large or small, should be washed immediately with soap and water. If the wound is deep, it may be best to leave the cleaning to trained medical personnel, who will use an antiseptic agent, such as Betadine™, and will irrigate the wound with sterile saline solution. Early cleansing can reduce the number of germs in and around the wound so that the body's natural defenses can ward off infection.

Because infection is a danger in all wounds, a tetanus shot is often given following a wound made with a dirty object. Because there are germs everywhere, it is a good idea to have a tetanus shot every ten years.

It is important to know how to recognize and treat an infected wound. Most infected wounds swell and become reddened. They may give off a sensation of heat and develop a throbbing pain and a pus discharge.

An infection that is not treated soon enough could cause more serious symptoms affecting other areas of the body. For example, the person with an infection may develop a fever. Lymph nodes near the infection may swell. If the infection is in the hand, lymph nodes in the armpit may swell. If the infection is in the leg, lymph nodes in the groin may swell. If the infection is in the head, lymph nodes in the neck may swell. Then, one or more red streaks may develop leading from the wound toward the heart. This is a serious sign that the infection is spreading and could cause death.

In the early stages of an infection, a physician may allow home treatment of applying warm, wet compresses; elevating the injured part; and taking antibiotics.

Some wounds are more likely to become infected than others. Special care should be given a wound received from a bite—either human or animal. Wounds of the hands and feet are susceptible to infection. Any head wound, especially of the scalp, has a high likelihood of infection and should be treated by a physician. Puncture wounds that are difficult to clean have a high incidence of infection, as do wounds made by dirty objects.

Many people have been led to believe that applying a medication such as an antiseptic or first aid antibiotic is important for preventing infections and promoting healing.

According to *Consumers Union,* using an antiseptic is usually superfluous. An antiseptic agent that can kill germs is also capable of killing living cells. Dead tissue in a wound provides an excellent medium in which bacteria can multiply.

Another problem with many antiseptics is that their efficacy or safety is unproved. Only two of the many products used as skin antiseptics were judged safe and effective according to the U.S. Food and Drug Administration. The two were ethyl alcohol (60% to 95% by volume) and isopropyl alcohol (50% to 91% by volume). The rest were not considered safe or effective.

The FDA also said that the familiar and commonly used antiseptics are not very good. For example, Mercurochrome™ makes a red dye mark on the skin but it does little else and kills few germs. Merthiolate™ does slow bacterial growth, but it does not kill bacteria, which then can grow again when the antiseptic wears off. It can be damaging to the skin and many people are allergic to it. Iodine kills bacteria, but its safety for use on the skin remains unproved.

If you feel you must use an antiseptic, choose isopropyl alcohol (rubbing alcohol) because it is cheaper than ethyl alcohol, but apply it only on the intact skin around a wound, not in the wound.

After cleaning a small wound, you should protect it from trauma and infection to allow normal healing. There are two ways of protecting a small wound:

1. Dressings and bandages
2. Skin-wound protectants with or without antibiotics

Most wounds need only cleaning and a dressing placed over the wound. If a skin protectant other than a dressing is desired, wash the wound first, then apply a small ribbon of the ointment on the wound, and then cover the ointment and the wound with a sterile bandage. The antibiotic can be replaced up to three times daily.

Many skin-wound protectants are available. This list is not all inclusive, but the following are recommended:

- Americaine™ and Vaseline Carbolated Petroleum Jelly™, which do not contain antibiotics
- Bacitracin™, Neomycin™, and Neosporin™, which do contain antibiotics

Remember that others are also deemed safe and effective according to *Consumers Union*.

TETANUS

A boy steps on a rusty nail. You receive a scratch from a rose thorn. Your child falls and scrapes a knee. These are three injuries that need first aid. Which of the three could carry the danger of tetanus? Surprisingly, all three. Tetanus is also called "lockjaw" because of its best-known symptom, tightening of the jaw muscles.

Tetanus is caused by a toxin produced by a bacterium. This bacterium forms a spore that can survive in a variety of environments for years. It has been found in soil and air samples throughout the world, on human skin, and in human and animal feces.

The bacterium by itself does not cause tetanus. But when it enters a wound that contains little oxygen (e.g., a puncture wound), it can produce a toxin, which is a powerful poison. The toxin travels through the nervous system to the brain and spinal cord. It then causes contractions of certain muscle groups (particularly in the jaw). There is no known antidote to the toxin once it enters the nervous system. In the industrialized world, because of good medical care, almost half of the victims survive the disease.

Tetanus is a killer. The World Health Organization reports 50,000 deaths each year from tetanus, but some authorities estimate that the disease may kill as many as one million people per year. About one hundred deaths a year are reported in the United States.

Prevention

Even though no specific therapy for tetanus exists, vaccination can completely prevent the disease. Vaccination is a way to prepare your body's immune system to defend against a specific disease by introducing in advance a small amount of the infectious agent and its products.

Everyone needs a series of vaccinations to prepare the immune systems to defend adequately against the toxin. Then a booster shot once every ten years is sufficient to jog the immune system's memory.

People who get wounds a long time after their last vaccination (i.e., ten years) or those who did not receive all the recommended vaccinations early in life may not be able to defend adequately against the tetanus toxin. In such cases, physicians administer solutions of tetanus antibodies that are collected from other people's blood.

Always clean wounds thoroughly with soap and water to eliminate tetanus and other bacteria that may contaminate wounds.

Tetanus is not contagious. With vaccination, it is preventable at low cost and at very low risk. Therefore, no one should get tetanus. However, tetanus remains an important health problem because the tetanus organism is found throughout the world.

AMPUTATION

As microsurgical procedure and instrumentation have improved, successful reimplantation of amputated body parts, especially of the extremities, has become common.

Blood loss in cases of complete amputations is often surprisingly quite minimal. Blood vessels at the injured ends tend to retract into the traumatized body parts and to contract in diameter as nature's mechanism of preventing life-threatening bleeding.

Bleeding control efforts should start with direct pressure along with elevation. Tissue, vessel, and nerve damage that could result from the application of a tourniquet will be avoided if these techniques are used.

The amputated part should be transported with great care. In most cases, the severed part should be recovered at the accident scene. But, in multicasualty cases, in reduced lighting conditions, or when untrained people transport the injured, someone may be requested to locate and transport the missing body part to the hospital emergency department after the victim's departure.

Studies have indicated that severed parts that have been without oxygen as a result of the loss of blood supply for more than six hours without cooling have little chance for survival; twenty-four hours is probably the maximum time allowable for an adequately cooled part (32–39°F). The severed part must not be packed in ice, however, as reimplantation of frozen parts is usually unsuccessful.

In caring for severed body parts, follow these procedures (*see* Figure 5-7):

1. Soak a clean gauze with clean water. If gauze is unavailable, use a clean towel, washcloth, etc.

2. Wrap the amputated part with wet gauze or towel. Do not immerse the body part.

Soft Tissue Injuries

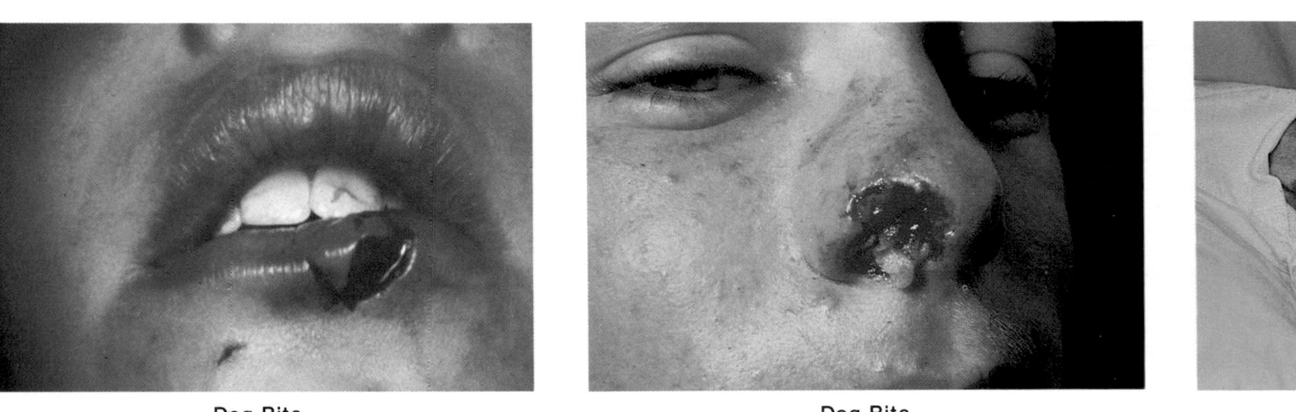

Dog Bite

Dog Bite

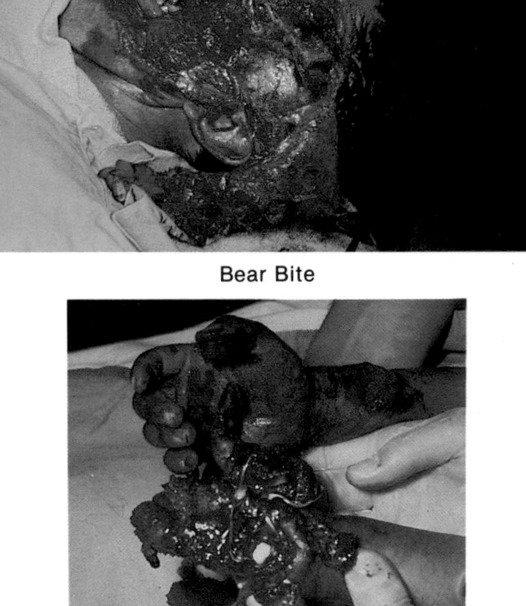

Bear Bite

Human Bite (Avulsed Ear)

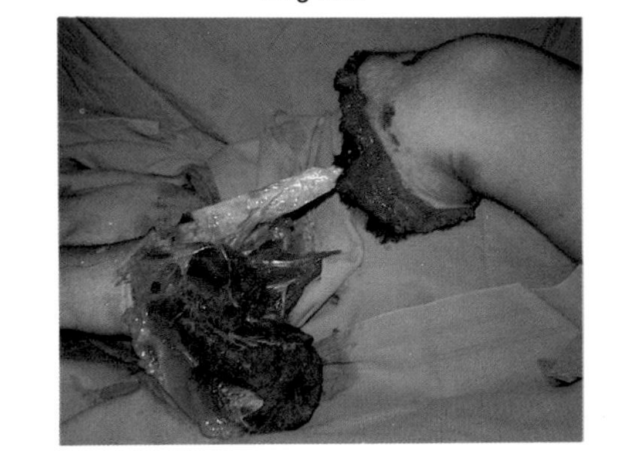

Shark Bite (Avulsed Leg)

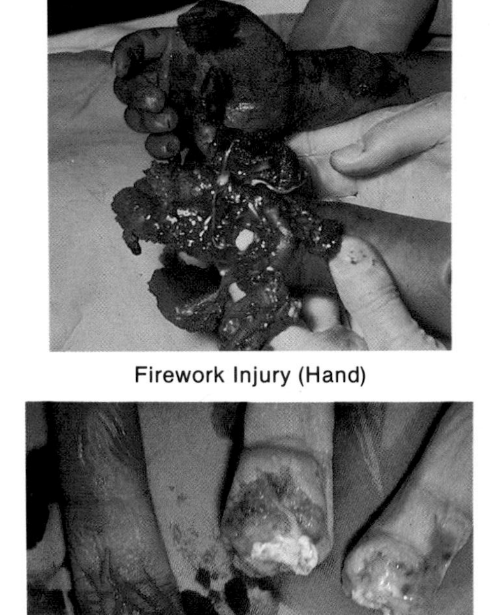

Firework Injury (Hand)

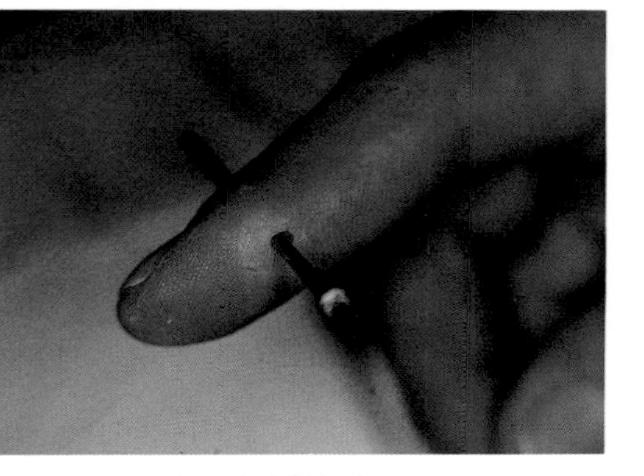

Impaled Object

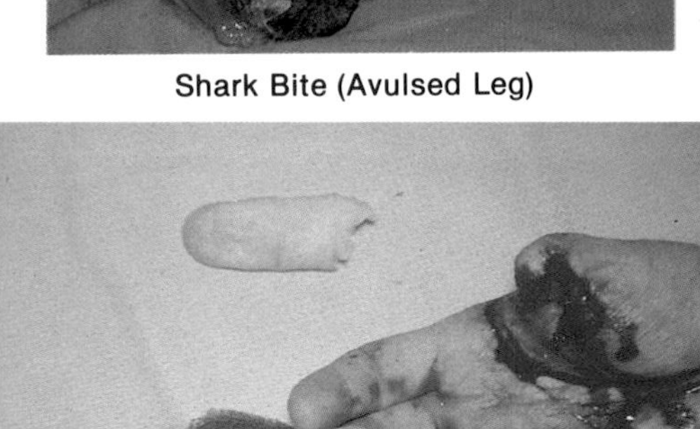

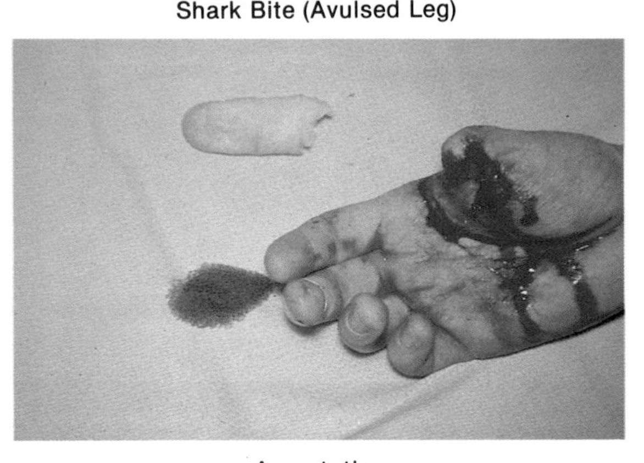

Amputation

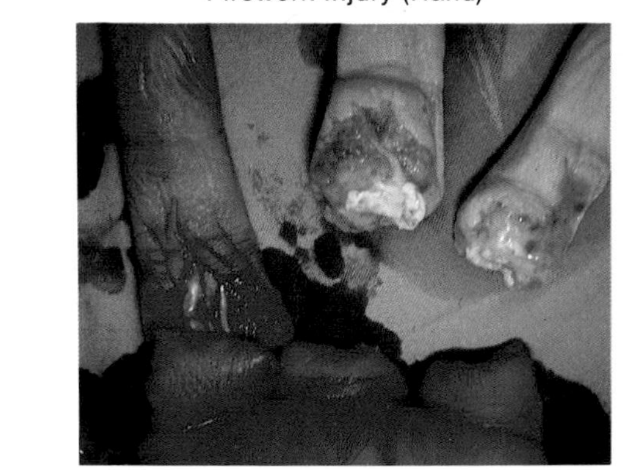

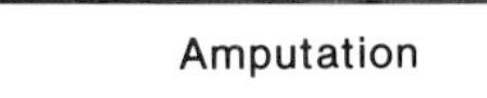

Amputation

Soft Tissue Injuries

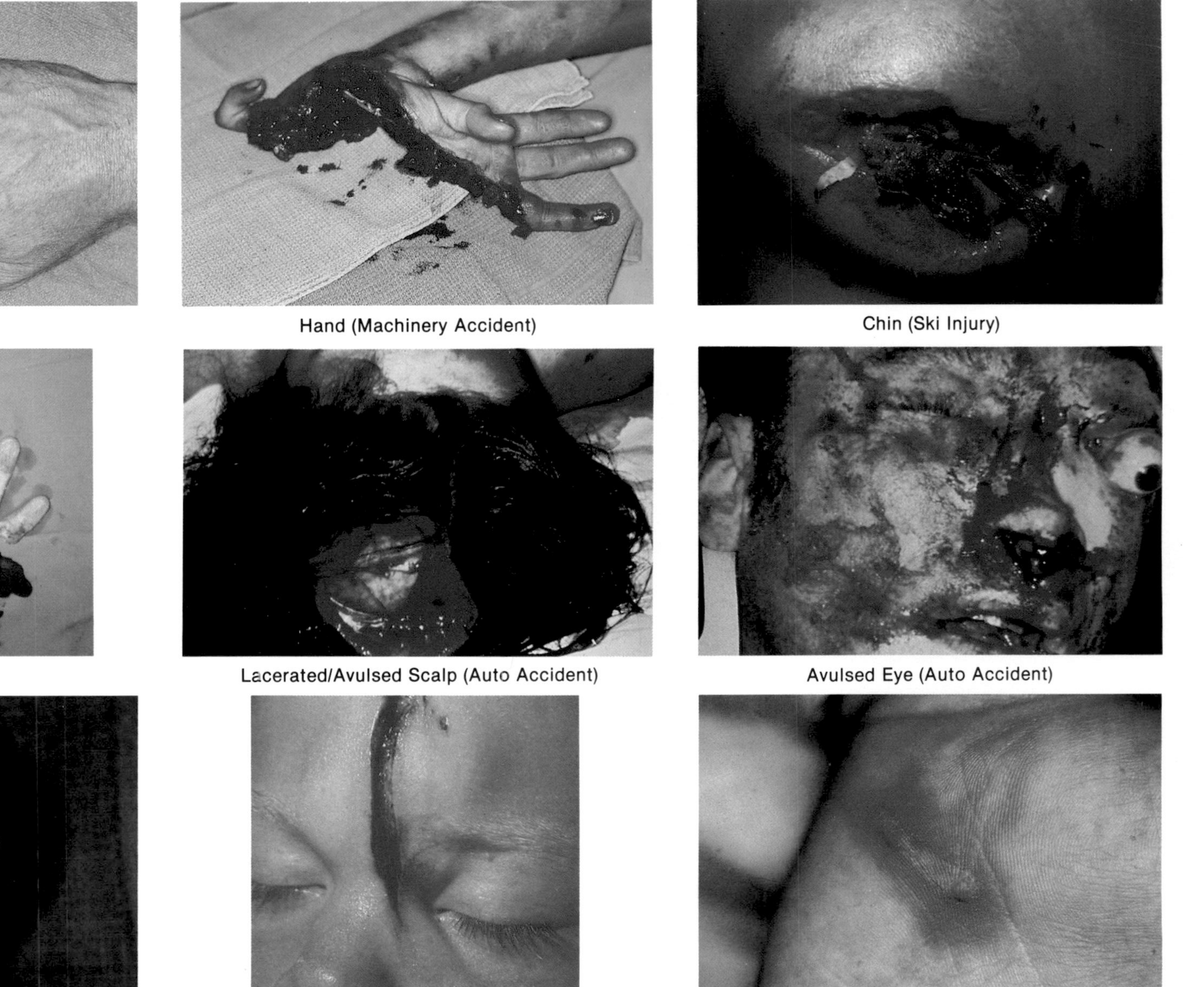

Ring Avulsion

Hand (Machinery Accident)

Chin (Ski Injury)

Amputation

Lacerated/Avulsed Scalp (Auto Accident)

Avulsed Eye (Auto Accident)

Laceration (Lawn Mower Accident)

Laceration

Infection

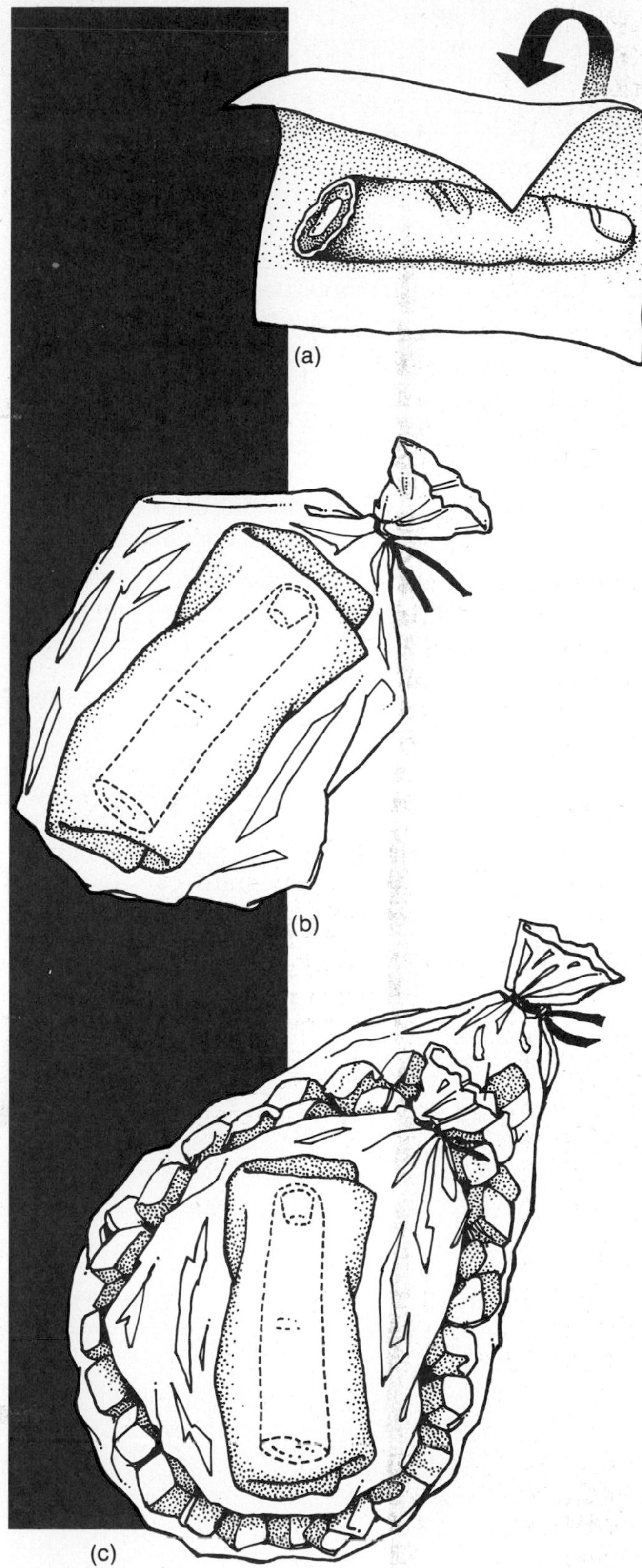

5-7. Care of amputated part
(a) Wrap the part completely in a wet gauze or towel.
(b) Place in a plastic bag or other type of water-proof container.
(c) Place bag or container inside larger bag or container filled with ice.

3. If a plastic bag or container is available, put the wrapped, severed part in it.

4. Place the bag or container with the amputated part on a bed of ice, but do not submerge it.

5. Transport the part immediately to the emergency department.

If the injured part is still partially attached to the stump by a tendon or small skin "bridge," the treatment is essentially the same. The part can still be wet-wrapped and ice placed on it after it is repositioned in the normal position. Do not sever the "bridge" attaching the part.

ANIMAL BITES

More than one million people are bitten by dogs each year. Such bites are responsible for 1% of all emergency room visits. About one bite in ten will need stitches, but all bites need complete cleaning, which may not be possible at home.

From a first aid standpoint, the main concerns in animal bites are bleeding and infection. There may be considerable bleeding because many dogs' jaws are powerful enough to puncture sheet metal. The crushing nature of a bite often deposits bacteria deep beneath the surface of the skin, where it is hard to clean.

A dog's mouth may carry more than sixty different species of bacteria, some of which are very dangerous to human. Cat bites are equally contaminated and dangerous.

The location of a bite is a critical factor in producing infection as well as in determining whether it needs professional medical treatment. Often the better the blood supply to the bitten area, the safer the bite because it is less like to get infected. (Only 4% of facial bites studied became infected, whereas 33% of the hand bites did.) Puncture wounds have the greatest chance of developing infection as compared to lacerations.

All bites of the face, neck, and head should be professionally treated for two reasons: the closeness of the brain and the fact that they often must be irrigated and stitched to prevent scarring.

First Aid

Wash the wound with soap and water and rinse it thoroughly under running water. This should take ten minutes.

Then control bleeding with direct pressure and elevation. Puncture wounds can be encouraged to bleed. This helps remove bacteria deposited deep in the tissues. Most bites should be treated in an emergency room or physician's office because of the danger of infection and the need for a tetanus shot.

Rabies

Rabies is an almost universally fatal disease in man and animal. Prevention remains the most significant factor in controlling the illness.

Rabies is caused by a virus found in warm-blooded animals. The rabies virus is spread from one animal to another usually through a bite that involves saliva from the affected animal.

Sources of rabies: Cases of rabies in animals remains high. Wild carnivores account for about 90% of the cases, and domestic pets representing the other 10%. Of all types of animals capable of carrying rabies, seven species were responsible for 97% of the documented cases. Of the wild animals, skunks were responsible for 62% of the reported cases; bats, 11.9%; raccoons, 6.7%; cattle, 6.4%; and foxes, 2.7%. Of the domestic animals, cats were responsible for 4% of the cases and dogs were responsible for 3%.

The prevalence of rabies in cats is interesting. This may be true because cats are frequent household pets, are not subject to prelicense vaccination laws as are dogs, and are not actively restricted by leash laws or other control measures. Stray cats roam frequently and are adopted into a household without much consideration for their immunization status.

Dogs are the other common source of rabies from domestic animals. Even though the incidence of the disease appears to be decreasing in this group, dog bites still constitute an estimated 1% of all hospital emergency department visits.

Treatment: If an animal does bite, try to capture it for observation without further endangering the captors. Every attempt should be made to avoid destroying the animal. If it is killed, the head and brain should be protected from damage so that they can be examined for rabies. If killed, it is best to transport the animal intact to prevent exposure to potentially infected secretions or tissues. If necessary, the animal's remains can be refrigerated. (Avoid freezing.)

Bites breaking the skin should be vigorously cleansed and washed with large amounts of soap and water. Medical care is of utmost importance, not only for repairing the wound, but also for consultation regarding further treatment.

Many people are still under the misconception that treatment for rabies involves a long, painful series of injections. Until 1980, it did take a series of twenty-three injections. A new vaccine has been found to be safer, less painful, and more effective than the old type.

Bites from domestic animals that are not warm blooded, such as birds, snakes, and other reptiles do not carry the danger of rabies. But these, too, may become infected. Such bites should be washed well and watched for signs of infection.

Although rabies is an infrequent disease in humans, greater efforts are needed to control potential carriers, including domestic pets. All adults, especially those with children and those with cats or dogs, should be well versed in the basic facts regarding rabies. If a wild animal bites a human, the only certain way to rule out rabies is to examine the animal's brain. If the animal cannot be found or the brain cannot be examined, the human who was bitten may have to take rabies injections.

Bleeding Control

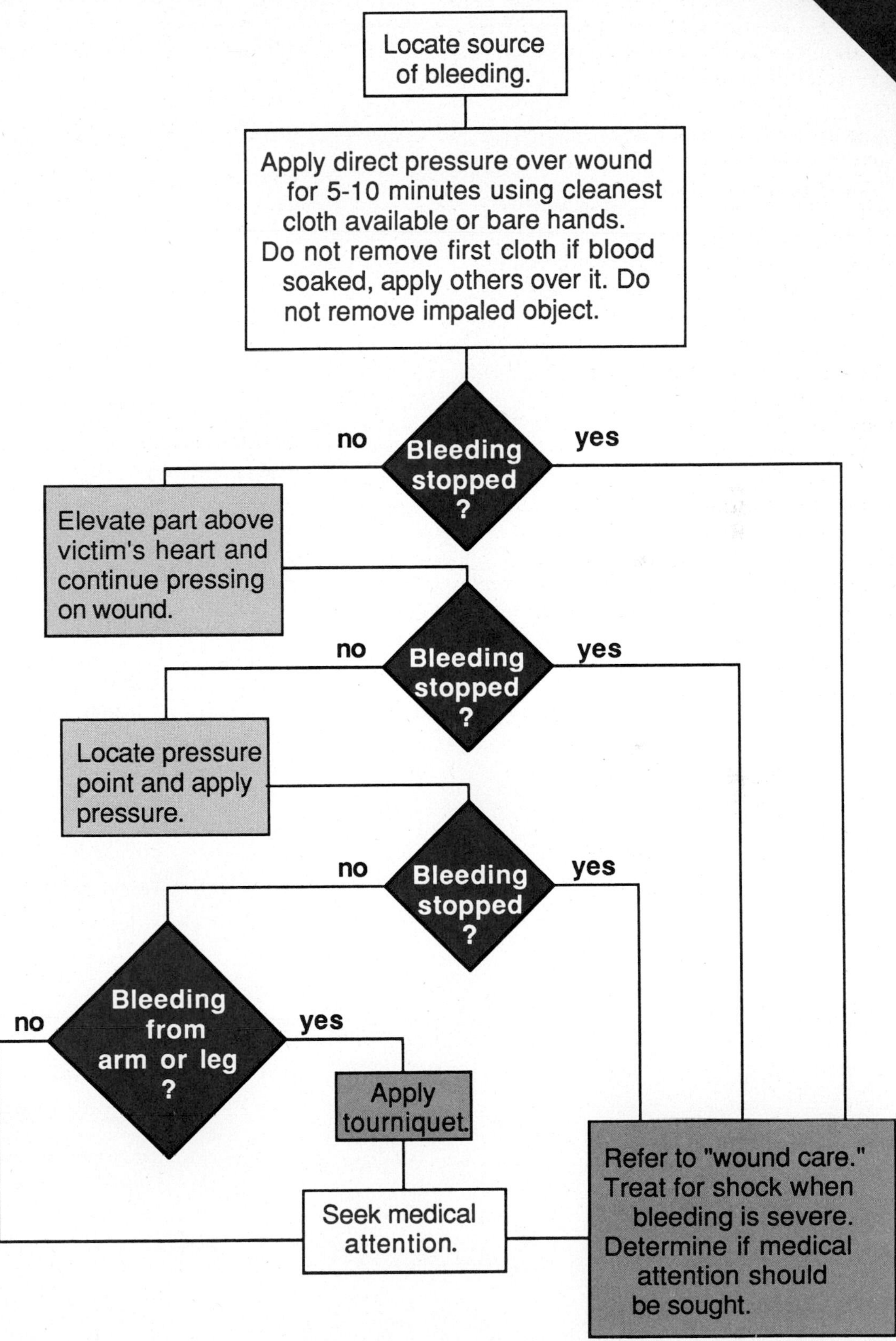

Amputation

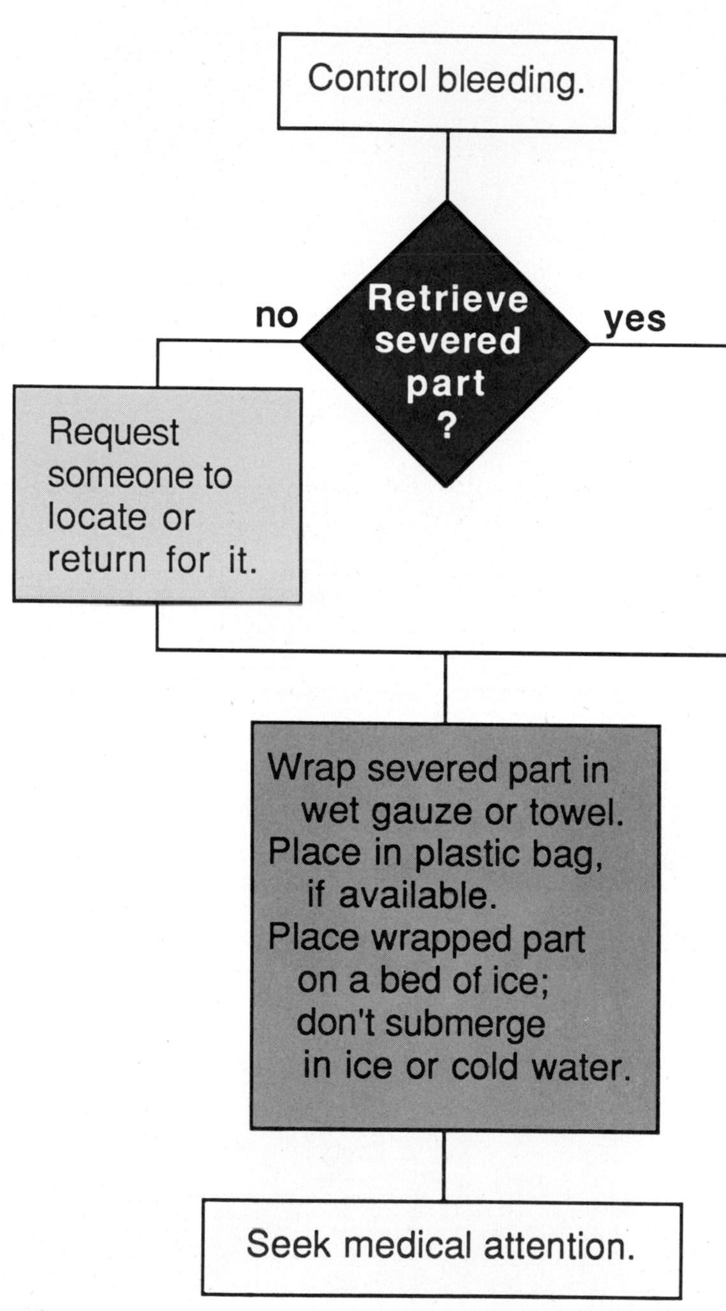

Control bleeding.
Retrieve severed part ?
no
yes
Request someone to locate or return for it.
Wrap severed part in wet gauze or towel.
Place in plastic bag, if available.
Place wrapped part on a bed of ice; don't submerge in ice or cold water.
Seek medical attention.

Animal Bites

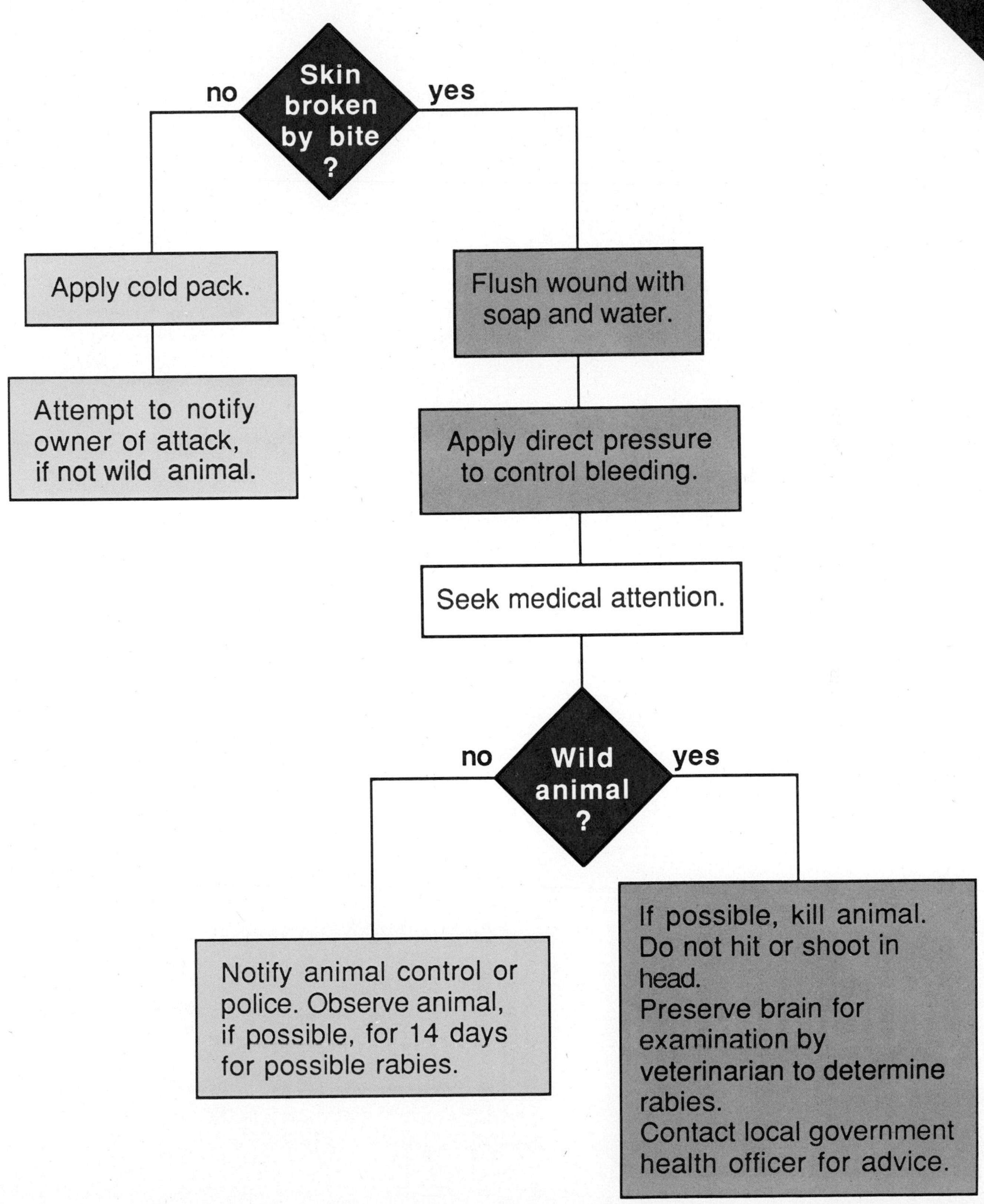

Bleeding

LEARNING ACTIVITIES

T F 1. Once a dressing becomes blood-soaked, it should be removed.
T F 2. If a body part is elevated to control bleeding, direct pressure is no longer needed.
T F 3. Use a pressure point when direct pressure and elevation fail.
T F 4. Tourniquets are a last-resort measure.
T F 5. A first aider should never loosen a tourniquet unless instructed by a physician.
T F 6. Tetanus can result only from puncture wounds.
T F 7. Arterial bleeding is usually more serious than venous bleeding.
T F 8. Infection may take only hours to develop.
T F 9. The loss of one pint of blood by an adult is serious.
T F 10. A tourniquet should be loosened every 15 minutes.
T F 11. Only two pressure points are recommended for first aiders to use in controlling severe bleeding.
T F 12. Blood oozes from an artery and is dark red in color.
T F 13. Direct pressure over the wound stops most cases of bleeding.
T F 14. Dressing is the name of the material placed directly on a wound.
T F 15. Abrasions are wounds that bleed freely.
T F 16. Loss of more than a quart of blood is a threat to an adult's life.
T F 17. Bleeding from veins is usually fast and in spurts.
T F 18. Tourniquets left on for a long time may cause gangrene.
T F 19. Blood normally clots in six to eight minutes.
T F 20. Puncture wounds are easily infected.
T F 21. Puncture wounds tend to bleed freely.
T F 22. Lacerations are more subject to infection than incised wounds.
T F 23. Swelling and redness of the affected part are major signs of infections.
T F 24. Completely severed arteries bleed more freely than partially severed arteries.
T F 25. Swollen lymph glands are a major sign of infection.
T F 26. The incidence of tetanus in the United States is usually high.
T F 27. A tetanus booster shot should be received every two years to ensure adequate protection.
T F 28. Mercurochrome™ or Merthiolate™ is preferred over soap and water in preventing infection in wounds.
T F 29. Rubbing alcohol kills germs and should be applied directly on the wound.
T F 30. There are several skin-wound protectants that can be used to protect small wounds.
T F 31. Cuts to eyelids and lips should be stitched by a physician.
T F 32. Stitches to close an open wound should be placed for most wounds within six to eight hours of the injury.
T F 33. A "butterfly" bandage can be used to bring small lacerations together.
T F 34. Hydrogen peroxide kills bacteria in a wound.
T F 35. If a dressing must be removed and part of the scab is sticking to it, soaking it in warm water can help soften the scab for easier removal.
T F 36. When washing a wound with soap and water, wash toward the wound.

Case 1: A person's right hand has been badly mangled by a rather powerful firecracker explosion. You arrive soon afterwards to find the victim's hand bleeding profusely.

1. What sequence of emergency care procedures would you provide in this situation?

   A. ______________________________
   B. ______________________________
   C. ______________________________
   D. ______________________________

2. What is the most effective method for controlling bleeding in this situation?

_______ A. Direct pressure over the wound
_______ B. Pressure point
_______ C. Tourniquet
_______ D. Run cold water over the bleeding area

3. What is the most effective method for controlling many types of bleeding other than that found in most other situations?

_______ A. Direct pressure over the wound
_______ B. Pressure point
_______ C. Tourniquet
_______ D. Run cold water over the bleeding area

4. Is the use of a tourniquet ever an appropriate method to control bleeding described in this case? Why? (Check your choice and explain your answer in the space provided.)

_______ A. Yes _______ B. No

____

____

5. What are the major symptoms and corresponding emergency care for the three types of external bleeding? (Write your answers in the following chart below.)

External Bleeding	*Signs/Symptoms*	*Emergency Care*
Capillary	A. Flow ________	C. ________
	B. Color ________	D. ________
Venous	E. Flow ________	G. ________
	F. Color ________	H. ________
		I. ________
		J. ________
Arterial	K. Flow ________	M. ________
	L. Color ________	N. ________
		O. ________
		P. ________

Case 2: A neighbor has walked through a sliding glass door. Blood is spurting from a wound in his lower left leg and is flowing from his left arm. Blood is oozing from many smaller abrasions on his body.

1. Match the type of bleeding observed in this victim with the involved blood vessel. Also indicate the color of the blood associated with each type of bleeding observed.

Vessel	*Type of Bleeding*	*Blood Color*
Arterial	A. _____	B. _____
Capillary	C. _____	D. _____
Venous	E. _____	F. _____

2. What is the preferred method of controlling the spurting blood?

3. List three other methods that could be used to control the spurting blood:

A. ____
B. ____
C. ____

4. List and describe the six major types of wounds.

A. ______________________________
B. ______________________________
C. ______________________________
D. ______________________________
E. ______________________________
F. ______________________________

5. The victim is unconscious and upon checking the pupils of the eyes, you notice they are dilated and respond slowly to light. What condition should you highly suspect?

____

____

Amputation

T F 1. A severed part should be submerged in ice after being protected.
T F 2. A part partially attached should be severed.
T F 3. Direct pressure should be attempted in controlling bleeding involving an amputation.
T F 4. Any severed part, regardless of size, should be located and taken to the medical facility.

Case: A wheat harvest worker caught his hand in a combine header drive shaft and had his hand torn off. He had been working about two hours when he came running from the field with blood running and his hand missing.

1. Blood loss in cases of amputation is often ______________________________
______________________________.

2. Explain why. ______________________________
____

3. If not adequately cooled, a severed body part has ______ hours for survival, whereas if adequately cooled, the part may survive for ______ hours.

Animal Bites

T F 1. Snakes and other reptiles can carry rabies.
T F 2. An animal's saliva will reveal rabies.
T F 3. A dog's mouth may carry more than sixty different species of bacteria.
T F 4. All bites of the head, face, and neck should be treated by a physician.
T F 5. Water and soap work well for an animal bite.

Case: A small girl complains of having been bitten by a stray dog. Upon examination you find only minor scratches.

1. How extensive is the dog bite problem?

____

____

2. What type of wound is most likely to become infected?

____

____

3. Why should all bites of the face, neck, and head be treated by a physician?

A. ______________________________
B. ______________________________

4. What are the two main concerns in animal bites?

A. ______________________________
B. ______________________________

5. How long should a wound be washed with soap and water? ______ minutes

6. The new rabies vaccine requires ______ injections, whereas the old vaccine required ______ injections.

6 Specific Body Area Injuries

- Head Injuries
- Eye Injuries
- Nosebleeds
- Dental Emergencies
- Larynx Injuries
- Chest Injuries
- Abdominal Injuries
- Foreign Objects
- Hand and Finger Injuries
- Blisters

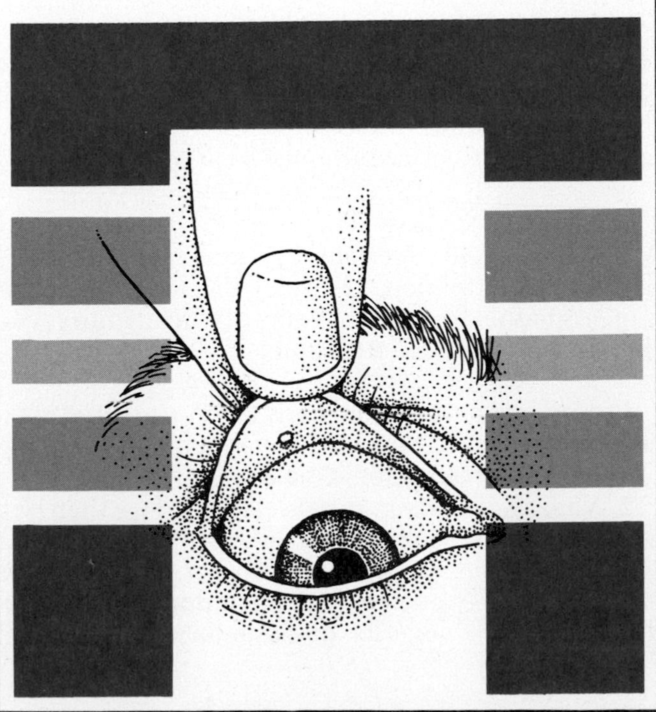

HEAD INJURIES

Head injury is the primary cause of death in accidents. Three types of injury that can occur to the head include skull fracture, concussion, and contusion.

A *skull fracture* is a crack in the cranium (bony case surrounding the brain). This crack may be small and visible only by x-ray (linear), or it may have many cracks radiating from the area of contact (comminuted). Even more severe is the *depressed* skull fracture in which the bone is driven inward into the brain. A fourth type is the *basal* skull fracture, where the base of the skull is damaged.

Signs and symptoms of a skull fracture include: pain at the point of injury, deformity of the skull, bleeding from ears and/or nose, cerebrospinal fluid leaking from ears or nose, discoloration under the eyes, and unequal pupils.

A second type of head injury is the *concussion*. The brain is surrounded by cerebrospinal fluid. When there is a blow to the head or the head flies forward and is then suddenly snapped back (whiplash), the brain may bang against the inside of the skull causing temporary loss of consciousness and a headache. Usually no permanent brain damage occurs. Sometimes, though, there may be short-term memory loss.

A more severe head injury is the *contusion*. It is caused by the same action as a concussion—the brain hitting the skull. It is a bruise of the brain—the blood vessels within the brain substance rupture and bleed. Inside the skull there is no way for blood to escape, and there is no room for it to accumulate.

All head injuries have the potential for stopping breathing and heartbeat. Therefore, the first step in aiding this victim is to check for breathing. If the victim's awkward position is closing the airway, you are justified in moving him or her; but it is important to try to keep the head, neck, and spine in the same alignment. Once you have the victim in a workable position:

1. Open the airway by the jaw thrust maneuver. Do not hyperextend the neck. Give mouth-to-mouth resuscitation if needed.

2. If the victim is breathing, check his or her pulse next. Count it for a full 60 seconds. If it is less than 55 or more than 125, the victim may be in serious condition.

3. Now check for bleeding. Cover any bleeding head injury with a sterile dressing. If fluid is flowing from the ears, *do not* stop it. Otherwise, it could put pressure on the brain. Instead, try to place the victim in the coma position (on his or her side, knees up, head supported on one arm). Do not remove any object embedded in the skull.

4. Try to maintain the victim's body temperature with blankets if necessary, but do not overheat. In head injuries, it is common for the body temperature to rise, so monitor temperature as well as breathing and pulse while you wait for an ambulance.

When head injury victims are conscious, it is important to find out if they are thinking clearly. You may ask their name, address, location, and age, for example. If they cannot answer these questions, suspect brain injury and administer first aid accordingly. Observe pupil size—they should be equal and react to light. Note any limb weakness or paralysis. Touch feet and hands and ask the victim if there is a sensation. If the victim loses consciousness, all this information will be very important to medical personnel. The length of time of unconsciousness is also important.

Occasionally, the effect of a blow to the head may be delayed. Some time later the victim faints or develops a headache. Again, knowing the victim has sustained a blow to the head may explain these symptoms. Head injuries that produce these symptoms should be promptly checked by a physician.

Recognizing Concussion

It is not necessary to be hit on the head to receive a concussion, which is what most first aiders look for. It can occur simply from sudden deceleration of the head (e.g., in an automobile crash).

In the absence of unconsciousness (one of the best signs), a glassy-eyed look, uncoordination, inability to walk correctly, or obvious disorientation provide clues. The victim may complain of dizziness, lightheadedness, blurred vision, and disorientation.

Headaches may or may not follow head injury. If the victim complains of a headache immediately after a head injury, that is a significant symptom. On the other hand, it is common for people suffering a concussion to develop a headache a day or two later and sometimes even as long as a week following injury.

Mental Status Tests

It is important to ask the victim simple questions, such as subtracting numbers, what food was eaten for breakfast, and other short-term memory tests. Studies show that deficits in short-term memory are the first to occur after concussion.

Also ask what day it is, where he or she is, and personal questions such as birthday and home address. If the victim cannot answer these questions, there may be a significant problem.

Another test that may be useful is to give the person a list of five or six numbers and ask him or her to repeat them back in that order. Lists of objects can also be used as short-term memory tests. If a person fails on these tests, you can be sure he has been concussed.

If the victim loses consciousness momentarily, he or she should remain inactive. Anyone who remains unconscious for more than several minutes should be transported immediately to the hospital.

Degrees of Concussion

Concussion is sometimes described as having several different degrees. The value of categorizing them is in deciding how to manage the victim. Those categories are mild, moderate, and severe. (Refer to Table 6-1.)

In a *mild* concussion, there is no loss of consciousness, but there is a disturbance of neurological function.

In the *moderate* concussion, there is a loss of consciousness for less than five minutes, usually with the inability to remember events after being injured.

In the *severe* concussion, there is a loss of consciousness for longer than five minutes, wandering eye movements, and a lack of purposeful responses.

A victim with a severe concussion must be seen immediately by a physician trained in managing head injuries and must be hospitalized. At the other end of the scale, the mild concussion does not require hospitalization but does require observation.

Head Injury Follow-Up

After a head injury, certain signs may indicate a need for medical attention. If any of the following signs appears within forty-eight hours of a head injury, you should seek medical attention:

1. *Headache.* A headache is to be expected. If it lasts more than one or two days or increases in severity, medical advice should be sought.

2. *Nausea, vomiting.* If nausea lasts more than two hours, you must seek medical advice. Vomiting once or twice, especially in children, after a severe head injury may be expected. Vomiting does not tell anything about the severity of the injury. However, if

TABLE 6-1. Concussion Guidelines

Type	Description	Guidelines
Mild	Momentary or no loss of consciousness.	Delay return to activity until medical evaluation has been made.
Moderate	Unconscious for less than five minutes.	Avoid vigorous activity for a few days or longer. Resume activity only when associated symptoms of headache, visual disturbances, etc. have been resolved.
Severe	Unconscious for more than five minutes.	Avoid rigorous activity for one month or longer. Clearance from a neurosurgeon is advised.

vomiting begins again hours after one or two episodes had ceased, consult a physician.

3. *Drowsiness.* If the victim wants to sleep, let him, but do wake him to check his state of consciousness and sense of orientation by asking his name, address, telephone number, and whether he can process information such as adding or multiplying numbers; if he cannot answer correctly or appears confused or disoriented, call the doctor. You will have to modify the questions for a small child.

Experts disagree on the time intervals for waking a sleeping victim to check consciousness. Some say every thirty minutes to an hour; others say every two to three hours. It would seem that on the night following a head injury, or during any nap, that the victim should be awakened at least every two hours to check for state of consciousness and the other signs in this list.

4. *Vision problems.* If the victim "sees double," if the eyes fail to move together, or if one pupil appears to be larger than the other, these are signs of possible trouble.

5. *Mobility.* The victim cannot use his arms or legs as well as previously or is unsteady in walking.

6. *Speech.* The victim slurs his speech or is unable to talk.

7. *Convulsions.*

EYE INJURIES

Correct treatment of an eye injury immediately following an accident can prevent loss of sight. However, because it is difficult to determine the extent of damage to the eye, medical help should be sought as soon as first aid is completed: call an ophthalmologist, your family physician or go to a nearby hospital emergency room immediately.

Specks In The Eye*

Never rub any speck or particle that is in the eye. Lift the upper lid over the lower lid allowing the lashes to brush the speck off the inside of the upper lid. Blink a few times and let the eye move the particle out. If the speck remains, keep your eye closed and seek medical help.

Blows To The Eye*

Apply an ice cold compress immediately for about 15 minutes to reduce pain and swelling. A black eye or blurred vision could signal internal eye damage. See your ophthalmologist immediately.

Cuts Of The Eye And Lid*

Bandage the eye lightly and seek medical help immediately. Do not attempt to wash out the eye or remove an object stuck in the eye. Never apply hard pressure to the injured eye or eyelid. (*See* Figure 6-1.)

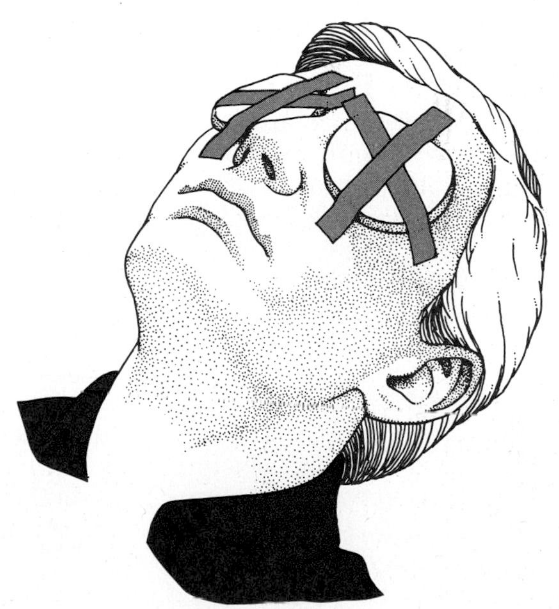

6-1. Cover both eyes to minimize eye movement (exception is chemical burns).

*American Academy of Ophthalmology, "Eye Injuries: Prevention and First Aid." Reprinted with permission.

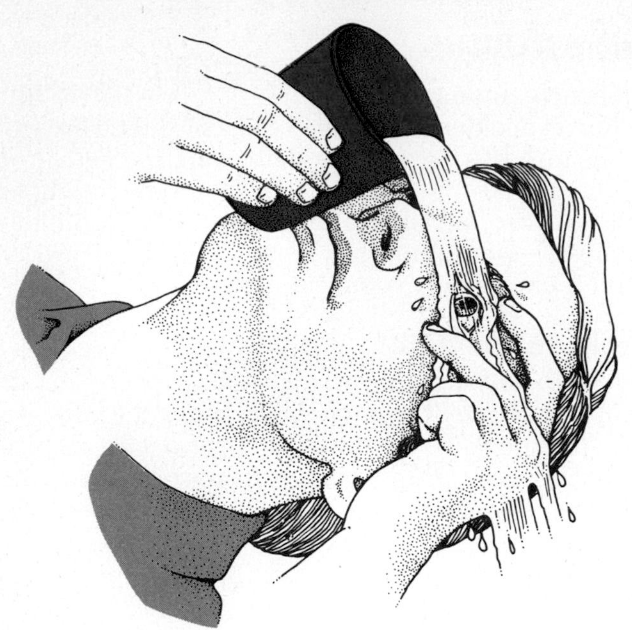

6-2. Immediately flush the eye in case of chemical burns.

Chemical Burns*

Flood the eye with warm water immediately, using your fingers to keep the eye open as wide as possible. Hold your head under a faucet or pour water into the eye from any clean container for at least 15 minutes, continuously and gently. (*See* Figure 6-2.) Roll the eyeball as much as possible to wash out the eye. Do not use an eye cup. Do not bandage the eye. Seek medical help immediately after these steps are taken.

Avulsion Of The Eye

A blow to the face can avulse an eye from its socket. If such an injury occurs, do not attempt to push the eye back into the socket. Cover the extruded eye loosely with a sterile dressing that has been moistened with clean water. Then cover the eye with a paper cup, just like the same procedure for an impaled object in the eye.

Contact Lenses

Determine if the victim is wearing contact lenses by asking him, checking on a driver's license, or looking for them on the eyeball by shining a light on the eye from the side. Lenses should be removed immediately only in cases of chemical eye burns.

Proper precautions should always be taken to protect the eyes. Knowing what to do and/or what not to do in the event of an eye injury can save the precious gift of eyesight.

*American Academy of Ophthalmology, "Eye Injuries: Prevention and First Aid." Reprinted with permission.

Though prompt, proper treatment of eye injuries can save vision, it is important to remember that first aid is just that. It is immediate treatment that is "first," until experienced medical help is available. When an accident involves the eye, it is always wise to be safe: seek medical help immediately if there is pain or any question of damage or impaired vision.

NOSEBLEEDS

Severe nosebleed is frightening to the victim, occurs at inopportune times, and often challenges the skill of the first aider. Minor nosebleeds are usually self-limited (about 90%) and seldom require medical attention, unless they become recurrent. Severe nosebleed episodes are high and death is not uncommon.

Types of Nosebleeds

Nosebleeds can be divided into anterior (front) and posterior (back) types—that bleed through the nose and those that bleed backward into the mouth or down the back of the throat. Anterior bleeding is by far the most common, occurring nine times out of ten.

Nosebleeds are most common in children, and the great majority of these cases, approximately 90%, originate in the vascular junction of three blood vessels located in the anterior septum of the nose. Nosebleeds that originate in this area generally resolve spontaneously and are easy to control.

In older persons, bleeding usually occurs in the posterior nose. Nearly all nosebleeds in children will be in the anterior part of the septum.

Stopping a Nosebleed

Most nosebleeds from the anterior nasal septum can be stopped by simple procedures (*see* Figure 6-3):

1. Reassure the victim that most nosebleeds are not serious. Keep him quiet. Though a large amount of blood may appear to have been lost, most nosebleeds are not likely to be serious.

2. The victim should be in a sitting position to reduce blood pressure. Keep the head in an upright position or tilted slightly forward so that the blood can run out the front of the nose, not down the back of the throat, causing either choking or nausea and vomiting dark clots. These clots may be aspirated into the lungs.

3. If a foreign object in the nose is suspected, look into the nose, but do not probe with finger or swab.

4. With thumb and forefinger, apply steady pressure to both nostrils for five minutes before releasing. Remind the victim to breathe through his mouth and to spit out any accumulated blood.

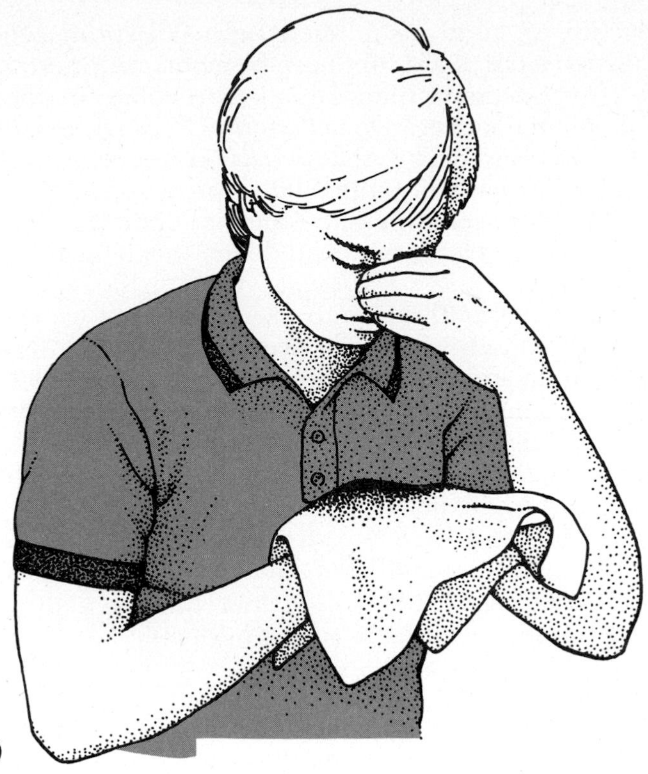

5. If bleeding persists, have the victim gently blow the nose to remove any clots and excess blood, and to minimize sneezing. This allows new clots to form. This is a new concept for most first aiders. Then press the nostrils again for five minutes.

6. Some experts recommend soaking a cotton ball in hydrogen peroxide, a nasal decongestant (nose drops or spray), or plain water; wring out the excess; and gently insert the cotton ball inside the bleeding nostril. Criticism against this step is the lack of time and/or materials. When five minutes are up, slowly and gently remove the cotton.

7. Place a roll of gauze between the upper lip and gum and press against it with your fingers.

8. Some experts recommend applying a cold compress over the nose.

9. If the victim is unconscious, place the victim on his side to prevent aspiration of blood and attempt the procedures in this list.

Seek Medical Care

You should seek medical attention if any of the following occurs:

1. The procedures do not stop the bleeding after a second attempt.
2. The signs and symptoms indicate a posterior source of bleeding.
3. The victim has hypertension.
4. The victim is taking anticoagulants (blood thinners) or large doses of aspirin.
5. The bleeding occurred after an injury to the nose.

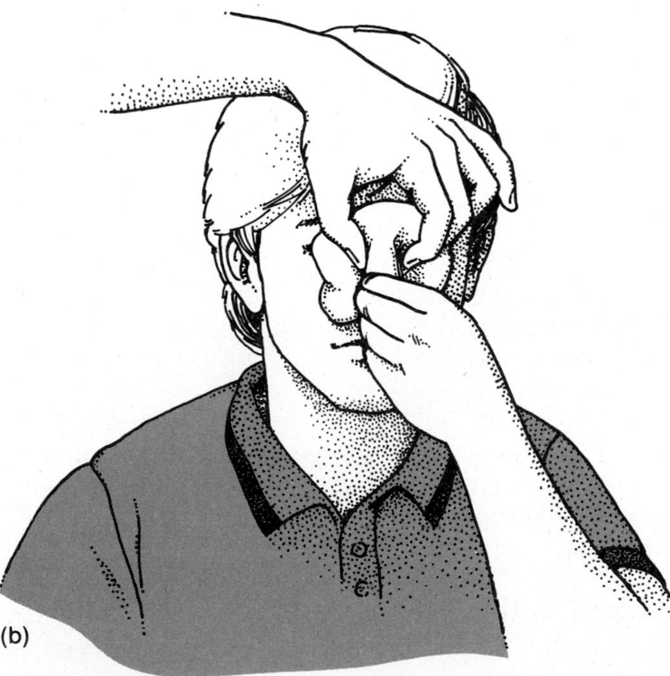

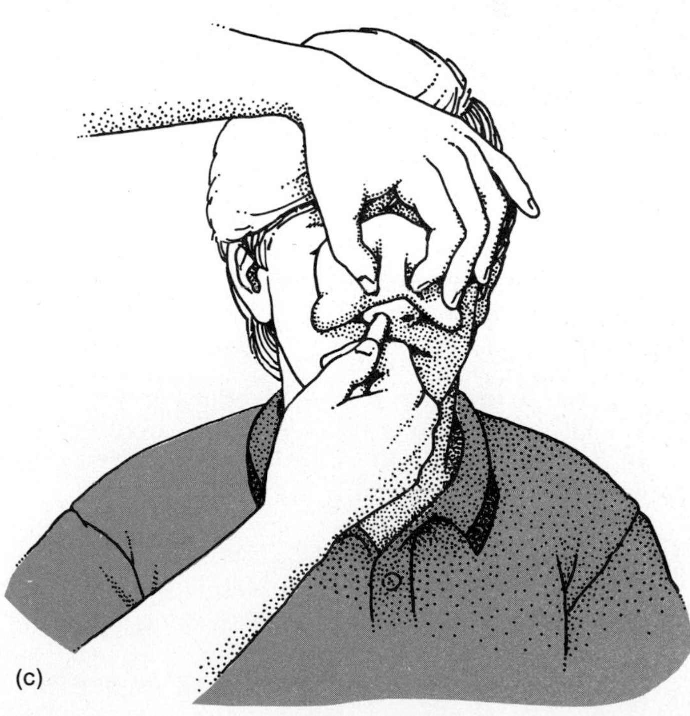

6-3. Nosebleeds
(a) Have the person sit leaning slightly forward to prevent blood from running down his throat. Have the person pinch his nose firmly for at least five full minutes.
(b) While the person is pinching, apply a cold compress to the nose and surrounding area.
(c) If pinching does not work, gently pack the nostril. Be sure that the end hangs out to aid in removing later. Then pinch the nose, with the gauze in it, for another five minutes.

Treatment of posterior bleeding is best left to a physician. It may involve cauterization with chemicals or an electric needle. A physician may pack the nose with sterile gauze or insert and inflate a small balloon to create pressure on the ruptured part. As a last resort the doctor may tie off the bleeding vessel.

Care After A Nosebleed

After a nosebleed has stopped, you should suggest that the victim:

1. Sneeze through an open mouth, if there is a need to sneeze.
2. Not stoop or exert physically.
3. When lying down, elevate the head with two pillows.
4. Keep the nostrils moist by applying a little petroleum jelly just inside the nostril for a week and increase the humidity in the bedroom during the winter months with a cold-mist humidifier.
5. Avoid picking or rubbing the nose. If a child has an uncontrollable habit, trim his fingernails frequently.
6. Avoid hot drinks and alcohol beverages for a week.
7. Not smoke or take aspirin for a week.

Most victims with nosebleeds never need medical care. Most nosebleeds are self-limited and the victim can control the bleeding himself.

DENTAL EMERGENCIES*

First aiders often deal with dental emergencies. The following first aid procedures are guidelines for providing temporary relief for dental emergencies, but it is imperative to consult with a dentist as soon as possible (*See* Table 6-2).

Objects Wedged Between Teeth

Attempt to remove the object with dental floss. Guide the floss in carefully so the gum tissue is not injured. Do not use a sharp or pointed tool to remove the object. If unsuccessful, take the victim to a dentist.

Bitten Lip or Tongue

Apply direct pressure to the bleeding area with a clean cloth. If the lip is swollen, apply a cold compress. Take the victim to a hospital emergency room if the bleeding persists or if the bite is severe.

Knocked-Out Tooth

When a permanent tooth is completely knocked out in an accident, save it and take it, along with the victim, to the dentist immediately. With proper first aid procedures, the tooth can be given an opportunity for successful reimplantation (placing the tooth back in the socket). Do not attempt to clean the tooth because this destroys necessary connective fibers which assist in the reimplantation process. Do *not* put the tooth in mouthwash or alcohol or scrub it with abrasives or chemicals. And do *not* touch the root of the tooth.

Place the tooth in a cup of milk or cool water or wrap it loosely in a clean, wet cloth or gauze. Take the victim and tooth to a dentist immediately (within thirty minutes). If in remote areas with no dentist nearby, replant a knocked-out tooth by first running cool water over it to clean away debris (do not scrub the tooth), and then by gently repositioning it into the socket, using adjacent teeth as a guide. Push the tooth so the top is even with the adjacent teeth. Successful replanting occurs best within thirty minutes of the accident. See a dentist as soon as possible.

Broken Tooth

Immediate attention is necessary when a child breaks a tooth or else it may need to be extracted. Attempt to clean any dirt, blood, and debris from the injured area with a sterile gauze pad and warm water.

Apply a cold compress on the face next to the injured tooth to minimize swelling. If a jaw fracture is suspected, immobilize the jaw by any available means—place a scarf, handkerchief, tie, or towel over and under the chin, and tie the ends on top of the child's head. In either case, immediately take the victim to an oral surgeon or hospital emergency room.

Although temporary relief can be provided in most dental emergencies, by all means, when in doubt, consult a dentist as soon as possible.

LARYNX INJURIES

Injuries to the larynx that compromise the airway have the potential to be life threatening, so first aiders should be able to recognize and care for such injuries.

Trauma to the Larynx

Occasionally, trauma results in a fractured larynx. A direct blow to the neck, for example, by a fist, a steering wheel, or a baseball can injure this structure, producing the following signs and symptoms:

- Hoarseness
- Shortness of breath
- A harsh vibrating sound during exhalation
- Bluish discoloration of skin
- Loss of voice; only whispered speech

*American Dental Association. Reprinted with permission.

- Cough
- Pain and tenderness

The possibility of accompanying vertebral fracture must always be kept in mind. Sports-related neck injuries involve less force and cause cervical vertebral fractures less frequently that those from auto crashes. If unconscious, the victim should be treated as though the neck is broken, and gentle, stabilizing traction to the head should be maintained. Until cervical fracture is ruled out, the airway should be maintained with as little extension of the neck as possible. More often, however, if the victim is experiencing obstructed breathing, the problem is one of restraining thrashing, agitated movements.

Emergency Care

When the victim does not have obvious signs of fracture, closed airway, or cervical vertebral fracture, the most important initial responses are reassuring the victim and positioning the victim's head in a chin-up position to straighten the airway. Sudden inability to breathe produces immediate panic, and the victim often physically resists the first aider and thrashes around. Reassurance that help is being provided, preferably by someone in whom he or she has confidence, is of primary importance.

If the degree of obstruction is great enough to make respirations difficult, you must act immediately. Airway obstruction for more than four minutes may cause brain damage or even death.

A tracheostomy is most desirable. This establishes an airway below the level of obstruction and avoids disruption of the injured area. However, it is a thirty-minute procedure, best done in a surgical environment by a medical specialist.

For clarification, a tracheotomy is the process of surgically opening the trachea, and a tracheostomy is the procedure in which a tube is placed into the trachea to permit breathing and to keep the passageway open for a period of time. Again, a tracheotomy should be performed only by a competent physician because there is a tremendous risk of cutting a laryngeal nerve or carotid artery, which are also in this area. Some experts recommend that a cricothyrotomy is a simpler, safer, faster alternative, but only by medical experts.

Laryngospasm

Laryngospasm is another type of upper airway obstruction that may result. Laryngospasm is the spastic closure of the larynx. Spasm of muscles of the vocal cords pulls the cords tightly together. The victim is agitated and may thrash about, clutch his or her throat, become cyanotic, and lose consciousness. These victims cannot cough or talk.

Closure of the larynx is a serious emergency. It is difficult to resist attempting to force oxygen into the severely cyanotic, struggling victim's lungs. However, this results in a greater spasm. Continued efforts frequently result in gastric distention. A more effective maneuver is to force the chin forward by strong pressure behind the angles of the jaw.

Another maneuver advocated by anesthesiologists is to grasp the base of the tongue, pulling it forward. As the spasm starts to relax, usually within forty-five to sixty seconds, a loud crowing sound will be heard.

Laryngospasms also occur in some drownings. In the process of drowning, a person can no longer keep afloat and starts to submerge. He or she tries to take and hold one more deep breath. As he or she does, water enters the mouth and nose. The victim inhales and swallows water. As the water flows past the glottis and enters the trachea, it contacts the larynx and triggers a reflex spasm or laryngospasm. The laryngospasm seals the airway so effectively that no more than a small amount of water ever reaches the lungs. An estimated 10% of all drowning victims die without aspiration of water because of a prolonged laryngospasm. However, it accounts for 90% of those successfully resuscitated.

CHEST INJURIES

Chest injuries are a leading cause of accidental death. For example, of all traffic fatalities in the United States, 35% to 40% of the victims have chest injuries; and the majority of these deaths were due to chest injuries alone. Chest injuries may also be the result of gunshot wounds, stab wounds, falls, or blows.

Signs of Chest Injuries

The important signs of chest injuries are:

1. Pain at the injury site
2. Painful breathing
3. Difficult breathing
4. Cyanosis (blueness of the lips, fingernails), indicating oxygen deficiency
5. Coughing up bright red frothy blood, indicating a punctured lung
6. Failure of one or both sides of the chest to expand normally when inhaling

Types of Chest Injuries

Rib fractures: These are usually caused by direct blows or compression of the chest. The upper four ribs are rarely fractured because they are protected by the collarbone and shoulder blade. The lower two ribs are hard to fracture because they are attached only on one end and have freedom to move (known as "floating" ribs). The victim can usually point out the exact injury site. There may or may not be a rib deformity, contusion, or a laceration of the area. Deep breathing, coughing, or movement is usually quite painful.

Simple rib fractures should not be bound, strapped, or taped. With multiple fractures of the ribs, the victim may be more comfortable with the arm strapped to the chest with a sling and swathe.

Flail chest: When three or more ribs are broken, each in two places, the segment of the chest wall will move independently of the rest of the chest wall when the victim attempts to breathe. Often the movement of the injured segment of the chest wall moves in the opposite direction to the rest of the chest wall. This is called paradoxical respiration.

The signs and symptoms of a flail chest include:

1. The same signs and symptoms of fractured ribs
2. The failure of a section of the chest wall to move with the rest of the chest wall when the victim is breathing.

The emergency care of a flail chest is to immobilize the ribs to improve breathing.

Penetrating wounds: Stab and gunshot wounds are examples of penetrating chest wounds. Sucking chest wounds, rib fractures, or laceration of the heart or blood vessels of the chest may result. The wound must be closed quickly because it can result in air outside the lung to enter the chest cavity. Do not remove or attempt to remove an impaled object penetrating the chest because bleeding and air in the chest cavity can rcsult. Stabilize the foreign object, and seek medical attention for the injured victim.

If the victim starts to get worse after the penetrating wound has been sealed, lift the dressing off the wound to allow air to escape from the chest cavity—immediate improvement should be shown. Then, reapply the seal over the wound and be prepared to relieve the build-up of air in the chest cavity by the same method.

Summary: Almost all types of chest injuries require the same initial care. Breathing should be checked and taken care of if needed. Open chest wounds must be covered. Broken ribs are usually immobilized by a sling and swathe, rather than by adhesive taping. Bleeding from the chest wall should be controlled, preferably by direct pressure. Embedded or protruding foreign objects (e.g., knives) should be bandaged in place and left alone. Medical care should be sought.

ABDOMINAL INJURIES

Abdominal injuries may be closed or open, and they may involve hollow or solid organs.

Closed injuries are those in which the abdomen is damaged by a severe blow (e.g., hitting a steering wheel or the dashboard of a car or being tackled in football), but in which there is no open wound or bleeding to the outside. *Open* injuries are those in which a foreign body has entered the abdomen, and bleeding to the outside is occurring. Examples are stab or gunshot wounds.

The rupture of hollow organs (e.g., organs of the digestive system such as stomach or intestines) spills the contents into the peritoneal cavity causing inflammation. Rupture of solid organs (e.g., the liver) may result in severe bleeding.

Signs and Symptoms

The signs and symptoms of abdominal injury can include:

1. Victim is in pain, often starting as mild pain then rapidly become severe.
2. Victim has cramps in the abdominal area.
3. Victim will be still, usually with legs drawn up.
4. Breathing will be rapid and shallow.
5. Skin wounds and penetrations may be evident.
6. Victim may be nauseated and may vomit.
7. Organs may protrude.
8. There may be blood in the urine.
9. Victim tries to protect his abdomen.

Types of Abdominal Injuries

Blunt wounds: Severe bruises of the abdominal area can result from a blow to the abdomen. Within the abdomen, the liver, spleen, or intestine may be lacerated or ruptured. In fact, any internal organ could be affected.

Place the victim on one side in a comfortable position. Vomiting may occur. Combat shock by maintaining body warmth, giving no liquids unless hours from a medical facility, and keeping the victim lying on his side in case of vomiting. Seek medical attention for the victim.

Penetrating injuries: This type of injury presents a special problem. Assume that major damage has occurred. In these injuries, hollow organs are usually lacerated.

If a penetrating object is still in place, leave it and bandage it so that external bleeding is controlled and the object is stable. Do not withdraw it. If there is vomiting, place the victim on his side. Make the victim as comfortable as possible and seek medical attention.

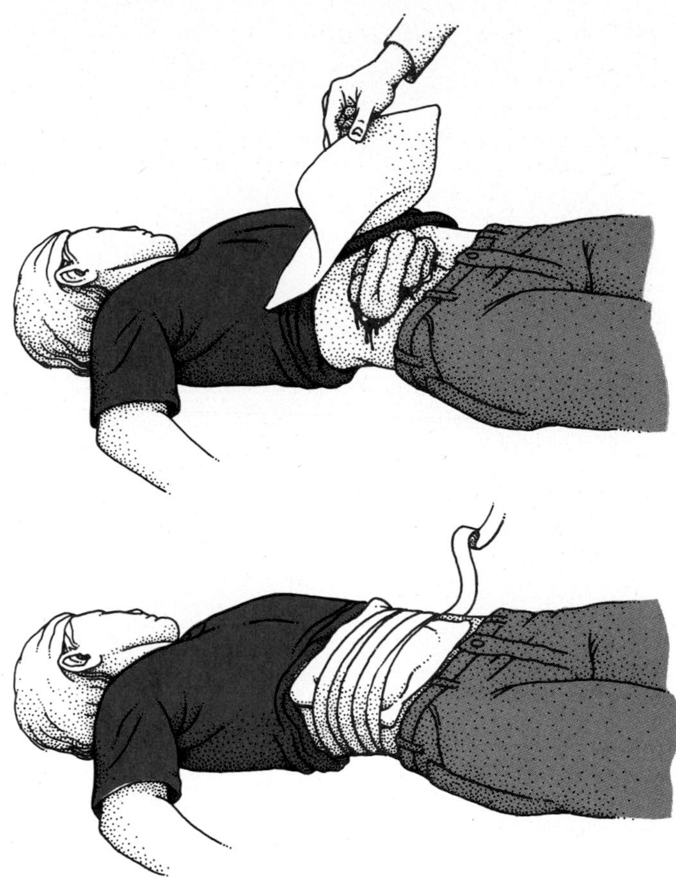

6-4. Protruding organs. Do not replace them. Cover them with a moist, sterile dressing.

Protruding organs: When an injury has resulted in the abdominal organs lying outside the abdominal cavity, do not try to replace them within the abdomen. Cover them with a moist, sterile dressing. It is important to cover extruding organs and to keep them moist and warm. Do not cover protruding organs with material that clings or loses its substance when wet (e.g., cotton). Time will be lost in surgery in removing the mess. (*See* Figure 6-4.)

Summary: For all abdominal injuries, suspect shock and work to prevent it. Be alert for vomitus and turn the victim on his side if it does occur. Afterwards, wipe the mouth out. Do not remove penetrating objects, but control bleeding and stabilize the object. Do not touch protruding organs, but cover them with a sterile dressing and keep the dressing moist. Do not give anything to eat or drink.

FOREIGN OBJECTS

Managing foreign objects in the body is relatively simple and straightforward as long as the first aider follows some basic treatment principles.

The most basic principle of emergency care is to keep things simple. You usually do not need a lot of supplies and equipment to care for a victim with a foreign object embedded somewhere in his or her body. Another basic principle that needs repeating is to treat the *entire* victim. Do not let the obvious injury lure you to overlook other possibilities such as prevention and care of shock.

Eyes

The most common eye injury may be due to a foreign body that has been blown onto the outer surface of the eye. Common foreign bodies include eyelashes, sand, soot, cinders, chips of rust, paint, and metal shavings.

Most foreign bodies are flushed out of the eye by a large amount of tears produced by the irritation. However, sometimes the foreign body remains and must be removed either by a first aider or someone with greater medical expertise.

Foreign bodies on the eye are often difficult to see and must be looked for carefully. Usually such foreign bodies lodge under the upper lid. In this case, the first method to try is to gently rinse the eye by pouring clean water over the eye. If this method does not work, the foreign body is probably stuck under the upper lid and the lid will have to be everted to get the foreign body out. To evert a lid, ask the victim to look down while you grasp the eyelash of their upper lid between your thumb and index finger. Place a smooth narrow object horizontally along the outer surface of the eyelid, and then pull the eyelid gently forward and upward so that it folds back on itself over the smooth narrow object. (*See* Figure 6-5.)

When the foreign object is found, try to remove it with a dampened (not dry) sterile gauze. Do not, however, use another object (i.e., toothpick, match stick) to remove the foreign body if it is lying on the surface of the eyeball. If you are unsuccessful, you should patch both eyes and transport the victim to a medical facility.

Do not try to remove an impaled foreign object. It should be stabilized in place. One way to do this is to take a stack of 4-inch gauze pads and cut a hole in the center of the stack large enough to fit over the object. Then carefully pass the stack of gauze pads over the object, so that the dressing is resting gently against the surrounding skin. To prevent the impaled object from being caught or jarred, position a paper cup or similar item over the gauze pads so that the object is enclosed within it but not touching it. Fasten the paper cup in place. (*See* Figure 6-6.)

When patching the injured eye, the uninjured eye should also be patched. The reason for patching the uninjured eye is that normally both eyes move together. If the uninjured eye starts looking around to

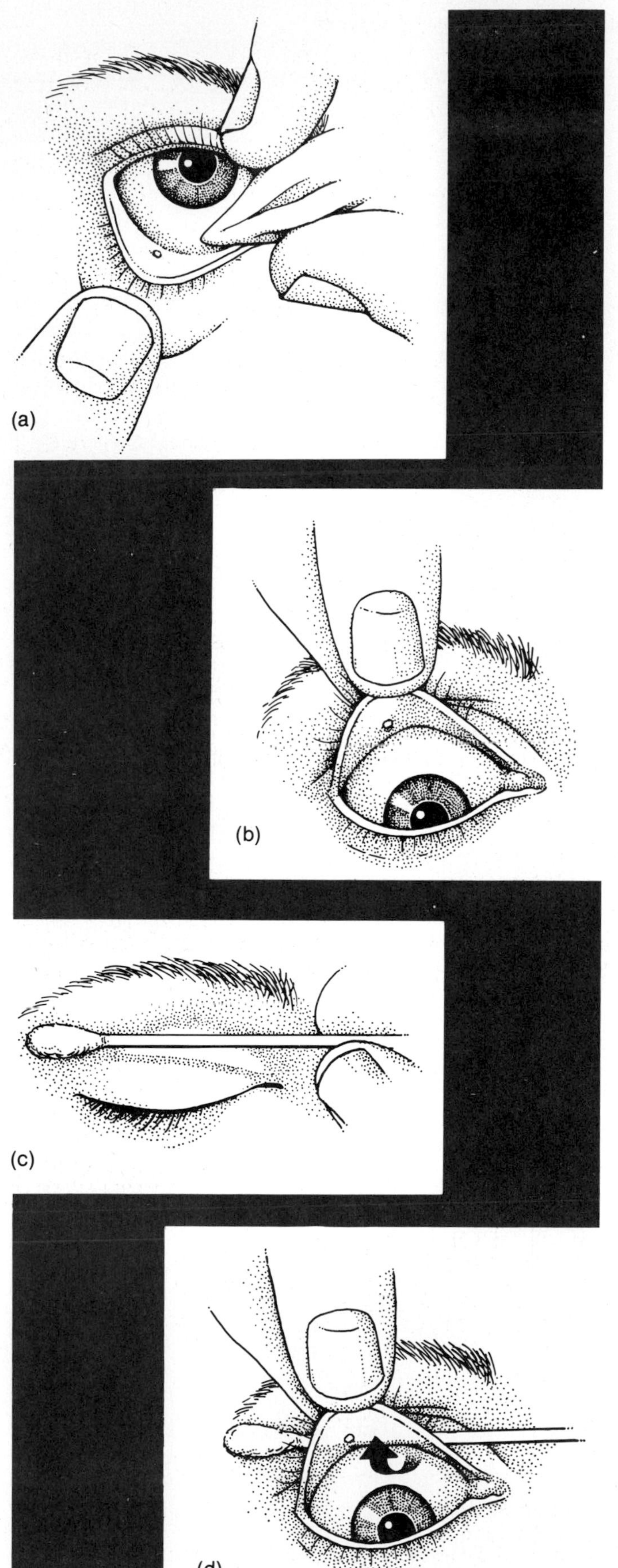

check out the scenery, the eye with the impaled object will move as well, and this can further damage the injured eye. When covering both eyes, take time to explain to the victim what you are doing and why the patch is necessary.

Nose

Foreign bodies in the nose are a problem mainly among small children who seem to gain some satisfaction from putting peanuts, beans, raisins, and similar objects into their nostrils.

A foreign object in the nose can usually be removed by one of several methods:

1. Sneeze out the foreign object by sniffing pepper or tickling the opposite nostril.

2. Blow gently as the opposite nostril is compressed.

3. Use tweezers to pull out an object that is easily visible. Be careful not to push on it and lodge it farther in the nostril. Some experts do not suggest this procedure because the object may have penetrated the nasal tissues.

4. Consult a physician if the object cannot be expelled. Probing into a nostril may jam the foreign body deeper into the nose.

Ears

Various foreign bodies such as insects, seeds, match sticks, and cotton can become lodged in the ear canal. This type of emergency most often occurs with young children.

Do *not* try to kill a lodged insect by poking something in the ear. Insects are attracted to light, so it may be coaxed out with light. If outdoors, pull the earlobe gently to straighten the canal and turn the ear toward the sun. If indoors, turn off all the lights and shine a flashlight into the ear while pulling gently on the earlobe. The insect might crawl out toward the light.

If the light method fails, inserting a little oil (mineral, baby, or olive oil) may cause the insect to float out when you turn the victim's ear down and allow the oil to run out. Do not use this method if you are not absolutely sure that the foreign body in the ear is an insect because, if it is a bean, popcorn, or other similar object, it may swell and be difficult to move.

◄ **6-5.** Loose or invisible object in eye
(a) If tears or gentle flushing do not remove object, gently pull lower lid down. Remove an object by gently flushing with lukewarm water or a wet sterile gauze.
(b) If no object is seen inside lower lid, check the upper lid.
(c) Tell the person to look down. Pull gently downward on upper eyelashes. Lay a swab or match stick across the top of the lid.
(d) Fold the lid over the swab or match stick. Remove an object by gently flushing with lukewarm water or a wet sterile gauze.

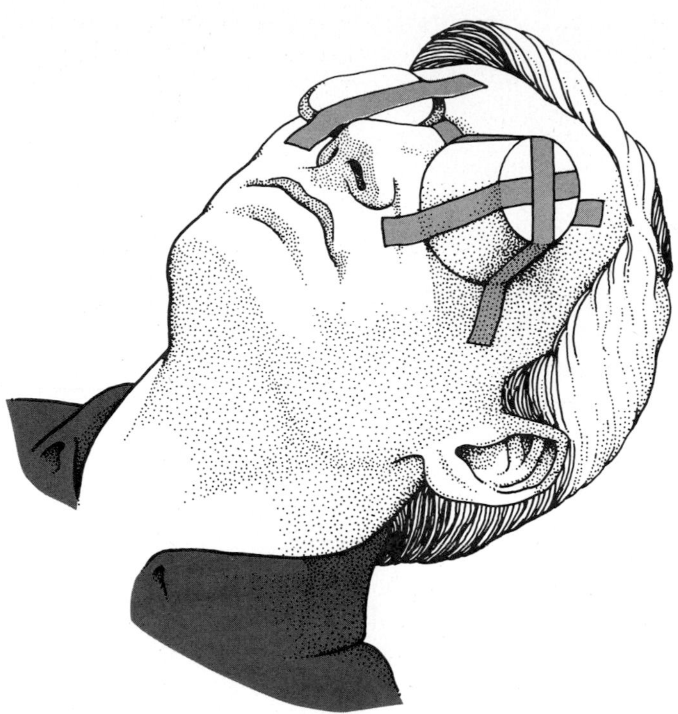

6-6. Use paper cup or make paper cone to cover the impaled object or an avulsed eye.

Do *not* go into the ear canal with a pin, toothpick, or other slender object to remove foreign bodies. These items may force the object farther into the ear and damage the lining of the ear canal or eardrum.

Some experts recommend that foreign bodies can occasionally be jarred loose from an ear canal by gently pounding with the hand on the opposite side of the head with the affected ear held down. Other experts do not recommend this procedure.

If the object cannot be seen or cannot be easily removed, seek medical attention.

Cheek

An impaled object in the cheek should be removed quickly. As long as the object remains impaled in the cheek, it will be impossible to control blood flowing into the mouth and throat and, if dislodged, the object may pose a threat as an airway obstruction.

Removal of an impaled object in the cheek represents the only situation where it is permissible for a first aider to remove an impaled object. If the cheek is perforated, carefully remove the impaled object by pulling it out in the direction it entered the cheek. If it cannot be easily done, leave the object in place.

Once the object is removed, pack the space between the cheek and gums with gauze pads and apply pressure against the packing with a dressing held against the outside of the cheek. Periodically check the packing inside because it could induce gagging or block the airway.

Abdomen and Chest

When an object is impaled in the abdomen or chest, do not remove the object because serious bleeding and further damage may occur to nerves, blood vessels, or other tissue.

If there is external bleeding, control it by direct pressure on the surrounding tissue but not on the impaled object.

Place bulky dressings around the object to immobilize it. Do *not* shorten the impaled object unless it is too long. It must be stabilized in place to prevent motion.

Most cases of foreign objects usually require medical attention. Obvious exceptions are small splinters embedded under the skin.

Most impaled objects can be treated in a similar way as shown in Figure 6-7.

Fishhook Embedded

When only the point and not the barb of a fishhook penetrates the skin, you can easily remove a fishhook by backing the hook out. However, if the barb of the hook enters the skin, follow these procedures:

1. If the medical care is near, transport the victim and have a physician remove the hook.

2. If in a remote area far from medical care, remove the hook by either the pliers method or the fishline method.

Pliers Method

You must have pliers with tempered jaws that will cut through a hook. Cut through an extra hook to ensure that the pliers are capable of cutting through a hook. If so, use cold or hard pressure to provide tem-

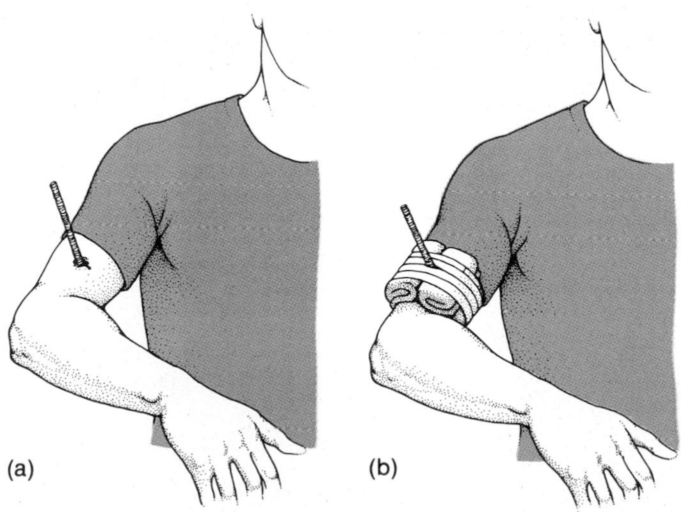

6-7. Impaled object
(a) Do not remove nor disturb.
(b) Control bleeding by applying direct pressure to the wound. Stabilize the impaled object.

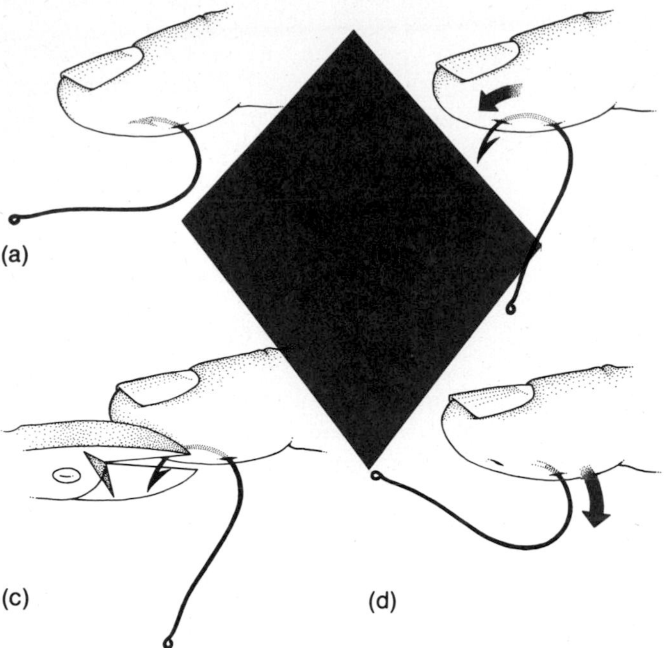

6-8. Pliers method

porary anesthesia. Then push the embedded barb further in, in a shallow curve, until the point and barb come out through the skin. Cut the barb off and back the hook out the way it came in. After removing the hook, treat the wound. Most of the time the proper kind of pliers is lacking or the barb is buried too deeply to be pushed on through. (*See* Figure 6-8.)

Fishline Method

Loop a piece of fishline over the eye of the embedded hook and bring it down to the middle of the hook's curve. Immobilize the victim's hand (or wherever the hook is embedded). Use cold or hard pressure to provide temporary anesthesia. With your other hand, press down and back on the eye of the hook as you sharply jerk the hook with the loop. The jerk movement should be parallel to the skin surface. The hook will neatly come out of the same hole it entered, causing little pain. After removing the hook, treat the wound. (*See* Figure 6-9.)

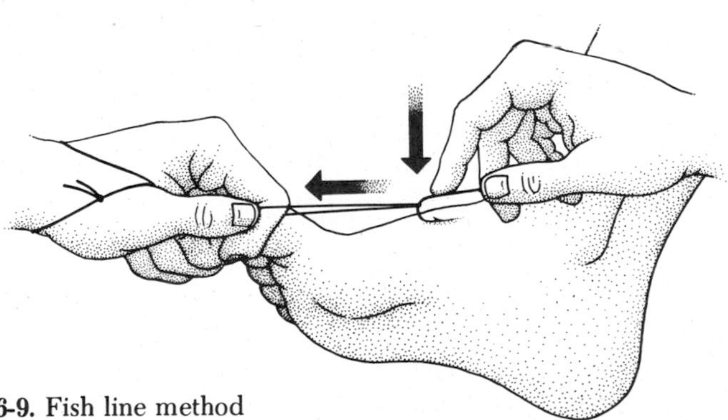

6-9. Fish line method

HAND AND FINGER INJURIES

The hand is a marvel of structural organization that, considering its complexity, is able to sustain considerable abuse. Nevertheless, hands may often be injured. Fractures, often the result of direct blows, are among the most serious injuries that occur to the hand and fingers and are discussed in Chapter Ten.

Fingernail Hematoma

Any direct blow to the fingertip or to the fingernail can cause the accumulation of blood directly beneath the nail. A purple discoloration is visible under the nail. This is a minor injury but is an extremely painful condition because of the accumulation of blood underneath the fingernail.

Emergency care: The victim should place the finger in ice water until the hemorrhage ceases. If painful, the pressure of blood should then be released from under the fingernail. The entrapped blood may be released in two different ways. One way is to use a sharp knife to drill by a rotary action drill a hole through the fingernail. A second way, which is faster, is to heat a paper clip to a red-hot temperature and to lay the red-hot paper clip on the surface of the nail with moderate pressure. This melts a hole through the nail to the site of the blood. The nail has no nerves, thus there will be no pain. Be sure not to pierce the nail unless a blood blister is really present. (*See* Figure 6-10.)

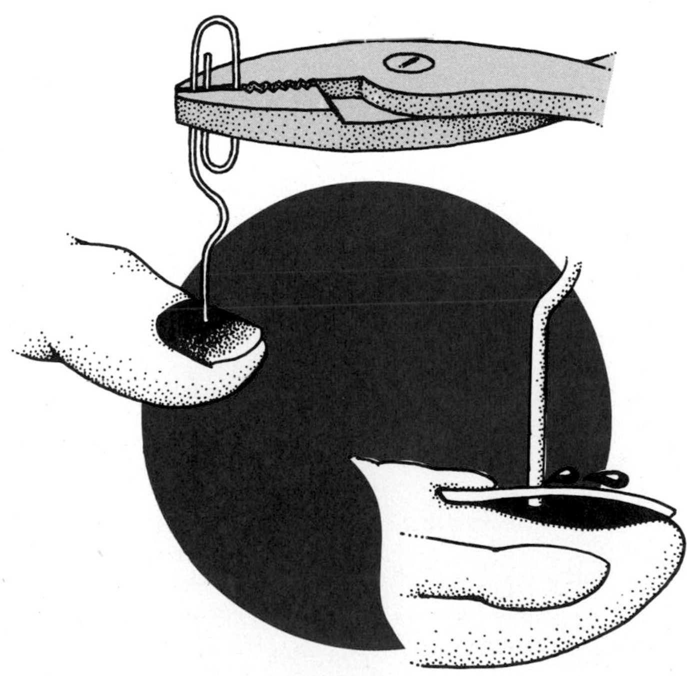

6-10. Making a hole in a fingernail

Laceration

A laceration that involves the hand should not be considered a minor injury. It should be taken seriously because nerve and tendon damage can accompany lacerations. If there is any doubt as to the damage, consult an orthopedic or hand surgeon immediately. Standard treatment of bleeding should be applied before referral.

Splinters

If a splinter passes under the nail and breaks off flush, you may remove it by grasping the end of it with tweezers, after cutting a V-shaped notch in the nail to gain access to the splinter.

Finger Avulsion

The finger is the body part that becomes avulsed or amputated most often.

Emergency care: Successful reimplantation of amputated body parts has become common. Blood loss in cases of complete amputations is often surprisingly quite minimal. Direct pressure controls most bleeding. You should retrieve the amputated part and follow these procedures:

1. Wrap the amputated part with a wet gauze or cloth. Do not immerse the part in water.
2. If possible, put the wrapped part in a plastic bag or container.
3. Place the wrapped, amputated part on a bed of ice, but do not submerge.
4. Seek medical attention immediately.

If the part is still partially attached by a tendon or a piece of skin, the part can still be wet-wrapped and placed on ice after it is repositioned in the normal position.

Ring Removal

Most rings stuck on fingers are removed with a combination of lubrication and gentle tugging. But sometimes a finger is too swollen for the ring to be removed in the usual manner. Removal is simple with a ring cutter—if it is available. If not, try the following techniques:

1. Slide the ring off after lubricating the finger with grease, oil, butter, petroleum jelly, or some other slippery substance.
2. Immerse the finger in ice water for several minutes in an effort to reduce the swelling. Move the ring to a point on the finger where it is loose. Gently massage the finger from tip to hand; this may move the fluid from the swollen area. After a few minutes of massaging, lubricate the finger again and try to slip the ring off.

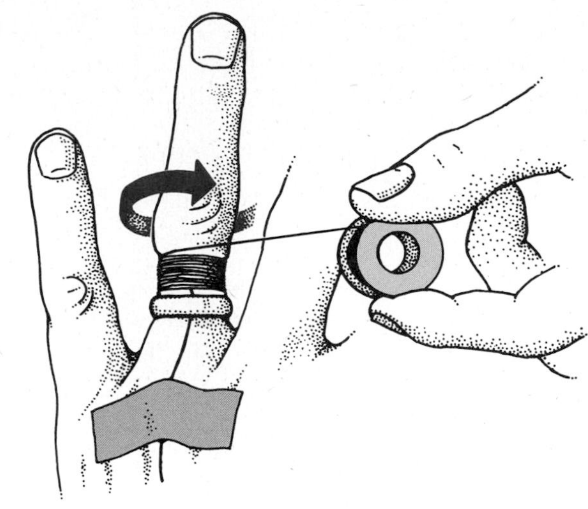

(a)

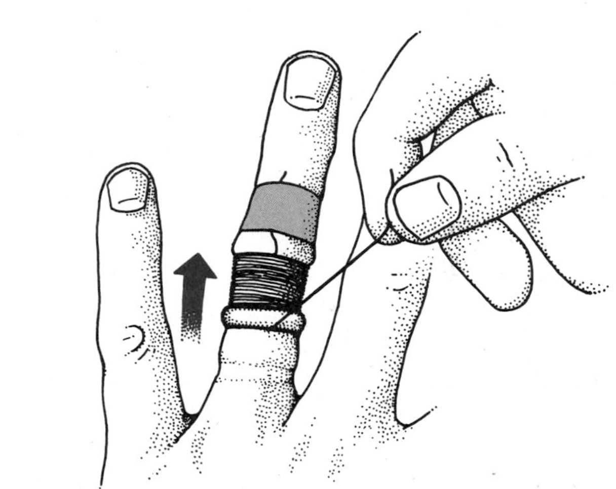

(b)

6-11. Ring removal with string

3. Slide three or four inches of thin string under the ring toward the hand. (*See* Figure 6-11.) The string may need to be pushed through with a match stick or toothpick. Then wrap the string tightly around the finger below the ring for about three-quarters of an inch, going toward the fingernail and away from the ring. Each wrap should be right next to the one before. While holding the wrapping snugly in place with the fingers of one hand, grasp the upper end of the string with the fingers of the other hand. Pull the string downward over the ring. This starts an unwrapping process. If the finger is not too badly swollen, the ring may slide over the string that is still wrapped around the finger and continue to move as you continue to unwrap. It may be necessary to repeat the procedure several times to get the ring completely off the finger.
4. Start about three-quarters of an inch to one inch from the ring edge and smoothly wind string around the finger going toward the ring with one strand touching the next. Continue winding smoothly and

tightly right up to the edge of the ring. The advantage of this method is that it tends to push the swelling toward the hand. Slip the end of the string under and through the ring. (You may have to push it through with a match stick or toothpick.) Slowly unwind the string on the hand side of the ring and the ring is gently twisted off the finger over the spiraled string.

5. Carefully cut the narrowest portion of the ring with a ring saw, jeweler's saw, ring cutter, or a fine hacksaw blade. If anything other than a ring saw is used, take care to protect exposed portions of the finger.

6. Inflate an ordinary balloon about three-quarters full. Tie the end. The slender tube-shaped balloons work best. Insert the victim's swollen finger into the end of the balloon so that the balloon rolls back evenly around the finger. In about fifteen minutes the finger should return to its normal size and the ring can be removed.

Ring strangulation can be a serious problem if it cuts off circulation long enough. Gangrene may result within four or five hours.

Bandaging

All hand and finger injuries can be effectively bandaged and dressed with a bulky hand dressing. The injured hand is formed into what is called the "position of function" (finger joints flexed moderately similar to the position in which one would most comfortably hold a baseball). A roller bandage is then placed in the palm of the hand. A padded board splint is applied to the palm side of the hand and secured with a roller bandage.

BLISTERS

Because many activities involve walking, running, jumping, and other such motions, it is not surprising that the feet have more than their fair share of skin injuries. Perhaps the most common skin injury are blisters due to friction. Blisters are most often caused by ill-fitting shoes or wrinkled socks.

Blisters can be avoided by buying properly fitting shoes or boots, breaking the shoes/boots in prior to their extensive use, putting adhesive tape over the areas that are prone to blister, or wearing two pairs of socks. The inner pair should be of form-fitting, thin material, and the outer pair should be made of bulkier wool or a wool blend. A person can also apply Vaseline™ to cut down on the friction.

Once a blister has formed, you should prevent further injury by covering the blister with tape, moleskin, or a doughnut of gauze or felt. It is best to leave blisters unbroken, whenever possible. If the pain is unbearable, then the blister can be broken.

When a blister must be broken, first wash the area with soap and water. Then make a small hole at the base of the blister with a sterilized needle. Sterilize the needle by either soaking it in rubbing alcohol or holding it over the top of a match flame. (*See* Figure 6-12.)

Drain the fluid and apply a sterile dressing to protect the area from further irritation. In some cases, the blister may have to be drained up to three times in the first twenty-four hours. Roofs of blisters should remain intact.

If a blister has ruptured and its roof is gone, apply a sterile dressing. All ruptured blisters should be cleaned with soap and water to prevent infection.

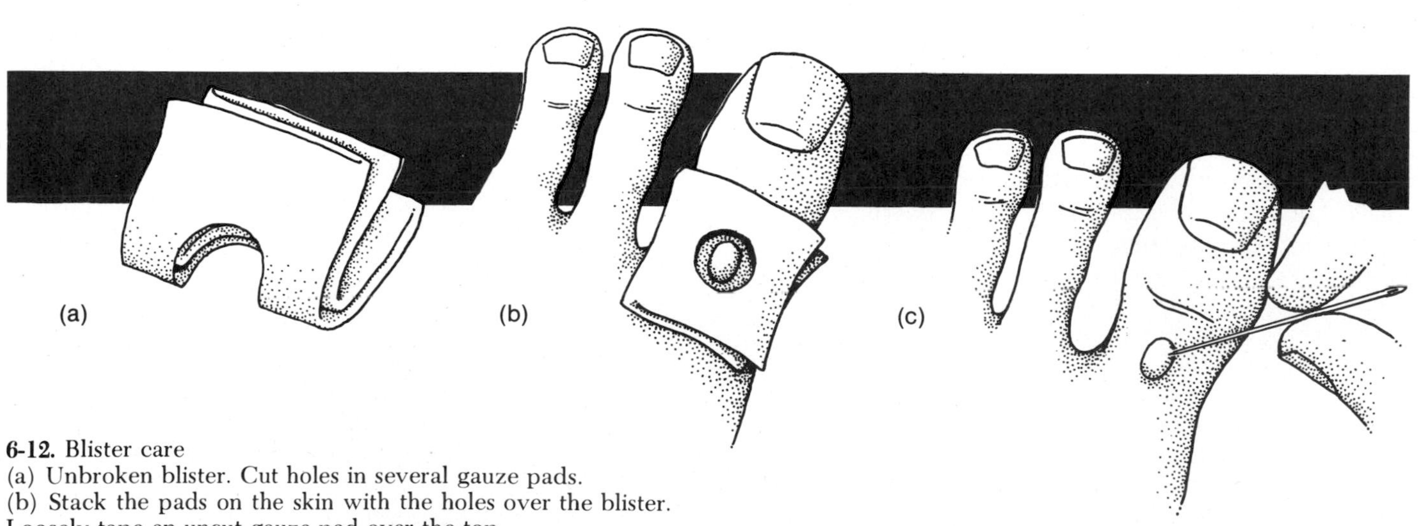

6-12. Blister care
(a) Unbroken blister. Cut holes in several gauze pads.
(b) Stack the pads on the skin with the holes over the blister. Loosely tape an uncut gauze pad over the top.
(c) Blister is painful or likely to break. With a sterilized needle puncture the blister's edge. Drain all the fluid. Tape a sterile or clean gauze pad or cloth over the flattened blister.

TABLE 6-2. Dental Emergency Procedures

Toothache	Rinse the mouth vigorously with warm water to clean out debris. Use dental floss to remove any food that might be trapped between the teeth. (*Do not place aspirin on the aching tooth or gum tissues.*) See your dentist as soon as possible.
Orthodontic Problems (Braces and Retainers)	If a wire is causing irritation, cover end of the wire with a small cotton ball, beeswax, or a piece of gauze, until you can get to the dentist. If a wire is embedded in the cheek, tongue, or gum tissue, do not attempt to remove it. Go to your dentist immediately. If an appliance becomes loose or a piece of it breaks off, take the appliance and the piece and go to the dentist.
Knocked-Out Tooth	If the tooth is dirty, rinse it gently in running water. *Do not scrub it.* Gently insert and hold the tooth in its socket. If this is not possible, place the tooth in a container of milk or cool water. Go immediately to your dentist (within 30 minutes, if possible). Don't forget to bring the tooth.
Broken Tooth	Gently clean dirt or debris from the injured area with warm water. Place cold compresses on the face, in the area of the injured tooth, to minimize swelling. Go to the dentist immediately.
Bitten Tongue or Lip	Apply direct pressure to the bleeding area with a clean cloth. If swelling is present, apply cold compresses. If bleeding does not stop, go to a hospital emergency room.
Objects Wedged Between Teeth	Try to remove the object with dental floss. Guide the floss carefully to avoid cutting the gums. If not successful in removing the object, go to the dentist. Do not try to remove the object with a sharp or pointed instrument.
Possible Fractured Jaw	Immobilize the jaw by any means (handkerchief, necktie, towel). If swelling is present, apply cold compresses. Call your dentist or go immediately to a hospital emergency room.

Source: Copyright by the American Dental Association. Reprinted by permission.

Head Injury

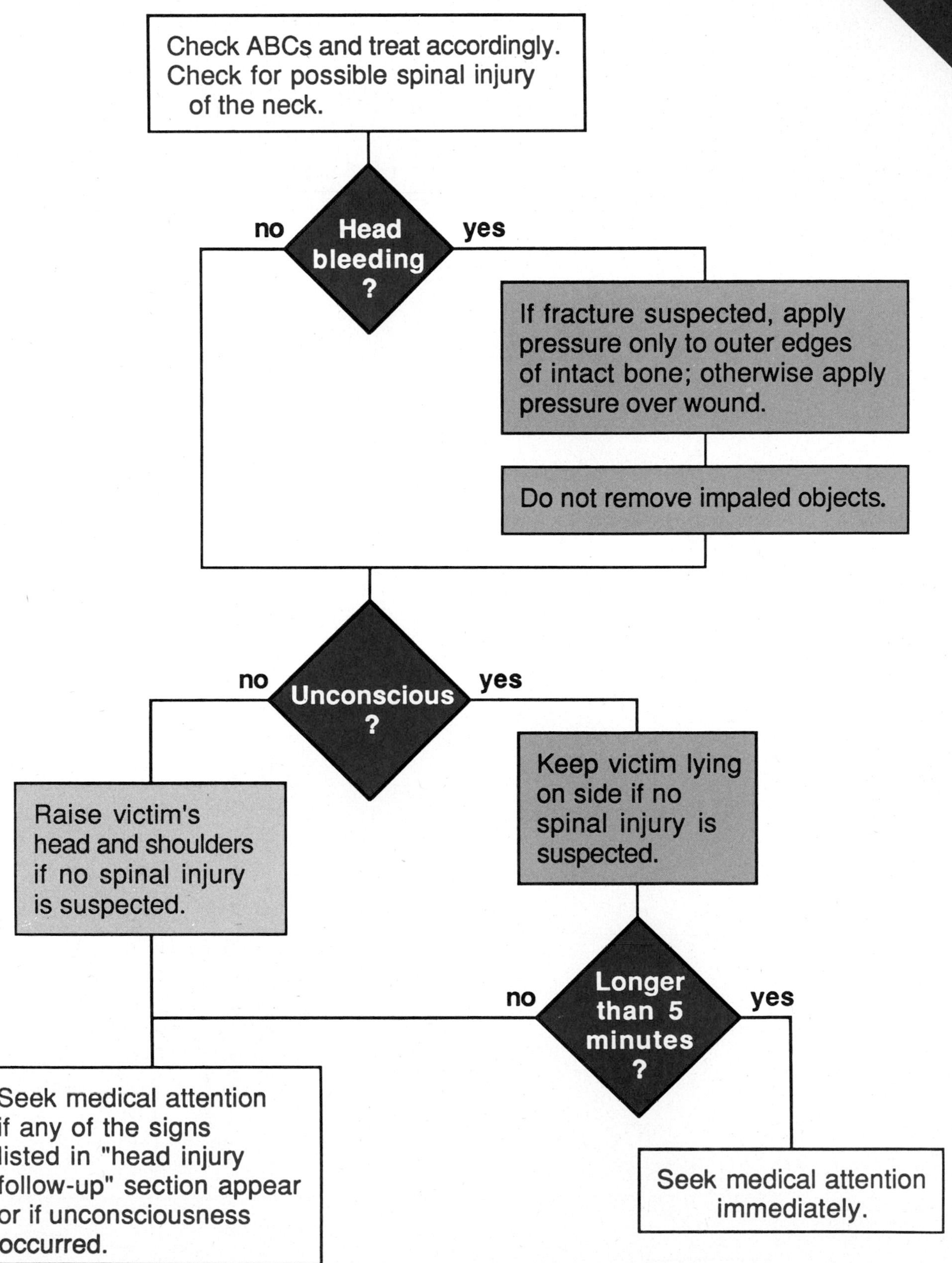

Check ABCs and treat accordingly.
Check for possible spinal injury of the neck.
no
Head bleeding ?
yes
If fracture suspected, apply pressure only to outer edges of intact bone; otherwise apply pressure over wound.
Do not remove impaled objects.
no
Unconscious ?
yes
Raise victim's head and shoulders if no spinal injury is suspected.
Keep victim lying on side if no spinal injury is suspected.
no
Longer than 5 minutes ?
yes
Seek medical attention if any of the signs listed in "head injury follow-up" section appear or if unconsciousness occurred.
Seek medical attention immediately.

Eye Injuries

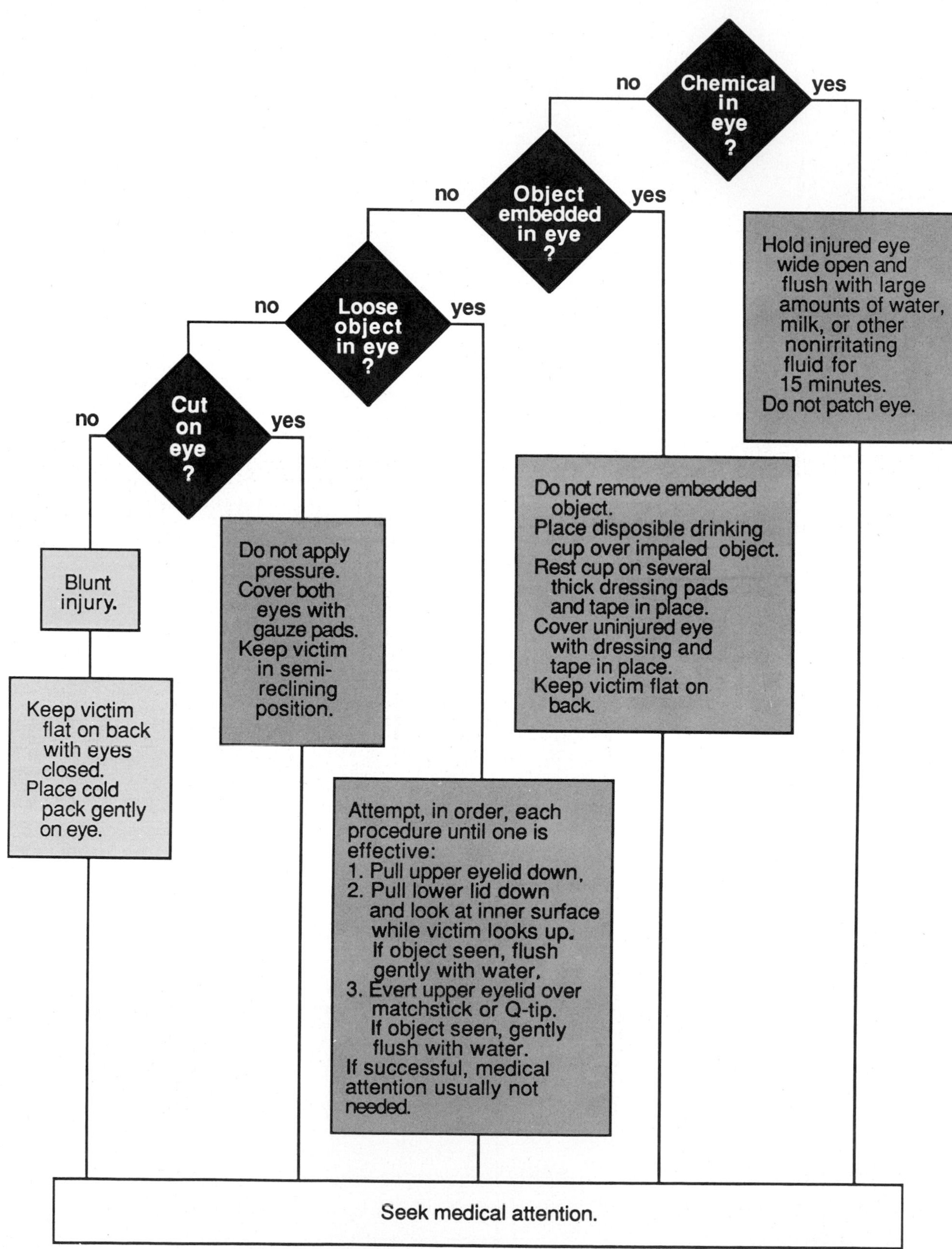

Nosebleeds

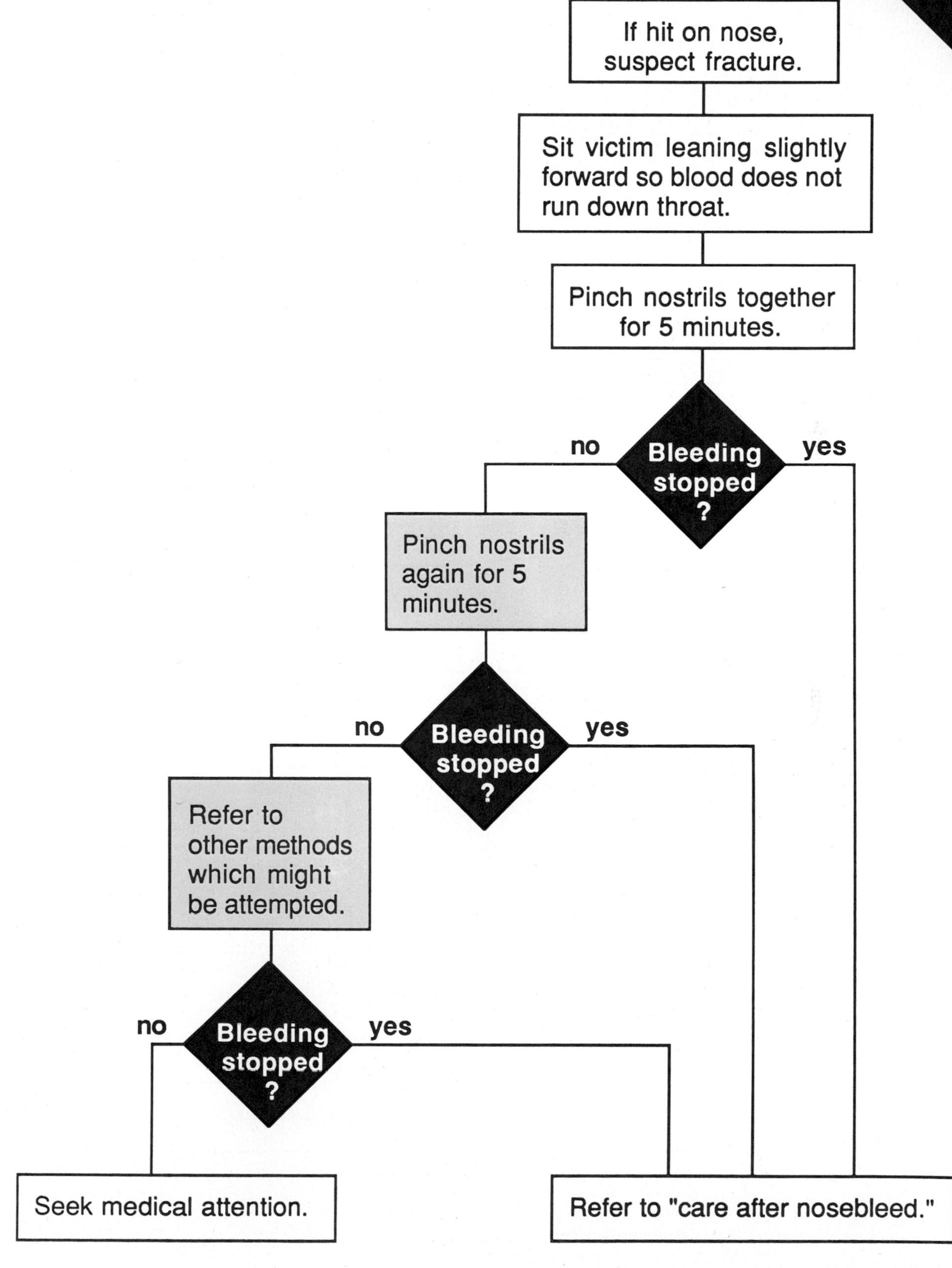
If hit on nose, suspect fracture.
Sit victim leaning slightly forward so blood does not run down throat.
Pinch nostrils together for 5 minutes.
no
Bleeding stopped ?
yes
Pinch nostrils again for 5 minutes.
no
Bleeding stopped ?
yes
Refer to other methods which might be attempted.
no
Bleeding stopped ?
yes
Seek medical attention.
Refer to "care after nosebleed."

Tooth Injury

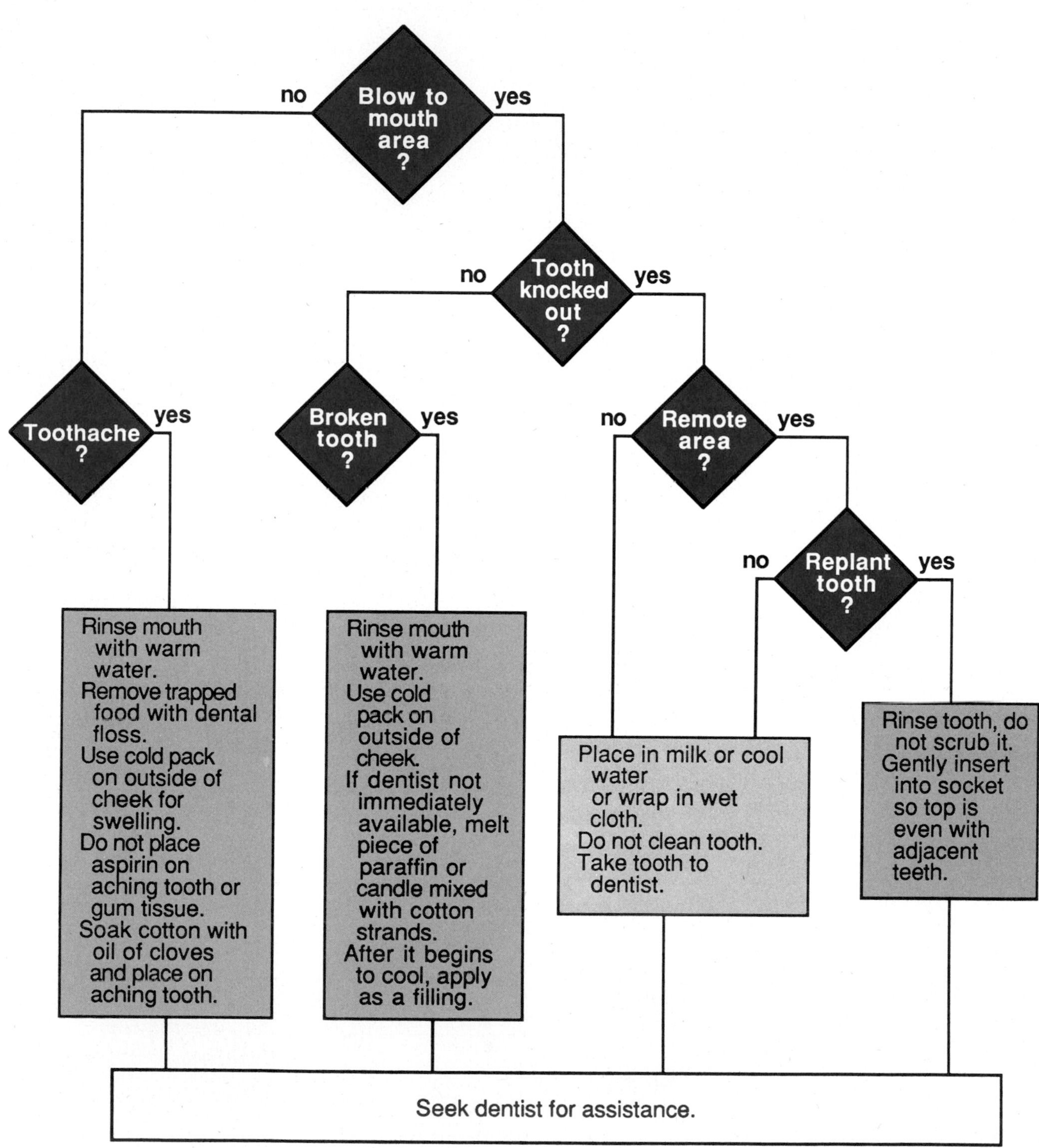

Larynx Injuries

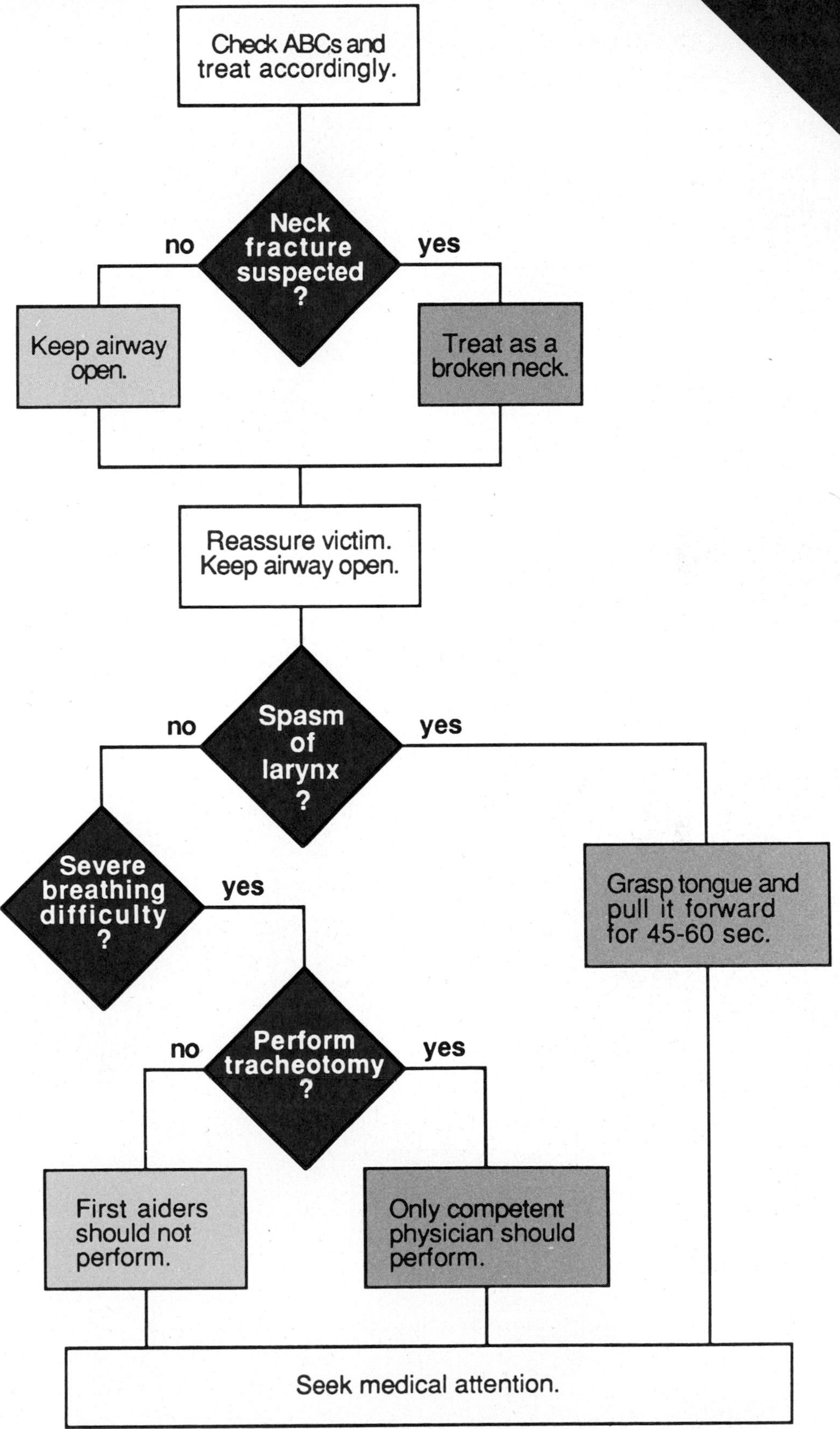

Chest Injuries

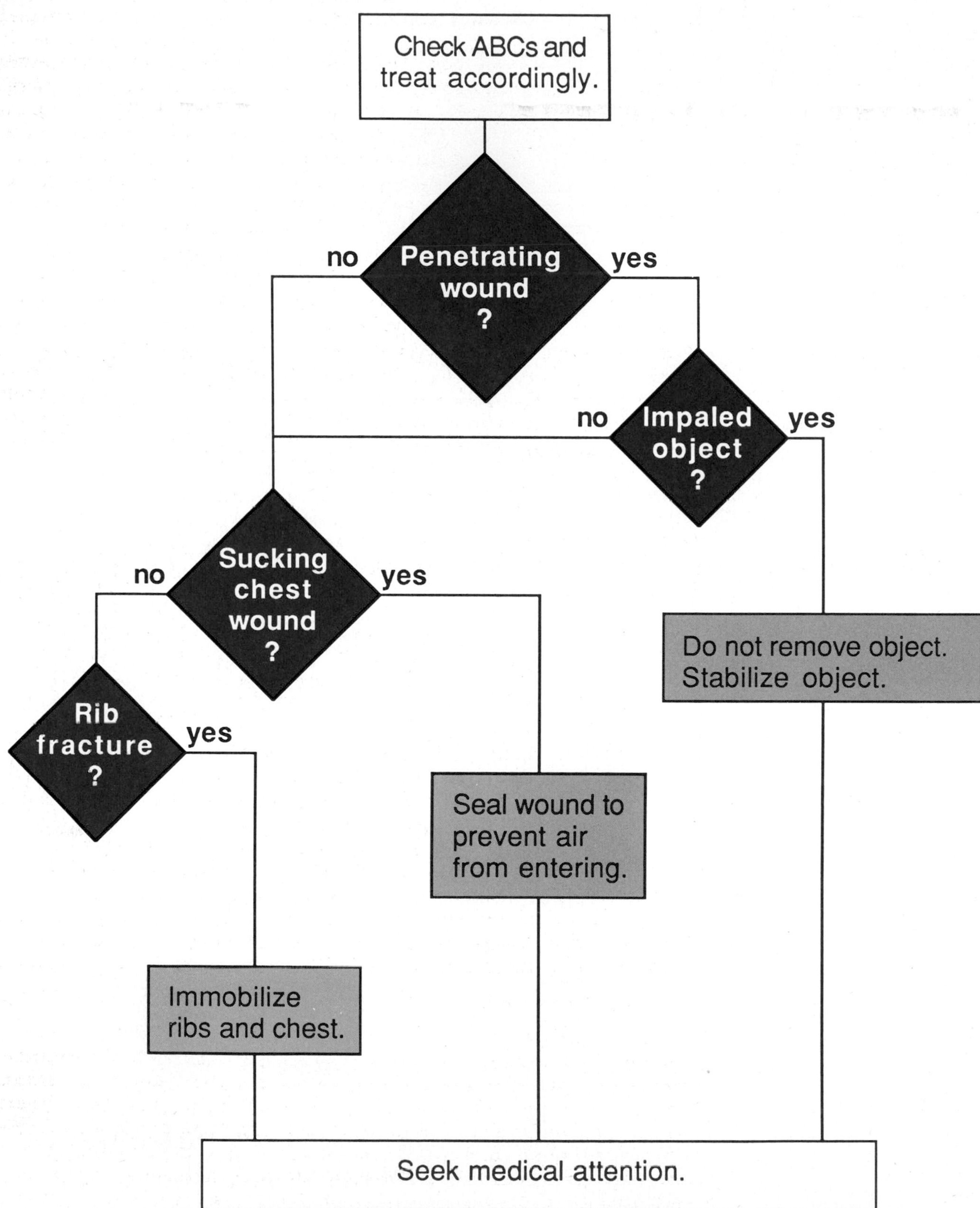

Abdominal Injuries

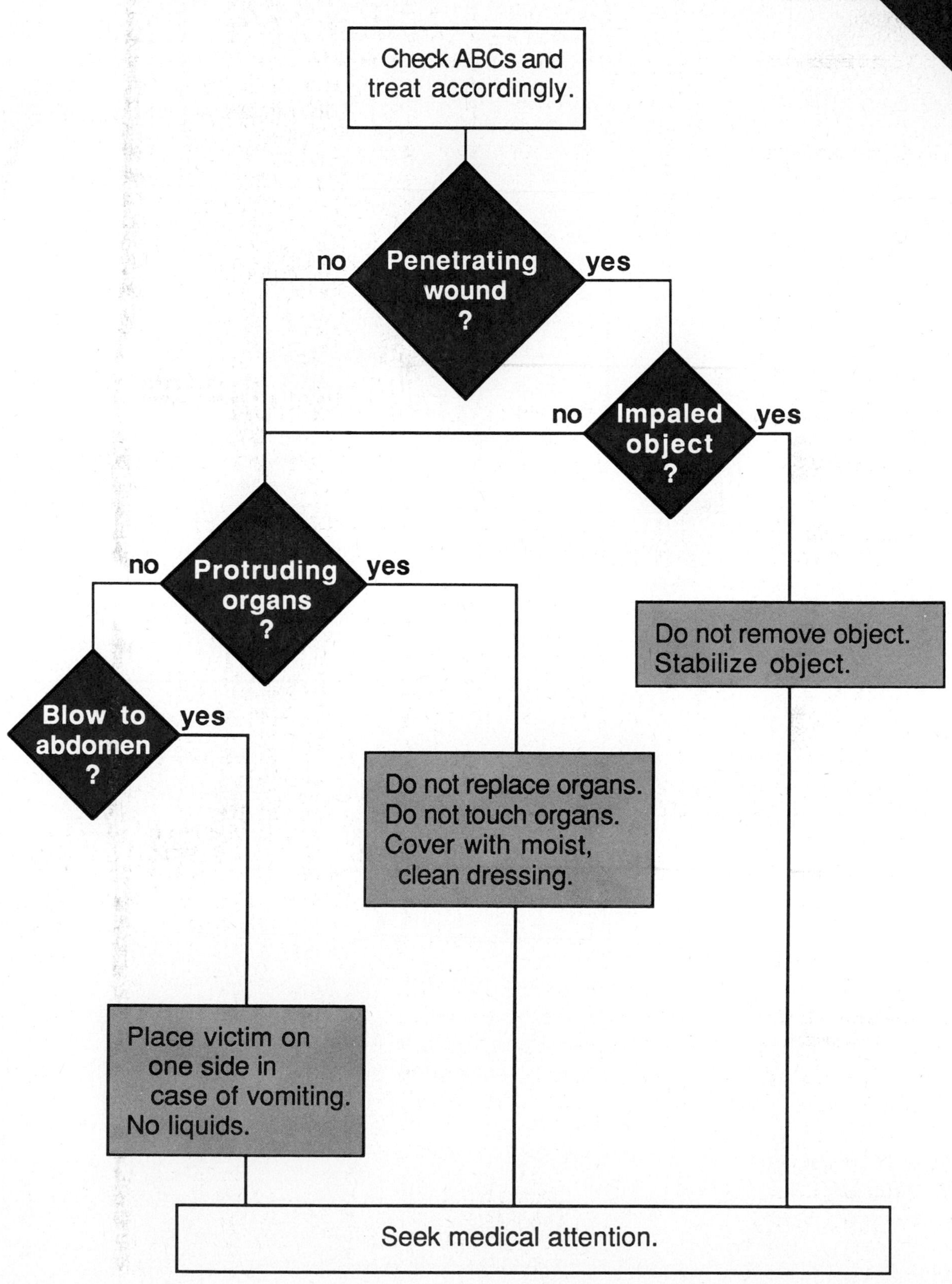

Object In Nose

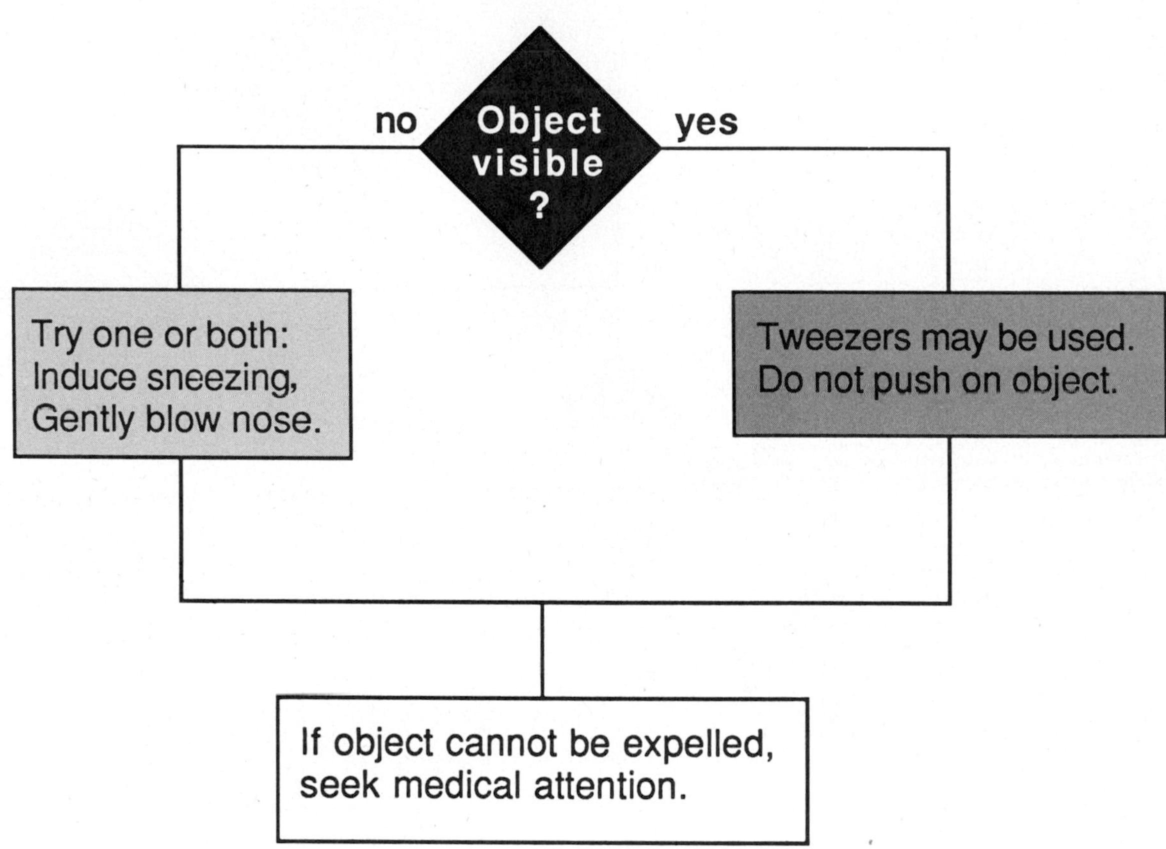

Object In Ear

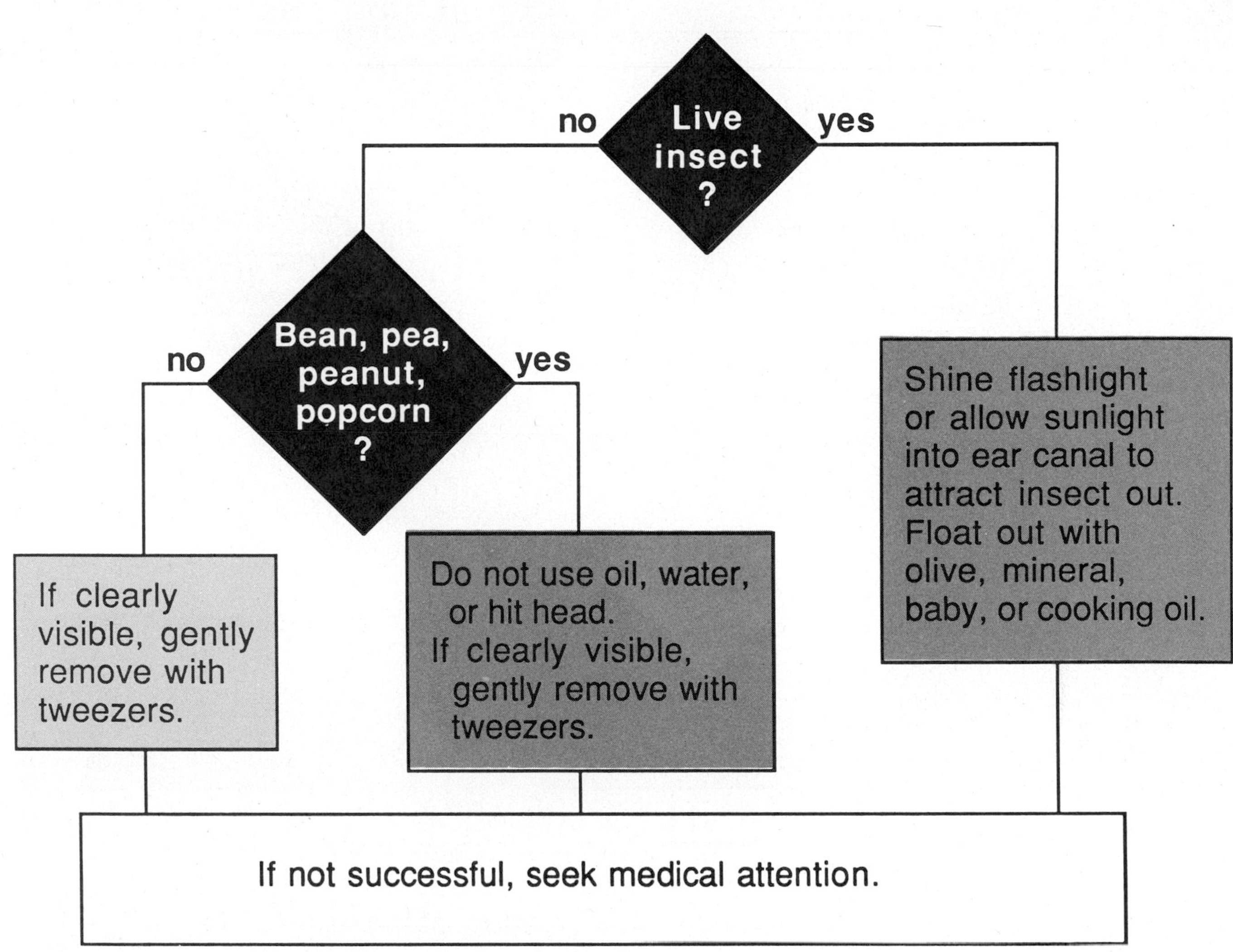

Fishhook Removal

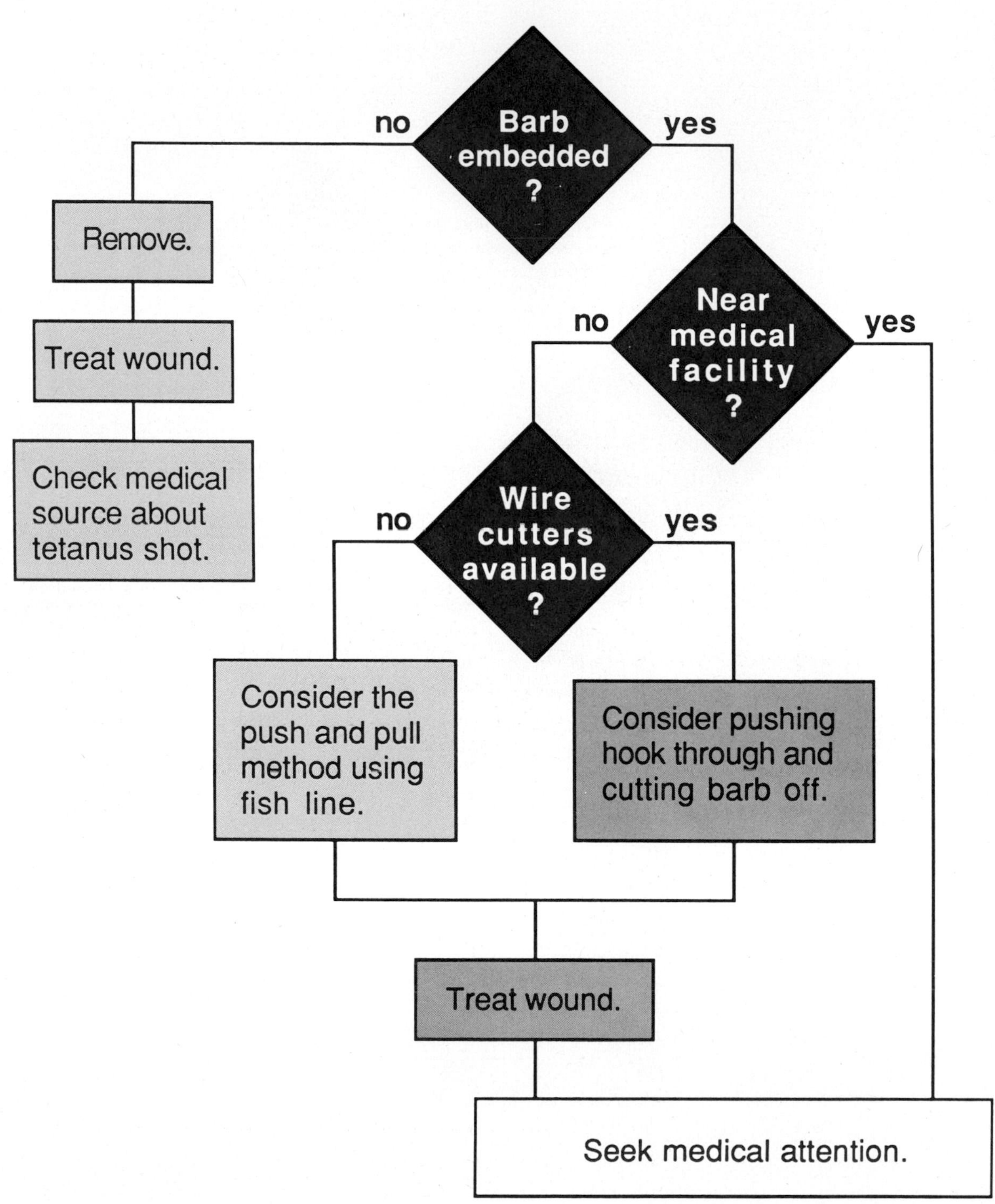

Blisters

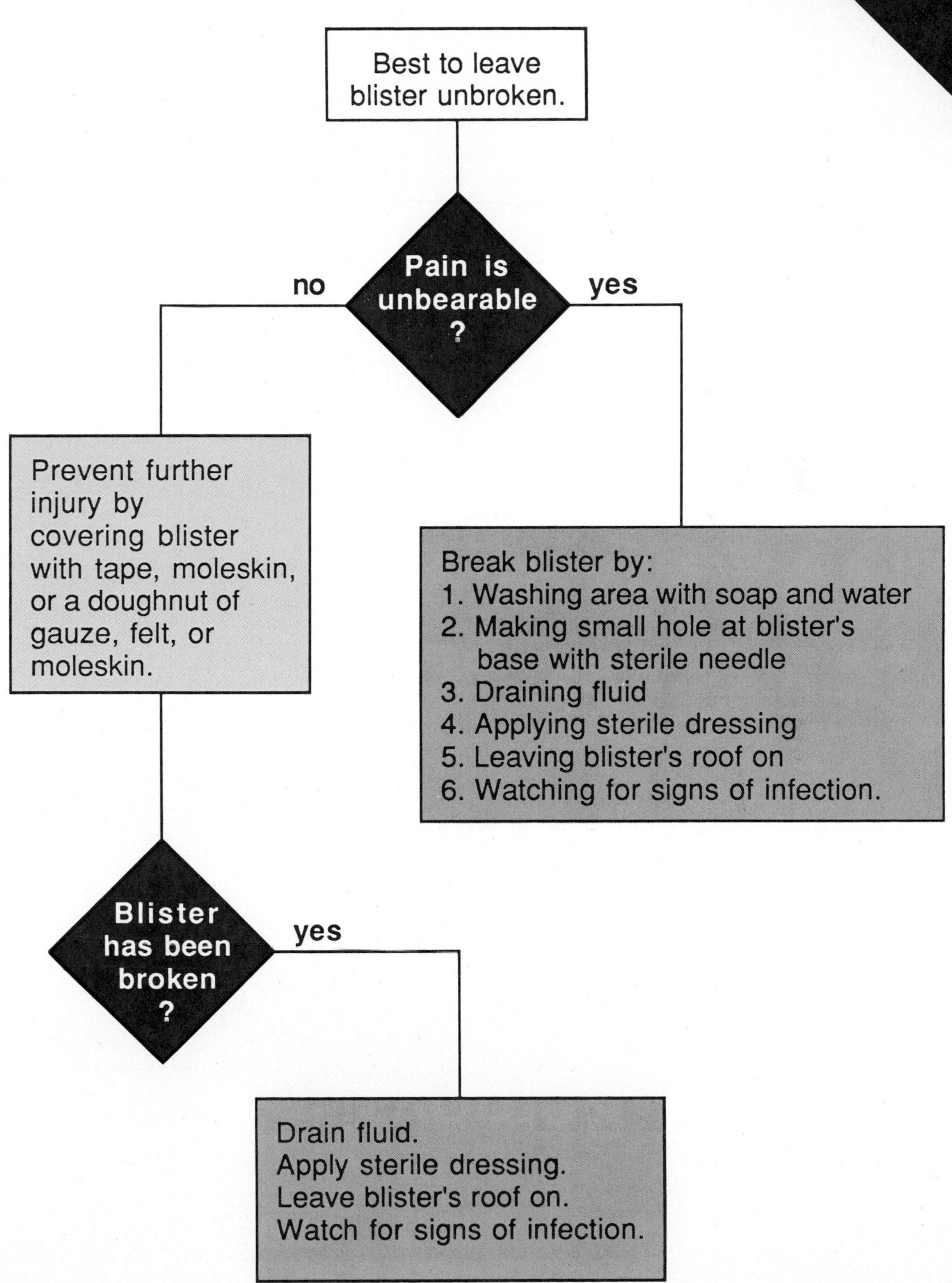

Best to leave blister unbroken.
Pain is unbearable ?
no
yes
Prevent further injury by covering blister with tape, moleskin, or a doughnut of gauze, felt, or moleskin.
Break blister by:
1. Washing area with soap and water
2. Making small hole at blister's base with sterile needle
3. Draining fluid
4. Applying sterile dressing
5. Leaving blister's roof on
6. Watching for signs of infection.
Blister has been broken ?
yes
Drain fluid.
Apply sterile dressing.
Leave blister's roof on.
Watch for signs of infection.

Head Injuries

LEARNING ACTIVITIES

T F 1. The face and scalp are richly supplied with arteries and veins, and wounds of these areas bleed heavily.
T F 2. Brain injury should be suspected when any injury about the head is noted.
T F 3. Cervical spine (neck) injury should be suspected when any injury about the head is noted.
T F 4. Cerebrospinal fluid is a clear liquid.
T F 5. If pupils are unequal in size, brain damage may exist.
T F 6. Bleeding from the ear should be stopped by cotton plugs.
T F 7. The first aider should raise the victim's head and shoulders when treating head injuries.
T F 8. Blood-colored fluid draining from the ears is a good indicator of a skull fracture.
T F 9. If the clear, water-like cerebrospinal fluid is coming from the ears and nose, the first aider should apply a snug pressure bandage.
T F 10. Vomiting can be expected after head injuries; however, if it begins again hours after one or two episodes have stopped, consult a physician.

Case 1: During a football game, a player is "knocked-out" for ten minutes.

1. Define concussion. ________________________________
____

2. List four signs of a concussion.
   A. ________________________________
   B. ________________________________
   C. ________________________________
   D. ________________________________

3. The best position for a concussion victim with a head injury is ______ without the neck flexed.

4. Give an example of a mental test you could use on a conscious victim. ________________________________
____
____

5. When should the victim be allowed to return to activity?
____
____

Case 2: You find an unconscious man "snoring" at the bottom of a flight of stairs. Witnesses say he fell about ten minutes before your arrival. You note a bleeding scalp laceration and a clear fluid coming from the nose.

1. All head injuries, regardless of apparent severity, may produce injury to the ________________________ .

2. A first aider's main concern in the unconscious victim must be to ________________________ .

T F 3. It is permissible to use direct pressure to control bleeding from a scalp laceration.
T F 4. A skull fracture must be present for a head injury to be fatal.
5. Watery liquid leaking from the head is a strong indication of ______. This liquid is probably ______ and will be leaking from the ______ or ______. Treatment of such a leak is by light application of a ______ .

Case 3: Several children had been playing on a swing set. One child had been hit on the forehead by another child who came back on the swing. The child was knocked several feet behind the swing set by the impact and appears dizzy, confused, and very weak. There was no bleeding. Pupils reacting slowly to light.

1. You would most likely suspect
   A. ______ skull fracture.
   B. ______ brain concussion.
   C. ______ both, as the signs and symptoms are almost identical.

2. Emergency care for this child would include:
   A. ________________________________
   ____
   B. ________________________________
   ____
   C. ________________________________
   ____
   D. ________________________________
   ____

E. ______________________________

____

3. With any head injury, always suspect:

A. ______ the worst; inform the parents the child may die.

B. ______ neck and back injury.

C. ______ the best; no real emergency care is needed if there is no bleeding or other major sign of injury.

Eye Injuries

T F 1. Direct pressure should be applied to a lacerated eyeball in order to control the bleeding.
T F 2. If it is necessary to bandage one eye, it is advisable to cover both eyes.
T F 3. The unconscious victim should have his or her eyes closed.
T F 4. In all chemical burns of the eye, irrigate with water and vinegar solution.
T F 5. In all chemical burns of the eye, irrigate for at least twenty minutes.
T F 6. If an eyeball is knocked out of the socket, gently and carefully replace the eyeball in the socket and cover with a dressing.
T F 7. In an unconscious victim with contact lenses in his or her eyes, slide each lens over to the side of the eye.

Case 1: A young woman passenger is thrown from the back seat into the windshield during an automobile accident. Her left eyelid is bleeding profusely and the left eyeball appears to be slightly extruded. Other sustained injuries include a laceration of the forehead and bruises on her arms and legs.

1. What emergency care should you provide to this victim?

A. ______________________________

____

B. ______________________________

____

C. ______________________________

____

D. ______________________________

____

2. What specific care should be directed to the eyelid?

____

____

3. Should both eyes be bandaged? (Circle one and explain your answer.)

Yes. Why? ______________________________

____

No. Why not? ______________________________

____

4. What special precautions should be taken in caring for the extruded eyeball?

A. ______________________________

____

B. ______________________________

____

5. What special precaution should be followed during transport?

____

____

Case 2: A woman has a piece of dirt in her eye. She tells you her eye has been tearing for thirty minutes but she can still feel the particle. She is also wearing contact lenses.

1. A small foreign object may be removed from the eye with ______________________________ .

2. What should be done about contact lenses in a victim's eyes?

____

____

Nosebleeds

T F 1. Cold compresses on the victim's nose and face may help control a nosebleed.
T F 2. Regardless of what a first aider may do, there are some nosebleeds that he or she cannot control.
T F 3. Neither gauze nor cotton should be inserted into the nostrils to control a nosebleed.
T F 4. If cerebrospinal fluid is present in the blood coming from the nose, an attempt to stop the flow should be made.
T F 5. Most nosebleeds have blood coming from both nostrils.
T F 6. In older persons, bleeding most commonly occurs in the posterior part of the nose.
T F 7. The nosebleed victim should tilt his or her head slightly back while attempting to control the bleeding.
T F 8. Nosebleeds are most common in children.
T F 9. Blood can flow from the nose without it having been hit.
T F 10. The most effective procedure to control a nosebleed is pinching the nostrils.

Case: While playing in a summer baseball league, a twelve-year-old boy receives a smashing blow to the nose when he fails to catch a baseball. He is bleeding from the nose.

1. What is the emergency care in this situation?

A. ______________________________

B. ______________________________

2. What should be looked for when caring for this victim?

A. ______________________________

B. ______________________________

3. What additional body areas might be injured? Select two from the following list.

______ A. Neck
______ B. Back
______ C. Brain
______ D. Chest

4. Is it necessary for this victim to be transported for medical attention?

______ A. Yes. Why? ______________________________

______ B. No. Why not? ______________________________

Dental Emergencies

T F 1. Permanent teeth can be successfully reimplanted.
T F 2. Scrub the tooth before attempting to reimplant.
T F 3. Put the knocked-out tooth in mouthwash or alcohol to preserve it.
T F 4. Attempt reimplantation only if in remote areas (no dentist nearby).

Case: While riding a bicycle, ten-year-old Mike hit a chuckhole and fell off his bike. During the fall, his two upper front teeth were knocked out and another tooth broken.

1. Cite the emergency procedures in this case.

A. ______________________________

B. ______________________________

C. ______________________________

D. ______________________________

2. Successful replanting is best when done within ______ minutes of the accident.

3. What can be done for the broken tooth?

A. ______________________________

B. ______________________________

C. ______________________________

Larynx Injuries

T F 1. A tracheostomy is the same thing as a tracheotomy.
T F 2. A first aider can perform a tracheotomy and should when circumstances warrant.
T F 3. Laryngospasm can close off the airway.
T F 4. Grasping the base of the tongue and pulling it forward is one method to start a laryngospasm to relax within 45–60 seconds.
T F 5. Some drowned victims will experience laryngospasm.
T F 6. A person who has been hit across the larynx should be suspected to have an accompanying vertebral fracture.

Foreign Objects

T F 1. A foreign object in an eye can be "sneezed" out.
T F 2. Foreign objects in the ears and noses are most common among children.
T F 3. An insect in the ear may be attracted out by shining a flashlight into the ear.
T F 4. If a little oil (mineral, baby, olive) is used to float a foreign object out of an ear canal and the object is a bean or other type of seed, swelling of the object could occur if not retrieved.
T F 5. Impaled object in the cheek can be removed.
T F 6. Impaled objects in the chest or abdomen should be removed.
T F 7. Most foreign objects in an eye can be flushed out with water.
T F 8. When patching the injured eye, the uninjured eye should also be patched.

Blisters

T F 1. The skin of a broken blister should be left intact.
T F 2. Cover a broken blister with a sterile dressing.
T F 3. If not broken, a blister should not be deliberately broken.
T F 4. Blisters can be prevented.

Case: While on a ten-mile hike, a blister appears on your foot. It is painful enough to prevent you from continuing.

1. What could you try first?

____
____
____

2. When can a blister be broken?

____
____
____

3. What are the procedures to break a painful blister?

A. ______________________________
____
B. ______________________________
____
C. ______________________________
____
D. ______________________________
____
E. ______________________________
____

7 Poisoning

- Poisoning by Ingestion
- Insect Stings
- Snakebites
- Spider Bites
- Scorpion Stings
- Tick Removal
- Poison Ivy, Sumac, and Oak
- Carbon Monoxide
- Marine Animal Injuries
- Alcohol
- Drugs

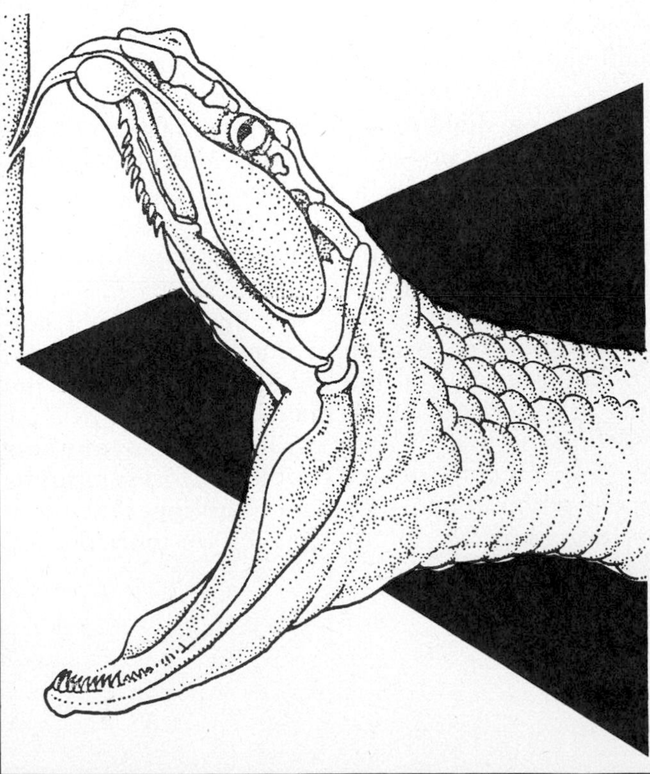

POISONING BY INGESTION

Poisoning is mainly a pediatric problem. Of the one million poisonings reported in the United States each year, about 75% occur in children under five, and most are caused by household products. Suicidal and homicidal attempts account for most adult poisonings.

It is beyond the scope of this book to provide an encyclopedia of poisons. Detailed information can be obtained from all local poison control centers, which are staffed by experienced people with access to information of the thousands of poisonous substances.

This section provides guidelines for the first aid and emergency care of poisoning in general. For each case, however, the first aider should seek advice from the local poison control center.

Poisons can enter the body through ingestion, inhalation, surface absorption, or injection. Ingested poisons usually remain in the stomach only a short time, and the stomach absorbs only small amounts. Most absorption takes place after the poison passes into the small intestine. Suspect poisoning in any person who suddenly has an onset of unexplained illness, especially an illness characterized by abdominal pain, nausea, and vomiting. Thus first aid is aimed at trying to rid the body of the poison before it reaches the intestines.

To manage a poisoned person, the first aider should obtain answers to the following questions:

1. What was ingested? The poison container and all its remaining contents, the plant, or a sample of what was ingested should be brought to the emergency department. If the person has vomited, save a sample of the vomitus in a clean, closed container and take it to the hospital with the victim.
2. When was the substance taken?
3. How much of the substance was taken?

The first aider should keep three basic principles in mind when managing the victim who has ingested a poison:

1. Maintain the airway.
2. If possible, identify the poison and answer the questions of when was the poison taken and how much was ingested. Then call the local poison control center (refer to Table 7-1 or telephone directory) for advice on proper procedures.
3. If inducing vomiting is advised by a medical authority, do so.

As a general rule, if the victim has ingested a poison within the past three to four hours, the stomach should be emptied, but there are important exceptions. Never induce vomiting in:

- The unresponsive, unconscious, or potentially unconscious victim
- The victim with seizures
- The pregnant woman
- The person with possible heart attack or a history of heart disease
- The victim who has ingested corrosives (strong acids or alkalies)
- The victim who has ingested petroleum products (e.g., kerosene, gasoline, lighter fluid, furniture polish)

For practically all other ingested poisons, the first aider should promptly empty the victim's stomach, if advised by a poison control center. Studies have shown that vomiting is the most effective way to empty the stomach of ingested poisons. To empty the victim's stomach in this way, you should:

1. Give syrup of ipecac—one tablespoonful (use the type used in cooking because household tablespoons hold less) with one to two glasses of water for a child over one year old, and two tablespoonfuls with two to three glasses of water to an adult. Other methods (e.g., salt water or gagging) are not reliable and may be dangerous.
2. Place the victim face down, with the head lower than the hips, to reduce the possibility of the victim's breathing in the vomitus.
3. If vomiting does not occur within twenty minutes, repeat the dose of ipecac and water once.
4. After vomiting stops, give activated charcoal.

The dose of charcoal should be eight to ten times the amount of the poison ingested. When the exact quantity of poison is unknown, a general guideline is to give about one-half of a lightly packed 8 ounce glass in about two cups of water for children. Double the amounts for an adult victim. The consistency should be similar to a thin milk shake so the victim can drink it. Mix the charcoal and water by shaking well in a jar. Children may require some persuasion to drink the mixture because of its uninviting appearance. A firm, positive approach generally works. Do not give activated charcoal with syrup of ipecac because the charcoal will inactivate the syrup of ipecac.

A shortcoming of ipecac is that it only removes 30%—40% of the poison, leaving the remaining 60%—70% to be absorbed and produce possible toxic effects. Therefore, the procedure for handling the remaining poison is the use of activated charcoal, which has a huge capability to bind chemicals. Ordinary charcoal is "activated" by heating it in carbon dioxide. This causes each grain of charcoal powder to expand like a sponge. Substances such as burnt toast, fireplace ashes, and charcoal briquettes are all ineffective in treating poisoning. Even though activated charcoal is effective and should be used more frequently, most pharmacies do not stock it because of a lack of demand.

Diluting poison with water or milk is often recommended. For many chemicals, especially those with corrosive effects (e.g., acids and alkalies), giving water or milk is appropriate. Water or milk dilutes the corrosive agent and decreases its potential for damaging tissues. However, dilution may actually increase the rate of absorption of tablets and capsules by causing them to dissolve more rapidly in the stomach. Also, large amounts of fluid can distend the stomach, which allows the contents to move into the small intestines faster, increasing the rate of absorption.

Therefore, dilution with water or milk should *not* be an automatic first aid procedure unless the poison control center advises, a corrosive is swallowed, or vomiting is to be induced immediately after dilution through the use of syrup of ipecac, which requires water to be effective.

Poisonous plants are the leading household poisoners, overtaking aspirin, which was once the leading child poisoner. Table 7-2 identifies some of the more prevalent poisonous plants. If the plant was ingested more than 12 hours earlier and no symptoms have appeared, there is no problem. Most symptoms appear within 4 hours of plant ingestion. Only with mushrooms are symptoms delayed for more than 12 hours.

TABLE 7-1. Certified Regional Poison Control Centers

Alabama

Alabama Poison Center
809 University Boulevard, East
Tuscaloosa, AL 35401
205/345-0600 (Administrative); 800/462-0800 (AL only)

Arizona

Arizona Poison Control System
AZ Health Sciences Center, Room 3204K
University of Arizona
Tucson, AZ 85724
602/626-6016; 800/362-0101 (AZ only)

California

Los Angeles County Medical Association
Regional Poison Information Center
1925 Wilshire Boulevard
Los Angeles, CA 90057
213/484-5151

San Diego Regional Poison Center
University of California Medical Center
225 Dickinson Street, H925
San Diego, CA 92103
619/294-6000 (Emergency)
619/294-3666 (Administrative)

San Francisco Bay Area Regional Poison Center
1E86, San Francisco General Hospital
1001 Potrero Avenue
San Francisco, CA 94110
415/666-2845; 800/233-3360

University of California Davis Medical Center
Regional Poison Control Center
2315 Stockton Boulevard
Sacramento, CA 95817
916/453-3414

Colorado

Rocky Mountain Poison Center
645 Bannock Street
Denver, CO 80204-4507
303/893-7774

District of Columbia

National Capital Poison Center
3800 Reservoir Road, NW
Washington, DC 20007
202/625-3333

Florida

Tampa Bay Regional Poison Control Center
P.O. Box 18582
Tampa, FL 33679
813/251-6995; 800/282-3171

Georgia

Georgia Poison Control Center
Grady Memorial Hospital
Box 26066
80 Butler Street, SE
Atlanta, GA 30335
404/589-4400

Illinois

St. John's Hospital, Springfield
Regional Poison Resource Center for
Central and Southern Illinois
800 East Carpenter Street
Springfield, IL 62769
217/753-3330; 800/252-2022

Indiana

Indiana Poison Center
1001 West Tenth Street
Indianapolis, IN 46202
317/630-7351; 800/382-9097
317/630-6382 (Administrative)

Iowa

University of Iowa Hospitals and Clinics
Poison Control Center
Pharmacy Department
Iowa City, IA 52242
319/356-2922

Kentucky

Kentucky Regional Poison Center
of Kosair Children's Hospital
P.O. Box 35070
Louisville, KY 40232-5070
502/562-7270; 800/722-5725 (KY only)

Louisiana

Louisiana Regional Poison Control Center
1501 Kings Highway
P.O. Box 33932
Shreveport, LA 71130
318/425-1524; 800/535-0525

Maryland

Maryland Poison Center
20 North Pine Street
Baltimore, MD 21201
301/528-7701

Michigan

Blodgett Regional Poison Center
Blodgett Memorial Medical Center
1840 Wealthy Street, SE
Grand Rapids, MI 49506
800/442-4571 (AC 616 only)
800/632-2727 (MI only)

Poison Control Center
Children's Hospital of Michigan
3901 Beaubien Boulevard
Detroit, MI 48201
313/494-5711

Minnesota

Hennepin Poison Center
701 Park
Minneapolis, MN 55415
612/347-3141

Minnesota Poison Control System
640 Jackson Street
St. Paul, MN 55101
612/221-2113; 800/222-1222
612/221-3096 (Administrative)

Missouri

Cardinal Glennon Children's Hospital
Regional Poison Center
1465 South Grand Boulevard
St. Louis, MO 63104
314/772-5200

Nebraska

Mid Plains Poison Control Center
Children's Memorial Hospital
8301 Dodge Street
Omaha, NE 68114
402/390-5434; 800/642-9999

New Jersey

New Jersey Poison Information
and Education System
201 Lyons Avenue
Newark, NJ 07112
201/926-8005; 800/962-1253 (NJ only)
201/926-8008 (TTY/TTD only)

New Mexico

New Mexico Poison & Drug Information Center
University of New Mexico
Albuquerque, NM 87131
505/843-2551; 800/432-6866

New York

Nassau County Medical Center's
Long Island Regional Poison Control Center
2201 Hempstead Turnpike
East Meadow, NY 11554
516/542-2323

New York City Poison Center
455 First Avenue, Room 123
New York, NY 10016
212/340-4494

North Carolina

Duke Poison Control Center
Box 3007
Duke University Medical Center
Durham, NC 27710
919/684-8111; 800/672-1697 (NC only)

Ohio

Central Ohio Poison Control Center
700 Children's Drive
Columbus, OH 43205
614/461-2012; 614/228-1323

Southwest Ohio Regional Poison Control System
Drug & Poison Information Center
University of Cincinnati
College of Medicine
231 Bethesda Avenue ML 144
Cincinnati, OH 45267-0144
513/872-5111

Pennsylvania

Pittsburgh Poison Center
125 DeSoto Street
Pittsburgh, PA 15213
412/647-5600

Rhode Island

Rhode Island Poison Center
593 Eddy Street
Providence, RI 02902
401/277-5906 (Administrative); 401/277-5727

Texas

North Central Texas Poison Center
at Parkland Memorial Hospital
P.O. Box 35926
Dallas, TX 75235
214/920-2586 (Administrative); 214/920-2400
800/441-0040 (TX only)

Texas State Poison Center
Eighth and Mechanic
The University of Texas Medical Branch
Galveston, TX 77550-2780
409/761-3332 (Administrative); 713/654-1701 (Houston)
800/392-8548 (TX only)

Utah

Intermountain Regional Poison Control Center
50 North Medical Drive, Building 428
Salt Lake City, UT 84132
801/581-2151

Washington

Seattle Poison Center
Children's Orthopedic Hospital
and Medical Center, Box 5371
4800 Sand Point Way, NE
Seattle, WA 98105
206/526-2121

TABLE 7-2. Common Poisonous Plants

Plant	Toxic Part	Symptoms and Comment
House Plants		
Castor bean	Seeds	Burning sensation in mouth and throat. Two to four beans may cause death. Eight usually lethal. Death has occurred in U.S.
Dieffenbachia (dumbcane), caladium, elephant's ear, some philodendrons	All parts	Intense burning and irritation of mouth, tongue, lips. Death from dieffenbachia has occurred when tissues at back of tongue swelled and blocked air passage to throat. Other plants have similar but less toxic characteristics.
Mistletoe	Berries	Can cause acute stomach and intestinal irritation. Cattle have been killed by eating wild mistletoe. People have died from "tea" of berries.
Poinsettia	Leaves, flowers	Can be irritating to mouth and stomach, sometimes causing vomiting and nausea, but usually produces no ill effects.
Vegetable Garden Plants		
Potato	Vines, sprouts (green parts), spoiled tubers	Death has occurred from eating large amounts of green parts. To prevent poisoning from sunburned tubers, green spots should be removed before cooking. Discard spoiled potatoes.
Rhubarb	Leaf blade	Several deaths from eating raw or cooked leaves. Abdominal pains, vomiting and convulsions a few hours after ingestion. Without treatment, death or permanent kidney damage may occur.
Ornamental Plants		
Atropa belladonna	All parts, especially black berries	Fever, rapid heartbeat, dilation of pupils, skin flushed, hot and dry. Three berries were fatal to one child.
Carolina jessamine, yellow jessamine	Flowers, leaves	Poisoned children who sucked nectar from flowers. May cause depression followed by death through respiratory failure. Honey from nectar also thought to have caused three deaths.
Daphne	Berries (commonly red, but other colors in various species), bark	A few berries can cause burning or ulceration in digestive tract causing vomiting and diarrhea. Death can result. This plant considered "really dangerous," particularly for children.
English ivy	Berries, leaves	Excitement, difficult breathing and eventually coma. Although no cases reported in United States, European children have been poisoned.
Golden chain (labumum)	Seeds, pods, flowers	Excitement, intestinal irritation, severe nausea with convulsions and coma if large quantities are eaten. One or two pods have caused illness in children in Europe.
Heath family (some laurels, rhododendron, azaleas)	All parts	Causes salivation, nausea, vomiting and depression. "Tea" made from two ounces of leaves produced human poisoning. More than a small amount can cause death. Delaware Indians used wild laurel for suicide.
Holly	Berries	No cases reported in North America, but thought that large quantities may cause digestive upset.

TABLE 7-2 continued

Jerusalem cherry	Unripe fruit, leaves, flowers	No cases reported, but thought to cause vomiting and diarrhea. However, when cooked, some species used for jellies and preserves.
Lantana	Unripe greenish-blue or black berries	Can be lethal to children through muscular weakness and circulatory collapse. Less severe cases experience gastrointestinal irritation.
Oleander	Leaves, branches, nectar of flowers	Extremely poisonous. Affects heart and digestive system. Has caused death even from meat roasted on its branches. A few leaves can kill a human being.
Wisteria	Seeds, pods	Pods look like pea pods. One or two seeds may cause mild to severe gastrointestinal disturbrances requiring hospitalization. No fatalities recorded. Flowers may be dipped in batter and fried.
Yew	Needles, bark, seeds	Ingestion of English or Japanese yew foliage may cause sudden death as alkaloid weakens and eventually stops heart. If less is eaten, may be trembling and difficulty in breathing. Red pulpy berry is little toxic, if at all, but same may not be true of small black seeds in it.
Trees and Shrubs		
Black locust	Bark, foliage, young twigs, seeds	Digestive upset has occurred from ingestion of the soft bark. Seeds may also be toxic to children. Flowers may be fried as fritters.
Buckeye, horsechestnut	Sprouts, nuts	Digestive upset and nervous symptoms (confusion, etc.). Have killed children but because of unpleasant taste are not usually consumed in quantity necessary to produce symptoms.
Chinaberry tree	Berries	Nausea, vomiting, excitement or depression, symptoms of suffocation if eaten in quantity. Loss of life to children has been reported.
Elderberry	Roots, stems	Children have been poisoned by eating roots or using pitty stems as blowguns. Berries are least toxic part but may cause nausea if too many are eaten raw. Proper cooking destroys toxic principle.
Jatropha (purge nut, curcas bean, peregrina, psychic nut)	Seeds, oil	Nausea, violent vomiting, abdominal pain. Three seeds caused severe symptoms in one person. However, in others as many as 50 have resulted in relatively mild symptoms.
Oaks	All parts	Eating large quantities of any raw part, including acorns, may cause slow damage to kidneys. However, a few acorns probably have little effect. Tannin may be removed by boiling or roasting, making edible.
Wild black cherry, chokecherries	Leaves, pits	Poisoning and death have occurred in children who ate large amounts of berries without removing stones. Pits or seeds, foliage and bark contain HCN (prussic acid or cyanide). Others to beware of: several wild and cultivated cherries, peach, apricot and some almonds. But pits and leaves usually not eaten in enough quantity to do serious harm.
Yellow oleander (be-still tree)	All parts, especially kernels of the fruit.	In Oahu, Hawaii, still rated as most frequent source of serious or lethal poisoning in man. One or two fruits may be fatal. Symptoms similar to fatal digitalis poisoning.

Poisonous Plants and Insects

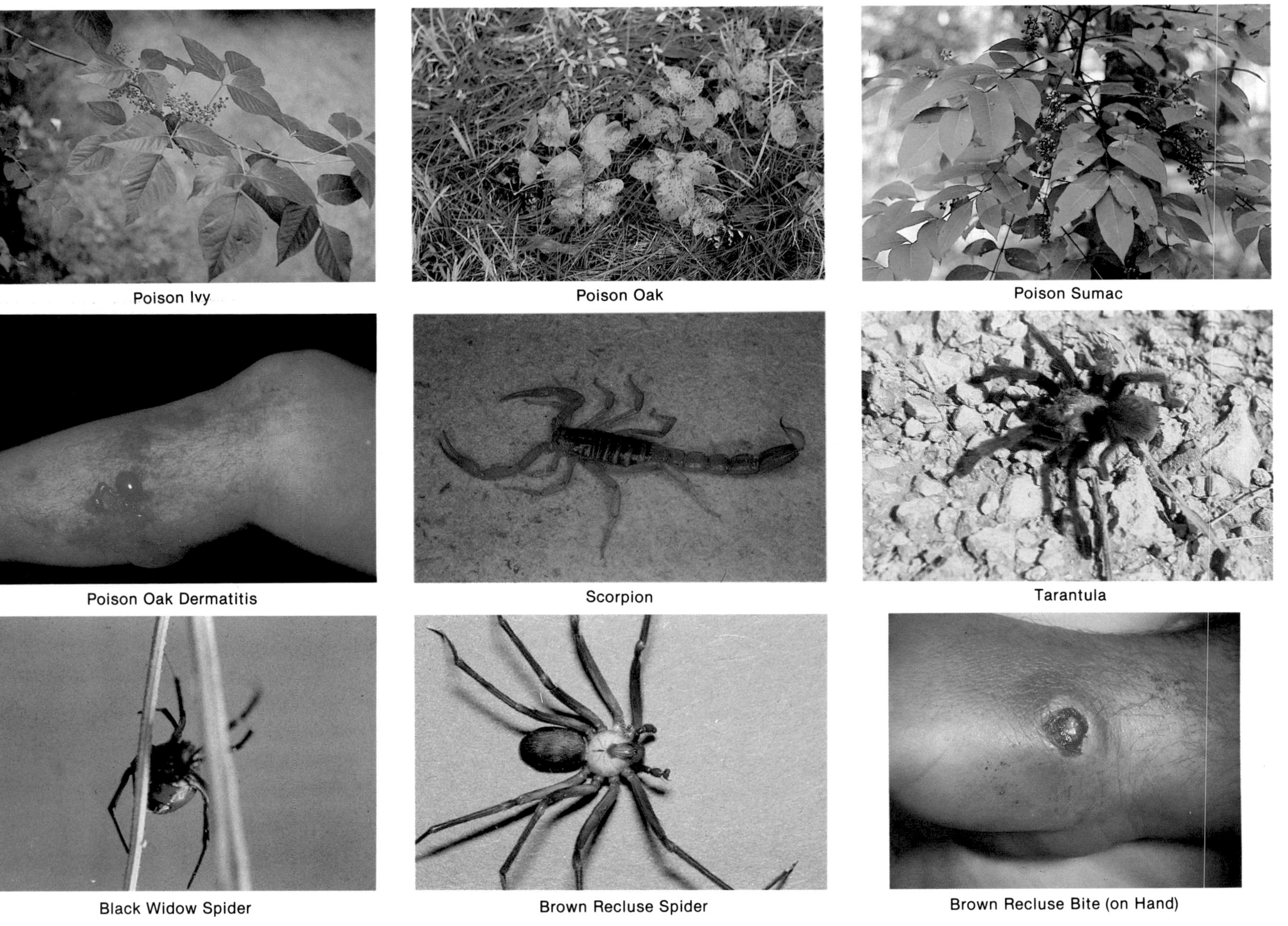

Poison Ivy

Poison Oak

Poison Sumac

Poison Oak Dermatitis

Scorpion

Tarantula

Black Widow Spider

Brown Recluse Spider

Brown Recluse Bite (on Hand)

Poisonous Snakes and Bites

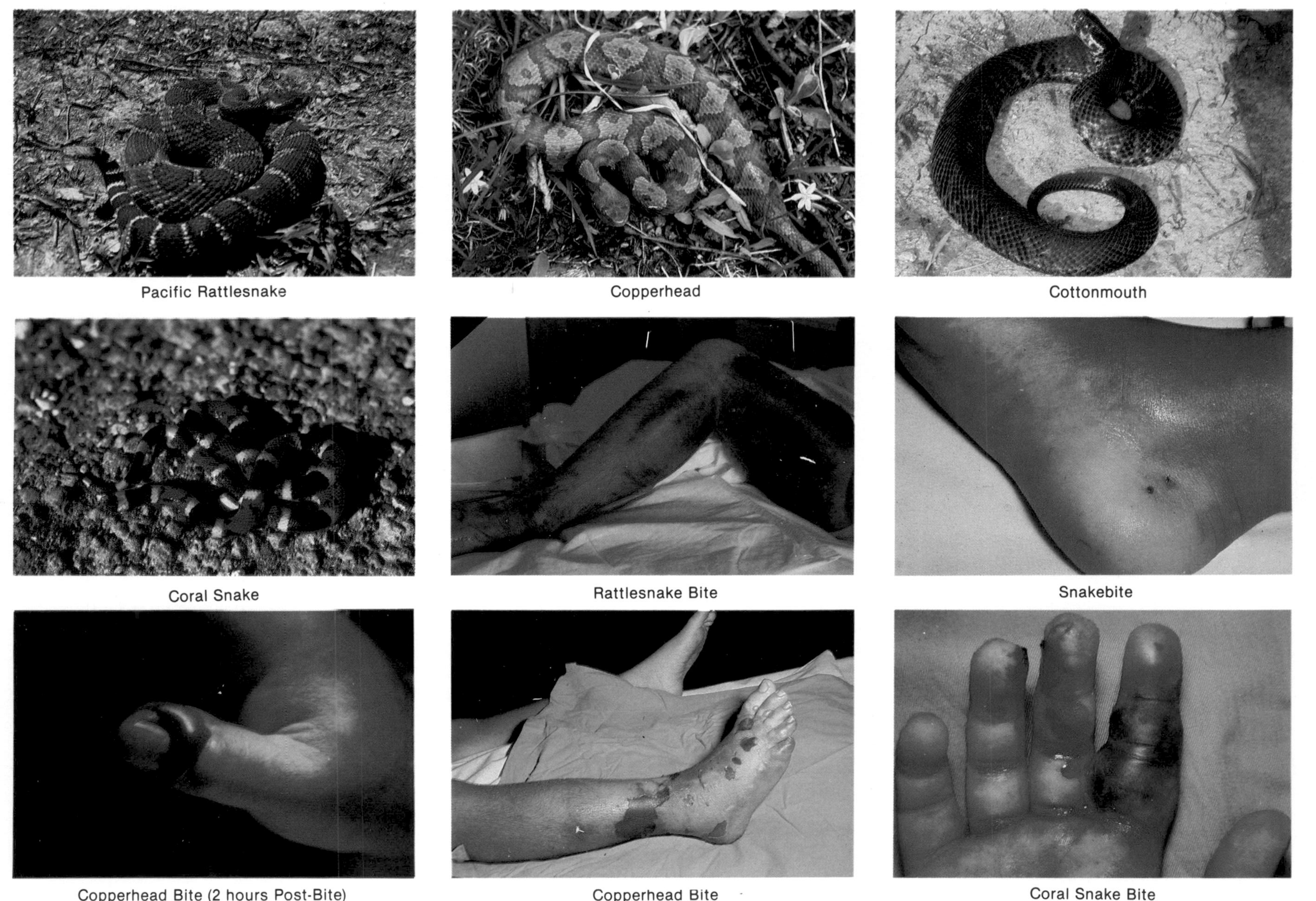

Pacific Rattlesnake

Copperhead

Cottonmouth

Coral Snake

Rattlesnake Bite

Snakebite

Copperhead Bite (2 hours Post-Bite)

Copperhead Bite

Coral Snake Bite

TABLE 7-2 continued

Flower Garden Plants		
Aconite, monkshood	Roots, flowers, leaves	Restlessness, salivation, nausea, vomiting, vertigo. Although people have died after eating small amounts of garden aconite, poisoning from it is not common.
Autumn crocus	All parts, especially bulbs	Burning pain in mouth, gastrointestinal irritation. Children have been poisoned by eating flowers.
Dutchman's breeches (bleeding heart)	Foliage, roots	No human poisonings or deaths, but a record of toxicity for livestock is warning that garden species may be dangerous.
Foxglove	All parts, especially leaves, flowers, seeds	One of the sources of the drug digitalis. May cause dangerously irregular heartbeat, digestive upset and mental confusion. Convulsions and death are possible.
Larkspur, delphinium	Seeds, young plant	Livestock losses are second only to locoweed in western United States. Therefore, garden larkspur should at least be held suspect.
Lily-of-the-valley	Leaves, flowers, fruit (red berries)	Produces glycoside like digitalis, used in medicine to strengthen the beat of a weakened heart. In moderate amounts, can cause irregular heartbeat, digestive upset and mental confusion.
Nicotiana, wild and cultivated	Leaves	Nervous and gastric symptoms. Poisonous or lethal amounts can be obtained from ingestion of cured smoking or chewing tobacco, from foliage of field-grown tobacco or from foliage of garden variety (flowering tobacco or nicotiana).
Wild Plants		
Baneberry (doll's-eyes)	Red or white berries, roots, foliage	Acute stomach cramps, headache, vomiting, dizziness, delirium. Although no loss of life in United States, European children have died after ingesting berries.
Death camas	Bulbs	Depression, digestive upset, abdominal pain, vomiting, diarrhea. American Indians and early settlers were killed when they mistook it for edible bulbs. Occasional cases still occur. One case of poisoning from flower reported.
Jack-in-the-pulpit, skunk cabbage	All parts, especially roots	Contains small needle-like crystals of calcium, oxalate and causes burning and severe irritation of mouth and tongue.
Jimsonweed (thornapple)	All parts, especially seeds and leaves	Thirst, hyper-irritability of nervous system, disturbed vision, delirium. Four to five grams of crude leaf or seed approximates fatal dose for a child. Poisonings have occurred from sucking nectar from tube of flower or eating fruits containing poisonous seeds.
Mayapple (mandrake)	Roots, foliage, unripe fruit	Large doses may cause gastroenteritis and vomiting. Ripe fruit is least toxic part and has been eaten by children—occasionally catharsis results. Cooked mayapples can be made into marmalade.
Nightshades, European bittersweet, horse nettle (solanum)	All parts, especially unripe berry	Children have been poisoned by ingesting a moderate amount of unripe berries. Digestive upset, stupefaction and loss of sensation. Death due to paralysis can occur. Ripe berries, however, are much less toxic.

TABLE 7-2 continued

Poison hemlock	Root, foliage, seeds	Root resembles wild carrot. Seeds have been mistaken for anise. Causes gradual weakening of muscular power and death from paralysis of lungs. Caused Socrates' death.
Pokeweed (pigeonberry)	Roots, berries, foliage	Burning sensation in mouth and throat, digestive upset and cramps. Produces abnormalities in the blood when eaten raw.
Water hemlock (cowbane, snakeroot)	Roots, young foliage	Salivation, tremors, delirium, violent convulsions. One mouthful of root may kill a man. Many persons, especially children, have died in United States after eating this plant. Roots are mistaken for wild parsnip or artichoke.

Source: National Safety Council, *Family Safety,* Spring 1979, pp. 18–19.

INSECT STINGS

The venom of Hymenoptera kills three to four times more people than that of snakebites. The number of deaths definitely known to have resulted from such stings averages about forty a year; however, many deaths identified as natural causes or heart attack may actually have been from insect stings.

For a severely allergic person, a single sting may be fatal within 15 minutes. Although there are accounts of individuals who have survived some 2,000 stings, generally 500 or more will bring about the death of those not allergic to stinging insects.

First aiders need to know more about this important problem. Refer to Table 7–3 for more information. First aiders need to know if a reaction is dangerous and when a victim should be seen by a physician. A knowledge of emergency care procedures, as well as preventive measures, is also important.

Fatalities from Hymenoptera most frequently occur during the summer months when exposure is maximum. Most stings are on the head, neck, or feet. About two-thirds of those who die from Hymenoptera stings die within one hour, which stresses the importance and the need for immediate medical treatment.

Types of Reactions

Dr. Claude A. Frazier,* a noted authority, identifies the symptoms of most stings. The normal reaction to an insect sting or bite is momentary pain; redness around the bite or sting site, surrounded by a whitish zone; itching; irritation; and heat. All traces are usually gone within a few hours.

Dr. Frazier cites the following as an allergic or systemic reaction to a sting or bite:

- Early reaction symptoms—itching around the eyes; dry, hacking cough; widespread hives; constriction of chest and throat; wheezing; nausea; abdominal pain; vomiting; dizziness
- More severe symptoms—difficulty in breathing; hoarseness and thickened speech; difficulty in swallowing; confusion, a sense of impending disaster
- Anaphylactic shock symptoms—cyanosis (bluish, purplish, or grayish coloring of the skin); collapse; unconsciousness.

Emergency Care

Carefully examine the sting site to determine whether a stinger is still embedded in the skin. If it is embedded, remove it to prevent further injection of toxin into the skin. If the stinger is left in the skin (only honeybees leave a stinger), it will continue to inject venom through spasmodic muscle contractions for two or three minutes unless immediately removed. Scrape off the stinger with your fingernail or a knife (*see* Figure 7-1). Removal with the fingers or tweezers exerts pressure on the venom sac, and the victim will get the full amount of venom.

After examining the sting site and removing any stinger, place an ice pack over the affected area to slow absorption of the toxin into the bloodstream. An ice pack relieves some of the pain associated with the sting. Wash the site with soap and water to cleanse the area of bacteria.

Full strength household ammonia or sodium bicarbonate (baking soda) paste usually helps control the pain. Some suggest smearing a paste of water and meat tenderizer on the sting site to reduce discomfort. An antihistamine may prevent some local symptoms if administered early, and an analgesic may be needed for pain relief. The victim should be observed for at least thirty minutes for signs of an allergic reaction.

*Claude A. Frazier and F.K. Brown, *Insects and Allergy and What To Do About Them* (Norman, Oklahoma: University of Oklahoma Press, 1980), pp. 57–58.

TABLE 7-3 Facts About Troublesome Insects

Description	Habitat	Problem	Severity	Treatment	Protection
Chigger Oval with red velvety covering. Sometimes almost colorless. Larva has six legs. Harmless adult has eight and resembles a small spider. Very tiny—about 1/20-inch long.	Found in low damp places covered with vegetation: shaded woods, high grass or weeds, fruit orchards. Also lawns and golf courses. From Canada to Argentina.	Attaches itself to the skin by inserting mouthparts into a hair follicle. Injects a digestive fluid that causes cells to disintegrate. Then feeds on cell parts. It does not suck blood.	Itching from secreted enzymes results several hours after contact. Small red welts appear. Secondary infection often follows. Degree of irritation varies with individuals.	Lather with soap and rinse several times to remove chiggers. If welts have formed, dab antiseptic on area. Severe lesions may require antihistamine ointment.	Apply proper repellent to clothing, particularly near uncovered areas such as wrists and ankles. Apply to skin. Spray or dust infested areas (lawns, plants) with suitable chemicals.
Bedbug Flat oval body with short broad head and six legs. Adult is reddish brown. Young are yellowish white. Unpleasant pungent odor. From ⅛- to ¼-inch in length.	Hides in crevices, mattresses, under loose wallpaper during day. At night travels considerable distance to find victims. Widely distributed throughout the world.	Punctures the skin with piercing organs and sucks blood. Local inflammation and welts result from anticoagulant enzyme that bug secretes from salivary glands while feeding.	Affects people differently. Some have marked swelling and considerable irritation; others aren't bothered. Sometimes transmits serious diseases.	Apply antiseptic to prevent possible infection. Bug usually bites sleeping victim, gorges itself completely in 3 to 5 minutes and departs. It's rarely necessary to remove one.	Spray beds, mattresses, bed springs, and baseboards with insecticide. Bugs live in large groups. They migrate to new homes on water pipes and clothing.
Brown Recluse Spider Oval body with eight legs. Light yellow to medium dark brown. Has distinctive mark shaped like a fiddle on its back. Body from ⅜- to ½-inch long, ¼-inch wide, ¾-inch from toe-to-toe.	Prefers dark places where it's seldom disturbed. Outdoors: old trash piles, debris, and rough ground. Indoors: attics, storerooms, closets. Found in Southern and Midwestern United States.	Bites producing an almost painless sting that may not be noticed at first. Shy, it bites only when annoyed or surprised. Left alone, it won't bite. Victim rarely sees the spider.	In 2 to 8 hours pain may be noticed followed by blisters, swelling, hemorrhage, or ulceration. Some people experience rash, nausea, jaundice, chills, fever, cramps, or joint pain.	Summon doctor. Bite may require hospitalization for a few days. Full healing may take from 6 to 8 weeks. Weak adults and children have been known to die.	Use caution when cleaning secluded areas in the home or using machinery usually left idle. Check firewood, inside shoes, packed clothing and bedrolls—frequent hideways.
Black Widow Spider Color varies from dark brown to glossy black. Densely covered with short microscopic hairs. Red or yellow hourglass marking on the underside of the female's abdomen. Male does not have this mark and is not poisonous. Overall length with legs extended is 1½ inch. Body is ¼-inch wide.	Found with eggs and web. Outside: in vacant rodent holes, under stones, logs, in long grass, hollow stumps, and brush piles. Inside: in dark corners of barns, garages, piles of stone, wood. Most bites occur in outhouses. Found in Southern Canada, throughout United States, except Alaska.	Bites causing local redness. Two tiny red spots may appear. Pain follows almost immediately. Larger muscles become rigid. Body temperature rises slightly. Profuse perspiration and tendency toward nausea follow. It's usually difficult to breathe or talk. May cause constipation, urine retention.	Venom is more dangerous than a rattlesnake's but is given in much smaller amounts. About 5% of bite cases result in death. Death is from asphyxiation due to respiratory paralysis. More dangerous for children; to adults its worst feature is pain. Convulsions result in some cases.	Use an antiseptic such as alcohol or hydrogen peroxide on the bitten area to prevent secondary infection. Keep victim quiet and call a doctor. Do not treat as you would a snakebite since this will only increase the pain and chance of infection; bleeding will not remove the venom.	Wear gloves when working in areas where there might be spiders. Destroy any egg sacs you find. Spray insecticide in any area where spiders are usually found, especially under privy seats. Check them out regularly. General cleanliness, paint, and light discourage spiders.
Scorpion Crablike appearance with claw-like pincers. Fleshy post-abdomen or "tail" has five segments, ending in a bulbous sac and stinger. Two poisonous types: solid straw yellow or yellow with irregular black stripes on back. From 2½ to 4 inches long.	Spends days under loose stones, bark, boards, floors of outhouses. Burrows in the sand. Roams freely at night. Crawls under doors into homes. Lethal types are found only in the warm desert-like climate of Arizona and adjacent areas.	Stings by thrusting its tail forward over its head. Swelling or discoloration of the area indicates a non-dangerous, though painful, sting. A dangerously toxic sting doesn't change the appearance of the area, which does become hypersensitive.	Excessive salivation and facial contortions may follow. Temperature rises to over 104°F. Tongue becomes sluggish. Convulsions, in waves of increasing intensity; may lead to death from nervous exhaustion. First 3 hours most critical.	Apply constriction. Keep victim quiet and call a doctor immediately. Do not cut the skin or give pain killers. They increase the killing power of the venom. Antitoxin, readily available to doctors, has proved to be very effective.	Apply a petroleum distillate to any dwelling places that cannot be destroyed. Cats are considered effective predators, as are ducks and chickens, though the latter are more likely to be stung and killed. Don't go barefoot at night.
Bee Winged body with yellow and black stripes. Covered with branched or feathery hairs. Makes a buzzing sound. Different species vary from ½ to 1 inch in length.	Lives in aerial or underground nests or hives. Widely distributed throughout the world wherever there are flowering plants—from the polar regions to the equator.	Stings with tail when annoyed. Burning and itching with localized swelling occur. Usually leaves venom sac in victim. It takes between 2 and 3 minutes to inject all the venom.	If a person is allergic, more serious reactions occur—nausea, shock, unconsciousness. Swelling may occur in another part of the body. Death may result.	Gently scrape (don't pluck) the stinger so venom sac won't be squeezed. Wash with soap and antiseptic. If swelling occurs, contact doctor. Keep victim warm while resting.	Have exterminator destroy nests and hives. Avoid wearing sweet fragrances and bright clothing. Keep food covered. Move slowly or stand still in the vicinity of bees.
Mosquito Small dark fragile body with transparent wings and elongated mouthparts. From ⅛- to ¼-inch long.	Found in temperate climates throughout the world where the water necessary for breeding is available.	Bites and sucks blood. Itching and localized swelling result. Bite may turn red. Only the female is equipped to bite.	Sometimes transmits yellow fever, malaria, encephalitis, and other diseases. Scratching can cause secondary infections.	Don't scratch. Lather with soap and rinse to avoid infection. Apply antiseptic to relieve itching.	Destroy available breeding water to check multiplication. Place nets on windows and beds. Use proper repellent.
Tarantula Large dark "spider" with a furry covering. From 6 to 7 inches in toe-to-toe diameter.	Found in Southwestern United States and the tropical varieties are poisonous.	Bites produce pin-prick sensation with negligible effect. It will not bite unless teased.	Usually no more dangerous than a pin prick. Has only local effects.	Wash and apply antiseptic to prevent the possibility of secondary infection.	Harmless to man, the tarantula is beneficial since it destroys harmful insects.
Tick Oval with small head; the body is not divided into definite segments. Grey or brown. Measures from ¼ to ¾ inch when mature.	Found in all United States areas and in parts of Southern Canada, on low shrubs, grass, and trees. Carried around by both wild and domestic animals.	Attaches itself to the skin and sucks blood. After removal there is danger of infection, especially if the mouthparts are left in the wound.	Sometimes carries and spreads Rocky Mountain spotted fever, tularemia Colorado tick fever. In a few rare cases, causes paralysis until removed.	Gently remove with tweezers so none of the mouthparts are left in skin. Wash with soap and water; apply antiseptic.	Cover exposed parts of body when in tick-infested areas. Use proper repellent. Remove ticks attached to clothes, body. Check neck and hair. Bathe.

Source: National Safety Council, *Family Safety*, Spring 1980, pp. 20–21.

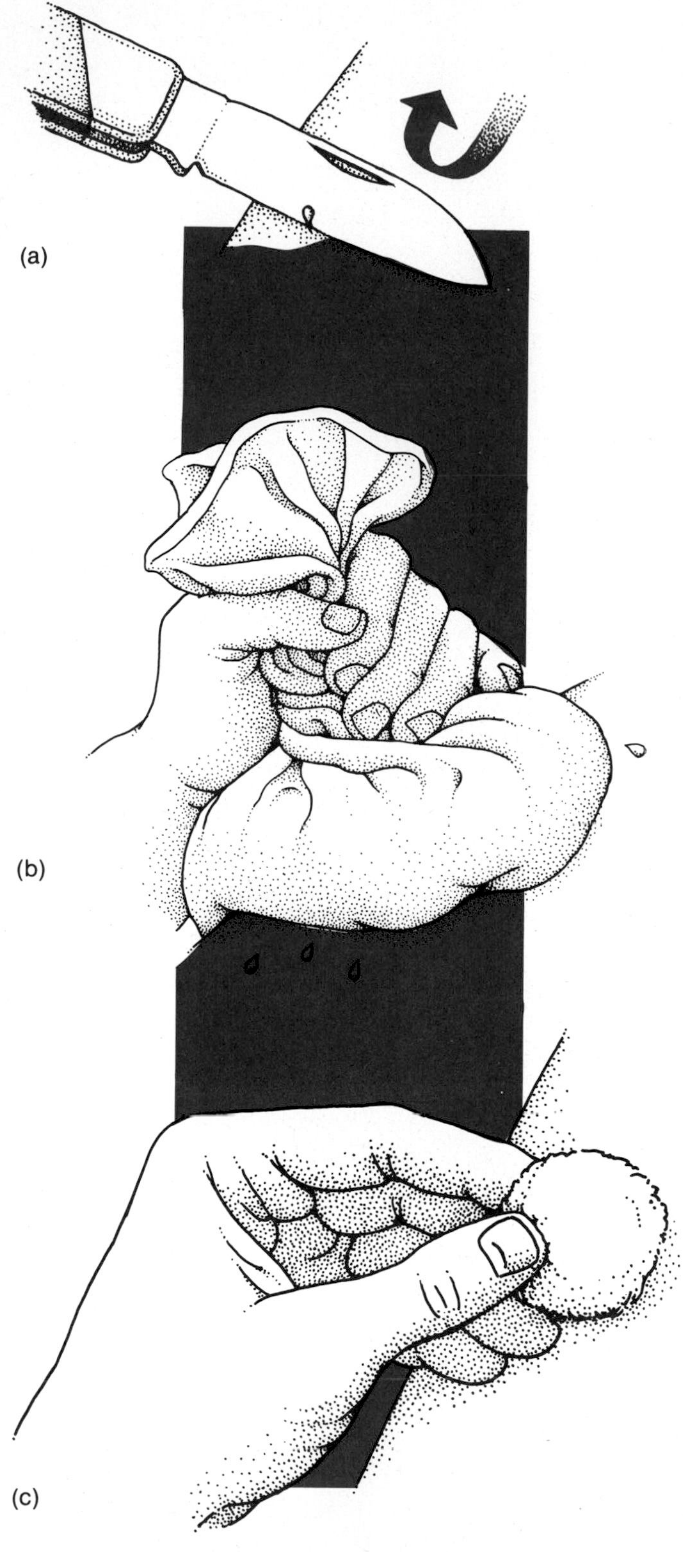

7-1. Bee stings
(a) If stinger is visible, carefully remove it with the edge of a knife or fingernail. Do not squeeze the stinger.
(b) Wash bee sting site with soap and water and put ice or a cold compress on the sting.
(c) Relieve the pain with a baking soda paste or full strength household ammonia.

The only effective treatment for insect sting anaphylaxis is the injection of epinephrine. Epinephrine should not be used to treat a sting unless anaphylaxis ensues, and on many occasions untrained persons might use the drug inappropriately. Finally, epinephrine has a limited shelf life of one to three years or when it has turned brown; therefore, over-the-counter kits would become outdated and ineffective. Such kits are, however, available through a prescription from a medical doctor.

These emergency insect sting kits contain a preloaded syringe of aqueous epinephrine and fast-acting antihistamine capsules or tablets. Antihistamines are of little value in treating the immediate and life-threatening reaction. The epinephrine (0.3 ml) is given subcutaneously at the sting site. Many kits also contain a constriction band. The kits contain simple instructions that almost any layman could follow.

Victims having had moderate to severe reactions with insect stings in the past should always be told to go to the nearest medical facility after a sting. Since epinephrine is short acting, the victim must be watched closely for signs of returning shock, and small doses of epinephrine should be injected as often as every fifteen minutes as needed.

SNAKEBITES

"Cut; don't cut." "Use a tourniquet; don't use a tourniquet."

"Capture the snake; don't capture the snake." "Use ice; don't use ice." "Use antivenin; don't use antivenin." "Apply mouth suction; don't apply mouth suction."

All these are offered in first aid and medical literature as proper first aid procedures for snakebite. With the maze of confusions about what to do in the event of a poisonous snakebite, it is amazing that only a dozen people die yearly from snakebite out of the 8,000 annually bitten by poisonous snakes. Rattlesnakes account for about 60% of venomous snakebites and for almost all the deaths.

Since opinions vary as to the correct first aid procedures, some of these opinions are misleading and occasionally dangerous.

Do not cool the bite site with ice: Some medical experts believe that cooling the bite with ice water or ice packs will slow the spread of the venom. The cold treatment of snakebite has fallen into disrepute. When it was thought that the only harmful substances in venom were enzymes, use of cold seemed reasonable. However, the more toxic effect of peptides in venom were overlooked, and it was found that they are not affected by cold temperatures.

A second problem with using ice is the freezing of tissue, thus the snakebite victim may receive frostbite as well. A third reason for not using a cold treatment is that the enzymes produced in any animal body generally are active at that animal's average body temperature. Snakes are cold-blooded animals. Thus, enzymes produced by cold-blooded animals are active at low temperatures.

Do not cut through the bite wound: Do not perform cuts if the victim is several hours from a medical facility—just quietly transport the victim. Since most bites occur at home, not in the wild, cutting should seldom be done. If thirty minutes has elapsed since the bite occurred, no cutting should be performed.

In situations other than the preceding ones, cutting over the fang marks should be done. The cut should be carefully done along the fang's path. Do *not* make cross cuts. Cuts should not be deeper (1/8 inch) than the skin because of the closeness of nerves and muscles. Cuts should be no more than 1/4 inch long. Cuts should not be made elsewhere. (*See* Figure 7-2.)

First aiders should not give antivenin: Only qualified medical personnel should administer antivenin because many people are allergic to it. Antivenin can be helpful if given within four hours, but it is of doubtful value if administered later than that.

Do not apply a tourniquet: A tourniquet is tight enough to stop arterial and venous blood flow which may result in the loss of the limb. Rather, you should apply a constriction band which allows a finger to be wedged under it in order to allow some arterial blood flow. Loosen the constriction band slightly as swelling appears, but do not release.

Do not capture the snake: The type of snake should be identified, but do not waste time if it is elusive. A pit viper bite can usually be identified by two large puncture wounds, blood oozing, and progressive swelling and discoloration.

Apply suction over the cut: Suction cups found in a snakebite kit are usually adequate. However, you could use mouth suction, but the danger of introducing infection to the wound is much greater. If you have sores or unfilled tooth caries, you could contract venom from the bite. Rinsing the mouth between suctions is suggested. Suction is only effective for about thirty minutes.

Other considerations in snakebite treatment are: immobilize the arm or leg below the heart; wash the wound thoroughly with soap and water; and carry the victim if possible, or have him move slowly if he must walk.

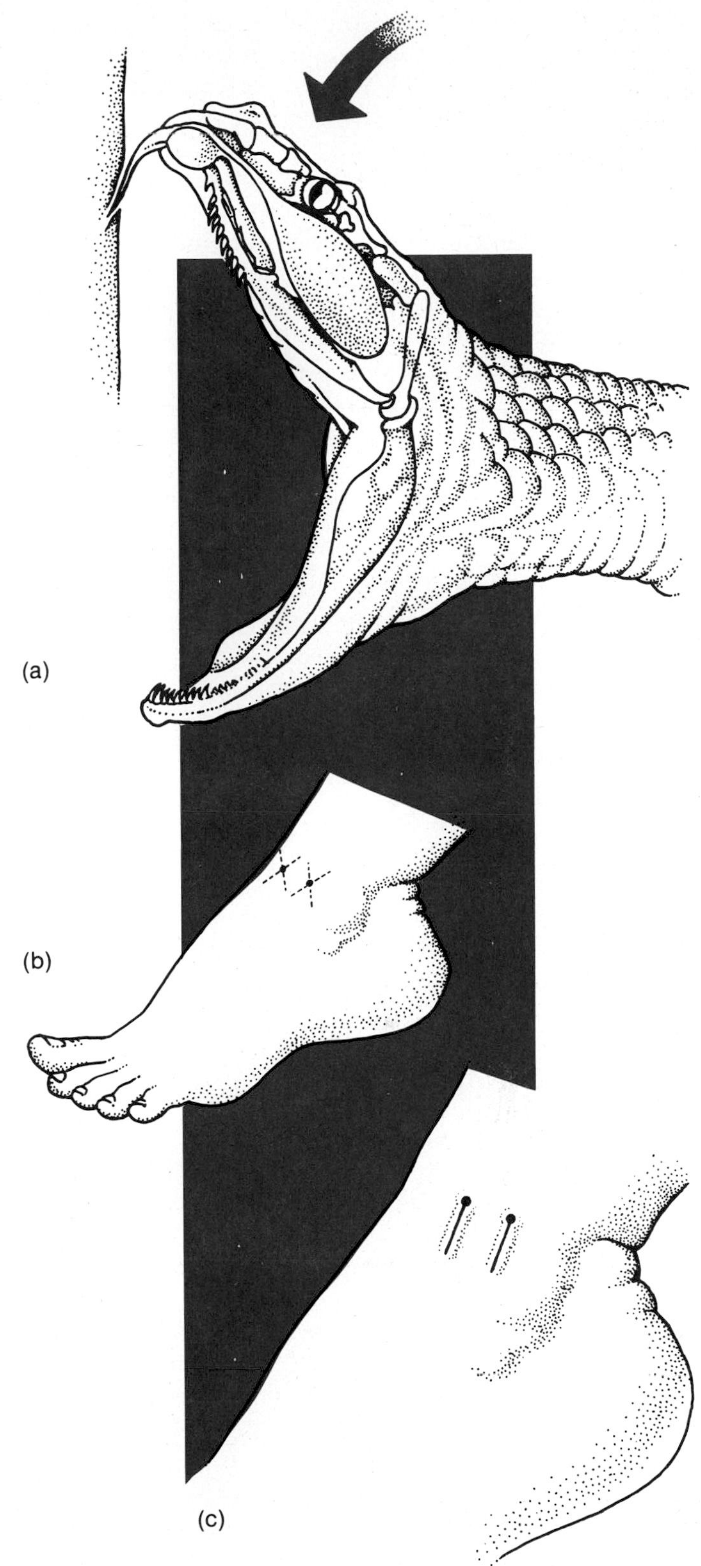

7-2. Snakebite
(a) Pit vipers inject their fangs in a slanting, shallow penetration.
(b) Do *not* use cross cuts when cutting and sucking are needed in snakebite cases.
(c) If incisions are to be used, make two parallel cuts starting at the punctures and extending along the presumed path of the fangs. Cuts are 1/8 inch deep and about 1/4 inch long.

Summary

- Get the victim away from the snake. Snakes have been known to bite more than once. Transport the victim to a physician or emergency department as rapidly and carefully as possible.

- Apply a constriction band above the bite area. Be sure that a finger can pass under the band, showing that it is not too tight. Do not periodically release it, unless you are one and one-half hours or more away from a physician.
- If feasible, do not allow the victim to walk, thus lessening the spread of the venom.
- If you are more than one and one-half hours from an emergency medical facility, or if a large snake is the offender, immediately use incision and suction. You can remove 22% to 50% of the venom with this method, if it is done within three minutes; a lesser quantity can be removed up to thirty minutes. A 1/4-inch incision going lengthwise through each fang mark, no more than 1/8 inch deep, is all that is necessary. Cross-cut incisions are not recommended. Use mouth suction if no other method is available.
- Transport the victim as rapidly as possible. If feasible, call ahead to report an extreme emergency.
- Perform CPR if the victim stops breathing or has no pulse.
- Use absolutely no form of cooling.
- Antivenin should not be used in the field due to a possible allergic reaction to horse serum.

Coral Snakebite

The coral snake is America's most venomous snake. This snake has short fangs and "chews" its venom into the victim. First aid includes washing the bitten area, transporting the victim to a hospital quickly, and not using a constriction band nor incision or suction.

SPIDER BITES

Just about all spiders are venomous—that is how they paralyze and kill their prey. Very few spiders, however, have fangs long enough to endanger the health of man.

The few fatal spider bites seen in this country are attributable to the black widow or to the brown recluse spider. (Refer to Table 7-3.) For a long time the black widow was thought to be the only highly poisonous spider in North America. In the late 1950s, reports began to appear about the bite of the brown recluse.

Black Widow Spider

Black widow spiders live in all states but Alaska. The female can be identified by a red spot on the abdomen—she is the one that bites. (Males do not have fangs large enough to puncture the site.) She has a coal black body. (*See* Figure 7-3.)

They hide in wood and brush piles, long grass, and under stones and logs. Most bites occur on the hands and forearms between April and October when humans are outside rooting around in seldom-used places.

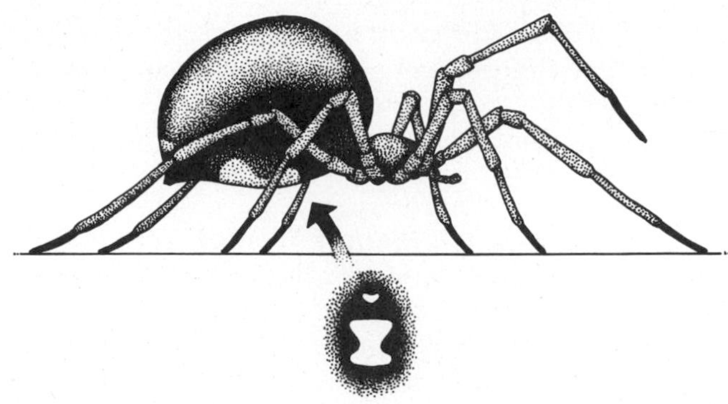

7-3. Female black widow spider with typical hourglass on the abdomen

Determining whether a person has been bitten by a black widow spider is difficult. After a sharp pinprick of the spider's bite is felt, it usually takes no more than fifteen minutes for a dull, numbing pain to develop in the bitten extremity. Muscle cramps occur next, usually affecting the abdomen when the bite is in the lower extremities and the shoulders, back, or chest when it is on the upper. Headache, heavy sweating, dizziness, nausea, and vomiting also can occur.

Even without treatment, most healthy adults will survive. However, black widow bites threaten the lives of children and the elderly.

By volume, black widow spider venom is more deadly than the rattlesnake's, but it is injected in much smaller amounts.

If possible, the spider should be caught to confirm its identify. Even if the body is crushed, save it for identification.

Victims of black widow spider bites should get medical help immediately. At the hospital, the wound is cleaned, muscle relaxants are given, and calcium gluconate is administered to relieve cramping. There is an antivenin for black widow bites. The antivenin brings relief of symptoms within one to three hours, especially if given as soon as possible after the victim was bitten.

The bitten area can be cleaned with alcohol. Do not apply a constricting band because the black widow venom's action is swift, and there is little to be gained by trying to slow absorption with a constriction band. In fact, it will hasten tissue death. An ice pack may be placed over the bite to relieve pain. Keep the victim quiet, and be alert for any respiratory difficulty.

Brown Recluse Spider

The initial pain felt from a brown recluse spider may be slight enough to be overlooked at first. The first signs are usually a blister at the bite site, along with redness and swelling. Pain, which may remain mild but can become severe, develops within two to eight hours. Days later the bite site hardens, and within a week the flesh forms an ulcer. Gangrene may develop in some cases.

First aid consists of cold packs and disinfecting the bite site. The victim should be transported to a medical facility as quickly as possible. If possible, the biting spider should be captured and taken with the victim for accurate physician diagnosis and treatment.

The brown recluse spider has a brown, possibly purplish, violin-shape figure on its back. (*See* Figure 7-4.) Brown recluse bites are rarely fatal, except for hypersensitive people, or for children, the elderly, or those with chronic health problems.

Tarantula Spider

The tarantula is far more ominous looking than the other two poisonous spiders, but its bite rarely produces symptoms other than mild to moderate pain. Clean the bite wound to prevent infection. (Refer to Table 7-3.)

SCORPION STINGS

Scorpions are nocturnal and live under buildings, logs, and debris in hot dry areas of California, Arizona, New Mexico, and Mexico. (*See* Figure 7-5.) Death from the sting of the scorpion is rare in the United States. Apply an ice pack over the wound and take the victim to a medical facility. (Refer to Table 7-3.)

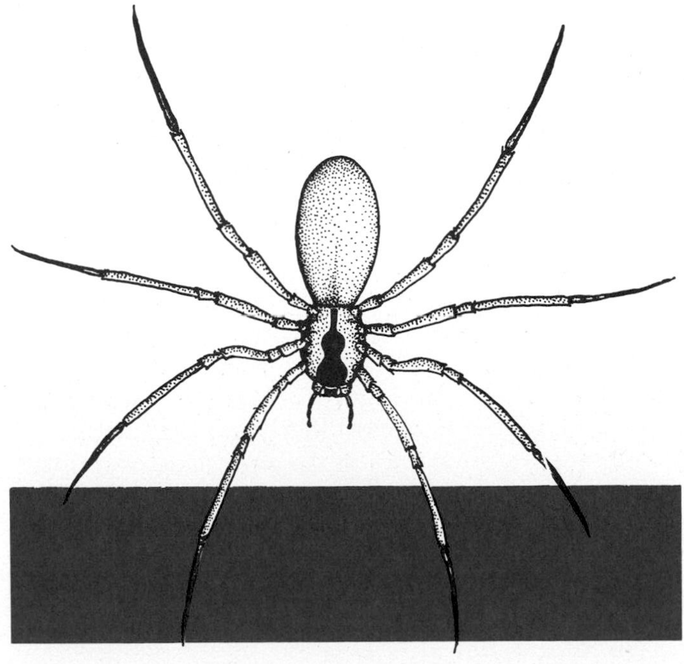

7-4. Brown recluse spider with typical violin-shaped marking on top

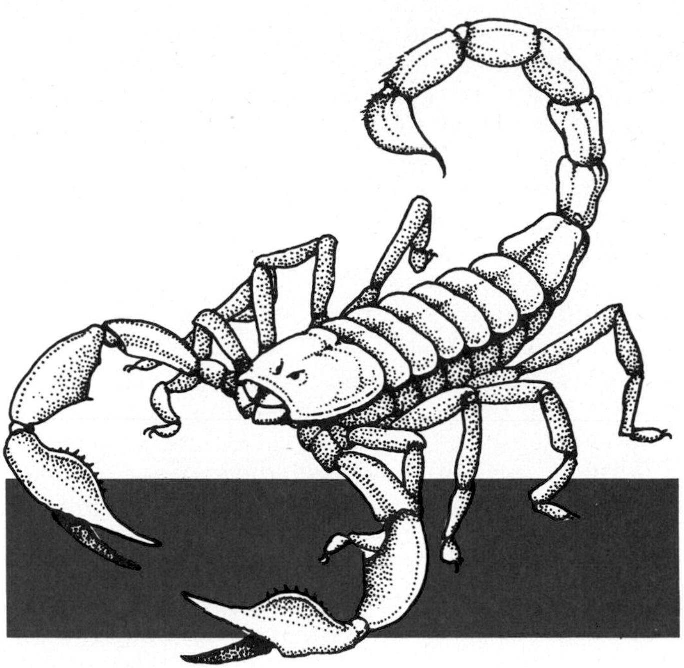

7-5. Scorpion

Its sting causes immediate pain around the sting site, followed by numbness or tingling. Severe cases may entail paralysis, spasms, or respiratory difficulties. Children are at greatest risk.

TICK REMOVAL

Of the infectious diseases that ticks carry, *Rocky Mountain spotted fever* can be one of the most severe and sometimes it can lead rapidly to death. Fortunately, only about 200 cases are reported yearly throughout the United States. Without specific antibiotic therapy, the mortality rate is more than 20%. Early medical treatment usually brings recovery; however, spotted fever has been mistakenly diagnosed as measles.

Colorado tick fever occurs only in the Rocky Mountain region. More ticks carry this disease than carry Rocky Mountain spotted fever, explaining why this disease is more common. In fact, the entire state of Colorado reports 200 cases yearly. The main difference between Colorado tick fever and Rocky Mountain spotted fever is the absence of a rash in the tick fever, and death has not been reported as a result of it.

Relapsing fever has occurred in the western part of the United States. The identifying mark of relapsing fever is recurrent fevers (lasting two to eight days with a rash), followed by a remission of three to ten days (no fever and the victim feels well), only to be followed by a relapse if the victim is not being medically treated.

Lyme disease is primarily found in the wooded vacation spots of the Northeast. Animals, such as deer, harbor the disease, which is transmitted by several tick species. The main sign of Lyme disease is a rash which appears an average of seven days after the tick bite. Arthritis is the major complication. Symptoms begin about a month after the rash and last from months to years. The heart and nervous system can also be affected.

In addition to being carriers of infectious diseases, ticks can produce several miserable conditions in human victims. A frightening looking granuloma (tumor or growth) can occur days or even months after the bite, even though all visible mouthparts have been removed. The cause is not completely known, but the granulomas are harmless and often disappear within a few months.

Tick paralysis can be quite serious especially if it occurs in the neck or spine area. The paralysis (occasionally fatal) begins in the legs, then moves upward. The paralysis is dramatically relieved when the tick is removed.

Four popular folk methods of tick removal—ways of inducing the tick to back out of the skin of its host—failed to work in a study carried out by Glen R. Needham.* Even if they worked, Dr. Needham says, the safest way to remove a tick is still to pull it off because that method lessens the likelihood of leaving behind tick secretions that later could lead to infection.

Dr. Needham tested the application of petroleum jelly, fingernail polish, 70% isopropyl alcohol, and a hot kitchen match as well as removal with tweezers or a protected hand as ways to remove ticks from a sheep.

After allowing a group of ticks to remain attached to the host for 72 to 96 hours, Dr. Needham attempted to remove them using the previously named methods. None of the ticks detached in a two-hour period.

To see whether any of these methods would work with ticks less firmly anchored, Dr. Needham applied them to a second group of sixteen that had been attached to the host for 12 to 15 hours. None of the ticks detached itself within 24 hours after application. Dr. Needham subsequently removed all of them intact by pulling with tweezers or protected fingers.

The strategy behind the use of petroleum jelly and perhaps behind the use of fingernail polish is presumably to deprive the tick of respiratory gas exchange, Dr. Needham says, but he points out that the tick breathes only a few times per hour when at rest and that a tick covered with fingernail polish probably cannot move on its own. The notion about getting ticks to back out persist, "probably because most people prefer not to touch them," he says.

Dr. Needham suggests the following removal method which you might want to use.

- Use tweezers or, if you have to use your fingers, protect your skin by using a paper towel or disposable tissue. Although few people ever encounter ticks infected with Rocky Mountain spotted fever or other disease, the person removing a tick may become infected by pathogens entering through breaks in the skin or through mucous membranes. For this reason, children should not be allowed to remove ticks from family pets.
- Grasp the tick as close to the skin surface as possible and pull away from the skin with a steady pressure or lift the tick slightly upward and pull parallel to the skin until the tick detaches. Do not twist or jerk the tick since this may result in incomplete removal. (*See* Figure 7-6.)
- Dispose of the tick by flushing it down a drain or wadding it in adhesive tape before placing it in the trash.
- Wash the bite site and your hands well with soap and water. Apply alcohol to further disinfect the area. Then apply a cold pack to reduce pain. Calamine lotion might aid in relieving any itching. Keep the region clean.

Dr. Needham says that in most instances you need not be overly concerned if the tick's cement is not removed or if the mouthpiece breaks off and remains in the skin.

Watch for signs of infection or unexplained symptoms, such as severe headaches, fever, or rash, which may develop three to ten days later. If these symptoms appear, seek medical care immediately.

POISON IVY, OAK, AND SUMAC

Two million Americans will suffer allergic contact dermatitis from poison ivy, poison oak, or poison sumac this year. (*See* Figure 7-7.) Young people are more susceptible than the elderly, and dark-skinned people seem somewhat less susceptible to dermatitis than others. It is estimated that at least 70% of the population of the United States would acquire dermatitis if casually exposed to the plants.

Resistance, or immunity, varies greatly from one person to another and even in the same person at different times, but probably no one is completely immune. Most people thought to be immune have just not been exposed under the right conditions.

*Glen R. Needham, "Evaluation of Five Popular Methods for Tick Removal," *Pediatrics*, Vol. 75, 1985, pp. 997-1002.

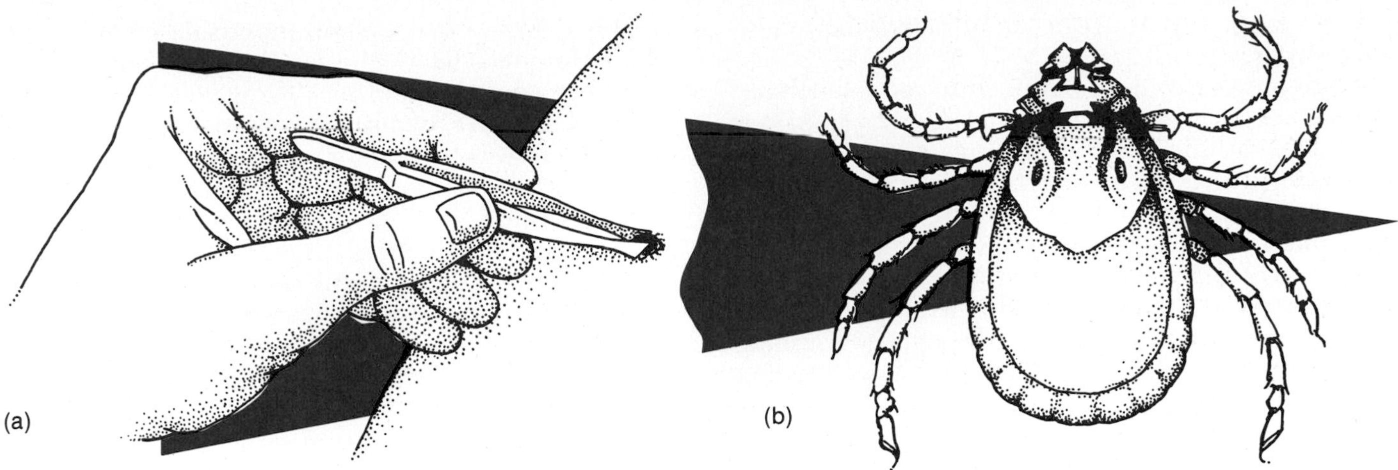

7-6. (a) Removing a tick with tweezers
(b) A Tick

Signs and Symptoms

Although the limbs, face, and neck are common sites of the dermatitis, all areas of the skin that come in contact with the sensitizing substance can be affected. However, different parts of the body may not have the same sensitivity; thus, the dermatitis may appear first in one area and later in another. The phenomenon is often called "spreading," but this description is inaccurate. Often, parts of the body that may sustain a heavy concentration of the allergen and exhibit more severe reactions will remain "hypersensitive" for years.

The characteristic burning, itching, rash, and swelling resulting from poison ivy, oak, or sumac contact may not follow for as long as ten days after exposure. A day or two is the usual interval between exposure and onset of signs and symptoms.

The rash first consists of streaks or patches of red discoloration of the skin associated with itching. Later, blisters develop which break down, resulting in oozing and crusting from the surface. Usually swelling of the tissue, burning, and itching are present. Avoid scratching because it can introduce infection or cause scarring. Scratching does not spread the rash. The blisters are filled with serum, not with urushiol, which causes the dermatitis.

Emergency Care

It has been demonstrated that washing delayed only five minutes after exposure does very little good.

Generally, the local treatment should be adapted to the stage or severity of the lesions. During the acute weeping and oozing stage, sodium bicarbonate (baking soda) solution should be used either as a soak, bath, or wet dressing for thirty minutes, three or four times a day. "Shake" lotions (calamine, zinc oxide) are used at night or when wet dressings are not desirable. Greasy ointments should not be used during active oozing. Unfortunately, there is no convincing evidence that any of the numerous over-the-

7-7. (a) Poison ivy
(b) Poison oak
(c) Poison sumac

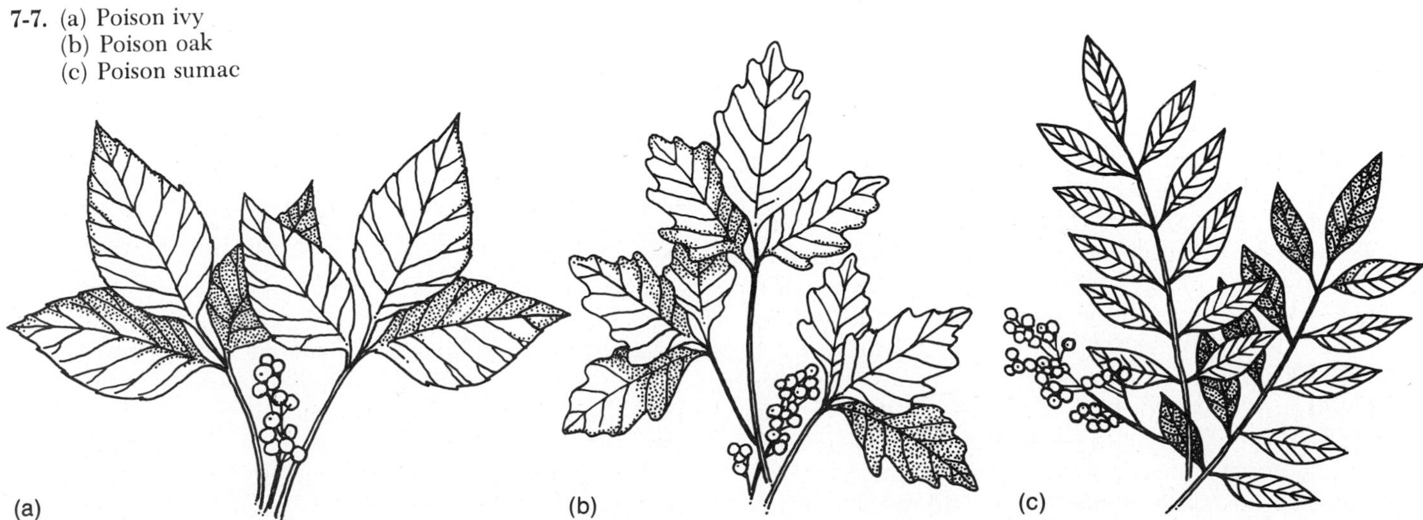

counter preparations are more effective than these few simple procedures.

Large blisters could be drained to reduce itching. Aseptic techniques should be used and the blister punctured at the edge. The tops of the broken blisters should be kept intact because they protect the underlying epidermis as they dry. Reassure the victim that the fluid from the blisters will not lead to spreading of the dermatitis, nor will touching someone with the dermatitis produce irritation. During the healing phase, application of a neutral soothing cream (such as cold cream) helps prevent crusting and scaling.

Studies indicate that not one medication tested was more effective than tap water compresses and "shake" lotions containing a soothing ingredient, such as zinc oxide or calamine. Antihistamines appeared to have no value taken by mouth or in ointments and lotions. In fact, ointments and lotions could even cause their own allergic reactions on top of the poison plant eruption.

When the dermatitis eruption affects a large part of the body, corticosteroids taken under the care of a physician may benefit most severely affected victims.

For severe itching, hot water—hot enough to redden the skin temporarily—may relieve discomfort. Heat releases histamine, the substance in the cells of the skin that causes the intense itching. Therefore, a hot shower or bath causes intense itching as the histamine is released. This depletes the cells of histamine and the victim will obtain up to eight hours of relief from itching. Using this method does not require frequent applications of ointment.

CARBON MONOXIDE

Carbon monoxide (CO) is produced by the incomplete combustion (burning) of any organic (carbon-containing) material. Incomplete combustion may occur with the burning of any fuel containing carbon, including coal, gas, kerosene, oil, wood, paper, and charcoal. Carbon monoxide is a nonirritating, colorless, tasteless, and odorless gas.

When you inhale air into your lungs, oxygen is transferred from the air to your blood. Oxygen attaches to a component of blood called hemoglobin; the hemoglobin carries the oxygen to the body's tissues. Carbon monoxide is also capable of attaching to the hemoglobin in the blood. The affinity of red blood cells (hemoglobin) for CO is more than two hundred times that for oxygen. When CO is attached to red blood cells instead of oxygen, the body is deprived. Therefore, a lethal concentration could be produced in as short a time as ten minutes.

The symptoms of carbon monoxide exposure include dizziness, headache, nausea, and vomiting followed or accompanied by loss of consciousness. In cases of massive exposures, consciousness may be lost with few or no other symptoms. Those who survive near lethal exposure will, if conscious, look and act intoxicated.

The traditionally cited sign of CO poisoning has been cherry-red color of the skin and lips. However, several studies indicate that the cherry-red color occurs at death and is, therefore, a poor initial indicator as to whether or not a person has been CO poisoned.

Children are affected worse than adults with CO poisoning. It is not unusual for a youngster, especially an infant, to have severe symptoms including unconsciousness, while adults subjected to exactly the same exposure may show little effect.

Women, because they are usually comparatively anemic, tend to fare less well than men. A person at complete rest is likely to be less affected than someone who was fairly active at the time of exposure.

Carbon monoxide poisoning can be fatal; all have probably heard of accidental deaths from carbon monoxide exposure. In such cases, the carbon monoxide level in the blood became so high that the person could not get enough oxygen to stay alive.

Sometimes people are exposed to carbon monoxide in amounts that do not threaten their lives but do make them feel dizzy or sick. Since the symptoms are indistinguishable from those of a viral infection such as the flu (headache, nausea, chills, dizziness, and tiredness), the person may not even realize what is causing the discomfort.

If you suspect carbon monoxide poisoning, remove the person from the source of the carbon monoxide and ventilate the area. Then, base your actions on the victim's condition:

- If the person is conscious, take him to a doctor who will perform a blood test to determine the level of carbon monoxide.
- If the person is unconscious, place him on his side with his head resting on his arm. Loosen tight clothing and maintain body heat with a blanket.
- If the person has stopped breathing, administer mouth-to-mouth respiration and CPR if you have been trained in cardiopulmonary resuscitation.

The *victim needs 100% oxygen as quickly as possible*. This will improve oxygenation and it also will disassociate the linkage between the carbon monoxide and the red blood cell. Therefore, either transport the victim to a hospital or call for an ambulance that carries oxygen.

Even when there are only mild symptoms, such as headache or nausea, it may be a good idea to check with a doctor if you suspect carbon monoxide poisoning.

MARINE ANIMAL INJURIES

Each year more than one million people are stung by jellyfish, corals, and anemones lying along the shallow ocean waters of the United States. Most will recover without medical attention; several will need emergency medical care for a period of time; some will die.

Jellyfish, anemones, and corals having stinging devices called nematocysts. These are tiny dart-like hairs lying coiled in small openings covering the surface of the tentacles and body. Each of the openings has a tiny trigger hair that protrudes and acts to "fire" the nematocysts in response to being touched.

Reactions to being stung by these ocean animals vary from mild dermatitis to almost instant death. When cast ashore or onto rocks, these animals can break into thousands of pieces. These detached pieces retain their ability to sting for a long period of time, usually until they are completely dehydrated.

The Portuguese man-of-war is probably the most familiar of the jellyfish specimens. It is not a single animal, but hundreds of small animals living together.

The Portuguese man-of-war is most abundant in warmer waters. It usually descends under the water during midday and darkness, returning to float on the surface in early morning and evening. The sting from the man-of-war is usually in the form of well defined linear welts or scattered patches of welts with redness and usually disappear within twenty-four hours.

Another ocean animal producing damage is the lion's mane jellyfish or sea nettle. Like that of the man-of-war, the sting of the lion's mane produces severe muscle cramping with multiple thin lines of welts crossing the skin in a zigzag pattern. Pain usually is a burning type lasting ten to thirty minutes. The welts on the skin usually disappear within an hour.

Emergency care for the sting of the jellyfish begins with immediate removal of any tentacles remaining on the skin. Use a towel, piece of clothing, or any material other than bare skin to scrape them off. Apply alcohol, suntan oil, or nearly any other solution directly to the welts to inhibit further activity by the nematocysts. Do not use water because it could cause the stinging cells to swell and become more difficult to remove. The victim must be kept warm and treated for shock. Be prepared to render mouth-to-mouth and/or cardiopulmonary resuscitation, if necessary.

There are hundreds of local remedies for jellyfish stings, each working with various degrees of success. Soap, sugar, vinegar, lemon juice, calamine lotion, meat tenderizer, ammonia, sodium bicarbonate, and boric acid are the most common.

The recovery period from stings of these ocean animals varies from hours to weeks. Note that recurrent stings may produce a sensitivity to the toxin, and subsequent stings could be fatal because of anaphylactic reactions.

ALCOHOL

Alcohol is a depressant, not a stimulant. Many people think alcohol is a stimulant because its first effect is to reduce tension and give a mild feeling of euphoria or exhilaration.

Alcohol affects a person's judgment, vision, reaction time, and coordination. In very large quantities, it can cause death by paralyzing the respiratory center of the brain.

The signs of alcohol intoxication are familiar to all. Some of them are:

1. Odor of alcohol on breath
2. Swaying and unsteadiness
3. Slurred speech
4. Nausea and vomiting
5. Flushed face

These signs can mean illnesses or injuries other than alcohol abuse (e.g., epilepsy, diabetes, or head injury). It is, therefore, especially important that you not immediately dismiss the person with apparent alcohol on his or her breath (which can smell like the fruity breath of a diabetic) as a drunk. Check the person carefully for other illnesses and injuries, and give the intoxicated victim the same attention you would give to those with other illnesses and/or injuries. The intoxicated victim needs constant watching to be sure that he or she does not aspirate vomitus and that respiration is maintained.

DRUGS

Drugs are classified according to their effects on the user:

1. *Uppers* are stimulants of the central nervous system. They include amphetamines, cocaine, caffeine, antiasthmatic drugs, and vasoconstrictor drugs.
2. *Downers* are depressants of the central nervous system. They include barbiturates, tranquilizers, marijuana, narcotics, and anticonvulsants.
3. *Hallucinogens* alter and frequently enhance the processing of sensory and emotional information in brain centers. They include LSD, mescaline, psilocybin, and peyote. Marijuana also has some hallucinogenic properties.

Amphetamines and Cocaine. These provide relief from fatigue and a feeling of well being. Blood pressure, breathing, and general body activity are increased. Some users take a "speed run" of repeated high doses. Results are hyperactivity, restlessness, and belligerence. Such persons need to be protected from hurting themselves and others. Acute cases need medical attention.

Hallucinogens. These produce changes in mood and sensory awareness—a person may "hear" colors and "see" sounds. They can cause hallucinations and bizarre behavior that can make the user dangerous to himself and others. Acute cases need medical attention. Users should be protected from hurting themselves.

Marijuana. Marijuana provides a feeling of relaxation and euphoria. Users report distortions of time and space. In some persons, use can result in a reaction similar to a bad LSD trip.

Barbiturates. These drugs result in relaxation, drowsiness, and sleep. Overdoses can produce respiratory depression, coma, and death. Withdrawal can cause anxiety, tremors, nausea, fever, delirium, convulsions, and ultimate death.

Tranquilizers. They are used to calm anxiety. High doses produce the same effects as barbiturates. Withdrawal may cause the addict problems similar to those occurring from withdrawal from barbiturates.

Inhaled Substances. A person who inhales glue or other solvents (gasoline, lighter fluid, nail polish, etc.) experiences effects similar to those of alcohol. The person can die through suffocation. In addition, some inhalants can cause death by changing the rhythm of the heartbeat.

Opiates (Narcotics). They are used medicinally to relieve pain and anxiety. Overdoses can result in deep sleep (coma), respiratory depression, and death. The pupils of opiate users are described as "pinpoint" in size. Withdrawal symptoms include, among others, intense agitation, abdominal discomfort, dilated pupils, increased breathing and body temperatures, and a strong craving for a "fix."

Emergency Care

Vomiting should be induced if the overdose was taken in the preceding thirty minutes and if advised by a medical authority. Hyperactive victims should be protected from hurting themselves and others. They should be reassured and treated calmly. Respirations should be monitored because overdoses of depressants can cause respiratory depression and death. The first aider should instill confidence. The victim should be assured that he or she will be all right. The first aider should be alert for possible allergic reactions and shock. Evidence should be preserved for the legal authorities. Prompt transportation is required to a medical facility.

Poisoning (Ingestion)

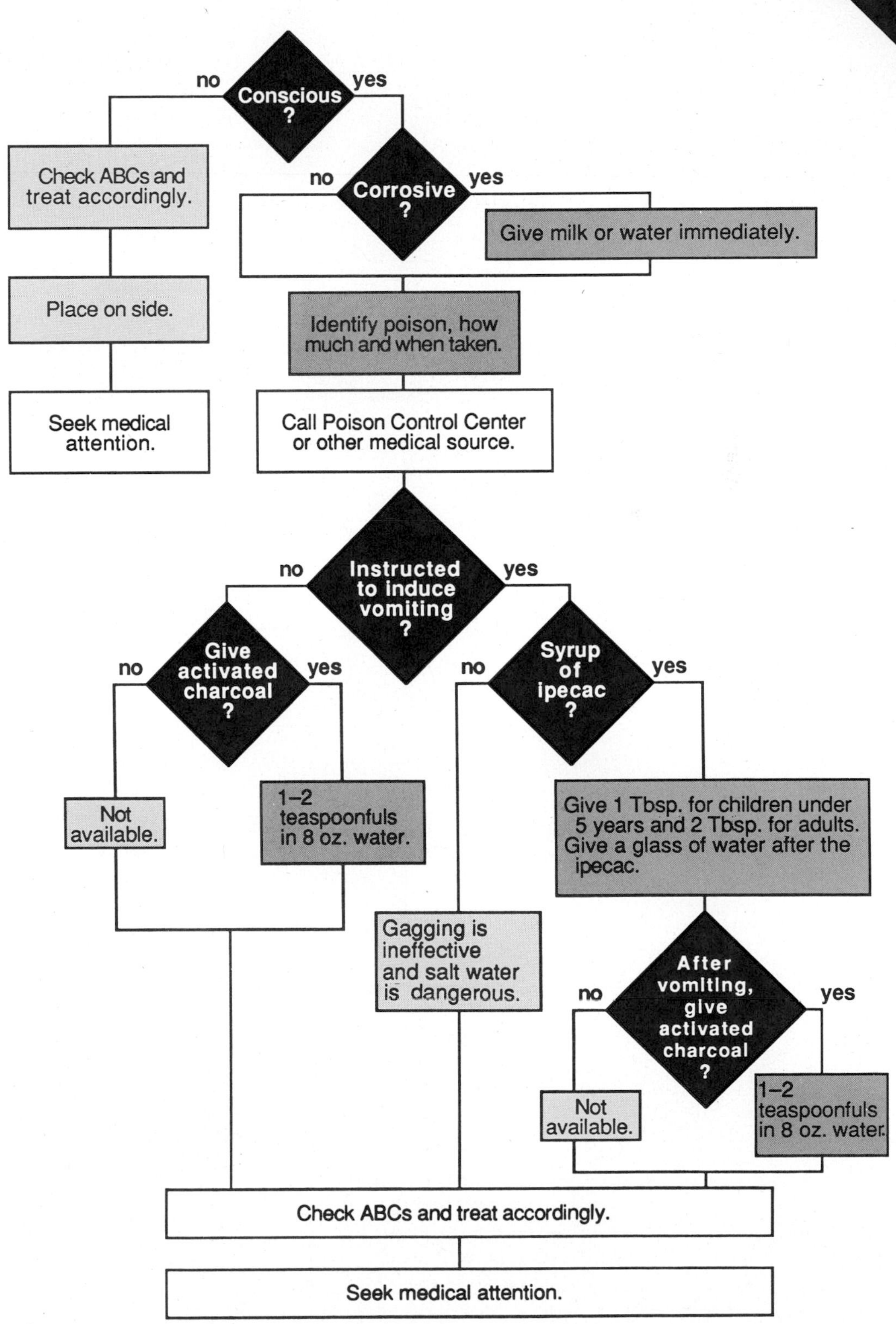

Poisoning (Inhaled)

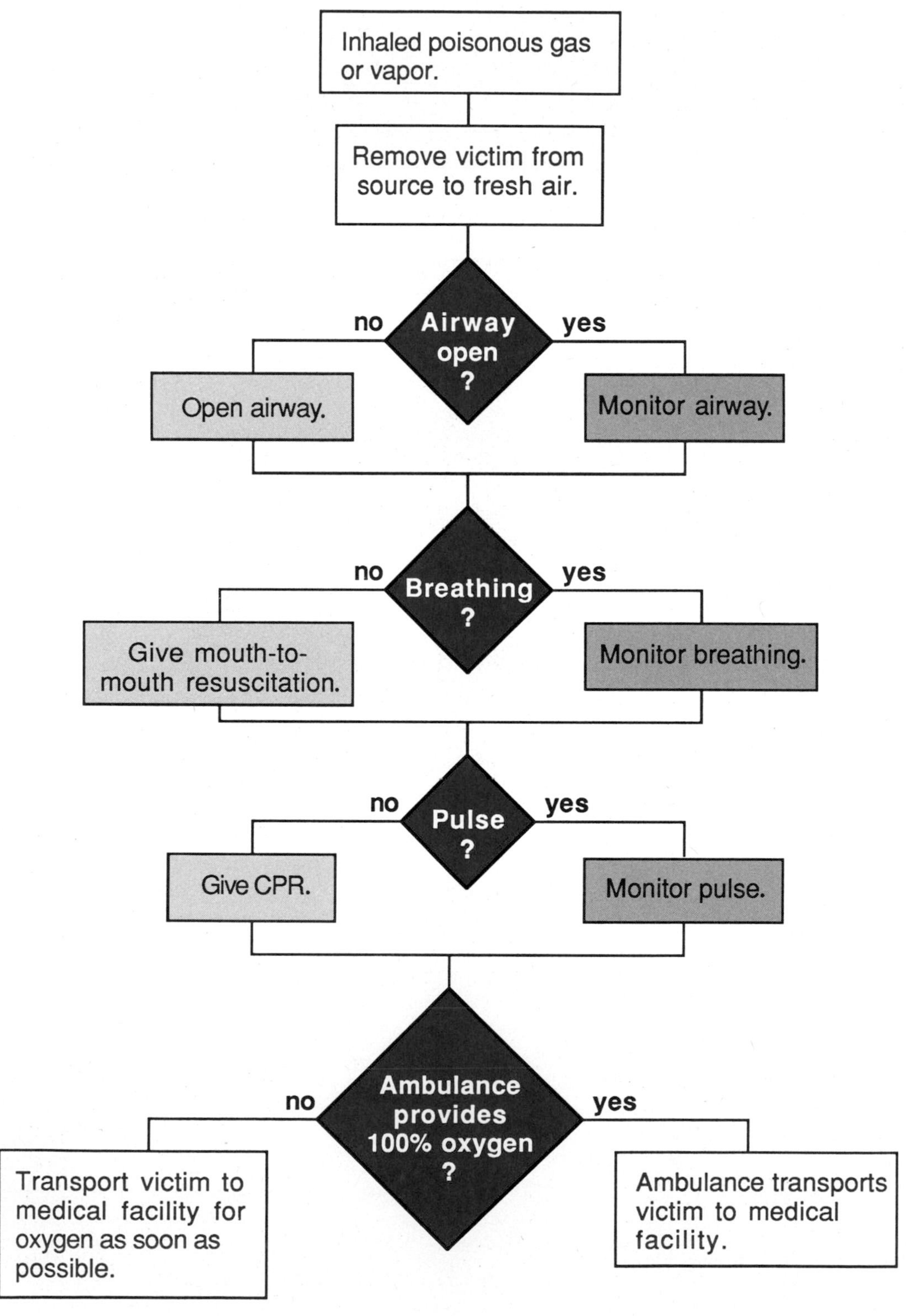

Insect Stings (Flying Insects)

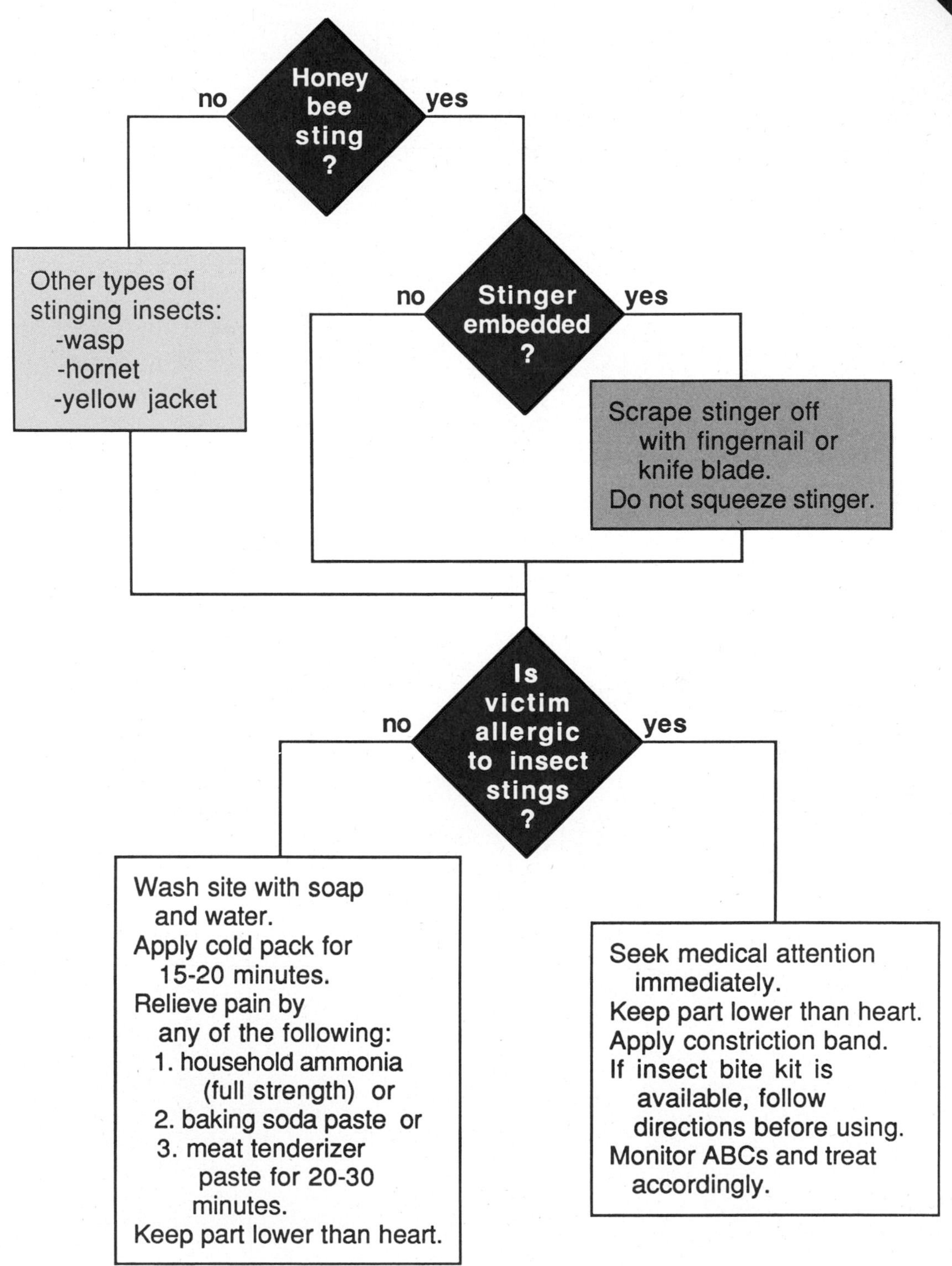

Snakebite

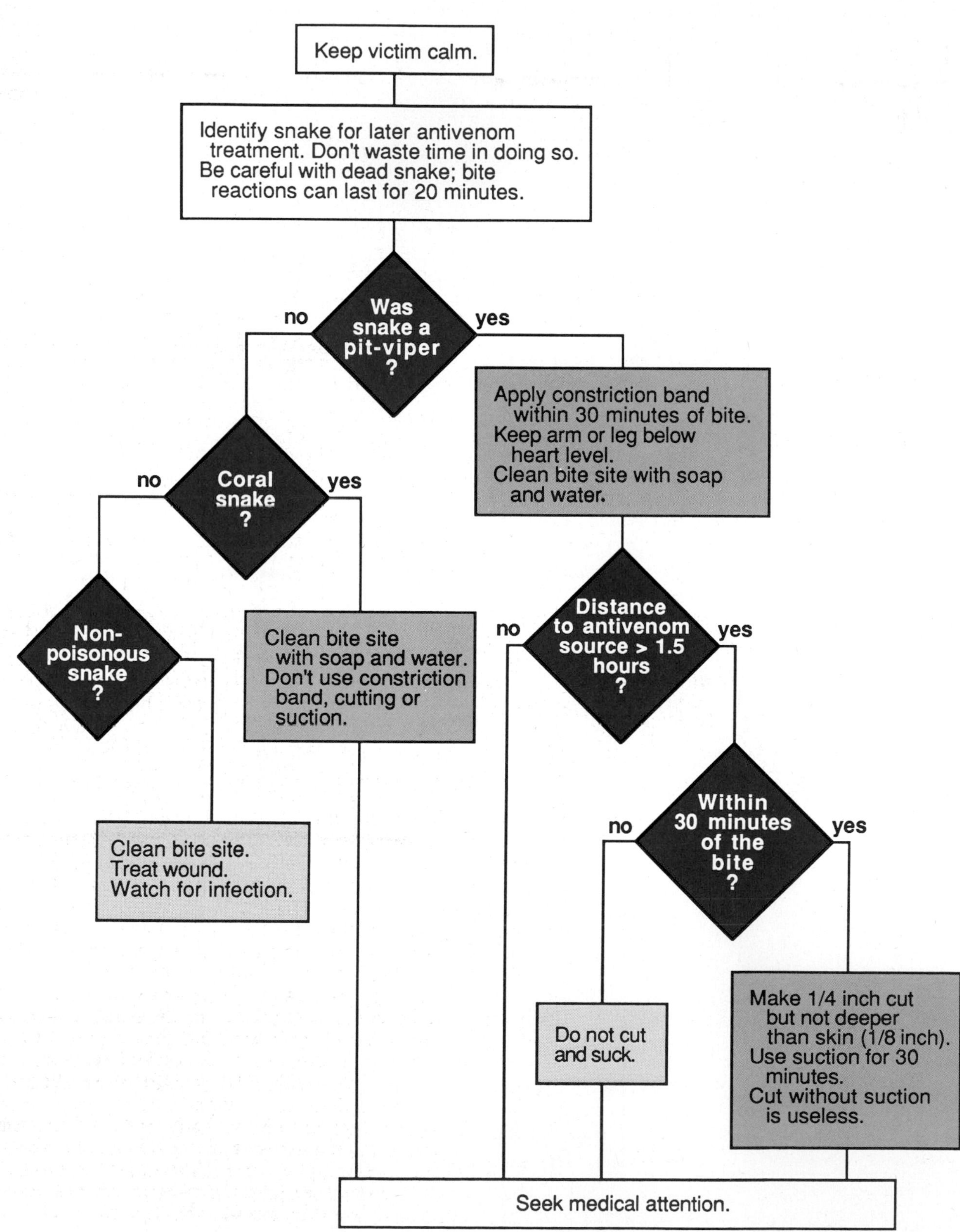

Keep victim calm.
Identify snake for later antivenom treatment. Don't waste time in doing so. Be careful with dead snake; bite reactions can last for 20 minutes.
Was snake a pit-viper ?
no
yes
Apply constriction band within 30 minutes of bite. Keep arm or leg below heart level. Clean bite site with soap and water.
Coral snake ?
no
yes
Non-poisonous snake ?
Clean bite site with soap and water. Don't use constriction band, cutting or suction.
Distance to antivenom source > 1.5 hours ?
no
yes
Within 30 minutes of the bite ?
no
yes
Clean bite site. Treat wound. Watch for infection.
Do not cut and suck.
Make 1/4 inch cut but not deeper than skin (1/8 inch). Use suction for 30 minutes. Cut without suction is useless.
Seek medical attention.

Spider Bites and Scorpion Stings

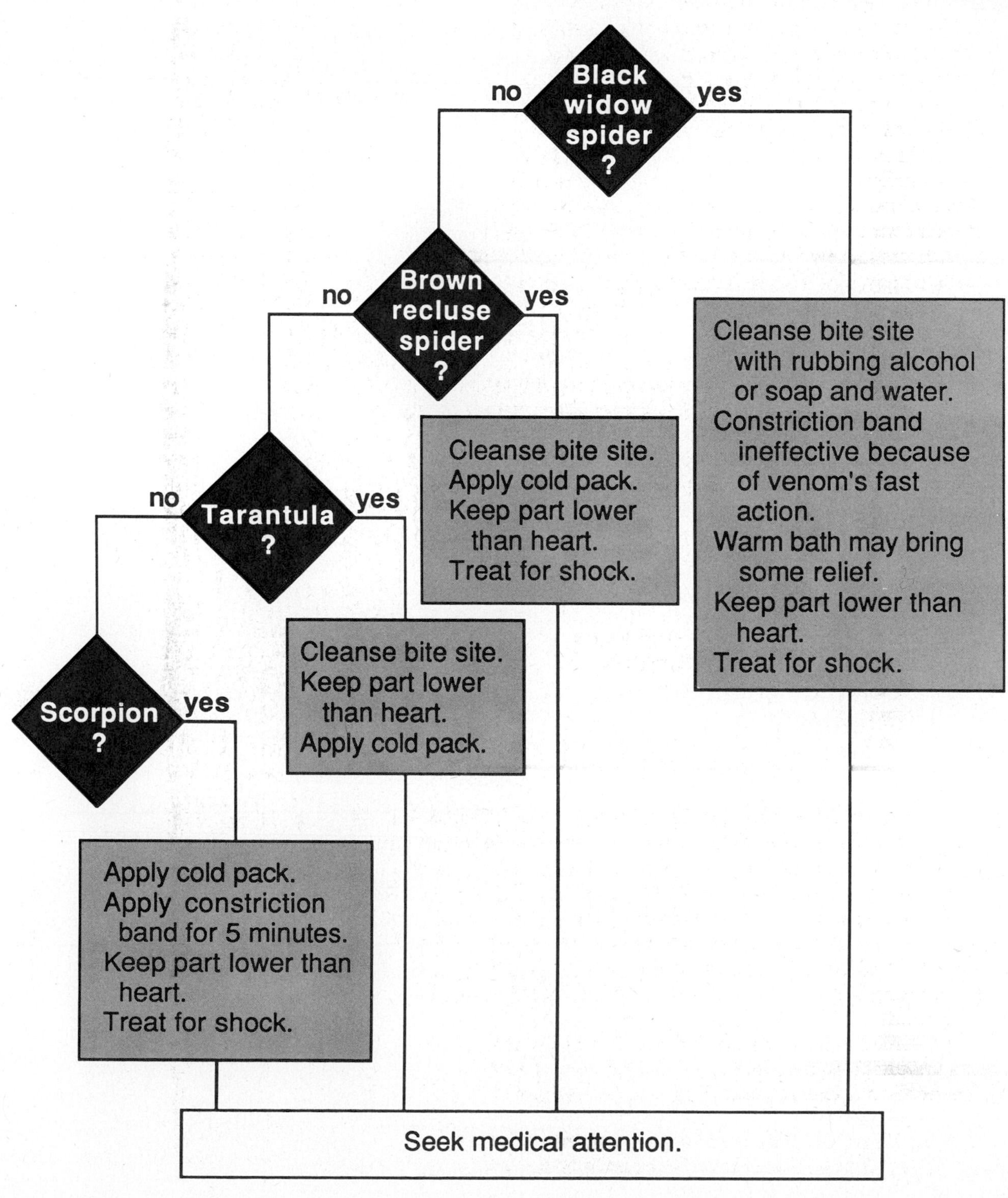

Tick Removal

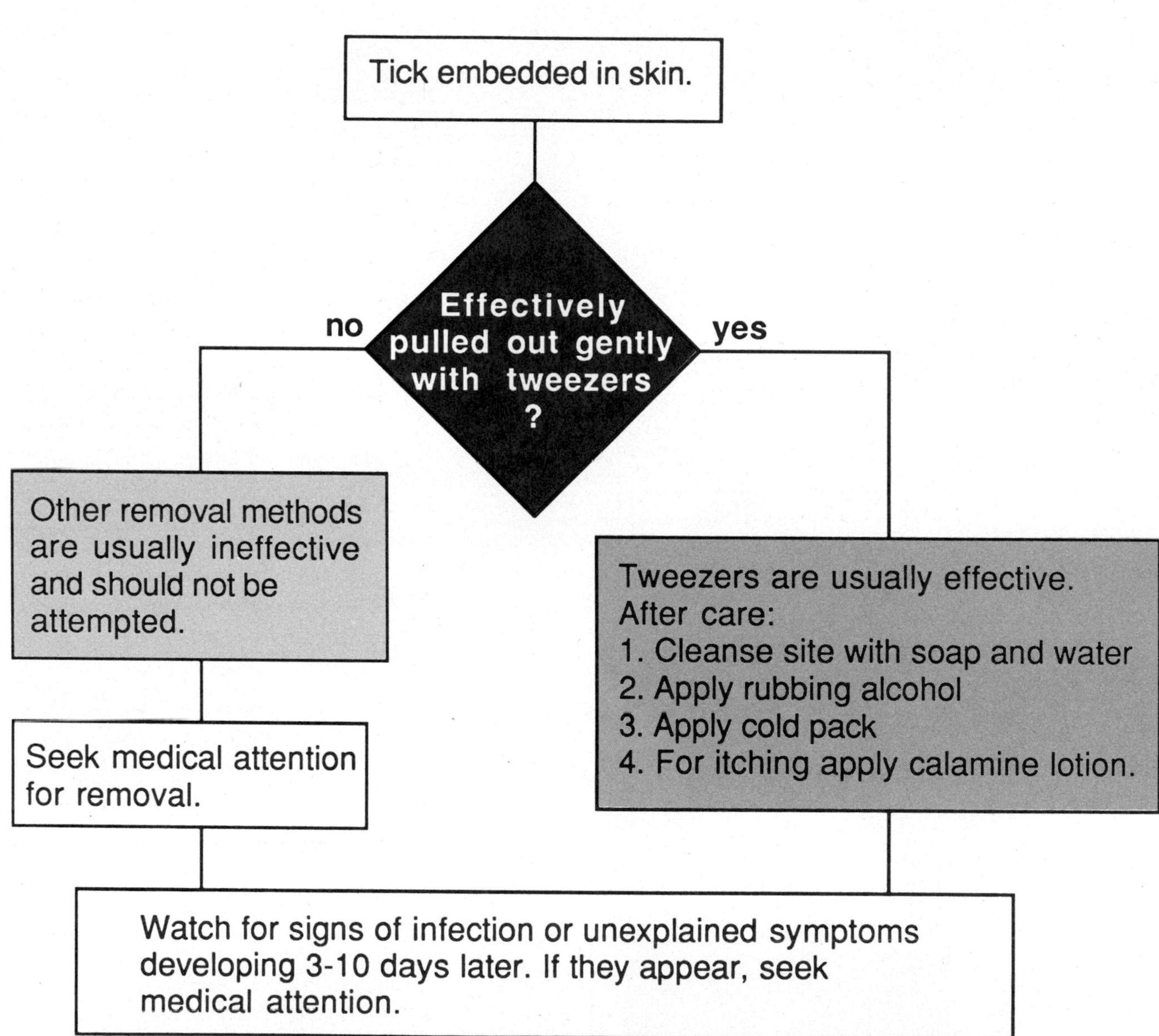

Poison Ivy, Poison Oak, and Poison Sumac

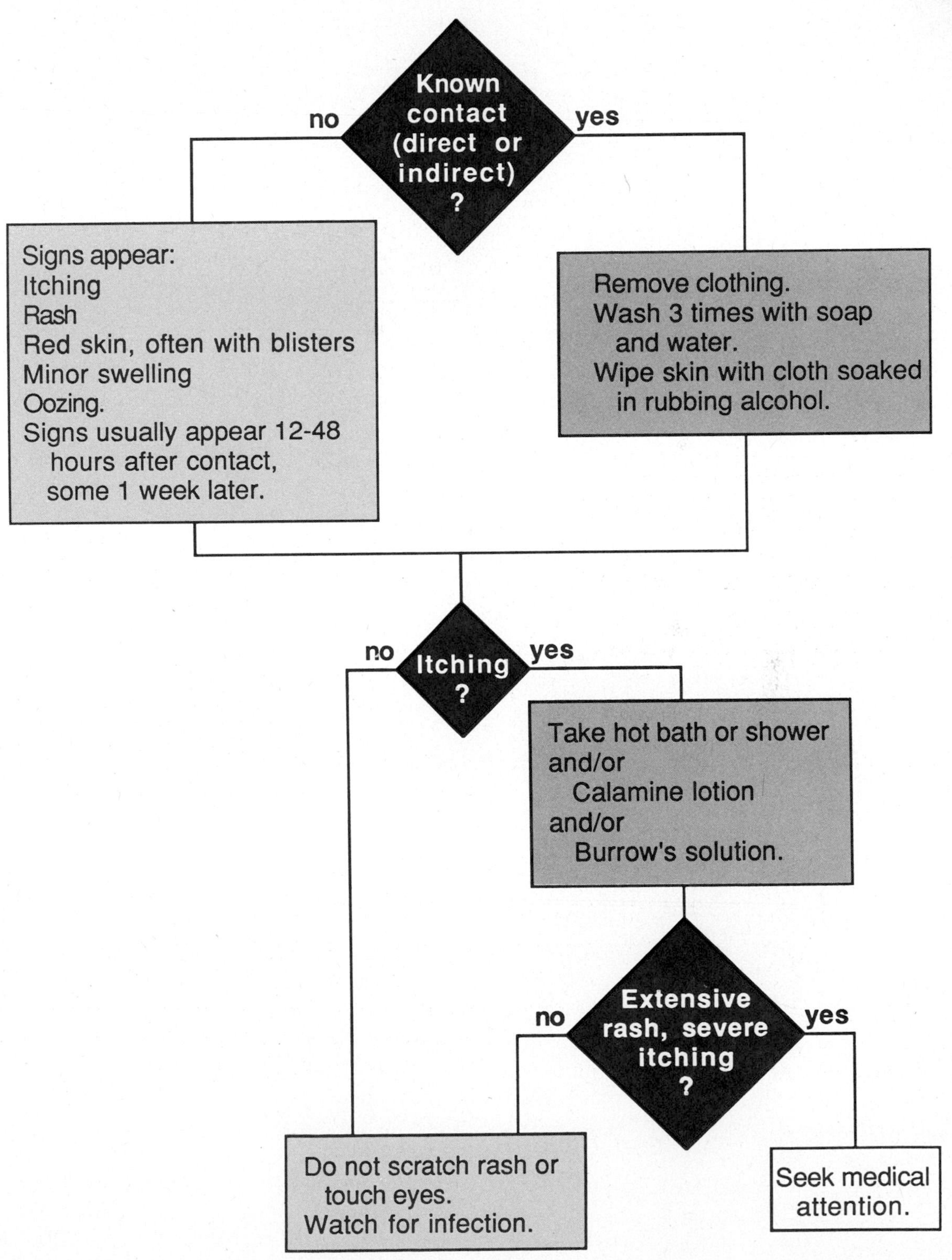

Poisoning (Ingestion)

LEARNING ACTIVITIES

T F 1. Burnt toast is a good substitute for activated charcoal.
T F 2. Activated charcoal can bind ingested poison.
T F 3. Any ingested poison should be diluted by a first aider.
T F 4. To induce vomiting by a poisoned victim, use a weak detergent soap.
T F 5. The best way to induce a vomiting in a poisoned victim is to gag them.
T F 6. Poisoning is classified as one of the urgent cases in first aid.
T F 7. The majority of accidental poisoning cases occur in children under five.
T F 8. Vomiting should be induced as quickly as possible in all poisoning cases.
T F 9. If a person swallows gasoline, kerosene, or furniture polish, he or she should be made to vomit immediately.
T F 10. If a victim has burns around the mouth and lips as a result of swallowing a corrosive agent, do not induce vomiting.
T F 11. If a victim has burns around the mouth and lips as a result of swallowing a corrosive agent, dilution with water or milk is recommended.
T F 12. If a person has a serious heart condition, do not induce vomiting.
T F 13. There is no specific antidote for most poisons.
T F 14. Fluids (water or milk) should be given immediately to dilute any poison swallowed.
T F 15. Carbonated beverages are recommended to use in the case of poisoning.
T F 16. Vomiting should be induced in poison cases involving lye or lye products.

Case 1: A frantic young mother fears that her two-year-old daughter has accidentally eaten some rat poison. Unfortunately, the toddler is too young to reliably tell what she has done. No unusual signs or symptoms are immediately present when you arrive at the scene.

1. For this apparent accidental poisoning, what action should the first aider take?

____

____

2. What should be done next?

____

____

3. What is the best method to administer the emergency care in Question 1?

____

____

4. What items should accompany the victim to the hospital?

A. ____

____

B. ____

____

5. What symptoms would you expect to appear eventually in this victim if she did in fact ingest some of the rat poison?

A. ____

____

B. ____

____

C. ____

____

6. Which of the following poisons should not be vomited? (Check *all* that apply.)

A. ______ Acids (hydrochloric, sulfuric, nitric)
B. ______ Alkalis (lime, potash, ammonia)
C. ______ Petroleum-based products (gasoline, kerosene, oil)
D. ______ Volatile liquids (lighter fluid, alcohol)

Case 2: You receive a call from an excited neighbor who explains that her three-year-old son is lying in pain on the bathroom floor. Upon arrival at the scene you find the boy still in pain. A quick look around reveals an empty aspirin bottle lying on the floor next to the youngster.

1. What is the very first action that you should take in this situation?

____

____

2. What should you do next?

____

____

3. What is a key point to remember when providing emergency care for ingested poisons?

____

____

4. Besides ingestion, what are three other ways poisons can enter the body?

A. ______________________________

____

B. ______________________________

____

C. ______________________________

____

Case 3: Each year there are approximately 1,000,000 poisonings in the United States. Although some of these are suicide attempts, many are the result of accidents. In any case, the poisoning problem is acute and one the first aider should be aware of. The following will test your knowledge of poison and response to various poisoning cases.

1. When transporting a poison victim to a medical facility, what items should you take with you and what information should you try to gather?

A. ______________________________

____

B. ______________________________

____

C. ______________________________

____

D. ______________________________

____

2. List the four ways poisons enter the body.

A. ______________________________

____

B. ______________________________

____

C. ______________________________

____

D. ______________________________

____

3. Match the following poisons with their signs or symptoms.

1. Corrosives ______
2. Drugs ______
3. Turpentine ______
4. Berries, plants ______

A. Breath odor
B. Tablets in vomitus
C. Burns around mouth
D. Stains around mouth

4. What is the preferred agent used to induce vomiting?

____
____
____
____

5. When inducing vomiting in children with the preferred agent, how much should be administered?

A. ______ One teaspoonful and then copious amounts of water
B. ______ One teaspoonful and then one drinking glass of water
C. ______ One tablespoonful and then copious amounts of water
D. ______ One tablespoonful and then one drinking glass of water

6. How soon after administering the agent should you expect vomiting to begin?

A. ______ Immediately
B. ______ 5–10 minutes
C. ______ 10–15 minutes
D. ______ 15–20 minutes
E. ______ Any time after 20 minutes

7. From the following poisons, check those that should *not* be vomited.

A. ______ Acids (hydrochloric, sulfuric, nitric)
B. ______ Alkalis (lime, potash, ammonia)
C. ______ Petroleum products (gasoline, kerosene)
D. ______ Volatile liquids (lighter fluid, alcohol)
E. ______ Strychnine

8. When should the agents in the preceding list not be given? (Check *all* that apply.)

A. ______ Comatose victim
B. ______ Volatile substances
C. ______ Caustic substances
D. ______ Two-year-old child

9. Are the following statements true or false regarding activated charcoal, suspended in water, which would be used in acute poisonings.

A. ______ It is safe to use and may be of value several hours after ingestion of poison.
B. ______ It is best used in tablet form rather than the powder form.
C. ______ It works by absorbing toxic substances directly onto the charcoal.

10. List the initial steps to take in treating the ingestion of a corrosive substance.

A. ______________________________
____
B. ______________________________
____
C. ______________________________
____
D. ______________________________
____
E. ______________________________
____

11. Are the following statements true or false regarding the initial treatment for the ingestion of a petroleum distillate?
   A. ______ It is often best treated by inducing vomiting.
   B. ______ It may best be treated by using a laxative.
   C. ______ It is an indication for activated charcoal.

Case 4: A two-year-old girl has ingested chlorine bleach from a kitchen cup. Upon your arrival the child is conscious, crying, and rubbing her abdomen.

1. List three factors that contributed to this situation and how each should have been avoided.
   A. ______
   B. ______
   C. ______

2. List the emergency care for a child poisoned by bleach.
   A. ______
   B. ______
   C. ______
   D. ______
   E. ______
   F. ______
   G. ______

3. What substance is recommended to induce vomiting if it is deemed necessary? What is the prescribed dose for a child?
   A. ______
   B. ______

4. What is the purpose of administering activated charcoal?
______

Case 5: You find your grandfather lying in the hallway between the bathroom and bedroom. Your grandmother explains that he went into the bathroom to take something for a persistent cough. You find an empty container with a faded label beside him; the label reads iodine. The man is unconscious and has brown stains around his mouth. Further examination reveals a weak rapid pulse.

1. What emergency care should you provide your poisoned grandfather?
   A. ______

B. ______________________________

____

C. ______________________________

____

D. ______________________________

____

E. ______________________________

____

2. What actions should be taken for a poisoned subject who begins to convulse?

A. ______________________________

____

B. ______________________________

____

C. ______________________________

____

D. ______________________________

____

E. ______________________________

____

3. Match the four ways in which poisons may be introduced into the body with the appropriate example.

A. ______ Ingestion
B. ______ Inhalation
C. ______ Absorption
D. ______ Injection

1. Insecticide sprays
2. Household cleaners
3. Snakebite
4. Rat poison

4. Under what circumstances would you not want to induce vomiting in a poisoned subject?

A. ______________________________

____

B. ______________________________

____

C. ______________________________

____

D. ______________________________

____

5. From the following list, check all the items that are categorized as poisons though they are commonly found in and around the home environment.

A. ______ Fingernail polish remover
B. ______ Aspirin
C. ______ Oven cleaner
D. ______ Leaves of rhubarb plant
E. ______ Turpentine
F. ______ Oil of wintergreen
G. ______ Weed killer

6. From the following list, check all the items that are categorized as possible symptoms or signs of poisoning.

A. ______ Unusual breath odor
B. ______ Irregular respirations
C. ______ Burns around the mouth
D. ______ Pinpoint pupils
E. ______ Empty container or bottle at subject's side
F. ______ Abdominal pain
G. ______ Rapid thready (faint) pulse
H. ______ Nausea and/or vomiting
I. ______ Anxiety and fear

7. When contacting your local Poison Control Center, list the information you must be prepared to provide them.
   A. ______
   B. ______
   C. ______

8. Where is your Poison Control Center located and how would you go about contacting it in your community?
   A. ______
   B. ______

Case 6: Your neighbor telephones you for help. Arriving at the home, you find your neighbor's wife lying on a sofa, disheveled, and in a state of relaxation. Her husband is berating her and almost forcibly pouring hot coffee down her throat. He explains that they had been at their local lodge drinking most of the night. When they returned home he noticed her taking a quantity of sleeping pills. The woman's pulse and respiration rate are slow but steady. Her pupils react to light slowly.

1. What is the appropriate emergency care for this apparent accidental poisoning?
   A. ______
   B. ______

2. What information should you attempt to provide to medical personnel?
   A. ______
   B. ______
   C. ______

3. What symptoms would you eventually expect to be present in this victim?
   A. ______
   B. ______
   C. ______

4. What are the two classes of corrosive substances that are ingested by mouth?
   A. ______
   B. ______

5. What symptoms would you expect to be present in a person who has ingested a corrosive substance?
   A. ______
   B. ______
   C. ______

Insect Stings

T F 1. Bee sting is not a serious health problem and should not be given undue attention.

T F 2. Some persons have been known to die within minutes after being stung by a bee.

T F 3. Do not squeeze the bee stinger with tweezers if attempting to remove the stinger.

T F 4. Remove bee stinger as quickly as possible from the victim.

T F 5. Bees are the only flying insect to leave its stinger embedded in its victim.

T F 6. A paste of meat tenderizer mixed in water can reduce the pain and itching from a bee sting.

T F 7. The victim of a bee sting that is causing anaphylactic shock needs epinephrine.

T F 8. Bee stings are responsible for more deaths than snakebites each year in the United States.

T F 9. A bee stinger can best be removed with a knife blade or similar object.

Case: A young child at a family picnic was stung several times by honeybees. The areas where he was stung are red andswollen with several stingers embedded in the skin. He complains of intense pain at each sting site.

Rank in order the proper first aid procedures for bee stings:

______ 1. Wash all sting sites with soap and water.
______ 2. Relieve pain with paste of meat tenderizer, calamine lotion, full-strength household ammonia or baking soda paste.
______ 3. Removc the stinger—by scraping with a knife blade or fingernail.
______ 4. Seek medical attention immediately if it is known that the victim is allergic to bee stings.
______ 5. Use the contents of an "emergency bee sting kit" if it is known that the victim is allergic to bee stings and if kit is available.
______ 6. Tie a constriction band above the sting site.
______ 7. Apply cold to the sting site.

Snakebites

T F 1. Always loosen a constriction band every ten minutes in cases of snakebite.

T F 2. Never use a constriction band.

T F 3. Pack the bitten extremity in ice.

T F 4. Apply incision and suction only if antivenin is more than an hour away or if the snake was large.

T F 5. Never attempt incision and suction.

T F 6. Attempt to identify the snake.

T F 7. Avoid all unnecessary movement.

T F 8. About a dozen deaths from poisonous snakebite are reported yearly in the United States.

T F 9. Death from snakebite usually occurs immediately after the bite.

T F 10. A first aider should administer antivenin.

T F 11. First aid for a nonpoisonous snakebite is the same as for any wound.

T F 12. In case of a poisonous snakebite to an extremity, a tourniquet should be applied.

T F 13. If a person is bitten by a rattlesnake, cross-cut incisions should be made over the fang marks.

T F 14. Coral snakes inject their poison through a chewing motion.

T F 15. Coral snakebite should be treated by application of a constriction band.

Case: A man bitten by a rattlesnake while hiking on Mt. Olympus was listed in critical condition at Valley Hospital. The victim was bitten on the leg while hiking with five companions in rugged Neff's Canyon. It was about eight hours later when rescuers took the victim to a rescue helicopter. The hiker was at the 9,000 foot level when bitten. Three companions stayed with him while two others went for help.

1. Rattlesnakes are classified as ____________ .
2. Other snakes included in this category are:

   A. ______________________________

   B. ______________________________
3. Which poisonous snake is not included in this classification? ______________________________
4. When would incision and suction be applied for poisonous snakebite?

   A. ______________________________

   B. ______________________________
5. What is wrong with using ice or cold on a snakebite?

   A. ______________________________

   B. ______________________________

   C. ______________________________
6. How tight should a constriction band be?

   ____
7. Draw the type of cut recommended for snakebites when a first aider needs to cut and suck:

Spider Bites

T	F	1.	Injected venom from the brown recluse spider may cause the death of tissue (gangrene).
T	F	2.	Application of ice may be beneficial in spider bites.
T	F	3.	Muscle cramps are characteristic of black widow spider bites.
T	F	4.	Tarantulas are America's most poisonous spider.
T	F	5.	Children and the elderly are at greatest risk from insect bites and stings.
T	F	6.	Always try to identify the biting spider.

Case: Your three-year-old daughter runs into the house crying and holding her arms. She complains about a "bug" on her. You look at her arm and notice a slight redness and swelling around what may be a bite.

1. A coal-black body with a red spot on its abdomen can be the identification of which poisonous spider?

   ____
2. The other poisonous spider that causes death and medical problems is the ____________ .
3. Which of the following first aid procedures are appropriate for spider bites and scorpion stings? (Check *all* that apply.)

   A. ______ Apply cold pack.

   B. ______ Seek medical attention immediately.

   C. ______ Capture the spider or have a definite identification.

   D. ______ Maintain open airway and restore breathing, if necessary.

   E. ______ Wash area with soap and water or rubbing alcohol.

   F. ______ Apply a constriction band 2 to 4 inches above the bite.

   G. ______ Apply calamine lotion to relieve discomfort.

Tick Removal

T F 1. Ticks can carry infectious disease which can be transmitted to humans.

T F 2. Signs of infection or other symptoms (e.g., headache, fever, and rash) may develop days later after a tick bite.

T F 3. Coating the tick with petroleum jelly (Vaseline™) is recommended as the method for removing an embedded tick.

T F 4. A drop or two of gasoline or kerosene will cause the tick to remove itself.

T F 5. The recommended procedure is to pull the tick out with tweezers.

Case: After a camping trip in a Colorado National Forest, you find a tick embedded in one of your children's legs. This surprises you because you thought you had taken all the precautions to prevent tick bites—inspecting for ticks two to three times each day, using a repellent an exposed skin and cloths containing DEET, and wearing tick repellent clothing (e.g., one-piece of outer garment tucked into high boots). Nevertheless, you are concerned and want to have the tick removed as soon as possible.

Which of the following methods are most likely to be successful in removing an embedded tick?

______ 1. Apply a substance that will smother the tick causing it to disengage its head (e.g., heavy oils or greases such as Vaseline).

______ 2. Apply fingernail polish and allow it to harden. Peel the polish off and the tick will come with it.

______ 3. Apply heat by holding a heated needle or a blown out, glowing match head to the tick.

______ 4. Pull the embedded tick out with tweezers.

______ 5. Pry a tick out with a needle.

______ 6. Put some gasoline or kerosene on a cotton ball and tape it loosely over the tick for 15 to 20 minutes.

______ 7. Apply an ice cube over the tick.

______ 8. Wash the tick and area with soap and water.

Poison Ivy, Sumac, and Oak

T F 1. Scratching spreads the rash from poison ivy.

T F 2. The rash related to poison ivy appears within the hour of contact with the plant.

T F 3. Washing the skin should be done immediately after contact with the poison ivy plant.

T F 4. Calamine lotion may be applied to relieve itching.

T F 5. A hot shower or bath will provide periods of relief from itching because of poison ivy.

Case: You hit a golf ball into the "rough." This area includes bushes, weeds, and other plants. The next day your skin on the arms is red with blisters. It starts to itch and burn. You also are experiencing headache and fever.

Check which of the following may be useful in alleviating the itching from poison ivy you are experiencing:

______ 1. Wash the rash and all affected areas with soap and water.

______ 2. Apply rubbing alcohol to the rash and all areas that may have been affected.

______ 3. Paint the rash with calamine lotion.

______ 4. There is no way to relieve the itching, thus any efforts other than a prescription for cortisone from a physician are useless.

______ 5. Take a hot shower or bath even though intense itching will initially result.

______ 6. Apply petroleum (Vaseline™) jelly to the affected area.

______ 7. Apply buttermilk or cream to the affected area.

Carbon Monoxide

T F 1. Cherry-red lips and skin are a sign of carbon monoxide poisoning only at autopsy.

T F 2. Carbon monoxide from automobiles is easily detected by its peculiar odor.

T F 3. Headache is a characteristic symptom of carbon monoxide poisoning.

T F 4. Treating the victim for shock is the initial emergency care procedure for inhalation poisonings.

T F 5. Carbon monoxide victims need pure oxygen as quickly as possible.

T F 6. A physician should be consulted whenever carbon monoxide poisoning is suspected.

Case: A man unaccustomed to drinking returns home, pulls into his garage, and falls asleep before he turns off the engine or leaves the car. A faulty exhaust system leaks carbon monoxide gas into the car. The wife, hearing the car running for an unusual length of time, is alerted and calls you. Upon arrival you find the victim cyanotic (blue) and with slow and irregular pulse and respiration rates.

1. What is the appropriate emergency care for carbon monoxide poisoning?

A. ______________________________

B. ______________________________

C. ______________________________

2. Poisons are categorized according to the route of entry into the body. List the four ways poisons can enter the body.

A. ______________________________

B. ______________________________

C. ______________________________

D. ______________________________

8 Burns

- Thermal Burns
- Sunburn
- Chemical Burns
- Electrical Burns

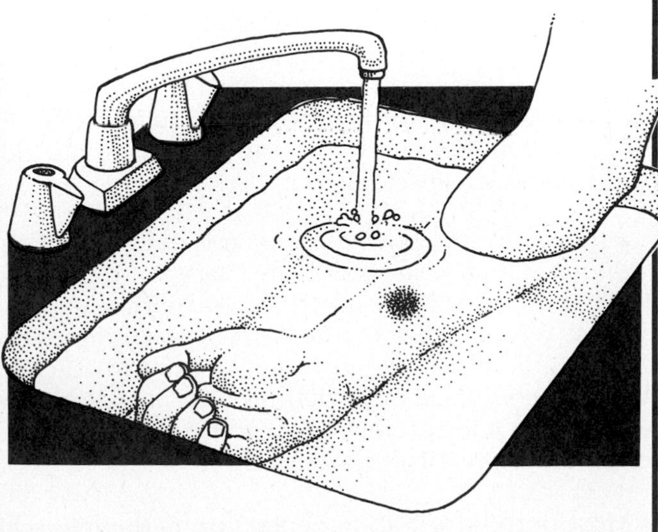

8-1. Applying cold water for a burn

THERMAL BURN

Burn injury often generates extraordinary anxiety, not only in the victim and bystanders but in the first aider as well. Inexperience may explain some of the apprehension felt by most first aiders. With two million people burned each year, most first aiders will eventually be called upon to treat this type of injury.

Initially, most burns are minor problems. But without aggressive emergency care, these injuries can progress to serious conditions. Early assessment and emergency care of the burn victim is critical in minimizing pain, long-term disability, and disfigurement.

Emergency Care

When a first aider encounters a burned victim, establish that the victim is not in any life threatening danger by quickly assessing the airway, pulse, and external bleeding and by treating any life threatening problems. The flames should be extinguished. During assessment, remove rings, bracelets, or other jewelry before edema (swelling) makes removal difficult. Take off burned clothing, cutting around and leaving fabric that adheres to wounds. Avoid unnecessary contamination, but since burn wounds are not life threatening at this point, cleansing is not recommended.

Quickly and carefully remove any of the victim's clothing. Do not pull a stuck fabric; cut around where it adheres to the skin. Later removal could be difficult and painful if swelling develops. A burn can be touched without causing further injury. Do not apply petroleum jelly, butter, or any burn medication. Ointments seal in the heat; may have to be scrubbed off in the hospital, causing unnecessary pain if the burn is serious; and offer little real pain relief.

For most minor burns, a continuous flow of cool tap water stops pain. (*See* Figure 8-1.) Prompt cooling may lessen local tissue destruction and the severity of the burn. In fact, if the burned skin has cold applied to it within thirty seconds of being burned, skin temperature drops to normal within three seconds. Cool water can help even when applied up to forty-five minutes after the burn. Have the victim immerse the burned area in cool water while keeping the tap on to maintain the cool temperature. If the site of the injury (e.g., the face) renders this awkward, cool compresses refreshed frequently under cool water will suffice.

The victim with a major burn—one involving more than 10% of the body surface or roughly the equivalent of the surface of one arm—should be transported immediately to the nearest emergency facility. Once a burn has been cooled, covering the area with a dry dressing will help control pain.

There is a controversy over whether to keep extensively burned areas wet or dry. One school of thought maintains that you should wrap the victim in sheets soaked with water. The other school of thought prefers to keep the victim dry because a wet victim easily becomes hypothermic in transport. Do not break any blisters because infection can be introduced.

When transporting the victim to an emergency facility, apply ice wrapped in several layers of towels. It takes from thirty minutes to three hours to stop the pain, depending on the depth and extent of the wound. Cooling is no longer necessary if pain does not recur when the compresses are removed from the burn for a five minute period.

TABLE 8-1. Burn Severity

Critical Burns
• All burns that are complicated by injuries to the respiratory tract, soft tissues, and bone structures.
• Third-degree burns that involve the critical areas of the body: hands, face, perineum.
• Third-degree burns that involve more than 10% of the body surface.
• Second-degree burns that involve more than 30% of the body surface.
Moderate Burns
• Third-degree burns that involve less than 10% of the body surface, excluding hands, face, and feet.
• Second-degree burns that involve 15% to 30% of the body surface.
• First-degree burns that involve 50% to 75% of the body surface.
Minor Burns
• Third-degree burns that involve less than 2% of the body surface, excluding the hands, face, and feet.
• Second-degree burns that involve less than 15% of the body surface.
• First-degree burns that involve less than 20% of the body surface.

Assessing the Burn

One of the first things for a first aider to do when confronted with a burned victim is to assess the severity of the burn. It should be stressed, however, that you should have already checked and taken care of breathing problems and severe bleeding.

In assessing a burn, you should appraise the following:

• *How large is the burn?* The extent of the burn is expressed as a percentage of the total body surface. The familiar "Rule of Nines" defines each hand and arm as 9% of the body surface. Each leg counts as 18% of the body surface. The front and back torso are each valued at 18% with the genital area at 1%. The victim's hand size is about 1% and this surface area can be used for calculating most burns. (*See* Figure 8-2.)

The Rule of Nines is accurate for adults, but it does not make allowances for the different proportions of a child. You will have to allow for that.

• *How deep is the burn?* If only part of the skin is damaged, the burn is called a partial-thickness burn or a first- or second-degree burn. These wounds will heal themselves. If all skin layers are destroyed, it is a full thickness burn or a third-degree. These injuries must be grafted for healing because the underlying tissue does not regenerate.

• *What parts of the body are burned?* Areas of most importance are the face (especially the eyelids), the hands, the feet, and the genitals. Burns of the respiratory tract are particularly serious if associated with the inhalation of fumes or blast effects.

• *How old is the burned victim?* A burn is considered more serious in a young infant and in an elderly person (over 65) than in other victims. Younger victims have poor antibody response to infection. In older victims, serious burns aggravate other health problems (e.g., heart disease).

• *Does the victim have any injuries or medical problems?* Burns can aggravate diabetes, rheumatic heart disease, chronic obstructive pulmonary disease, as well as other medical problems. Injuries received (other than the burn) such as extensive lacerations can complicate the victim's recovery. With this information and reference to Table 8-1, you can determine the severity of a burn on a victim.

Most burn information centers upon the immediate care of the damaged tissue rather than instruc-

Ticks, Fractures, and Dental Emergencies

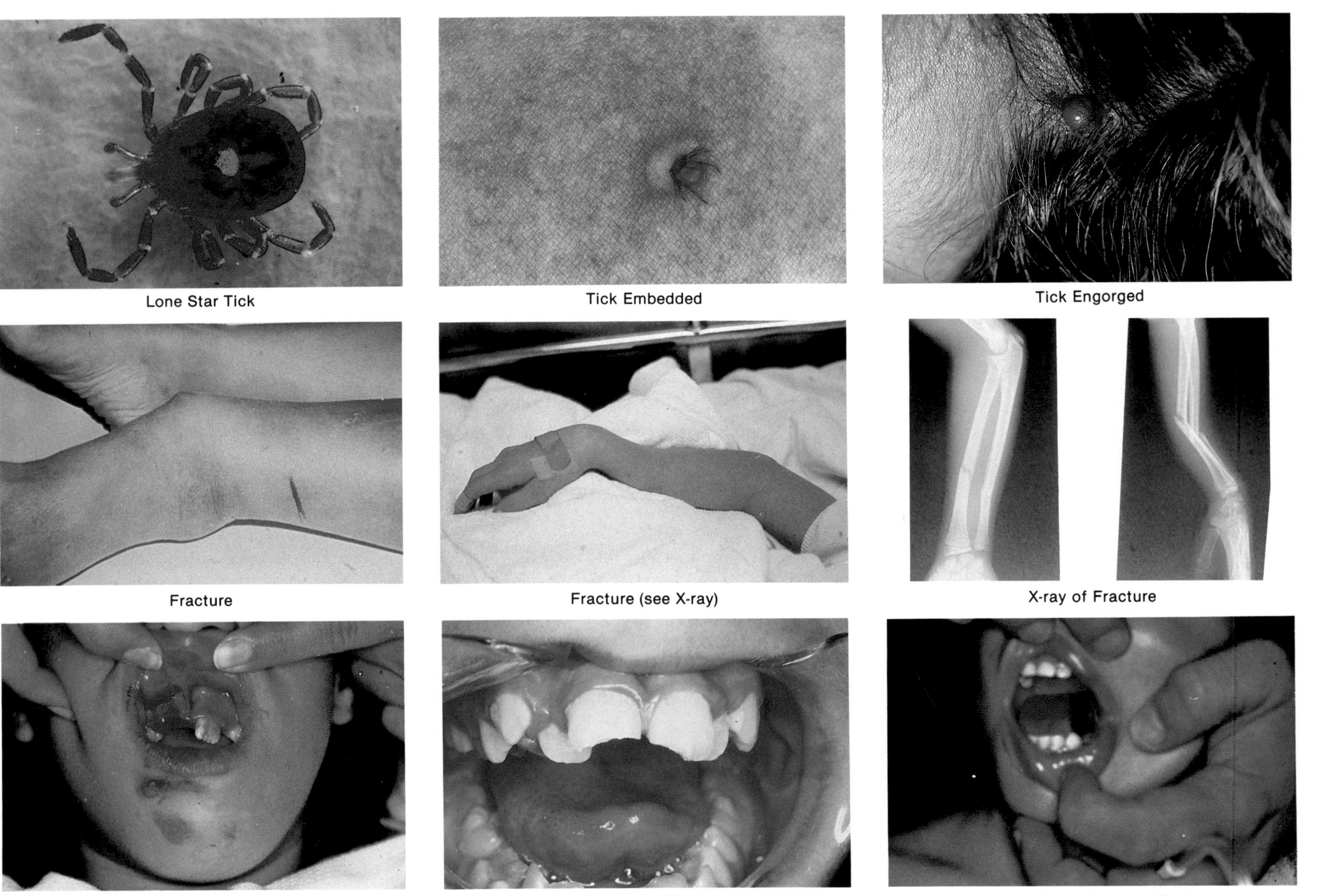

Lone Star Tick

Tick Embedded

Tick Engorged

Fracture

Fracture (see X-ray)

X-ray of Fracture

Tooth Avulsion (Baseball Injury)

Fractured Teeth

Penny Stuck Between Teeth

Burns and Frostbite

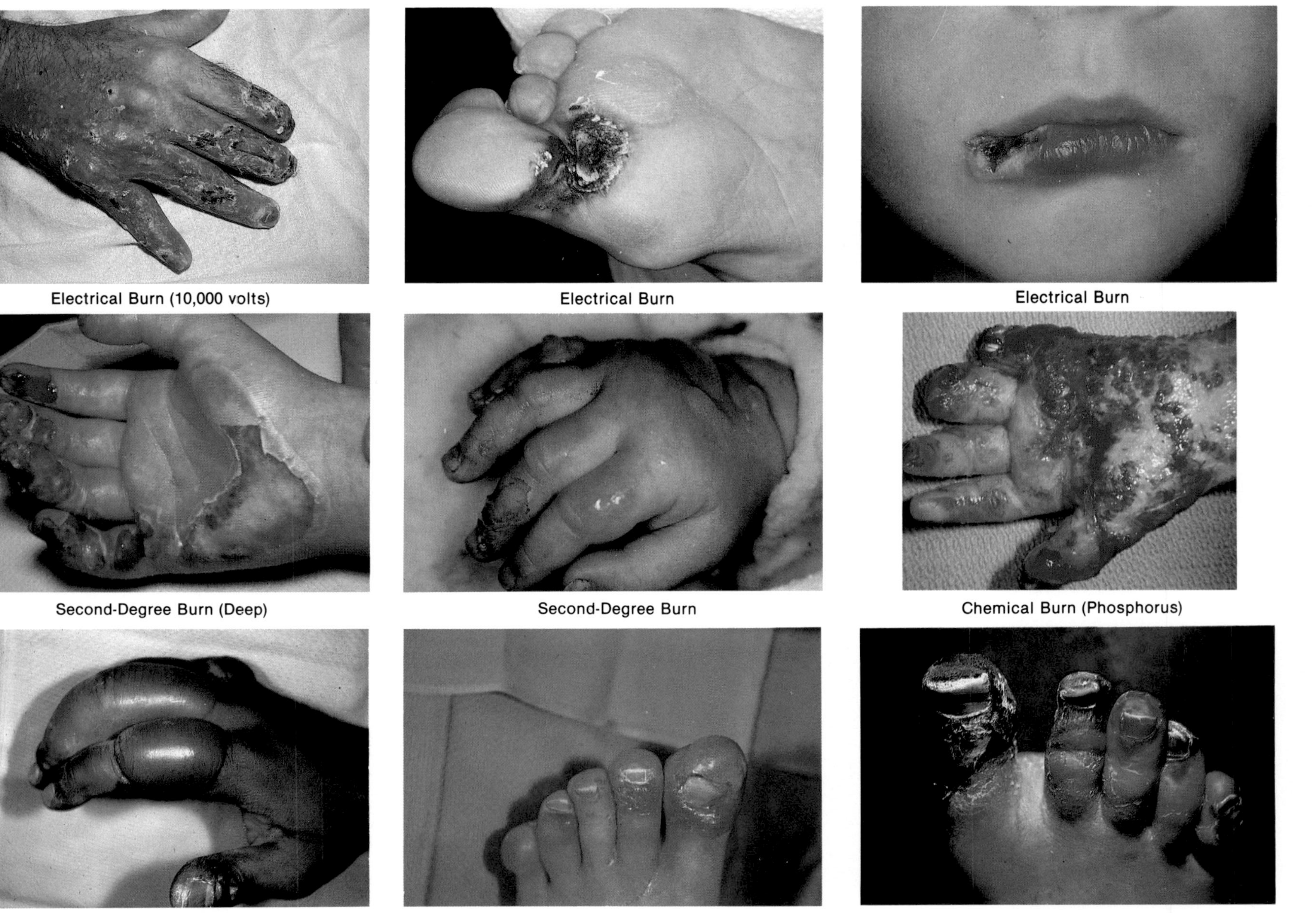

Electrical Burn (10,000 volts)

Electrical Burn

Electrical Burn

Second-Degree Burn (Deep)

Second-Degree Burn

Chemical Burn (Phosphorus)

Frostbite (Blisters)

Deep Frostbite

Deep Frostbite (3 Weeks Post-Thaw)

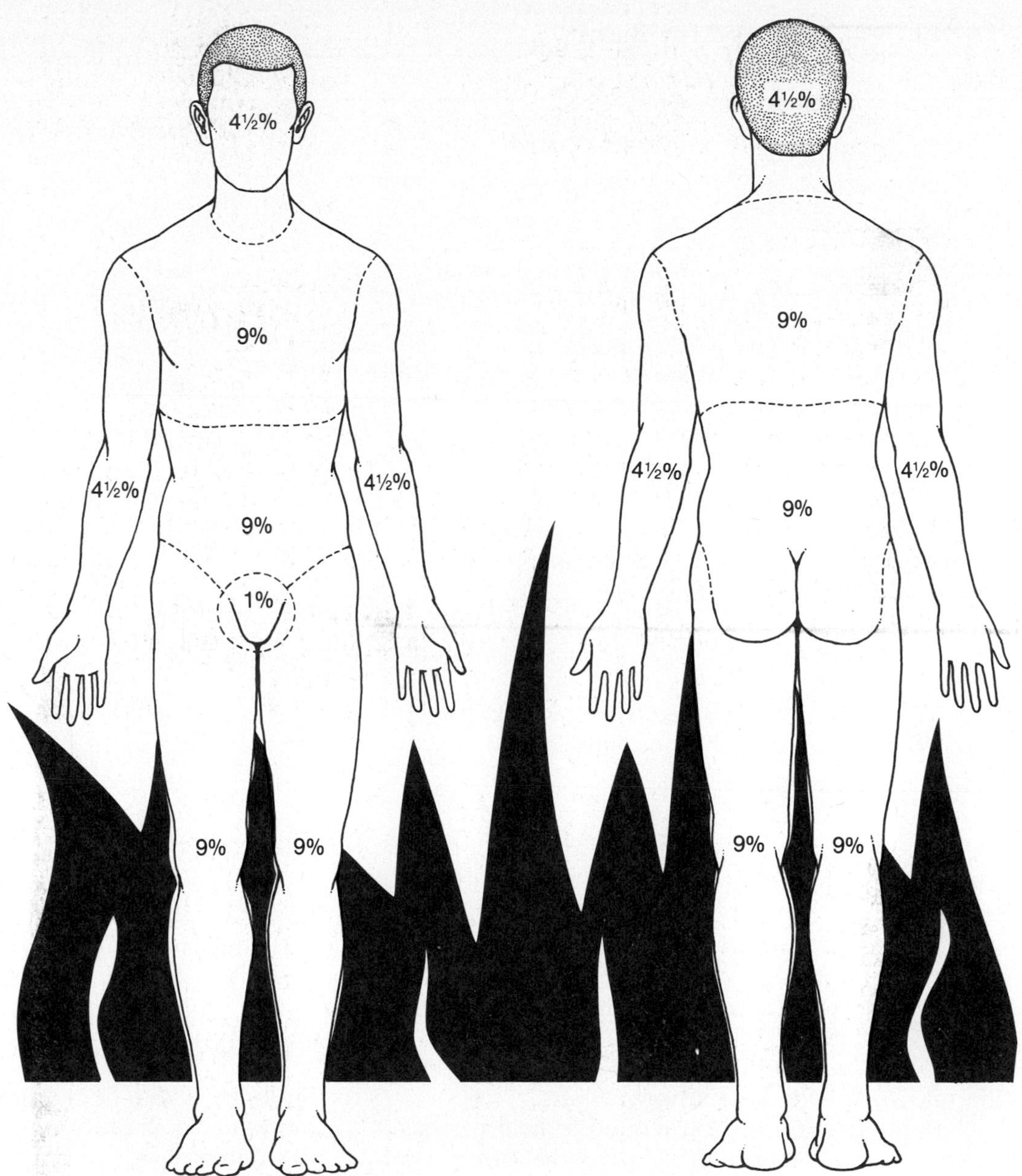

8-2. The "Rule of Nines"

tions about caring for that tissue during the subsequent days. Use of information in Table 8-2 serves as a guide to proper first aid for burns.

The quality of burn care has a definite impact on the eventual outcome. One should certainly follow a physician's recommendations about caring for the burn, but many burns are never seen by a doctor.

That is why the following suggestions are so relevant:

1. Wash hands thoroughly before changing any dressing.

2. Attempt to leave unbroken blisters intact.

3. Change dressings two times a day unless otherwise specified by a physician.

4. Change a dressing by:

a. Removing old dressings. If it adheres, soak it off with cool, clean water.

b. Cleanse area gently with mild soap (e.g., Ivory™) and water.

c. Pat dry with clean, dry cloth.

d. Apply a thin layer of antibacterial cream to the burn.

e. Apply clean dressings.

5. Watch for signs of infection. Call a physician if any of these appear:

a. Increased redness, pain, tenderness, swelling, or red streaks near burn

b. Pus

c. Elevated temperature (fever)

TABLE 8-2. First Aid for Burns

Burn	Do	Don't
First Degree (redness, mild swelling, and pain)	Apply cold water and/or dry sterile dressing.	Apply butter, oleomargarine, etc.
Second Degree (deeper; blisters develop)	Immerse in cold water, blot dry with sterile cloth for protection. Treat for shock. Obtain medical attention if severe.	Break blisters. Remove shreds of tissue. Use antiseptic preparation, ointment spray, or home remedy on severe burn.
Third Degree (deeper destruction, skin layers destroyed)	Cover with sterile cloth to protect. Treat for shock. Watch for breathing difficulty. Obtain medical attention quickly.	Remove charred clothing that is stuck to burn. Apply ice. Use home medication.
Chemical Burn	Remove by flushing with large quantities of water for at least 5 minutes. Remove surrounding clothing. Obtain medical attention.	

Source: U.S. Coast Guard.

6. Keep the area and dressing as clean and dry as possible.

7. Elevate the burned area, if possible, for the first twenty-four hours.

8. Administer a pain medication, if necessary.

Proper burn care will decrease the chance of infection and speed the healing process.

The time needed for the wound to heal varies according to the wound. A relatively minor partial-thickness burn may close in five to seven days; a deep partial-thickness burn may take up to thirty days to heal. When the wound is closed, apply moisturizing cream as needed to prevent excessive drying and itching.

Damaged skin cannot tolerate daily wear and tear even though it appears healed. An injury on an exposed area of the body is especially vulnerable. Total healing requires up to eighteen months, and the burned area may be hypersensitive to heat and cold for a long time after the injury occurred.

Vitamin E ointment has been promoted by some as useful for treating superficial burns; yet there are no known controlled studies to support the claim.

Extracts of the Aloe vera plant are widely believed by the public to be useful in the treatment of first-degree burns (e.g., sunburn). This is supported by a long history of use in Mexico. Even though scientific documentation of its effectiveness is extremely limited, researchers are finding support for its use in the treatment of minor burns after the burned part has been first cooled.

SUNBURN

Sunburn is one of the most common injuries to the human skin. A sunburn is caused by overexposure to ultraviolet rays, causing damage to the tissues of the skin. The nerves become inflamed, causing pain; the small blood vessels become injured, causing redness, swelling, and leakage of plasma, which result in blister formation.

It is difficult to gauge accurately the amount of ultraviolet light the skin has received. It is not until after exposure (four to twelve hours later) that the redness, tenderness, and discomfort of sunburned skin confirm the person's error of judgment.

If you have become sunburned:

1. Avoid any further exposure to the sun.

2. If your eyes are affected, contact your doctor.

3. Keep the sunburned area cool. Do not apply ice because this may result in frostbite. Cool water constricts blood vessels which reduces swelling and pain. If a cold shower makes you feel better, there is no reason to discourage it for first-degree sunburn.

4. Aspirin is extremely effective in relieving the inflammation and pain and should be used unless your doctor instructs you to the contrary.

5. If blisters break, thoroughly wash the area twice daily with soap and water and then cover with sterile gauze to prevent infection.

6. Apply a cream (Noxema™, Nivea™, etc.) after the pain has stopped to help keep the skin moist. Avoid topical burn ointments and sprays. They are generally ineffective and may cause allergic reactions.

7. It is important to drink lots of water during the acute period of sunburn and to eat only light foods.

8. If the burn becomes infected, contact your doctor. Infection seldom happens with sunburn unless there is also an abrasion or contact dermatitis, such as poison ivy.

CHEMICAL BURNS

You need not have training in toxicology to treat all of the common chemical burns, because emergency care is the same for all except a few special burns for which something has to be added to neutralize the chemical.

All acids, alkalies, and caustic agents are best treated by washing with large quantities of water. In acid and alkali burns, damage is practically set within three minutes after the victim comes in contact with the chemical, so if you get the victim in the water in the first minute or two after the injury, the damage will be substantially reduced.

Nevertheless, prolonged washing may do a great deal of good, even when it is started late. Prolonged washing means washing for no less than twenty minutes. That is a long time and it is difficult to do, even in the best of circumstances.

Try to avoid applying water under any type of pressure because it drives the chemical deeper into the tissue. Use a faucet or a hose under low pressure and simply wash with a gentle flow for long periods of time.

The washing technique must be modified for dry lime and white phosphorus burns. Before washing, the lime should be brushed away gently. Water mixed with lime reacts chemically to produce heat, which may further burn the skin. White phosphorus continues to burn as long as it is exposed to oxygen. The only way to stop the burning is to close off the air supply to the affected area. This can be done by submerging it in water or covering with an airtight wet dressing.

Do not attempt to neutralize a chemical because the neutralization process may produce heat, which can cause further damage. Additional treatments would be the same as for any thermal burn of the same extent and depth.

ELECTRICAL BURNS

When electrical current passes through tissue, it creates heat, causing internal burns. These burns are actually worse than they look from the outside. Third-degree burns will be seen where the current entered and exited the body. The current can travel along blood vessels and nerves as well as muscles.

If a person grabs hold of a "hot" wire, the electrical current causes the muscles in the hand to contract (fingers close around the cord), making it impossible for the person to remove his or her hand. The only safe way to "free" such a person is to stop the current. In addition, the current may paralyze the nerves and muscles that control breathing and heartbeat. Unconsciousness and death can occur even from house current.

When someone is in contact with electrical current, it is not safe to touch him or her until the current has stopped. You may unplug the appliance if the plug is not damaged, or turn off the power at the switch box if you are afraid to touch the cord. *Do not touch the appliance or the victim until the current is off.*

The first priority at the scene of an electrical injury is prevention of injury to rescuers and bystanders. If there is a fallen wire at the scene, treat it as live. Do not approach the victim until the power is disconnected, the wire removed from the victim, or the wire is dead. Do not attempt to remove the wire with ropes or wooden poles or to cut the wire. Wait until the electric company or qualified rescue unit arrives to handle the situation.

If the victim is involved in a motor vehicle accident and the downed wire is making contact with the car, do not let the victim get out of the car or let bystanders try to help the victim out of the car. The only exception to this rule is when there is a potential of the car igniting. In this case, instruct the victim to jump out of the car carefully without making contact with the car or wire.

Once the danger of causing injury to the rescuers has passed, treatment can begin. The first priority is to check the ABCs—airway, breathing and circulation. Give mouth-to-mouth resuscitation and/or cardiopulmonary resuscitation, whichever is needed. The two most common causes of death from electrical injury are asphyxiation and cardiac arrest.

Asphyxiation results from the muscular contractions produced by alternating current. The spasms not only affect the victim's ability to let go of the energized object, but also they impair the victim's ability to breathe.

Electrical current may result in loss of consciousness lasting from several minutes to hours. If the current passes directly through the brain, it may cause a seizure.

When vital signs are stable, you can check for burns. You may relieve the pain of first- and second-degree burns by applying cold water, but most electrical burns are third-degree burns. If the skin is charred or white, cover with sterile material, elevate the part, and treat for shock by elevating the legs about twelve inches and keeping the victim warm. Seek medical aid for the victim.

The victim should be transported to the nearest hospital capable of handling such an injury.

The severity of electrical burns often is difficult to determine because the deeper layers of the skin, muscles, and internal organs may be involved.

Thermal Burns

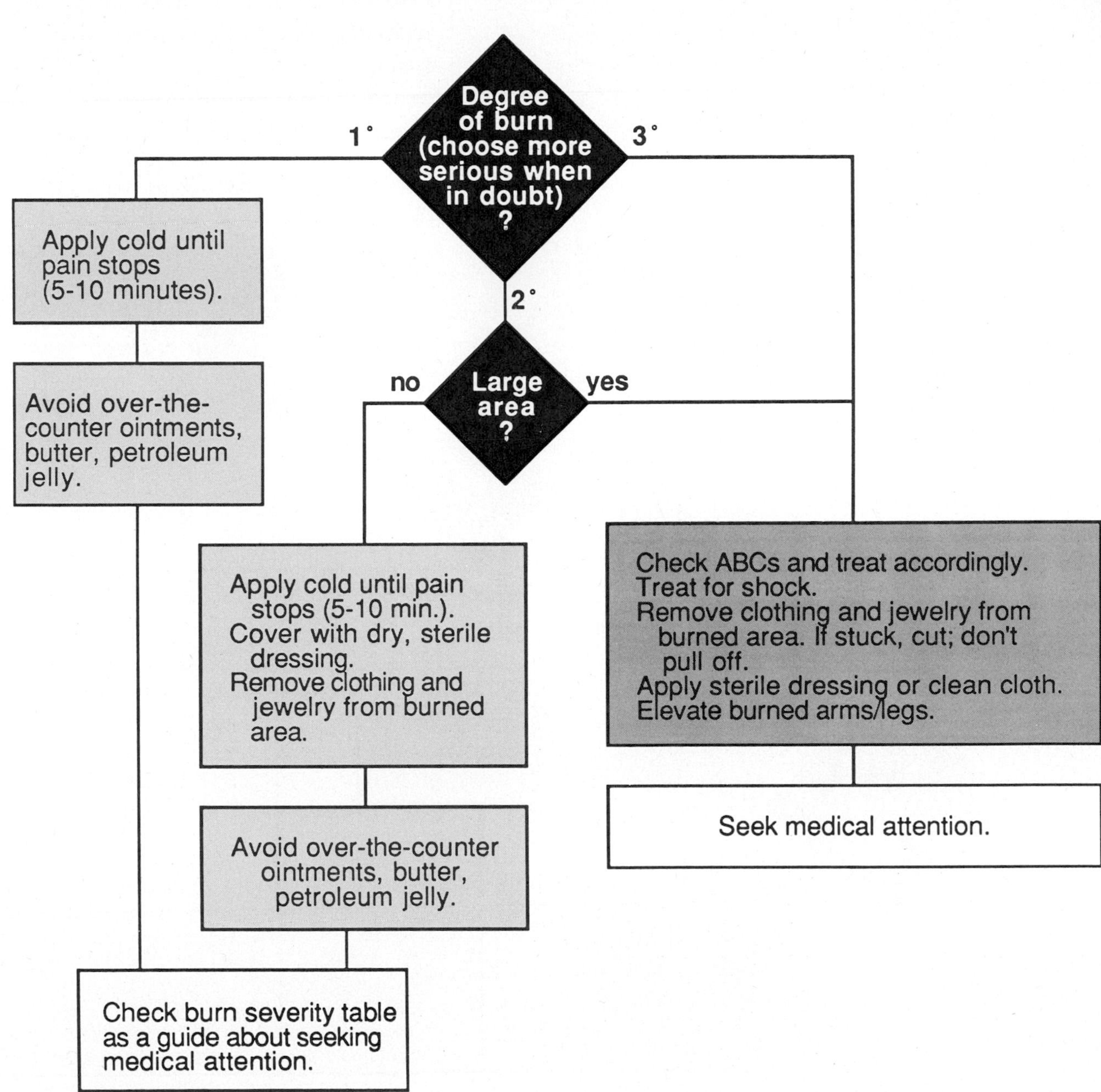

Chemical Burns

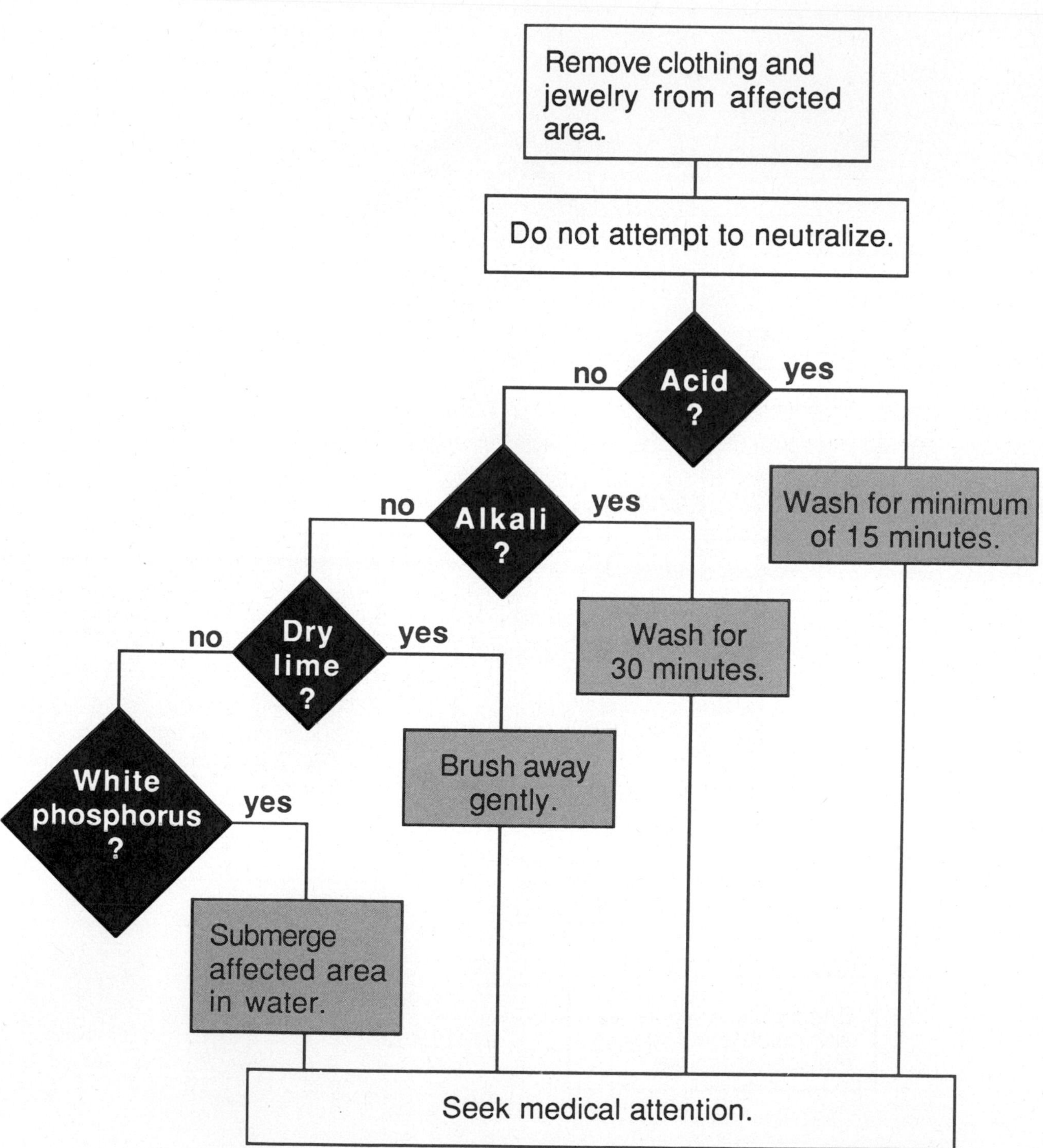

Electrical Burns

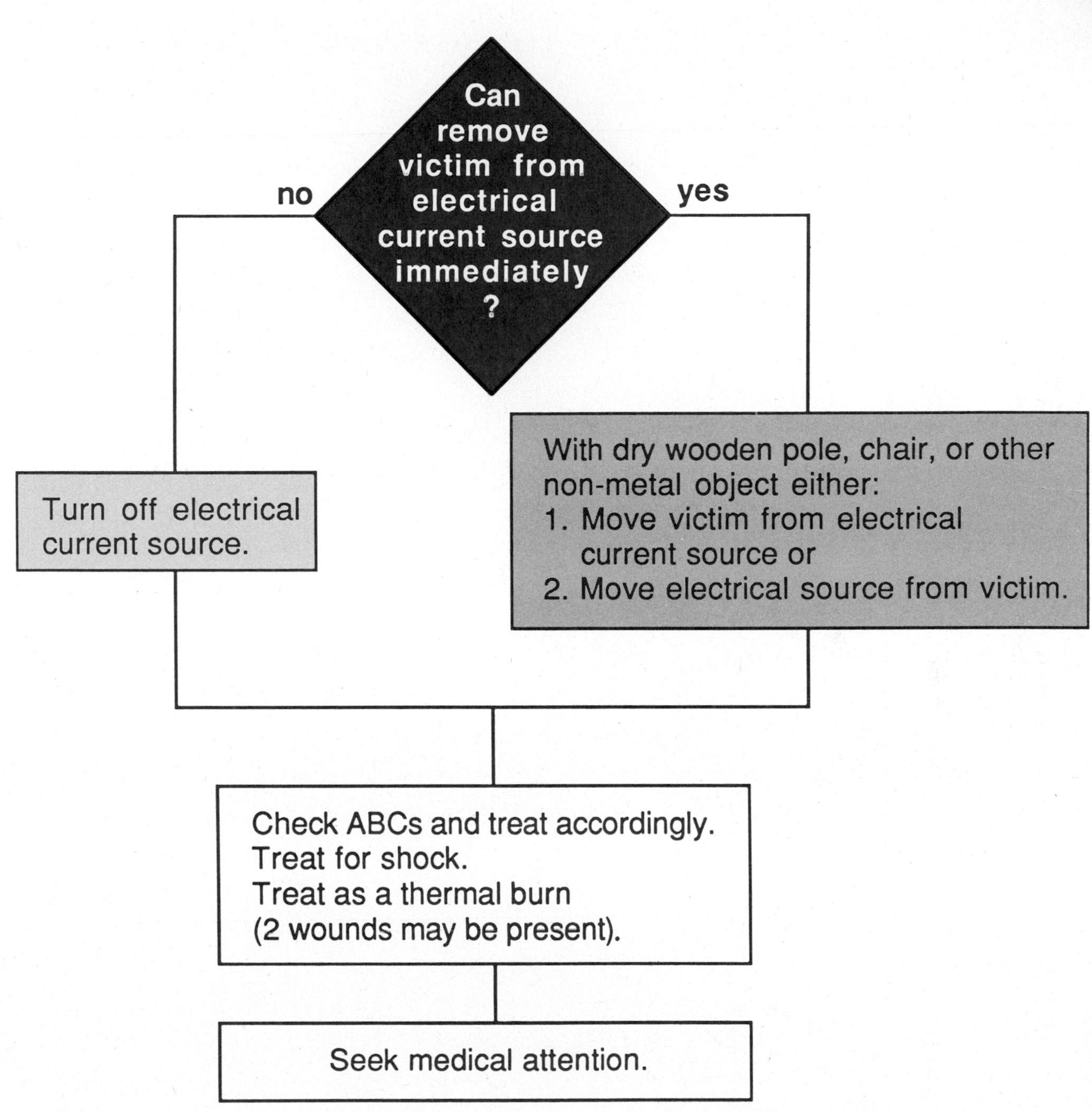

Thermal Burns

LEARNING ACTIVITIES

T F 1. A first-degree burn is characterized by blisters.
T F 2. A third-degree burn results in a loss of sensation in the burned area due to destruction of nerve endings.
T F 3. In an adult, a third-degree burn of one leg is considered critical.
T F 4. In a child, a third-degree burn of one leg is considered critical.
T F 5. Burns should be covered with grease to relieve pain.
T F 6. Cold water is suggested for first-degree and small second-degree burns.
T F 7. Commercial burn ointments, sprays, and home remedies are permissible for small second-degree burns.
T F 8. An entire leg represents 18% of the adult body.
T F 9. The depth of a burn can be easily determined by merely looking at the burn.
T F 10. The "Rule of Nines" is a general guide for measuring the size of a burn in terms of a percentage of a person's total body surface.
T F 11. Blisters caused by burns should be opened to relieve pressure.
T F 12. Third-degree burns are usually accompanied by the other degrees of burns.
T F 13. Third-degree burns are charred or whitish in appearance.
T F 14. The first aider can immediately determine the depth or degree of a burn.
T F 15. Dry dressings are preferable to wet dressings for covering burns.
T F 16. Fluids should not be given to burn victims.
T F 17. The first aider should apply butter or margarine to sunburn to relieve pain.
T F 18. A good index of the severity of the burn is the extent of the pain.
T F 19. The first aider should remove any clothing that sticks to a victim's burn.
T F 20. First-degree burns are more severe than third-degree burns.
T F 21. Second-degree burns are usually more painful than third-degree burns.
T F 22. Infection is major concern in burn treatment.
T F 23. In chemical burns, the first aider should neutralize the offending chemical.
T F 24. Generally, the best treatment of chemical burns is prolonged rinsing with water.
T F 25. Alkali burns are less serious than acid burns.
T F 26. Aloe vera can be useful in the care of a first-degree burn.
T F 27. Sunburns do not cause blistering of the skin.
T F 28. Burn ointments are ineffective on sunburns.
T F 29. Most electrical burns cause third-degree burns.
T F 30. Electrical burns will be seen where the current entered and exited the body.
T F 31. A burn that reddens the skin but does not cause blistering is a first-degree burn.
T F 32. According to the "Rule of Nines," one arm is estimated to constitute 9% of the body area.
T F 33. Tell victims to jump from a vehicle that has a downed power line lying across it.

Case 1: Upon arriving at a neighbor's home, you find two distraught parents trying to undress a screaming youngster. You learn that the child pulled a pan of hot grease off the stove onto himself.

1. What is the immediate emergency care in this situation? ______________________

____

2. What are three secondary emergency care procedures that should be initiated?

A. ______________________

____

B. ______________________

____

C. ______________________

____

Case 2: A 29-year-old male sustains burns on the front of both arms as a result of fall leaf fire getting out of control. On arrival at the scene of the fire, you assess the depth of the burn and the extent of body surface involvement.

1. His burns have a reddened appearance and blisters are present. Classify this type of burn and describe appropriate emergency care to provide for the victim.

____

____

____

____

2. What is the "Rule of Nines" and how is it useful to a first aider?

____

3. How would you describe the burns sustained by this man in terms of the "Rule of Nines?"

____

4. Describe each of the following burn classifications:

A. First degree: ____________________

B. Second degree: ____________________

C. Third degree: ____________________

5. List the body area percentages covered by the "Rule of Nines" for an adult.

A. Head ______
B. Arms ______
C. Legs ______
D. Anterior (front) torso ______
E. Posterior (back) torso ______
F. Genitals ______

6. Describe the appropriate medical treatment for a third-degree burn.

A. ____________________

B. ____________________

C. ____________________

D. ____________________

Case 3: A 15-year-old male was joy riding in his parent's car, driving on the wrong side of the road, when he met an oncoming vehicle head-on. The driver of the other car was killed on impact. The youth was trapped in the wrecked car when the gasoline tank exploded. Initial examination revealed minor lacerations and abrasions as a result of the impact. No fractures were detected. Burns were sustained on the back of the legs, thighs, buttocks, and back. The burns also involved the left side of his chest and abdomen, left arm, forearm, and hand.

1. What emergency burn care should the first aider administer once the victim has been removed from the vehicle?

____

2. You would expect this victim to have burns of what degree?

A. ______ first-degree
B. ______ second-degree
C. ______ third-degree
D. ______ all degrees would probably be exhibited

3. Using the "Rule of Nines," what is the extent of the victim's burns?

____

Case 4: A victim has been pulled from the burning wreckage of a car by a passerby. She has burns on the front of both lower portions of the legs and the palms of both hands.
Directions: Choose the letter of the correct answer to each of the following questions:

1. First aid for burns that do not cover a large area of the body is as follows:

A. ______ Soak in hot water until pain subsides.
B. ______ Apply a commercial ointment.
C. ______ Submerge in cold water.
D. ______ Apply butter and/or petroleum jelly (Vaseline™)

2. Heat is applied to burns:

A. ______ until the pain is relieved
B. ______ that do not cover a large area
C. ______ to reduce swelling
D. ______ to kill germs and reduce infection
E. ______ never

3. When covering a painful burn, use:

A. ______ a burn ointment
B. ______ first-aid cream
C. ______ a dry dressing
D. ______ a warm, moist dressing

4. A victim has burns covering the front of both arms, his neck, face, and chest. What percentage of his body is burned?

A. ______ 22%
B. ______ 36%
C. ______ 18%
D. ______ 27%

Sunburn

Case: While on vacation, your 16-year-old daughter has spent all day at the beach. She is unable to move because of severe pain. Her back and legs are bright red.

1. Sunburn should be treated with:

   A. ______ warm, moist dressings
   B. ______ a burn ointment with a painkiller
   C. ______ cold packs
   D. ______ first-aid cream

2. A first-degree burn is characterized by:

   A. ______ deep reddening and blistering
   B. ______ reddening
   C. ______ charring
   D. ______ reddening, blistering, and charring

Chemical Burns

Case 1: A 24-year-old female working as a research chemist in a large industrial plant has spilled acid on her left hand. She has started to flood her hand with a large amount of water.

1. What is the normal emergency care for the majority of chemical burns?

   ____
   ____

2. In dealing with powdered forms of chemicals, particularly lime, the initial emergency care procedure would be to

   A. ______ wash with large amounts of water
   B. ______ do nothing, but transport immediately
   C. ______ brush the powdered chemical off, wash with large amounts of water

3. What class of chemical inflicts the deepest and longest lasting burns?

   A. ______ acids
   B. ______ alkalies

4. In chemical burns affecting the eyes, what should be done before starting any emergency care?

   ____
   ____

5. Complete the following chart, giving the appropriate percentage of total body surface affected. Write the answer on the line beside each letter.

Severity/ degree	First degree	Second degree	Third degree
Minor	A. ______	B. ______	C. ______
Moderate		D. ______	E. ______
Critical		F. ______	G. ______

6. Exceptions to determining severity of burns would involve the following body areas or injuries:

   ____
   ____

Case 2: At a chemical manufacturing company, an alkali product is accidentally splashed onto the left upper body of a 47-year-old male. His left eye is also splashed with the solution.

1. What emergency care would you provide this worker?

   A. ______________________________________
   ____
   B. ______________________________________
   ____
   C. ______________________________________
   ____

2. How long is it necessary to flush an acid- or alkali-burned area with water? ______________
   ____

3. Would the above treatment be indicated for an alkali burn of the eye? ______________
   ____

Electrical Burns

Case 1: An 18-month-old child has bitten through a household electrical cord. He has a third-degree burn around his mouth.

1. What is the severity of this burn?
____
____

2. Electrical burns may result in paralysis of the breathing center and ventricular fibrillation. It may be necessary to start:
____
____

3. After basic life support is started and accompanying burns extinguished, victims sustaining an electrical burn should be examined for ______
______________________________ .

Case 2: A crane, which is being used to unload lumber from a railroad flat car, accidentally comes into contact with overhead power lines which run parallel to the railroad tracks. When you arrive, the crane appears to be energized and the crane operator, although conscious and in the cab, shows signs of being injured.

1. What is the first step to take in rescuing the crane operator? (Choose the best response.)

   A. ______ Tell him to jump clear of the crane.
   B. ______ Enter the crane and attempt to operate the controls to free the crane from the wires.
   C. ______ Help him out of the crane.
   D. ______ Contact the utility company.
   E. ______ None of the above.

2. What instructions should you give the crane operator in this situation?
____
____

3. The presence of which additional factor in this situation would cause you to alter drastically the instructions given the crane operator?
____
____

4. What is a general guideline that all emergency crews should follow when confronted with rescue attempts involving electrical power?
____
____
____
____

5. What two types of injuries could you expect the crane operator most likely to suffer?

   A. ______ Stroke
   B. ______ Electrical burns
   C. ______ Dislocations
   D. ______ Cardiac arrest
   E. ______ Fractures

6. When a person has contacted electrical sources, the heart may stop beating and have electrical activity (as would be seen on a cardiac monitor) in a completely disorganized manner. What term describes this kind of heart activity?
____
____
____

9 Exposure to Cold and Heat

- Frostbite
- Hypothermia
- Heat-Related Emergencies

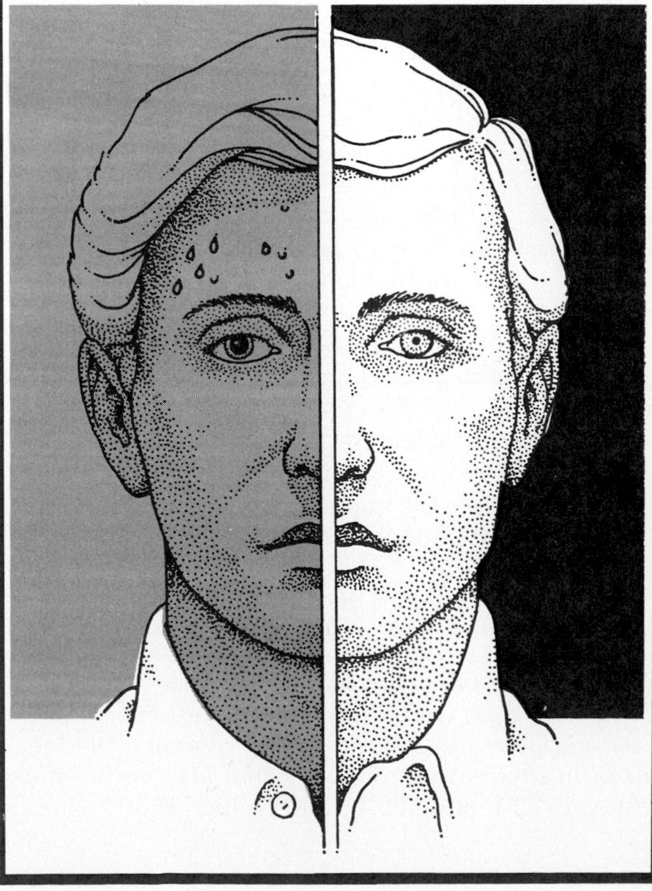

FROSTBITE

To most Americans, frostbite may seem like a remote risk. Yet, as more and more people venture outdoors in winter—skiing, hiking, hunting, snowmobiling—frostbite has become an increasing health hazard.

As the body tries to conserve heat for vital internal organs in bitter cold, the flow of warming blood to the extremities is reduced. Eventually, if the temperature in the tissue drops low enough, tiny ice crystals begin to form in the watery spaces between the cells. Expanding outward in all directions, the ice ruptures cell membranes and kills the tissue, which turns white, stiff, and insensitive to the touch. Furthermore, the reduced blood flow (due to sludging and clotting of blood inside small blood vessels) raises the possibility of gangrene occurring.

The extent of the injury depends on such factors as temperature, duration of exposure, wind velocity, humidity, lack of protective clothing, and the presence of wet clothing. Use Tables 9-1 and 9-2 as aids in determining actual temperatures. Also, the harmful effects of exposure to cold are intensified by fatigue, individual susceptibility, existing injuries, emotional stress, smoking, and drinking alcoholic beverages.

Types of Frostbite

The extent of injury is not usually known at first glance. At one time, some effort was made to describe frostbite injury in terms of degrees, as is presently done with burns (e.g., first, second, third degree). Frostbite injuries are now classified as either superficial or deep. Even these designations are somewhat limited because it is difficult initially to tell the extent of injury. Classifying may not matter, however, because the treatment for both types is basically the same.

TABLE 9-1. Wind-Chill Factor

Estimated Wind Speed (in MPH)	Actual Thermometer Reading (°F.)											
	50	40	30	20	10	0	-10	-20	-30	-40	-50	-60
	Equivalent Temperature (°F.)											
calm	50	40	30	20	10	0	-10	-20	-30	-40	-50	-60
5	40	37	27	16	6	-5	-15	-26	-36	-47	-57	-68
10	40	28	16	4	-9	-24	-33	-46	-58	-70	-83	-95
15	36	22	9	-5	-18	-32	-45	-58	-72	-85	-99	-112
20	32	18	4	-10	-25	-39	-53	-67	-82	-96	-110	-124
25	30	16	0	-15	-29	-44	-59	-74	-88	-104	-118	-133
30	25	13	-2	-18	-33	-48	-63	-79	-94	-109	-125	-140
35	27	11	-4	-20	-35	-51	-67	-82	-98	-113	-129	-145
40	26	10	-6	-21	-37	-53	-69	-85	-100	-116	-132	-148
(Wind speeds greater than 40 mph have little additional effect.)	Little danger (for properly clothed person.) Maximum danger of false sense of security.				Increasing danger. (Flesh may freeze within 1 minute.)				Great danger. (Flesh may freeze within 30 seconds.)			

Superficial: Fingers, cheeks, ears, and nose are the most commonly affected body parts. If the exposure is prolonged, the freezing may extend up the arms and legs. Ice crystals in the skin and other tissues cause the area to appear a white or grayish-yellow color. Pain may occur early and subside. Often, the part will feel only very cold and numb; and there may be a tingling, stinging, or aching sensation. The victim may not be aware of frostbite until someone mentions it. When the damage is superficial, the surface will feel hard and underlying tissue soft when depressed gently and firmly. After thawing, the part becomes flushed and sometimes deep purple in color. It later sheds by flaking.

Deep: In deep, unthawed frostbite, the area (mainly the hands and feet) will feel hard, solid, and cannot be depressed. It will be cold, pale, and numb. Blisters will appear on the surface and in the underlying tissues in twelve to thirty-six hours. After thawing, it may be blue, purple, or black in color. The area will become swollen when it thaws, and later gangrene may occur. There will be a loss of tissue. Time alone will reveal the kind of frostbite that has been present.

Emergency Care

All frostbite injuries follow the same sequence in treatment: initial care, rapid rewarming, and post care. You should also assess the victim for hypothermia because it is a life-threatening condition for which priority treatment should be given.

Initial Care: The principles of emergency care for frostbite injury are relatively few. The two most important aspects are getting the victim to a place of permanent treatment as soon as possible, and then rewarming.

If the victim is out in the field—but not too far away from a medical facility—and the part is still frozen, transport the victim as he is and make with no attempt to thaw the injured part. Be sure that the part is kept frozen. If partial thawing and refreezing occurs, ice crystals formed the second time are larger, and therefore, tissue damage is more severe.

If the injury occurs in a remote area and the victim's feet are frostbitten, you can allow the victim to walk on frostbitten feet only if the feet have not started to thaw. Otherwise, do not allow the victim to walk. Once rewarming has started, warming must be maintained. Refreezing or walking on a partially thawed part can be very harmful.

During transportation and initial treatment, do not permit the use of alcoholic beverages because they dilate capillaries and cause a loss of body heat. Do not let the victim smoke because smoking constricts capillaries and thus provides poor circulation.

Do not rub the affected part to restore circulation, and especially do not rub it with snow. Rubbing or massage increases the injury to frozen tissue; rubbing it with snow just intensifies the damage.

Rapid Rewarming: There are two techniques of rapid rewarming: wet and dry.

1. *The wet rapid rewarming technique* is preferred because it preserves the greatest amount of tissue. It is accomplished by completely immersing the local part in an adequate amount of water at a temperature between 102°F and 106°F. Different authorities have

TABLE 9-2. Estimating Wind Velocity from Simple Observations

If you see . . .	The wind is probably blowing
Flags or pennants hanging limp from their staffs; smoke rising vertically from chimneys and open fires	0–1 mph
Flags and pennants barely moving; leaves moving slightly on trees; smoke drifting lazily with the wind	0–3 mph
Flags and pennants moving slightly out from their staffs; leaves rustling in trees; if you feel wind on your face	4–7 mph
Flags and pennants standing out from their staffs at an angle of 30° to 40°; or leaves and twigs in constant motion	8–12 mph
Small branches moving in trees; dust and paper being blown about	13–18 mph
Flags and pennants flying at 90° angle; small trees swaying	19–24 mph
Flags and pennants standing straight out from their staffs and fluttering vigorously; large tree branches in motion; or if you hear whistling in power lines	25–31 mph
Flags and pennants whipping about wildly on the staffs; whole trees in motion; loose objects being picked up and blown about; or if you find it somewhat difficult to walk when facing the wind	32–38 mph
Twigs being broken from trees; drivers having a problem in controlling their vehicles; or if you hear power lines whining loudly	39–46 mph
Trees bending sharply; structural damage occurring in buildings; the progress of vehicles and pedestrians alike being seriously impeded	47–54 mph
Trees being uprooted; considerable structural damage occurring	55–63 mph
Buildings suffering severe damage	63–72 mph
Widespread destruction; or if walking is virtually impossible	more than 72 mph

suggested temperatures as low as 90°F to as high as 108°F. The water bath should be tested frequently with a thermometer. If a thermometer is not available, pour some of the water over the inner portion of your wrist or arm to make sure the water is not too hot. Discontinue warming when the part becomes flushed, usually within twenty minutes with the wet method. Further rapid wet rewarming is not necessary. For injuries involving the face or ears, you can apply warm moist cloths (frequently changed to maintain heat).

The thawing process is quick but usually quite painful. As thawing proceeds, a pink flushing progresses down the extremity; continue thawing until the tip of the thawed part flushes, is warm to the touch, and remains flushed when removed from the warm bath.

2. *The dry rapid rewarming technique* takes three to four times as long as the wet technique and is best accomplished by the use of natural body warmth as exemplified by putting the victim's hands in another person's axilla (armpit) or sharing warm clothing. Also, the victim can be exposed to warm room air.

The first aider should remember certain procedures *not* to take:

1. Do *not* allow the victim to walk nor massage a body part.
2. Do *not* use water hotter than 110°F (may cause massive tissue destruction).
3. Do *not* expose the extremity near an open flame or fire.

Post-Care: After rewarming frostbite of a lower extremity, treat the victim as a litter case. Remove any of the victim's constricting clothing, maintain total body warmth, and encourage sleep. Protect the injured part(s) from direct contact with clothing, bedding, and so on.

After rewarming, take care to leave any blisters intact. Place dry, sterile gauze between toes and fingers to keep them separated. Elevate the affected part(s), and protect them from being bumped or rubbed.

Depending on circumstances, anyone exposed to temperatures below 32°F is a candidate for frostbite.

This means that a large portion of the population are potential victims of frostbite injury. When dealing with frostbite, remember to "treat for the worst—and hope for the best."

HYPOTHERMIA

The *Guinness Book of World Records* reports two cases of victims surviving body temperatures as low as 60.8°F. One example is Dorothy Mae Stevens who was found alive in an alley in Chicago on February 1, 1951. In 1956, Vickie Mary Davis of Milwaukee, Wisconsin, at age two years and one month, was found unconscious on the floor of an unheated house and the air temperature had dropped to 24°F. Her temperature returned to normal after twelve hours, but it may have been as low as 59°F when she was first found.

Hypothermia (low body temperature) occurs when the body loses more heat than it produces. Subfreezing temperatures are not needed for hypothermia to occur. If body temperature falls to 80°F, most people die.

Types of Hypothermia

Mild hypothermia in the range of 90° to 95°F, may have few or no symptoms, but they can include uncontrollable shivering, abnormal drowsiness, slurred speech, memory lapses, incoherence, and fumbling hands. Persons suffering from mild hypothermia can walk but will frequently stumble and stagger. They are usually conscious and can talk. In healthy persons, there is almost no mortality. Though many people have cold extremities in winter, a hypothermic person has a cold abdomen and back. The hands and feet are the first body parts to get cold and the last to warm up.

Persons suffering from *severe* hypothermia with a temperature below 90°F must be considered at serious risk of dying. The following may be present: coldness to touch; pulselessness; cyanotic appearance; unresponsiveness to pain; and fixed, dilated pupils. Shivering usually stops. Muscles may become stiff and rigid, similar to rigor mortis.

Such findings make it difficult to distinguish a dead person from the hypothermic person who has a chance for complete recovery. The victim should not be considered dead unless he fails to respond to cardiopulmonary resuscitation after being rewarmed.

The victim's temperature should be taken rectally because oral and axillary temperatures reflect shell rather than core temperature. The standard clinical thermometer is calibrated from 94° to 108°F. A rectal thermometer reading from 84° to 108°F is available, though not commonly found.

TABLE 9-3. Treatment for Hypothermia by First Aiders and the General Public

1. Treat the victim very gently.
2. Remove wet clothing. Replace with dry clothing or dry coverings of some kind.
3. Insulate from the cold.
4. Add heat to the head, neck, chest, and groin externally (hot water bottles, warm bodies, warm packs—taking care not to burn the victim) or internally, if a system for breathing warm moist air is available. Avoid attempts to warm the extremities.
5. Do not rub or manipulate extremities.
6. Do not give coffee or alcohol.
7. Do not put victim in a shower or bath.
8. Warm fluids can be given only after uncontrollable shivering stops and the victim has a clear level of consciousness, the ability to swallow, and evidence of rewarming already.
9. If *severe hypothermia* is present, treat as above and transport to a medical facility.
10. If there is no way to get to a better medical facility, rewarm the victim slowly, cautiously, and gradually.

Treatment for Severe Hypothermia with No Life Signs (CPR Required)

1. Provide basic treatment as indicated above.
2. Carefully assess the presence or absence of pulse or respiration for one to two minutes.
3. If no pulse or respiration, start CPR.
4. Use mouth-to-mouth breathing.
5. Obtain a rectal temperature, if possible.
6. If you are less than fifteen minutes from a medical facility, do not bother trying to add heat.
7. If you are more than fifteen minutes from a medical facility, add heat gradually and gently.
8. Reassess the physical status (pulse and respirations) periodically.
9. Transfer to a medical facility in all cases.

Treatment for Severe Hypothermia with Signs of Life Pulse and Respirations Present (CPR Not Required)

1. Provide treatment as indicated in the first section.
2. If you are more than fifteen minutes from a medical facility, add heat gradually and gently.
3. Transfer to a medical facility.

Source: "State of Alaska Hypothermia and Cold Water Near Drowning Guidelines." Emergency Medical Services Section, Alaska Department of Health and Social Services. Reprinted with permission.

Types of Exposure

The different types of exposure are based on heat loss rate.

Acute exposure occurs when the individual loses body heat very rapidly, usually in a water immersion. Acute exposure is considered to be six hours or less in duration. An individual who plunges into cold water that causes his body care temperature to drop swiftly is an example.

Subacute exposure is defined as longer than six hours, but less than twenty-four hours, and it involves a land based experience or immersion in water warmer than 70°F. For example, a person who is lost in a sparsely populated area, or incapacitated for some reason elsewhere, who lies exposed much of the night to snow, rain, or cold, with insufficient clothing or shelter to maintain body core temperature.

Chronic hypothermia implies long-term cooling, generally occurring on land and lasting more than twenty-four hours. For example, a person could suffer from this as a result of drugs, disease, or failure of the body's temperature-regulating mechanism, perhaps combined with age. The person experiences a slow cooling over a period of days. This might occur without ever leaving a house where room temperatures are lower than the person can safely tolerate.

What You Need To Know About Hypothermia

Remember that subfreezing temperatures are not required for a person to succumb to hypothermia. It may develop within a few minutes by immersion in cold water, in a matter of hours by exposure to cold weather, or in a matter of days by continuous exposure to milder cold temperatures.

In the United States, hypothermia is most frequently seen among alcoholics, victims of drug abuse, and the elderly. One of the most common problems in the emergency care of hypothermia is the failure to recognize it. This is due, in part, to the inadequacy of standard thermometers. Oral thermometers (those found in most homes) register only as low as 94°F. Lower reading thermometers are used by emergency response teams and hospital emergency departments.

Emergency Care

The emergency care of hypothermia is aimed at rewarming the victim as well as treating complications that may arise. The hypothermic victim's heart is very susceptible to ventricular fibrillation which, therefore, is usually the ultimate cause of death in hypothermia. Keep this in mind while handling the hypothermic victim.

Guidelines (refer to Table 9-3) have been established and published for use by rescuers dealing with cold problems in Alaska. They evolved from a conference conducted by the State of Alaska Emergency Medical Services Section.

HEAT-RELATED EMERGENCIES

Heat afflicts people of all ages. However, the severity of the reaction tends to increase with age—heat cramps in a 17-year-old may be heat exhaustion in a 40-year-old and heat stroke in a person over 60.

The body tries to adapt to varying temperatures by adjusting the amount of salt in its perspiration. In hot weather, the idea is to lose enough water to keep the body cool, but to create the least possible chemical disturbance. Salt helps body tissues retain water, and if the body loses too much salt through perspiration, the person may be subject to dehydration and the further overheating that follows.

You should know the signs and symptoms of heat-related injuries and be able to administer first aid to others. Refer to Table 9-4 and see Figure 9-1. You must deal with heat exhaustion and heat stroke quickly or the victim can be in real trouble.

Heat Cramps

Heat cramps—muscle spasms occurring in the arms or legs after exertion—are the most painful, but least dangerous heat-related injury. They may occur when an excessive amount of body fluid is lost through sweating. The sodium and potassium lost from excessive sweating creates low amounts of these important minerals in the fluid surrounding the muscle cells. This changes the electrical sensitivity of the muscle, sometimes causing it to contract without warning and stay contracted, which can be very painful.

Cramping may recur because the mineral imbalance that caused the problem cannot be corrected immediately. A diet of fresh fruit and vegetables can help prevent potassium and sodium shortage. Dehydration must be prevented by drinking enough water to keep the body weight constant. Commercial exercise drinks contain the necessary minerals and fluids, but they should be used after exercising, rather than before or during it, when water is best.

Massage rarely provides relief and sometimes actually worsens pain; gentle stretching occasionally may be helpful. A salt water solution (one teaspoon per quart of water) provides the proper balance. About one-half glassful should be given every 15 minutes for an hour. Discontinue if the victim vomits. A soft drink mix (e.g., Kool-Aid) can help the drink's taste. For the next few days, the victim should avoid the activity that brought on the cramps.

Heat Exhaustion

Heat exhaustion implies the inability of the circulatory and thermoregulatory systems to keep pace with the demands of work in the heat. It is less critical

TABLE 9-4. Heat Exposure Emergencies

Indicators	Heat Cramps (Least Serious)	Heat Exhaustion (Serious)	Heat Stroke (Most Serious)
Cause	Salt and water loss	Salt and water loss	Failure of heat-regulating mechanisms
Cramping	Present	May be present	Absent
Skin	Cool, moist	Cool, pale, moist	Hot, flushed, dry
Temperature	Normal	Normal or low	Very high
Pulse	Rapid	Rapid, weak	Rapid, bounding
First aid	Salt water solution, unless on medical restriction. Commercial exercise drinks may be used.	Cooling Reclining position, elevate legs. If conscious, cold liquids may be used.	Rapid cooling Semireclining position Obtain medical care immediately.

than heat stroke, but it requires prompt attention because it can progress to heat stroke if left untreated.

The skin is pale, cool, and wet. Heat exhaustion is especially serious and may be fatal in older people and people with heart problems. The victim must discontinue physical activity and be cooled immediately by applying cold and ice to the skin, giving cold liquids by mouth, and exposing the skin to air (especially fans or air conditioners). The need for hospitalization is rare.

Heat Stroke

Heat stroke is the most dangerous heat emergency likely to be encountered. The death rate from this condition approaches 50%, even with appropriate therapy. Victims most commonly die of complications such as brain damage, shock, or liver or kidney failure. It occurs when heat exhaustion is not controlled.

Most victims are unconscious. The best sign of heat stroke is the victim's hot, dry skin and high body temperature. Heat stroke victims do not sweat because of severe electrolyte imbalance and impaired hypothalamus function. In addition, some experts believe that sweat glands actually become "fatigued" following periods of excessive perspiration. The victim may also reveal fixed, unreactive pupils of the eyes, blotchy redness of the face and skin.

Simply moving the person with heat stroke to a cooler environment is not usually enough to reverse

TABLE 9-5. Apparent Temperature

	Air Temperature										
	70	75	80	85	90	95	100	105	110	115	120
Relative Humidity	Apparent Temperature*										
0%	64	69	73	78	83	87	91	95	99	103	107
10%	65	70	75	80	85	90	95	100	105	111	116
20%	66	72	77	82	87	93	99	105	112	120	130
30%	67	73	78	84	90	96	104	113	123	135	148
40%	68	74	79	86	93	101	110	123	137	151	
50%	69	75	81	88	96	107	120	135	150		
60%	70	76	82	90	100	114	132	149			
70%	70	77	85	93	106	124	144				
80%	71	78	86	97	113	136					
90%	71	79	88	102	122						
100%	72	80	91	108							

*Degrees Fahrenheit.
Source: National Weather Service.

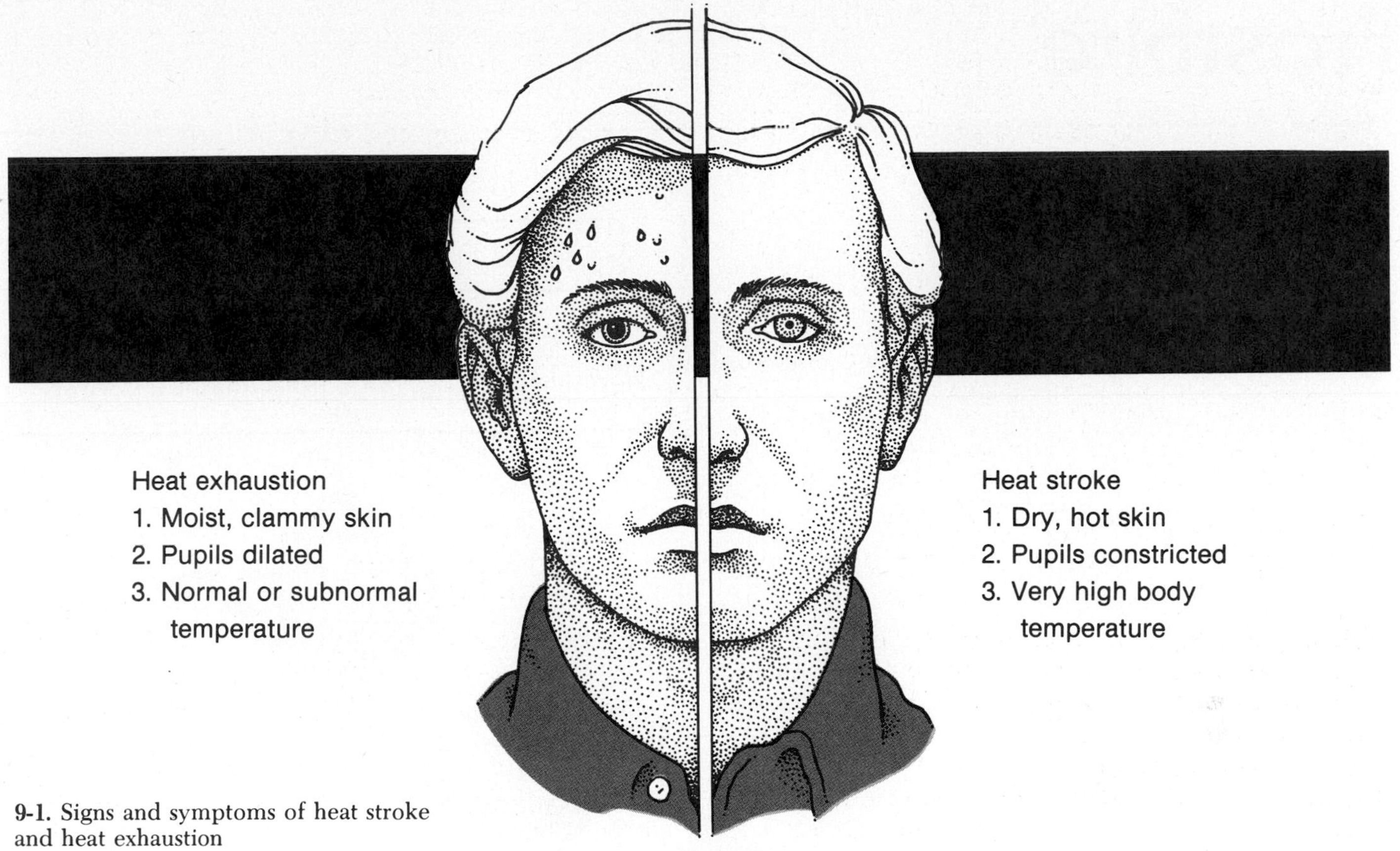

9-1. Signs and symptoms of heat stroke and heat exhaustion

the internal overheating. Quick action must be taken to lower the core body temperature. Immersion in tubs of ice water used to be the standard treatment for heat stroke victims. Many experts now recommend a simpler and more effective treatment. It can be started quickly and applied while transporting the victim to a medical facility.

Undress the heat stroke victim to allow air to circulate around his body (keep modesty in mind), and wrap him in wet towels. Then place ice packs at areas with abundant blood supply (e.g., neck, armpits, and groin). If driving to the hospital, leave the car windows open and have someone fan the victim, if possible. These maneuvers facilitate evaporation and begin the cooling process.

In addition to cooling the victim, check and treat accordingly any breathing stoppage and protect the victim during seizures, if they occur. Continue cooling the victim until his temperature drops to 102°F. Stop at this point in order to prevent seizures from occurring. All heat stroke victims should be hospitalized.

It is important to prevent heat-related injuries through adequate water and mineral intake to prevent the dehydration and chemical imbalances. If a heat-related injury occurs, prompt and adequate treatment are even more important to keep the condition from becoming a life-threatening one.

Table 9–5 shows the apparent temperature (how hot the weather feels) at various combinations of temperature and humidity. When the apparent temperature rises above 130°F heat stroke may be imminent. Between 105° and 130°F, heat cramps or heat exhaustion are likely. With prolonged exposure and physical activity, heat stroke is also possible. Between 90° and 105°F, heat cramps and heat exhaustion are possible with lengthy exposure and activity. Between 80° and 90°F fatigue occurs during prolonged activity and/or exposure. Heat stress varies with age, health, and body characteristics.

Frostbite

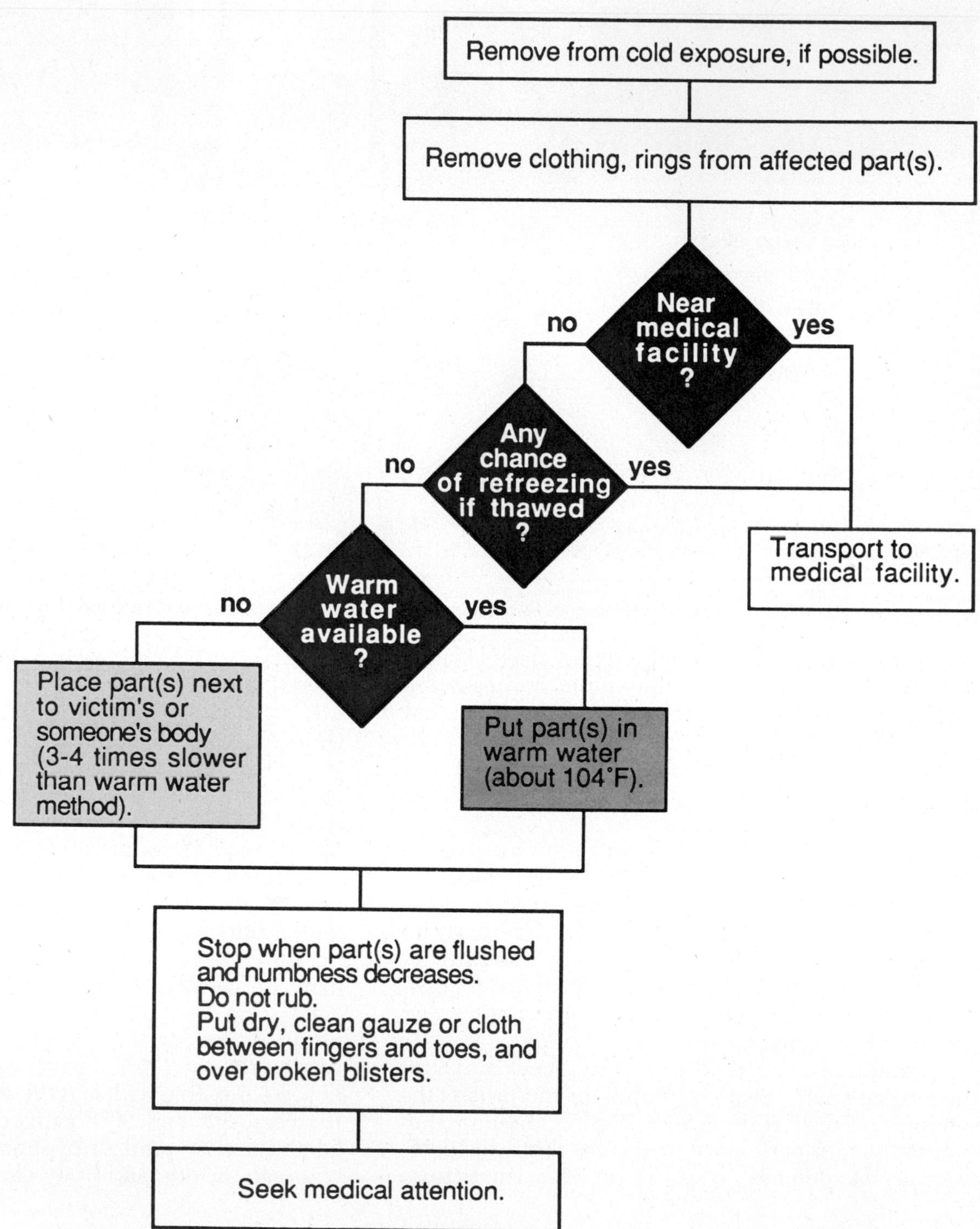

Remove from cold exposure, if possible.
Remove clothing, rings from affected part(s).
Near medical facility ?
no
yes
Any chance of refreezing if thawed ?
no
yes
Transport to medical facility.
Warm water available ?
no
yes
Place part(s) next to victim's or someone's body (3-4 times slower than warm water method).
Put part(s) in warm water (about 104°F).
Stop when part(s) are flushed and numbness decreases.
Do not rub.
Put dry, clean gauze or cloth between fingers and toes, and over broken blisters.
Seek medical attention.

Hypothermia

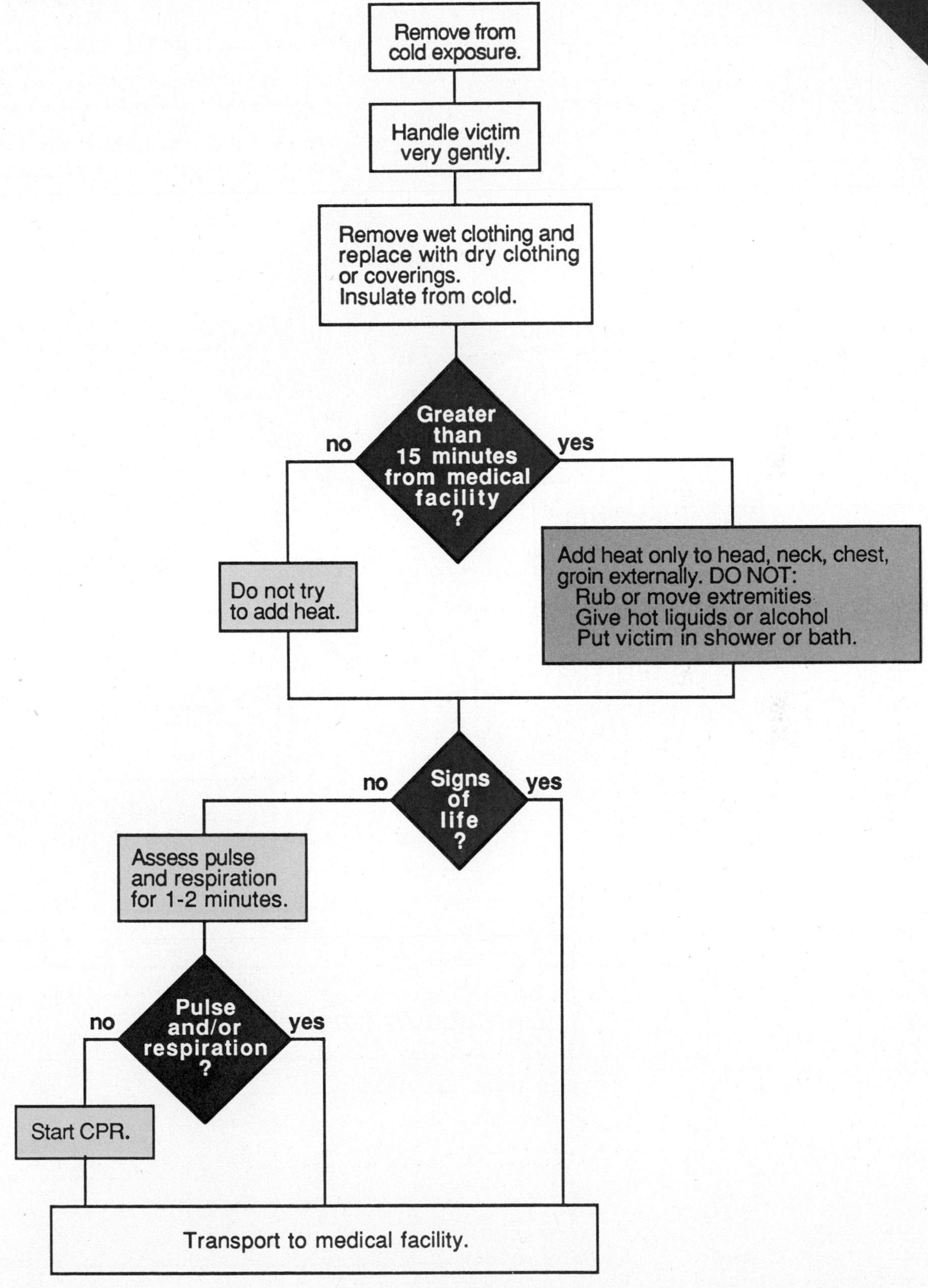

Cold Water Drowning

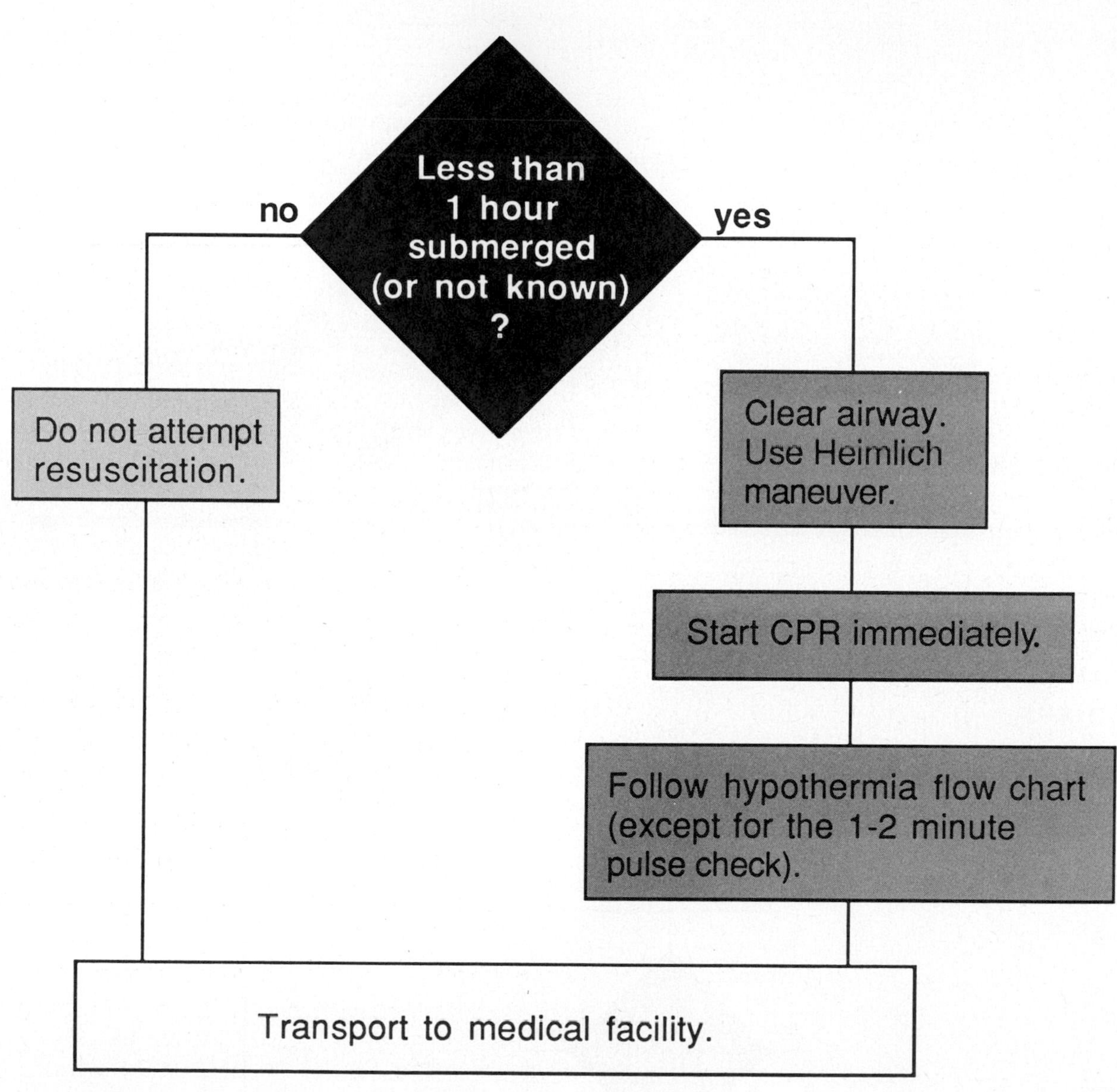

Heat-Related Injuries

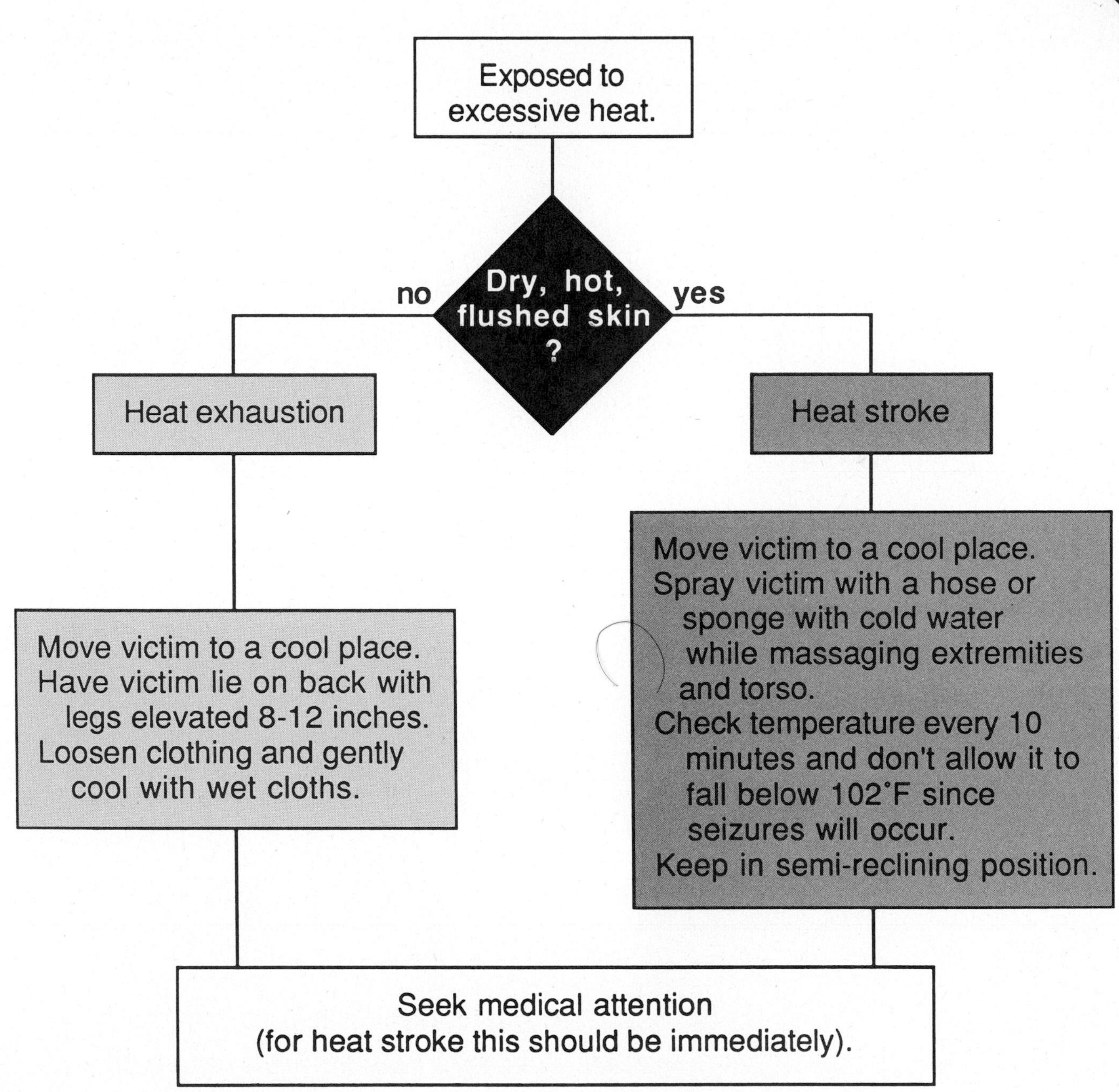

Frostbite and Hypothermia

LEARNING ACTIVITIES

T F 1. Shivering is an attempt by the body to generate heat.
T F 2. In cold weather, water or fluid between the body's cells can freeze.
T F 3. A frostbitten part should be massaged.
T F 4. Rewarm the frostbitten parts slowly because of the pain that will result.
T F 5. Blisters may form as a result of frostbite.
T F 6. Once the frostbitten part is rewarmed, the victim should exercise.
T F 7. Heat is lost more from cold air than cold water.
T F 8. Smoking and drinking alcoholic beverages intensify the harmful effects of cold.
T F 9. Rubbing frostbitten parts with snow is recommended.
T F 10. The effects of frostbite are more severe if the injured area is thawed and then refrozen.
T F 11. Temperatures below freezing are needed for frostbite to occur, but not for hypothermia.
T F 12. A frozen part should be warmed gradually.
T F 13. Stop rewarming a frostbitten part once it appears flushed.
T F 14. Gangrene may result from severe frostbite.
T F 15. The first aider should immediately break the blisters that may develop in frostbite because it reduces the pain.
T F 16. In hypothermia, CPR may be a necessary first aid procedure.
T F 17. In case of frostbite, it is best to rewarm the affected part(s) rapidly by immersing in water between 102° and 105°F.
T F 18. If no warm water is available, use of body warmth can be useful.
T F 19. People have survived over thirty minutes of submersion in cold water.
T F 20. Handle the hypothermic victim very gently.
T F 21. An individual who plunges into cold water is involved with subacute exposure.
T F 22. Giving a victim hot liquids (coffee, chocolate) may help psychologically but little physiologically.
T F 23. Victims of hypothermia are extremely prone to ventricular fibrillation.

Case 1: A middle-aged male is found beneath a railroad car on a cold night. He is semi-responsive and you detect an alcohol smell about his body. The temperature is 10°F with a wind speed of 25 miles per hour. His hands and feet are noted to be cold, pale, and solid. There is no evidence of other injury.

1. What is the injury suspected?

____

____

2. What is the emergency care for this condition?

A. ______________________________

____

B. ______________________________

____

C. ______________________________

____

D. ______________________________

____

3. If you were unable to transport the victim to a medical facility immediately for further treatment, what basic equipment would you need for the emergency care of the victim at this time?

A. ______________________________

____

B. ______________________________

____

C. ______________________________

____

4. In warming frostbitten extremities, what water temperature range must be maintained?

A. ______ 98.5°—98.7°F
B. ______ 95°—100°F
C. ______ 100°—105°F
D. ______ 105°—110°F

5. What should the color of the victim's skin be at the conclusion of the warming process? (Check *all* that apply.)

   A. ______ Purple
   B. ______ Flushed
   C. ______ Gray
   D. ______ Blue

6. What precautions should be kept in mind when bandaging frostbitten extremities?

   A. ________________________________
   ____
   B. ________________________________
   ____
   C. ________________________________
   ____

Case 2: A young hunter is found lying in the woods after being lost for two days. The weather has been windy and wet with occasional snow flurries. Temperatures have ranged between 20° and 30°F. The victim is found unconscious. There are no signs of other injuries.

1. What is the initial description of this man's condition?

   ____
   ____

2. What is the emergency care for this condition?

   A. ________________________________
   ____
   B. ________________________________
   ____
   C. ________________________________
   ____

3. What is a readily available source of heat for warming a person found in this condition?

   ____
   ____
   ____
   ____

4. What is a major judgment error that the first aider must be careful to avoid with a victim who has been exposed to cold weather?

   ____
   ____
   ____
   ____

Case 3: A middle-aged male is found beneath a park bench. He is poorly clothed with no hat nor coat in overnight weather temperatures around 25°F. He is conscious and tells you he is destitute with no family and was outside overnight.

1. How much body heat can be lost through an uncovered head? ________ percent

2. Hypothermia occurs when the core body temperature falls below ______ degrees Fahrenheit.

3. One of the first signs of hypothermia he may be showing is ________________________________
   ________________________________.

4. The type of exposure identified in this case is
   ________________________________.

   Name the other two types of exposure:

   A. ________________________________
   ____
   B. ________________________________
   ____

5. What is the cause of death in hypothermia victims?

   ____
   ____
   ____

Case 4: A young girl has just been pulled out of a cold river. The girl has no pulse and is not breathing. You are told that she has been in the river for about thirty minutes.

1. The case is an example of which type of exposure?

   ____

T F 2. People have survived similar situations.

3. What body mechanism may account for such survivals?

   ____
   ____
   ____
   ____

4. What triggers the reflex identified in question #3?

   ____

T F 5. Cardiopulmonary resuscitation can be given to this victim.

Heat-Related Injuries

T F 1. The signs of heat cramps are similar to those of shock.
T F 2. Victims of heat exhaustion have a hot, dry skin.
T F 3. Heat exhaustion results in a very high body temperature.
T F 4. Heat stroke is an immediate life-threatening problem.
T F 5. The first aid for heat stroke should be directed toward immediate measures to cool the body quickly.
T F 6. Heat exhaustion is more serious than heat stroke.

Case 1: A group of children summon you to a playground on a hot, humid summer day. You find a young girl sitting on the ground. She is breathing normally but is complaining of a headache and dizziness. Her skin is cool and she is sweating heavily.

1. From what condition is this child suffering?

   A. ______ Heat cramps
   B. ______ Heat exhaustion
   C. ______ Heat stroke

2. What is the appropriate emergency care?

   A. ____
   ____
   B. ____
   ____

3. Match the following heat conditions with their symptoms. Each symptom may be associated with more than one heat condition. 1 = heat cramps; 2 = heat exhaustion; 3 = heat stroke.

   A. ______ Skin—flushed, hot, dry
   B. ______ Skin—pale, cool, sweaty
   C. ______ Skin—pale, clammy
   D. ______ Profuse sweating
   E. ______ Absence of sweating
   F. ______ Breathing—normal
   G. ______ Breathing—rapid and usually shallow
   H. ______ Dizziness

Case 2: On a hot, humid summer day you respond to a call for help at a local park. A middle-aged man, apparently a jogger, has collapsed. His skin is hot to the touch and very dry. He is unconscious.

1. From what major heat condition is this man apparently suffering?

   ____
   ____

2. What is another major heat condition?

   ____
   ____

3. Following are signs and symptoms of the two major heat conditions you should have listed above. Write the name of the heat condition that corresponds to each sign or symptom.

   A. ____________ skin—flushed, hot, dry
   B. ____________ skin—pale, clammy
   C. ____________ profuse sweating
   D. ____________ absence of sweating

4. For the apparent heat condition described in this case, what is the appropriate emergency care?

   A. ____
   ____
   B. ____
   ____
   C. ____
   ____

5. What is the emergency care for the other common heat condition?

   A. ____
   ____
   B. ____
   ____
   C. ____
   ____

Case 3: On your vacation you spend a day at a large amusement park. It is an extremely hot and humid day. During the afternoon you decide to rest a while and watch one of the special shows. Soon after you have been seated, an elderly man in front of you suddenly falls forward out of his seat. When you reach him, his wife reports that they have been walking around the park without stopping practically all day. His skin feels cool and clammy.

1. What emergency condition is this man most likely suffering from?

   ____
   ____

2. What emergency care should you provide to this man?

A. ______________________________

B. ______________________________

C. ______________________________

3. The other major heat condition is heat stroke. Although not as common as heat exhaustion, heat stroke is more serious and a true medical emergency. What are the three major signs and symptoms of heat stroke?

A. ______________________________

B. ______________________________

C. ______________________________

4. What three steps constitute the emergency care for heat stroke?

A. ______________________________

B. ______________________________

C. ______________________________

5. How can you tell the difference between heat exhaustion and heat stroke by examination of the victim's skin?

A. Heat exhaustion ______________________________

B. Heat stroke ______________________________

10 Bone, Joint, and Muscle Injuries

- Fractures
- Spinal Injuries
- Joint Injuries
    - Shoulder Injuries
    - Knee Injuries
    - Finger Injuries
    - Ankle Injuries
- Muscle Injuries

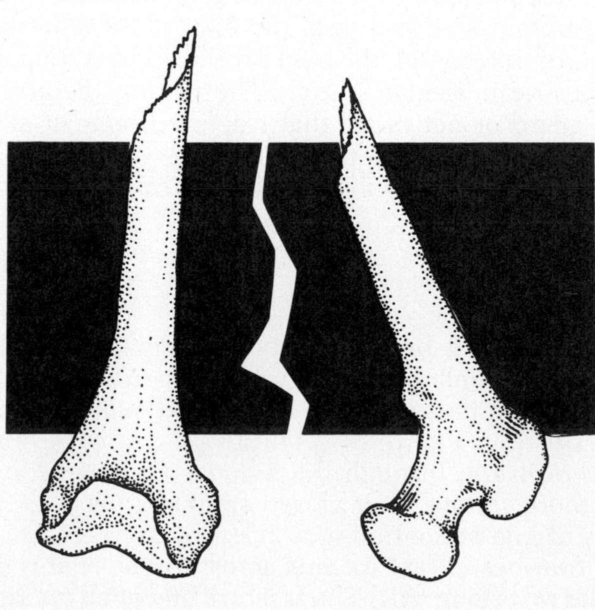

Bones, muscles, ligaments, tendons, and cartilage make up the musculoskeletal system. When the body is exposed to trauma, such as a motor vehicle accident, one or more of these parts are frequently damaged. To recognize and properly treat an injury requires an understanding of the system's composition and organization. To help this understanding, we discuss each major part separately.

Skeletal System

The human skeleton is composed of about 206 bones of many shapes and sizes. Each bone has its own characteristic structure. Bone is one of the strongest materials in nature. Yet, bones do get broken. It takes about 10 tons per square inch to fracture a bone. See Figure 10–1 for the names of the most common bones.

Joint

A joint is where two bones come together. The joint provides stability but, more important, allows for motion between the two bones. A typical joint is composed of two bone ends covered with cartilage that allows movement of the two ends with minimal friction. A thin tissue, the synovial membrane, covers this structure and secretes a fluid that lubricates the joint. Strong bands of tissue called ligaments help to hold the bone ends together.

Muscle

Muscle is a special kind of tissue that has the ability to contract or shorten.

Assessment

To evaluate a person with possible musculoskeletal damage you must examine the scene of the accident to determine what caused the injury, obtain an accurate victim history, and give a thorough physical examination.

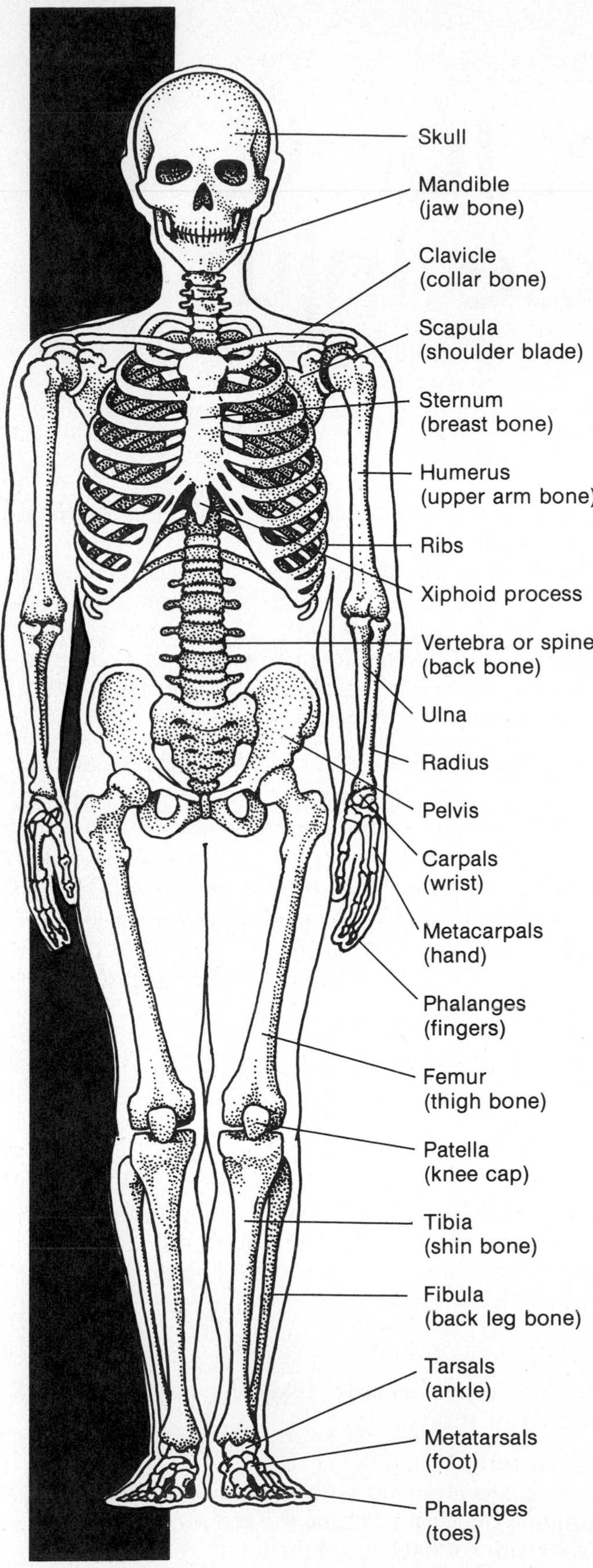

10-1. Bones of the body

Most victims with significant musculoskeletal injury will complain of pain. Usually the pain is well localized to the area of injury. Sometimes the person who has sustained a fracture will report having felt something snap.

With rare exceptions, fractures and other orthopedic injuries are not life threatening. In the victim with multiple injuries, fractures may be the most obvious and dramatic, but may not necessarily be the most serious. Therefore, the first aider should do the primary survey and manage any life threatening conditions first. Management of orthopedic injuries fit in their appropriate place in the secondary survey.

Look

Swelling and a black-and-blue mark indicate escape of blood into the tissues. Shortening or angulation between joints, deformity, or angulation in unusual direction around the joints, shortening of the extremity, and internal or external rotation when compared with the opposite extremity indicate a bony defect. Lacerations or even small puncture wounds near the site of the bony fracture are considered open fractures.

Feel

Feeling (palpation) along the length of a bone can help detect deformities, bony protuberances, or angulation that is not visible.

Always take the person's pulse below the fracture both before and after application of splints. In the arm, you should test the radial arteries, and in the leg, the pedal pulses. If there is no pulse, try to restore the blood flow with two or three gentle manipulations of the extremity. Do not make prolonged attempts.

It is difficult many times to distinguish between fractures and sprains without x-ray. If there is a question, immobilize and treat the injury as if it were a fracture. In general, the pain produced by a fracture will cause muscular spasm. The victim, therefore, will guard or not move that fractured bone at all.

Table 10-1 gives the signs and symptoms of common orthopedic injuries—fractures, dislocations, and sprains.

FRACTURES

A *fracture* is a break in a bone. It may either be closed, in which case the overlying skin is intact, or open, in which case there is a wound over the fracture site. (*See* Figure 10-2.) In an open fracture, bone may protrude through the wound. Open fractures are more serious than closed fractures because the risks of contamination and infection are greater.

A *transverse* fracture cuts across the bone at right angles to its long axis. The fracture line of an *oblique*

TABLE 10-1. Common Orthopedic Injuries—Signs and Symptoms

Fracture	Dislocation	Sprain
Pain, tenderness	Pain	Pain on movement; tenderness
Deformity or shortening.	Deformity	No deformity
Loss of use	Loss of movement	Painful movement
Swelling	Swelling	Swelling
Black-and-blue mark	Black-and-blue mark	Redness
Grating	Located at joint	
Guarding		
Exposed bone ends		

fracture crosses the bone at an oblique angle, or in a slanting direction. The *greenstick* fracture is an incomplete fracture that commonly occurs in children, whose bones (like green sticks) are still pliable. *Spiral* fractures usually result from twisting injuries, and the fracture line has the appearance of a spring. In *impacted* fractures, the broken ends of the bone are jammed together and may function as if no fracture were present. A *comminuted* fracture is one in which the bone is fragmented into more than two pieces (splintered, shattered, or crushed). (*See* Figure 10-3.)

Fractures—even open fractures—seldom present an immediate threat to life, and thus their treatment should be deferred until any life threatening conditions have been handled, for example, an airway established or hemorrhage controlled.

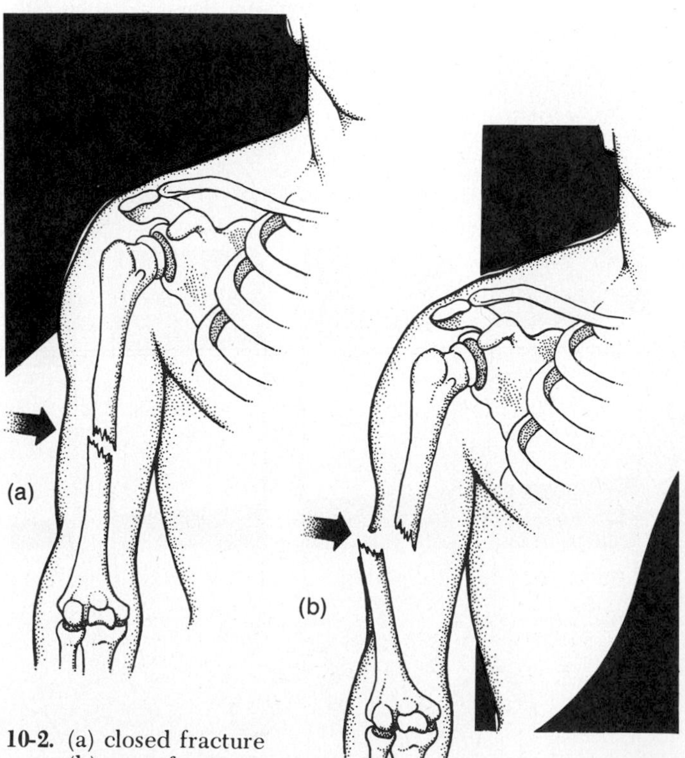

10-2. (a) closed fracture
(b) open fracture

Immobilization is commonly done by splinting for the following reasons:

- To prevent a closed fracture from becoming an open one
- To prevent damage to surrounding nerves, blood vessels, and other tissues by the broken bone ends
- To lessen bleeding and swelling
- To diminish pain

You should remember the following splinting and immobilization principles:

- Straighten severely angulated fractures of long bones before splinting. Explain to the victim that straightening the fracture may cause momentary pain, but that it will abate significantly once the fracture is straightened and splinted. Any overlying clothing should be cut away.
- Do not straighten dislocations and any fractures involving the spine, shoulder, elbow, wrist, or knee.
- The adage "splint them as they lie" should be changed to "immobilize them where they lie."
- In open fractures, do not attempt to push bone ends back beneath the skin surface. Simply cover them with a sterile dressing.
- Immobilize the joints above and below the fracture (e.g., at the wrist and elbow for fractures of the radius and ulna).
- Splinting should be done firmly, but not so tightly as to hinder circulation. Check pulses (radial or pedal) after the splint is in place to be certain that the circulation is still adequate. If the pulse disappears, loosen the splint until you feel the pulse again.
- For fractures of the femur or about the hip, a traction splint is best.
- All fractures should be immobilized before moving the victim.
- The fingers and toes should be exposed even though they are included within a splint.

Types of Splints

Any device used to immobilize a fracture or dislocation is a splint. This device may be improvised, such as a rolled newspaper, pillow, or virtually any other object that can provide stability; or it may be one of the several commercially available splints.

A rigid splint is an inflexible device attached to a limb to maintain stability. It may be a padded board or a piece of heavy cardboard. Whatever its construction, it must be long enough to be secured well above and below the fracture site.

To apply a rigid splint, grasp the extremity above and below the fracture site and apply gentle traction. While one first aider maintains traction, the other wraps the limb and splint with bandages, tight enough to hold the splint firmly to the extremity but not so tight as to hinder circulation.

Refer to chapter 13 for illustrations and an explanation on splinting various body parts.

SPINAL INJURIES

The incidence of spinal cord injuries has been escalating for many reasons. One is the increased use of motorcycles. Another is the change Americans have made to smaller motor vehicles that provide less protection in an accident. Even the increase in participation in recreational sports is partly responsible for more spinal cord injuries. A mistake in handling such victims may mean the victim spends the rest of his or her life in a wheelchair or bed.

When a person has damage that paralyzes the legs only, he or she is called a paraplegic and will probably be confined to a wheelchair. If the spinal cord damage is farther up, causing paralysis in all four limbs, the person is said to be quadriplegic and may require a device that is activated by mouth to move the wheelchair.

A first aider can tell if spinal damage may have occurred by first checking the circumstances of the accident, such as bent steering wheel and shattered windshield glass. Victims suspected of spine damage should not be moved except by professionally trained personnel with special equipment.

A second clue is a head injury. If a victim has been hit hard enough to cause head injury, the head has probably snapped suddenly in one or more directions. This endangers the spine. About 15% to 20% of victims with head injuries also have neck and spinal cord injuries.

The position of the victim's body may also suggest spinal damage. If the victim's head is at an unnatural angle or deformity along the spine is noticed, these are other clues to possible spine damage. Also, pain in the neck may be another symptom. Other symptoms of spinal damage may include loss of bowel or bladder control or paralysis.

If you are involved as a first aider at an accident scene and you are evaluating the victim for a possible spinal cord injury, ask the following questions:

1. *Is there pain?* A conscious victim should be asked about the presence of pain. Neck injuries (cervical) radiate pain to the arms; upper back injuries (thoracic) radiate pain around the ribs into the chest; and lower back injuries (lumbar) usually radi-

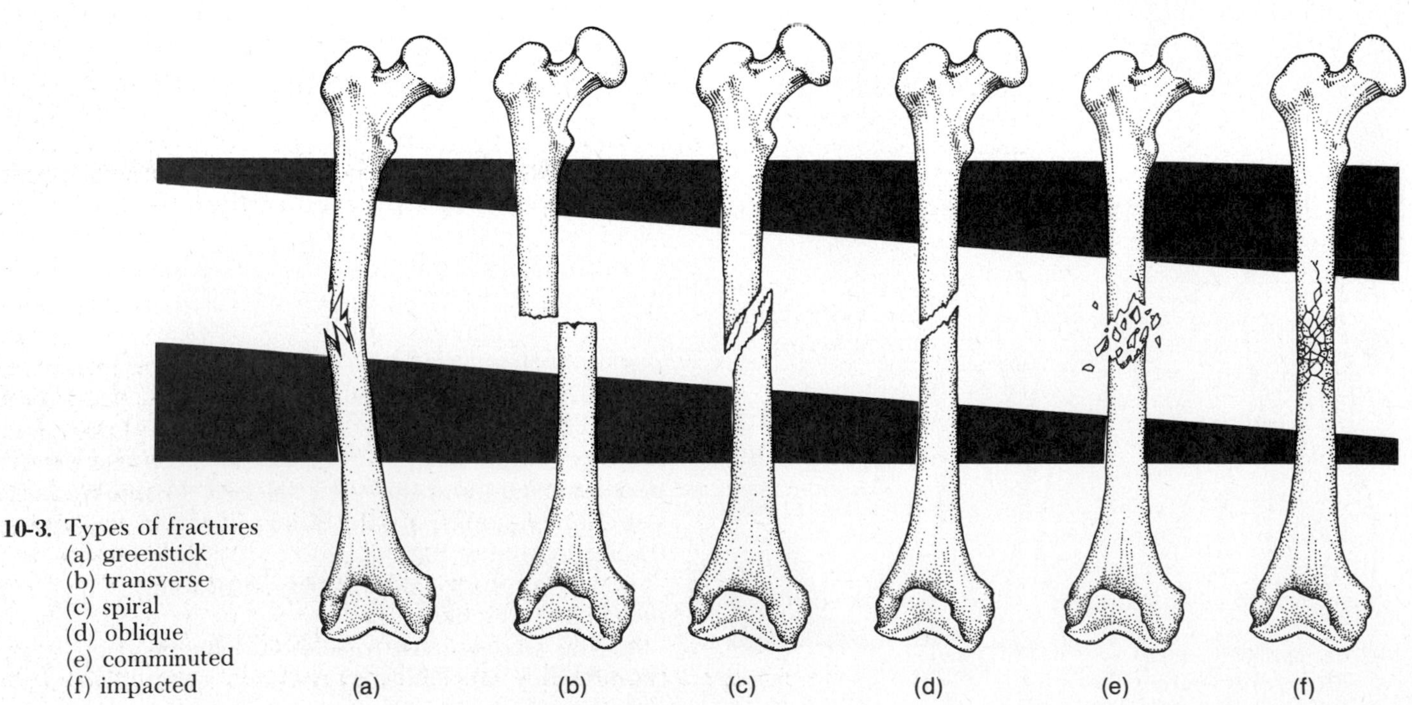

10-3. Types of fractures
(a) greenstick
(b) transverse
(c) spiral
(d) oblique
(e) comminuted
(f) impacted

ate pain down the legs. Often the victim describes the pain as "electric"—much like the pulsating pain that occurs when a dentist's drill exposes the nerve root of a tooth.

2. *Can you move your feet and legs?* Ask the victim to move his foot upward against the force of your hand. If the victim cannot perform this movement or if the movement is extremely weak against the pressure of your hand, the victim may have injured his spinal cord; the injury may be present anywhere along the spinal column.

3. *Can you move your fingers?* Moving the fingers is a sign that nerve pathways are intact. Ask the victim to grip your hand in his. Note the force of the grip. A strong grip indicates that a spinal cord injury is unlikely. If any one of these signs or symptoms is positive, spinal injury must be suspected. If you are not sure, assume that the victim has a spinal cord injury until proved otherwise.

First aiders should normally wait for paramedics or other rescue squads to transport the victim because of their training and equipment. Whatever you do, stabilize the victim against any movement.

If you determine that the victim may have spinal damage, the victim must be immobilized. Sometimes this just means telling the victim not to move. On other occasions, when the victim is unconscious, place objects on either side of the head to prevent it from rolling from side to side. If the victim is unconscious, determine if he or she is breathing and has a pulse.

If the victim is not breathing, give mouth-to-mouth resuscitation in the position in which the victim was found. The head tilt cannot be used because it would move the neck. Instead, jut the jaw forward by placing the fingers on the corners of the jaw and pushing forward. Keep the head and neck still and give mouth-to-mouth with the jaw held forward.

Victims with potential neck or back injury who are in water must be floated gently to shore. Before removal from the water, the victim must be secured to a backboard.

First aiders should remember to move the victim only if further injury is likely—such as in a smoking car or burning building. Bring help to the victim, not the victim to the help.

JOINT INJURIES

Shoulder Injuries

As the interest and participation in sports increase, the frequency of shoulder injuries also increases.

Assessment

The shoulder region is one of the most difficult areas of the body to evaluate. The person who complains of pain in the shoulder region may be reflecting conditions other than in that area. Pain could be referred from a neck nerve root irritation or from an intrathoracic problem coming from the heart, lungs, gallbladder, spleen, or other internal organs.

It is essential to know whether the condition was produced by sudden trauma or was of slow onset. The following questions can help determine the nature of the injury:

1. Can the radial pulse be felt for impaired circulation?
2. What is the duration and intensity of the pain? Where is the pain located?
3. Is there grating sensation (crepitus) on movement, numbness, or distortion in temperature, such as a cold or warm feeling? A cold temperature can be an indication of blood vessel constriction, whereas an overly warm temperature may indicate an inflammatory condition.
4. Is there a feeling of weakness?
5. What movement or body positions seem to aggravate or relieve the pain?
6. If the complaint has happened before, what, if anything, provides pain relief (e.g., cold, heat, massage, or analgesic medication)?

Shoulder Separation/Dislocation

Three bones come together at the shoulder: the scapula, clavicle, and humerus. The shoulder is the most freely movable joint in the body. The extreme range of all its possible movement makes the shoulder joint highly susceptible to dislocations. Shoulder dislocation is second only to finger dislocations.

Many muscles and tendons pass over the shoulder joint. A dislocation occurs at the shoulder when the different bones of the shoulder come apart as a result of a blow or a particular movement. This is a severe medical problem and must be seen by a physician. The physician will probably x-ray the area to confirm the diagnosis and then reduce the dislocation (set the bones back in place).

Emergency Care: Emergency care is to immobilize the injured part and adjacent joints by keeping the upper arm close to the body (not all shoulder dislocations allow this) and limiting further movement. Place a pillow between the arm and chest, and then place the arm in a sling with a swathe. Use ice and some compression if it relieves the victim's pain and discomfort. The physician will generally reset the dislocation (first aiders should never try to reset) and, depending on the severity, strap the injured arm so that no further harm comes to it. After a period of rest and rehabilitation (about three weeks), the victim can return to normal activity.

Fracture of the Clavicle
The clavicle is one of the most frequently fractured bones in the body. Fractured clavicles are caused by either a direct blow or a transmitted force resulting from a fall on the outstretched arm.

The victim usually supports the arm on the injured side and tilts his or her head toward that side, with the chin turned to the opposite side. The injured side appears a little lower than the uninjured side. Palpation may also reveal swelling and mild deformity.

Emergency Care: Care for this fracture immediately by applying a sling and swathe bandage and by treating the victim for shock, if necessary. Refer the victim to a physician, who will perform an x-ray examination of the area and continue to immobilize the injured area.

Contusions, Strains, and Tendonitis
Contusions: Blows about the shoulder that produce injury are most prevalent in collision and contact sports. Bruises of this area result in pain and restricted arm movement.

The most vulnerable part of the clavicle is the enlarged end near the shoulder. Contusions of this type are often called "shoulder pointers" and may cause the victim severe discomfort.

Strains: Throwing and swimming place great stress on the shoulder rotating mechanisms and can lead to an injury.

Tendonitis or Painful Shoulder: A painful shoulder is any irritation of the tendons or muscles surrounding the shoulder area. The cause of the painful shoulder is generally continuous overuse. Sports that involve repeated arm movement, like many of the throwing sports (e.g., baseball) or any other sports in which the shoulder is used extensively (e.g., swimming), often report painful shoulders.

Emergency care for contusions, strains, tendonitis: Begin cold therapy immediately after an injury. The best results are achieved if ice is applied for twenty minutes about three or four times during the first twenty-four hours after the injury. Continue this for twenty-four hours after the injury. After applying ice, you should immobilize the joint. Resting the joint is important.

The use of ice for extended periods is discouraged. Thermal damage, including damage to local blood vessels, may occur with prolonged applications of ice. The initial application of heat in an acute injury is not recommended because it increases swelling, thereby complicating the inflammatory process.

Post-Emergency Care
Topical analgesics: Some pain relief during the few days after the ice treatment may be necessary. External analgesics such as menthol, camphor, and eucalyptus oil act as counter-irritants and decrease the pain associated with minor muscle and joint injuries. Examples of brand names are Ben-Gay™ lotion, Mentholatum™ rub, and Infra-Rub™ cream.

These analgesics are applied to the skin over the source of the pain. The feeling of warmth from the topical analgesic has been proposed to crowd out pain perception and therefore divert the victim's attention. Be careful to avoid swelling and blistering of the skin. The recommended topical dosage to the affected area is no more than three to four times a day.

Analgesics and anti-inflammatory agents: For the pain and swelling of many injuries, the use of analgesics with anti-inflammatory properties may be appropriate. Aspirin is both inexpensive and as effective as any of the other currently available nonsteroidal anti-inflammatory agents. The FDA Arthritis Advisory Committee has recommended approval of Ibuprofen as an over-the-counter drug, which will provide an alternative anti-inflammatory analgesic for musculoskeletal pain.

Because of its lack of anti-inflammatory ability, acetaminophen is usually not as effective as aspirin for injuries producing inflammation, such as those found in joint injuries.

Knee Injuries

Knee injuries can be serious and of many types. There are many reasons for the large number of injuries to the knee, with automobile crashes and athletic participation leading the list.

Assessment of the Injured Knee
A physician is responsible for diagnosing the severity and exact nature of a knee injury. Usually a first aider is the first person to observe the injury and may be responsible for the initial assessment and immediate care of an injured knee. Also the first aider often relates pertinent information to a physician.

To determine the history and major complaints involved in a knee injury, use the following questions:

1. Was it a contact or noncontact injury? If contact, from what direction was the force applied?
2. In what direction did the knee go?
3. Did you hear a noise or feel any sensation at the time of injury, such as a pop or crunch?
4. Could you move the knee immediately after the injury? If not, was it locked in a bent or extended position? After being locked, how did it become unlocked?

5. Did swelling occur? If yes, was it immediate or did it occur later?

6. Where was the pain? Was it local, all over, or did it move from one side of the knee to the other?

7. Have you hurt the knee before?

You have probably seen a physician or an athletic trainer performing stress tests on a knee on the sidelines at a football game. There is still controversy as to the exact meaning and interpretation of many of the ligament stress tests. First aiders should not perform such testing due to lack of training and experience.

Various Knee Injuries

Fractured knee: A fracture of the knee generally occurs as a result of a fall or a direct blow. There will be an inability to kick the leg forward, and the leg will drag if an attempt is made to walk.

Fractures involving the knee may happen at the end of the femur, the end of the tibia, or in the patella. Such fractures may be confused with dislocations if deformity appears or with ligament damage if swelling and tenderness accompanies the injury.

To prevent further damage to nerves and blood vessels, immobilize the leg in the position found. If the leg is straight, use a padded board splint under the leg to keep it straight, or place two board splints (one on the inside and the other on the outside) on the leg. If bent, the knee should be immobilized in the bent position. When splints are not available, use a pillow or a blanket to immobilize the knee.

Check the pedal pulse for signs of circulatory impairment. If there is no pulse, try moving the leg (only once or twice) to a straight anatomical position. Do not force the leg. Stop if there is any resistance or an increase in pain.

Dislocation of the knee: This is a very serious injury. Deformity will be grotesque. Most concern should be for injury to the major artery supplying the leg below the knee (popliteal artery just behind the knee joint) rather than for ligament damage. Always check the pedal pulse for circulation before taking any other steps.

If pedal pulses are absent, the first aider should make an attempt to realign the limb in order to reduce the pressure on the artery. This is done by gently straightening the deformity with gentle traction along the axis of the limb. Continue to do this if no additional pain occurs. During straightening the joint may be relocated and the blood supply restored. Immobilize the limb with a rigid splint or pillow.

One attempt at gently straightening the knee should be attempted and no more. Then the knee should be immobilized in the position of deformity. No attempt to straighten any knee injury should be made when strong pedal pulses are present or when one attempt to realignment produce severe pain. In these cases, immobilize the knee in the position found.

Waiting longer than eight hours to reduce a knee dislocation can ultimately result in loss of the leg.

Dislocated patella: A dislocated patella most often is due to a blow or a very forceful unnatural contraction. Youth and young adults are most often the victims because of their participation in athletics where such injuries are most often found.

The kneecap moves to the side of the joint. It can be a very painful injury and must be treated immediately. Some people have repeated kneecap dislocations, just as other have a tendency for shoulder dislocations.

The emergency care for a dislocated patella is to reduce the dislocation as quickly as possible. Sometimes the victim can attempt to straighten the knee. Splint the leg so it cannot bend at the knee, and seek medical attention. The first aider should attempt to straighten the knee gently if additional pain is not produced. Sometimes the knee cap will relocate itself as the knee is straightened. If pain results while straightening the leg, immobilize the leg and knee in the deformed position.

Ligament injuries: The knee is quite prone to ligament injury from mild sprain to complete tearing. These injuries are quite common in athletics.

There are many tests to determine the stability of the knee after it has been hit. Some of these tests involve attempting to move the knee and applying certain stresses in different directions in an attempt to determine which ligament has been stretched or ruptured. Such testing should be reserved for physicians and experienced athletic trainers, not first aiders. In fact, some physicians and athletic trainers should not stress test a knee due to inexperience and lack of training.

Very often pain and tenderness are present in the area, and normal movement is not allowed because of the pain. Locking of the knee joint may also occur. These are all indications of serious ligament damage to the knee. Check the pedal pulse for signs of circulatory impairment.

Emergency care is the ICE procedure: I stands for ice or cold application; C means compression with elastic bandage; E represents elevation of the knee. The first aider can gently straighten the knee to apply a splint. If pain occurs, the knee should be immobilized in the position as it is. A qualified physician should be sought to determine if a ligament injury has taken place and, if so, if a cast should be applied, followed by rest, or if surgery is needed.

Cartilage injuries: Cartilage injuries in the knee can be incapacitating. Such injuries can result from a traumatic event or long-term wear and tear of the cartilage. A trained orthopedic physician should be sought.

Though knee injuries are not life threatening, they are common and pose a concern for the victim and the first aider. The first aider will not be able to identify the type of injury, yet the emergency care for most knee injuries is quite similar.

Finger Injuries

Finger Dislocation

Dislocations of the fingers have a high rate of occurrence in sports and are caused mainly by being hit on the tip of the finger by a ball.

Emergency care: The victim of a dislocated finger often attempts to pull the joint back in place. This is not recommended. The dislocation should be reduced by a physician after x-rays are taken to see that no other injury is involved. Broken bone chips can also be seen in the x-rays.

Taping to prevent another occurrence of the injury should be considered. The finger that was dislocated may be splinted to an adjacent, good finger to immobilize and protect it in future activity. To ensure the most complete healing, splinting should be maintained for about three weeks with the fingers flexed because inadequate immobilization could cause an unstable joint and/or excessive scar tissue and, possibly, a permanent deformity.

Since the thumb is necessary for hand dexterity, any traumatic injury to the thumb should be considered serious. Special consideration must be given to dislocations of the thumb.

Mallet Finger

The mallet finger is common in sports, especially baseball and basketball. It is caused by a blow from a thrown ball that strikes the tip of the finger. The victim is unable to extend the finger, and there is also tenderness at the site of the injury.

Emergency care: A physician should determine whether the tendon is actually ruptured and whether surgical repair is necessary. An x-ray is needed to determine any damage. The finger should be immobilized and splinted.

Fractures of the Fingers

The presence of swelling and tenderness are involved in fractures of the fingers.

One of the most useful ways to differentiate between a contusion and a fracture is by using the "percussion" or "hammer" test. In this test the victim holds the fingers in full extension. The ends of the fingers are firmly "hammered" toward the hand transmitting force down the shaft of the metacarpal and producing pain if a fracture is present.

Finger alignment should also be checked, but most important is nail alignment. If the normal fingernail alignment is disturbed, you should suspect a fracture. An x-ray will conclusively determine a broken bone.

Emergency care: Immediately place cold, apply compression, and elevate the arm. Seek medical attention.

Fingernail Avulsion

When a nail is partly torn loose, do not trim away the loose nail. Instead, secure the damaged nail in place with an adhesive bandage. If part or all of the nail has been completely torn away, apply an adhesive bandage coated with antibiotic ointment. Alleviate the victim's fears by telling him that a new nail will appear but it will take a month or more.

Ankle Injuries

A sprained ankle is a very common injury. Because of the frequency of this injury, anyone trained to render emergency care should understand the nature of the injury itself and how to deal with it effectively. A sprained ankle should not be handled casually. It can have consequences that include a lifelong disability. In some cases, the damage requires surgical correction.

It is usually impossible for a first aider to determine the exact nature of an ankle injury. The injury could be a sprain, dislocation, or fracture. Identification cannot be made on the basis of appearance or the amount of pain. A mild sprain often is considerably more painful than a severe one. A severe sprain frequently presents very little swelling.

The first aider can ask the victim three important questions:

1. Which way did the ankle turn? Most (over 80%) ankle sprains are of the lateral or inverted type.

2. At the time of the injury, did you hear or feel anything snap or pop?

3. Have you ever had problems with this ankle before?

It is often difficult to distinguish between a severe sprain and a fracture. The injury should be treated as a fracture until the advice of a physician can be obtained.

Emergency care: Initial care consists of elevating the ankle, applying cold compresses or ice packs to the injury site, and supporting the ankle with an elastic bandage. Remembering the mnemonic ICE—*I*ce, *C*ompression, *E*levation—is a guide to sprained ankle injuries.

The application of cold initially causes vasoconstriction of blood vessels. This decreases blood flow, thereby diminishing the amount of bleeding in the injured ankle. Cryotherapy (use of cold) is effective in diminishing bleeding and edema (accumulation of fluid) by the combined effect of a decrease in blood flow and a reduction in metabolic function of the cell.

Cold is available from ice, commercially prepared ice packs, frozen food cans, drinking fountains, etc. The earlier cold is applied, the better.

Never place ice directly on the skin except for intermittent ice massage because it can cause frostbite. Provide a towel between the ice bag and skin.

Applying cold for short periods of time does not cool deeper tissues—it only lowers skin temperature. Thus, the application of cold should be continued for at least twenty, and preferably thirty, minutes. This should occur about three times during the first twenty-four hours after the injury. Cold application will not only decrease the swelling, but also relieve the pain.

Some precautions about the use of cold, other than never applying cold directly to the skin, include the warning not to use salt water (it is too cold) or chemical ice (liquid nitrogen or solid carbon dioxide, also called dry ice). Be aware that some victims may have rheumatic conditions, Raynaud's phenomenon, or cold allergy which can be adversely enhanced in a victim to whom cold is applied.

A common error is the early use of heat. Heat results in swelling and pain if applied too early. A minimum of twenty-four hours, and preferably even seventy-two hours, should pass before any heat is applied to the injured ankle.

Swelling is like glue and can lock up a joint within a matter of hours. It is vitally important not only to prevent swelling by using cold promptly, but it is even more important to make the swelling recede as quickly as possible with a compression bandage (elastic bandage).

Experts disagree on the use of elastic bandages. Some believe that elastic bandages are often misused, especially on ankle injuries. The bandage should be applied firmly, but not too tightly. Toes should be checked periodically for blue or white discoloration, indicating that the bandage has been applied too tightly. Comparing the toes of the injured foot with those of the uninjured foot is also suggested. Pain, tingling, loss of sensation, and loss of pulses indicate impaired circulation. The elastic bandage should be loosened if any of these signs or symptoms are present.

Apply the elastic bandage (3 or 4 inch width) carefully to avoid hindering circulation. Apply the bandage in a figure-of-eight wrap around the ankle, and then continue up the leg with a closed spiral wrapping at least to mid-calf.

Check the pulse at the juncture of the big toe and the second toe. When in doubt as to the extent of the injury, splint the foot as you would a fracture by immobilizing the ankle with a pillow splint and then refer the victim to a physician.

To further reduce swelling and curtail bleeding, instruct the victim to elevate his or her ankle on two or three pillows for the first 24 to 48 hours. Some medical specialists say, "Keep the foot higher than the knee and the knee higher than the heart." Avoid any weight on the ankle. Some experts recommend crutches for the victim.

Swelling and pain should begin to subside within forty-eight hours, and the ankle should be nearly normal within ten days. If the injury is not healing on schedule, see a physician.

If a fracture is suspected, immobilize the foot using a pillow splint.

MUSCLE INJURIES

Muscle injuries are hard to explain because little solid information is available, and there are misconceptions and disagreement on proper emergency care. Though muscle injuries pose no real emergency, first aiders have ample opportunities to care for them.

Muscle Strains

Another term often used for muscle strain is muscle pull. Skeletal muscles have the capability to stretch and contract. However, if the muscle is stretched while attempting to contract or stretched beyond its normal range of motion, a tear of the muscle fibers may occur. There are various degrees of severity of muscle strains, depending on the degree of the actual muscle tear.

Signs of muscle strain include:

- The victim may have heard a snap when the tissue was torn.
- A sharp pain may have been felt immediately after the injury.
- There was a spasmodic muscle contraction of the affected part.
- Extreme joint tenderness occurs upon palpation.
- Disfigurement may be seen either in the form of an indentation or cavity where tissues have separated, or a bump indicating contracted tissue.

• There is a severe weakness and loss of function of the injured part.

Muscle Contusions

Another category of muscle injury is the blow to the muscle, or contusion. This injury is also known as a "charley horse." The term "charley horse" was derived from baseball players who experienced blows to muscles in the early twentieth century. At that time, the outfield grass of some of the major league ball parks was mowed by horses pulling lawnmowers. At Ebbit's Field in New York, the horse doing this chore was known as "Charley." Charley had a continual limp. When a baseball player was hit in the leg with a ball or received a blow to the leg muscle sliding into the base, which subsequently caused him to limp, it was said that the baseball player was limping like Charley, the horse. Consequently, the muscle blow and contusion to the athlete which caused pain and limping was referred to as charley horse injury. This term is still quite popular in America today.

Emergency Care of Muscle Strains and Contusions

Muscle injuries must receive proper and early care to avoid delay in recovery. This is especially true of muscle strains. It is well known that a severely injured muscle does not regenerate itself. Healing is by scar formation.

Even though the ice, compression, and elevation (ICE) procedure is used universally for immediate care of acute muscle strains and contusions, many first aiders and even emergency room personnel continue to treat new muscle injuries erroneously with heat packs.

Ice: The first initial in the acronym ICE stands for ice. Ice is applied to the injured area. Methods of applying cold include the use of crushed ice, immersion in ice water, or the application of cold towels. The application of ice should continue for twenty to thirty minutes of each hour for the first day, if possible. This procedure may be done into the second day of injury.

Placing towels or elastic wraps between the ice packs and the body insulates against the full effects of the cold. Frostbite will not occur if cold packs are applied for limited time periods. Constant use of an ice pack is not necessary because of the lasting effect of cold. For example, it takes two to four hours for the forearm and ankle to gradually return to pre-application temperatures.

The use of cold to an injured area reduces pain, hemorrhage, swelling, and muscle spasm following a muscle strain or contusion.

Compression: The second initial, C, stands for compression. In an attempt to limit internal bleeding, a compression bandage is applied to the injured area. Often, the compression bandage is applied directly to the site, ice is placed over the first layer of elastic bandage wrap, and more compression elastic wrap is put over the ice. The ice, together with the compression, serves to limit internal bleeding, which is associated with all acute muscle injuries. Compression of the injured area may also aid in squeezing some fluid and debris out of the injury site. The victim should wear the elastic wrap continuously for eighteen to twenty-four hours.

Elastic bandages may be applied too tightly, thus inhibiting circulation. Leave fingers and toes exposed to allow observation of possible color change. Pain, pale skin, numbness, and tingling are all signs of a bandage that is too tight.

Elevation: The E stands for elevation. Elevating the injured area limits circulation to that area and, hence, further limits internal bleeding. It is simple to prop up an injured leg or upper extremity to limit bleeding. The aim of this step is to get the injured part up to about the level of the heart, if possible. This should aid venous blood return to the heart.

Muscle Cramps

Another category of muscle injuries is the muscle cramp, in which the muscle goes into uncontrolled spasm or contraction, resulting in severe pain and a restriction or loss of movement. Muscle cramps can occur in any skeletal muscle that is overworked.

When the cramp occurs in the leg or hand muscles, the victim may attempt to relieve the spasm or cramp by gradual stretching or massaging of the muscle. Since a muscle cramp is really an uncontrolled spasm or contraction of the muscle, a gradual lengthening or kneading of the muscle may help to lengthen those muscle fibers and relieve the cramp. Other experts have implicated diet or lack of fluids as some of the possible reasons that an individual suffers from muscle cramps.

Fractures

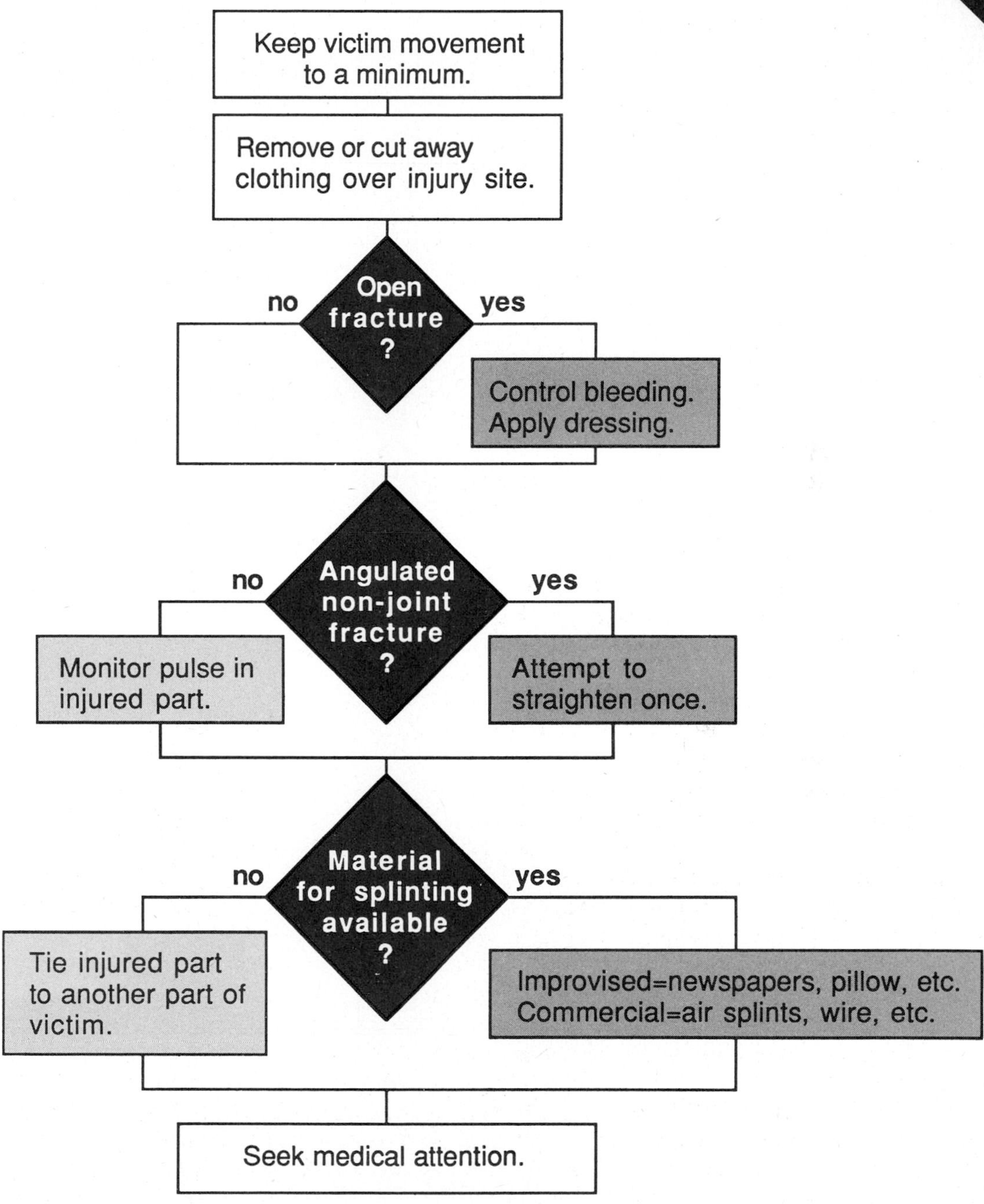

If a back or neck injury is suspected, immobilize victim in the exact position found by placing rolled blankets, clothing, etc. next to victim's head, neck, torso. Do not move unless victim is in immediate danger. In most cases, wait for trained rescuers with special equipment.

Spinal Injury

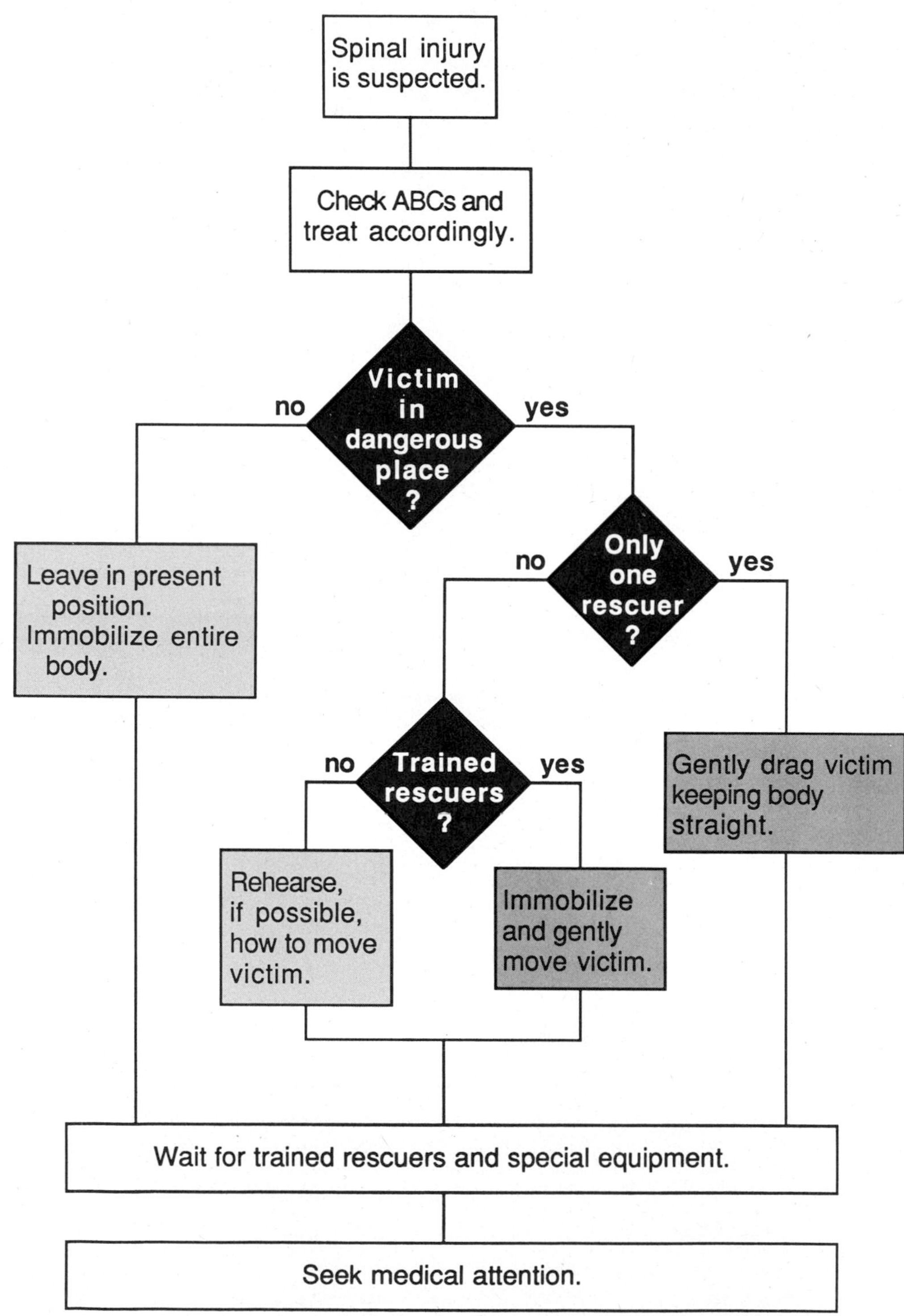

Shoulder Injuries

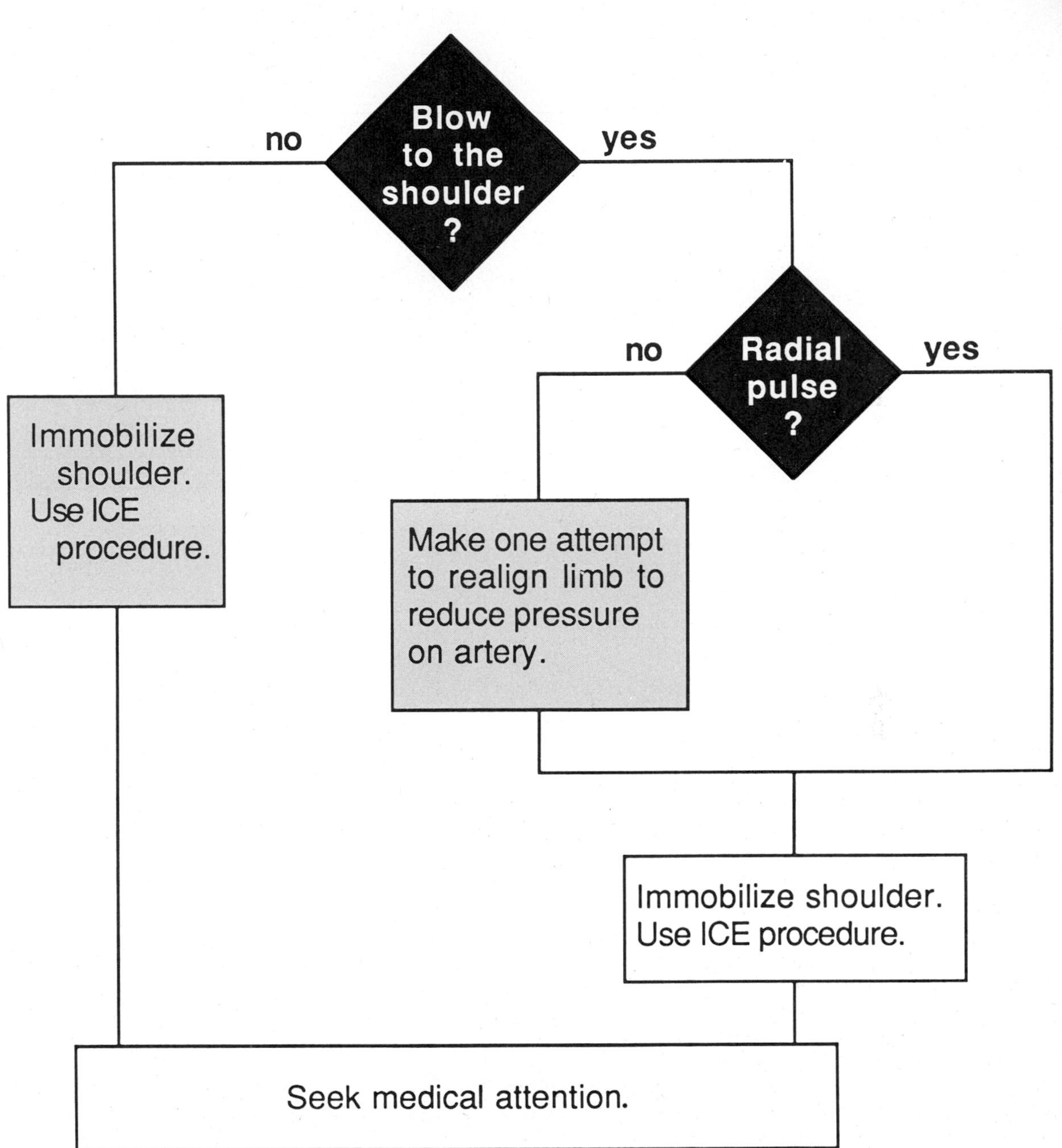

Knee Injuries

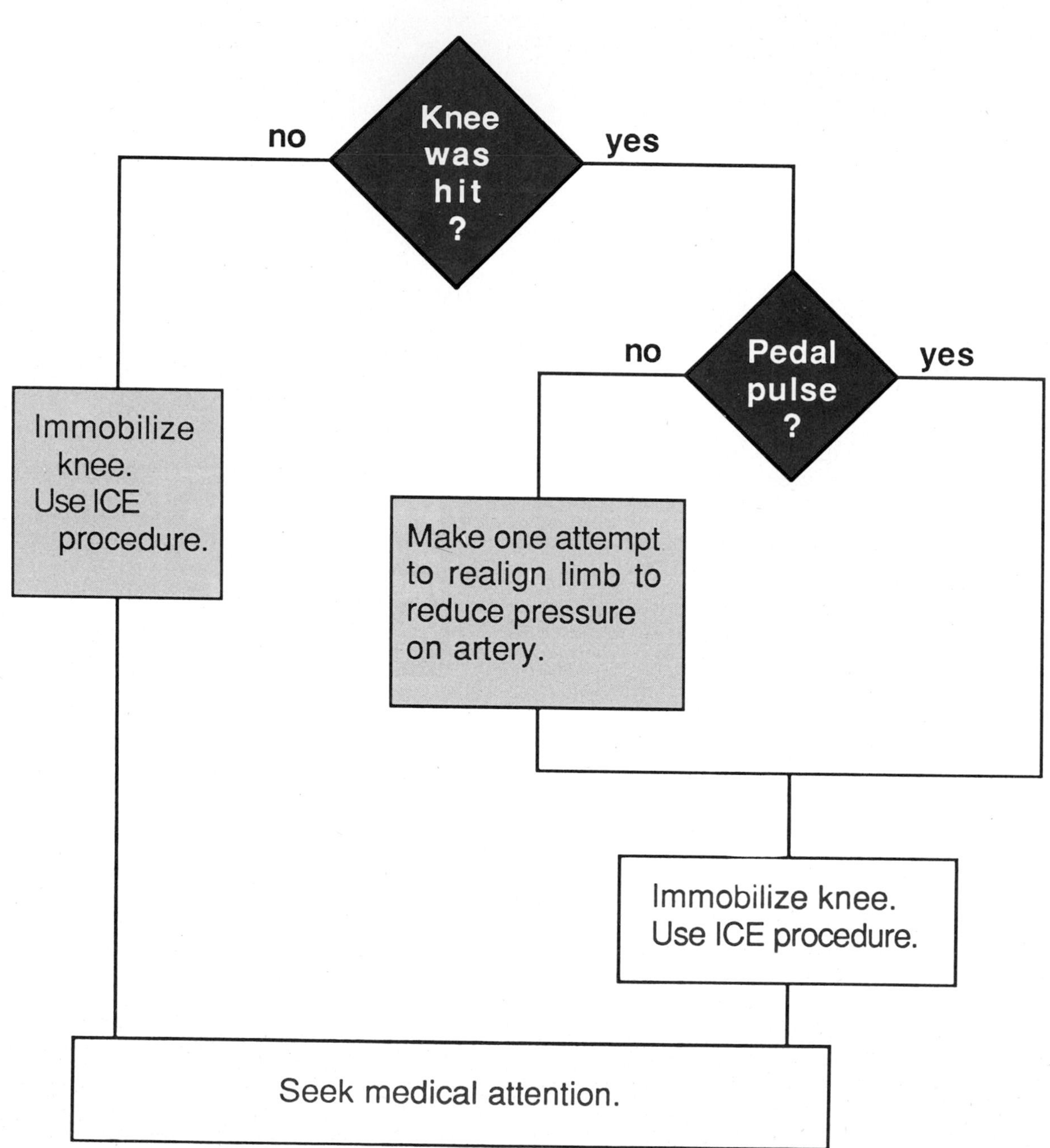

Ankle Injuries

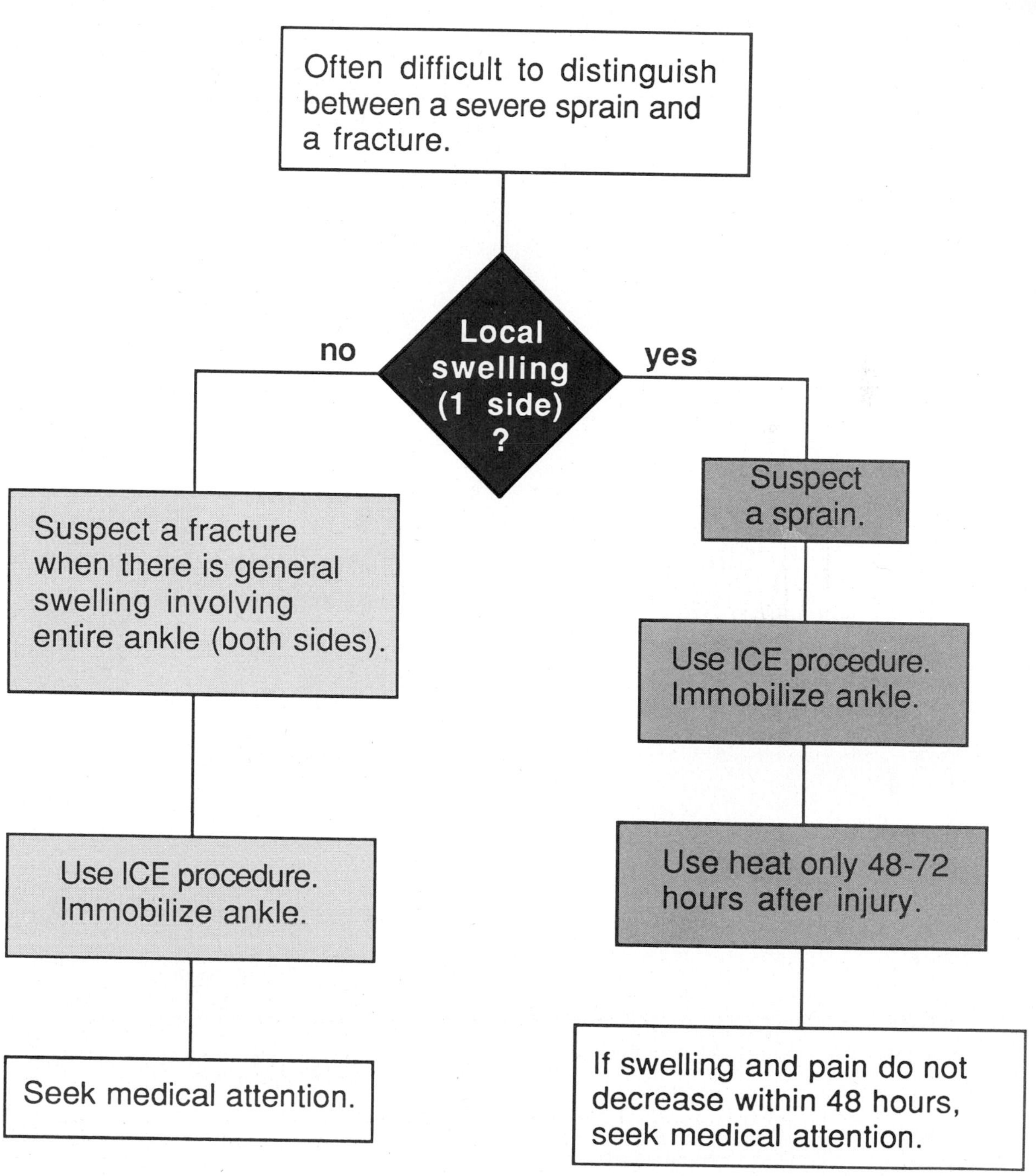

Muscle Injuries

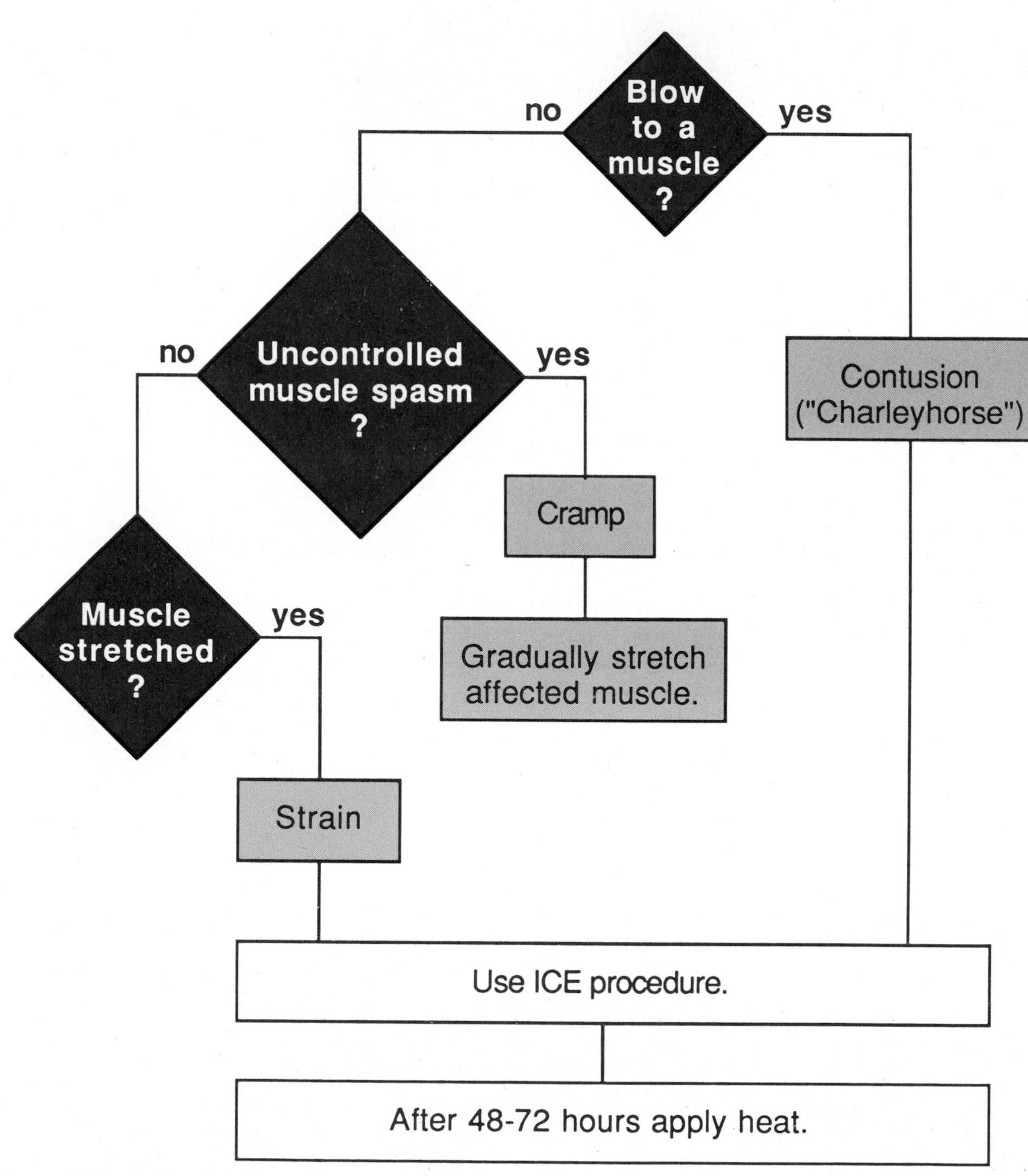

Sprains, Strains, Contusions, Dislocations

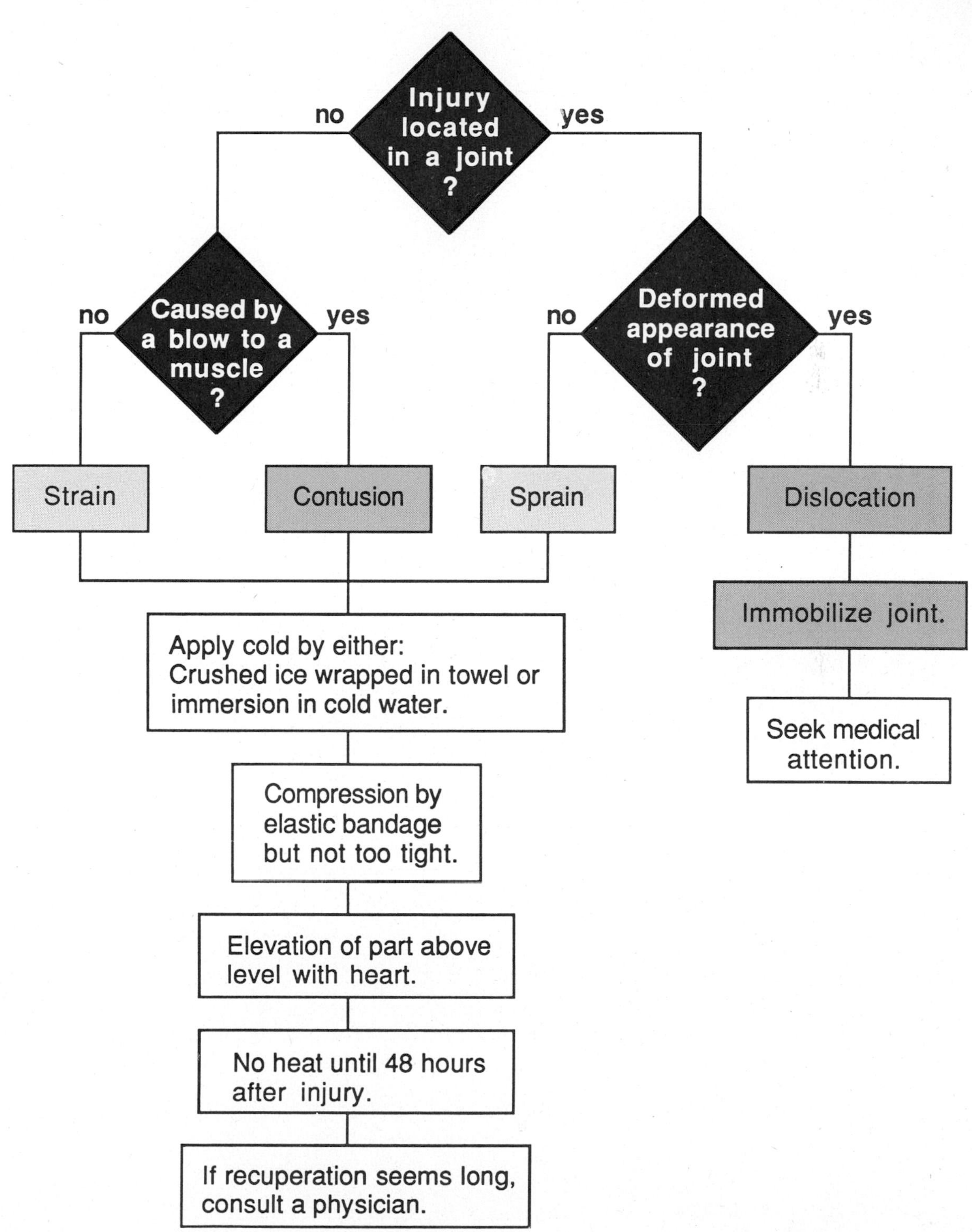

Fractures

LEARNING ACTIVITIES

T F 1. A fracture is a break in a bone.
T F 2. In an open fracture, the bone has not penetrated the skin.
T F 3. Closed fractures are more serious than open fractures.
T F 4. Most fractures do not present a threat to life.
T F 5. It is good first aid procedure to immobilize all fractures and suspected fractures before moving the victim.
T F 6. In open fractures, the first aider should wash the wound before splinting.
T F 7. It is easy to determine if a person has a fracture.
T F 8. Severely angulated long-bone fractures should be straightened.
T F 9. It is easy to differentiate between an ankle sprain and a fracture.
T F 10. A fracture in which the break is straight across the shaft of the bone is called a comminuted fracture.
T F 11. The type of fracture that twists around and through the bone is an impacted fracture.
T F 12. A greenstick fracture is found most often in infants and small children.

Case 1: A young boy falls out of a tree during a family picnic. The child exhibits no immediate evidence of a broken leg but complains of pain below his knee and is unable to walk.

1. What type of fracture would you suspect?

____

____

2. What is the other major classification of fractures?

____

____

3. What is the key word in treating fractures of any type?

____

____

4. When splinting fractures, where should the splints be applied? ______________

____

Case 2: A 5-year-old child falls off his two-wheeler onto the cement sidewalk. When he tries to get up he falls down again; it is obvious that he cannot put any weight on the leg.

1. You suspect a closed fracture. What signs and symptoms would you look for in this child to verify your diagnosis?

A. ______________________________

____

B. ______________________________

____

C. ______________________________

____

2. Which kind of closed fracture is most common in accidents like this? ______________

____

3. What emergency care would you provide this youngster?

A. ______________________________

____

B. ______________________________

____

C. ______________________________

____

4. Match the lettered types of the fractures with their numbered signs and symptoms.

A. ______ Impacted
B. ______ Closed
C. ______ Greenstick
D. ______ Comminuted
E. ______ Open

1. Bone broken in many pieces
2. Fracture with break of skin
3. Bone broken and one end driven into another
4. Bone bends and cracks but the crack is not all the way through the bone
5. Fracture without break of skin

Case 3: A 27-year-old male is unable to maneuver his truck under a lower clearance bridge, forcing the truck to stop suddenly. In attempting to brace himself, he gets his left hand caught between the steering wheel and the windshield. On arrival at the scene, you find his left hand is swollen, discolored, and deformed. He is complaining of pain and unable to move his fingers.

1. What would you do initially to assess this injury?

A. ______________________________

B. ______________________________

C. ______________________________

D. ______________________________

2. If you suspect a fractured hand, what bones might be involved?

A. ______________________________

B. ______________________________

3. How do you classify a fracture as open as opposed to closed?

____

4. What is the purpose of the initial emergency treatment for a fractured hand?

____

5. Specifically, what emergency care would you provide?

____

Case 4: One winter evening a 53-year-old woman parked her car and, while walking toward the entrance of a store, slipped and fell. On arrival at the scene you find her injuries consist of a minor abrasion of the right elbow and forearm and a swollen, deformed, tender right ankle.

1. What would your first action be before immobilizing this injury?

A. ______________________________

B. ______________________________

2. If nerve impairment is found, what actions should you take?

A. ______________________________

B. ______________________________

3. Describe two techniques to immobilize an ankle injury effectively.

____

4. Explain the difference between a sprain and a strain.

____

Case 5: An elderly woman has fallen and possibly broken her arm. When you arrive you find her seated on a bed. She explains she fell while getting a drink of water. She cannot move her left arm and it causes her a great deal of pain whenever you touch it. There are no obvious deformities or breaks in the skin.

1. What possible injuries should you suspect with this woman?

A. ______________________________

B. ______________________________

C. ______________________________

2. How should you treat this woman's injury?

A. ______________________________

B. ______________________________

C. ______________________________

Case 6: A young girl bicyclist has glanced off a moving car and is now lying in the street. The child is bleeding from her right forearm and a portion of bone can been seen protruding from the open wound.

1. What type of fracture does this child have?

____

2. What is the other major type of fracture?

____

3. What are other types of fractures?

A. ______________________________

B. ______________________________

C. ______________________________

4. Unless there is presence of some immediate danger, what is the key word in treating fractures of any type? ______________

5. When splinting fractures, the splint should be applied

A. ______________________________

and

B. ______________________________ the adjacent joints.

Spinal Injuries

T F 1. Victims of suspected spinal neck or back injuries should be moved as quickly as possible to a medical facility.
T F 2. Victims who are unable to move both their arms and legs should be suspected of having a spine fracture.
T F 3. First aiders should usually wait for trained rescuers to handle a victim of spinal injury.
T F 4. The head tilt can be used for the nonbreathing victim with a suspected spinal neck injury.
T F 5. Circumstances of the accident can be a clue to spinal damage.

Case: The victim of a motorcycle accident is found with loss of sensation in both lower extremities. He is found lying on his back with no other obvious injury. He is still wearing a helmet.

1. What should be suspected in this case? ______________________________

2. What leads you to suspect this? ______________________________

3. What is the correct first aid for this victim? ______________________________

4. Should a first aider move this victim? ______________________________

5. When would moving be justified by the first aider? ______________________________

Shoulder Injuries

T F 1. First aiders should immobilize a shoulder dislocation and never try to reset it.
T F 2. Using a sling and swathe will immobilize a fractured clavicle.
T F 3. Most shoulder dislocations result when the victim falls on an outstretched hand and arm.
T F 4. An injury in which ligaments are torn is known as a strain.
T F 5. The best emergency care for a dislocation is to massage the area immediately.
T F 6. Sprains occur around a joint.
T F 7. The best care for a strain is to apply heat.
T F 8. Displacement of a bone end from a joint is called a dislocation.
T F 9. The main signs of a dislocation is deformity.
T F 10. Emergency care for a dislocation is to transport the victim and do *not* reduce or splint.

Knee Injuries

T F 1. Stress testing a knee can be done by a first aider.
T F 2. Checking the pedal pulses is a method of checking for nerve damage.
T F 3. If an attempt is made without success to straighten a knee, no other attempt should be made.
T F 4. The initials ICE represent the treatment for knee injuries.

Hand and Finger Injuries

T F 1. For a finger dislocation, attempting to pull the joint back in place is recommended.
T F 2. An accumulation of blood directly beneath the nail and the pain from it can be relieved by using a red-hot paper clip to produce a hole in the nail.
T F 3. A broken finger can be detected by using the "hammer" test.
T F 4. An amputated finger should be placed directly in a bag of ice and taken with the victim to a medical facility.
T F 5. Removing a ring from a finger when a ring cutter is not available requires the use of a hacksaw.
T F 6. The "position of function" is with the fingers in a straightened position.

Ankle Injuries

T F 1. It is often difficult to distinguish between a severe sprain and a fracture.
T F 2. Cryotherapy is the use of heat on an injury.
T F 3. A pillow can serve as an ankle splint.
T F 4. A figure-of-eight wrap around the ankle is suggested for the elastic bandage application.
T F 5. A common error is the early use of heat on an ankle sprain.
T F 6. Place ice directly on the skin for cooling.
T F 7. A poorly cared for sprained ankle can allow the victim to be more susceptible for future ankle sprains.

Case: While retrieving a rebound during a basketball game, a player collapses to the floor. The pain is severe and he complains of "turning" his ankle.

1. Three questions asked of the victim are

A. ______________________________ ?

B. ______________________________ ?

C. ______________________________ ?

2. What three injuries could have occurred?

A. ______________________________

B. ______________________________

C. ______________________________

Muscle Injuries

T F 1. A tear in the muscle fibers is known as a muscle cramp.
T F 2. A blow to the muscle is sometimes known as a "charley horse."
T F 3. A muscle cramp has a uncontrolled spasm.
T F 4. Cold applications follow heat for muscle injuries.
T F 5. Elastic bandages can be used but can be applied too tightly.

Case: Those engaging in various types of sports may experience one of three different muscle injuries. Match the lettered types of muscle injury with their numbered definitions.

1. ______ Strains — A. Results from a blow

2. ______ Contusion — B. Uncontrolled spasm

3. ______ Cramp — C. A tear

4. All muscle injuries can follow the ICE procedures.

I = ____________
C = ____________
E = ____________

5. How can compression be applied?

____
____

6. Give two sources of ice or cold.

A. ______________________________
____

B. ______________________________
____

7. How long should cold be applied? ______ minutes

8. Cold will decrease the swelling and relieve the
____
____
____

9. It is best not to apply heat for ______ to ______ hours.

10. What is the best width for an elastic bandage on the ankle? ______ inches

11 Medical Emergencies

- Heart Attack
- Stroke
- Diabetic Emergencies
- Epilepsy
- Asthma
- Abdomen Pain
- Constipation
- Cough
- Diarrhea
- Earache
- Fever
- Headache
- Sore Throat
- Vomiting
- Hyperventilation
- Bleeding (Respiratory and Digestive Tracts)

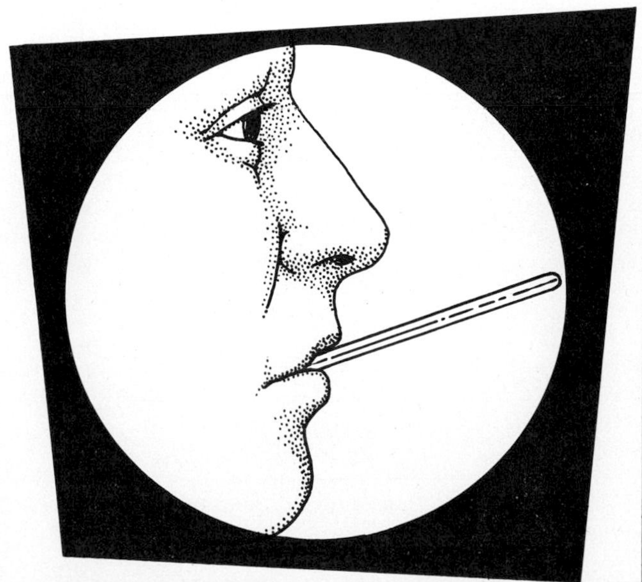

HEART ATTACK

Sudden death from heart attack is the most important medical emergency today. "Heart attack," though not a scientific term, is commonly used to describe the symptoms of an acute myocardial infarction (AMI) and of several other heart conditions. A heart attack occurs when the blood supply to some portion of the heart is either cut off or reduced to such low levels that cells in the area cannot survive.

The dead heart muscle area is called a myocardial infarction. In other instances, the sudden inability to supply enough blood to a portion of the myocardium (heart muscle) causes the heart to develop an abnormal or ineffective form of beating, called ventricular fibrillation. Because the heart muscle simply twitches and does not contract, effective circulation stops and death is imminent unless the normal beating mechanism of the heart is restored at once.

Signs and Symptoms

Difficulty in determining a heart attack from the character of the pain is understandable because as many as one third of all myocardial infarctions are either painless or produce so little discomfort that the pain is ignored. The character of heart pain is highly variable and there are a number of medical conditions that produce similar pain patterns. The typical forms of heart pain are usually easily recognized, but heart pain or similar pain from another cause may tax the skills of the most expert cardiologist. Because treatment at the onset of a heart attack is vital to survival and how well a person recovers, the rule to follow is that if you suspect a heart attack for any reason, seek medical attention at once rather than delaying a decision.

The classic symptom is often described as a pressure rather than a pain, or as a sensation of a clenched fist. The pressure, squeezing sensation, or dull pain is usually located in the center of the chest, sometimes a little to the left of the sternum, but usually not confined to the left side of the chest near the nipple. The pain may be in the pit of the stomach and may even present as abdominal pain causing the person to think he has indigestion. That symptom, along with vomiting which sometimes occurs with the onset of a heart attack, often leads to an initial suspicion of indigestion rather than of acute heart attack.

The pain may be in the upper sternum, traveling into the left or right shoulder or both, into the neck and jaw, and down the arm (more often the left arm), and it may follow a course along the inner aspect of the arm into the ring and little finger. It does not go into the thumb and index finger. The discomfort may rarely radiate into the back.

The main difference between the pain of angina and that of myocardial infarction is its duration (refer to Table 11-1). If the pain persists over fifteen to thirty minutes, it is more likely to be a myocardial infarction. The pain of infarction may last for hours and may be more severe. Also, the pain of myocardial infarction can occur at rest. Many such attacks occur at night, waking a person from sleep. Myocardial infarction pain can and does occur during exertion as well as at rest.

The medical disorder that is perhaps the most difficult to separate from myocardial pain is spasm of the esophagus. The muscular cramp of the esophagus causes a squeezing pain behind the sternum so similar to heart pain that only medical tests can really separate the two. Pleurisy causes chest pain, but it is sharp, not dull, and it occurs with respiration and movement of the chest wall. A variety of musculoskeletal pains resemble heart pain but they, too, are associated with chest wall movement.

Besides chest pain, other symptoms are commonly associated with an acute myocardial infarction. These include the following:

1. Sweating, often quite profuse (The victim may soak through his clothing and complain of a "cold sweat.")

2. Respirations are usually normal but may be rapid and shallow.

3. Nausea and/or vomiting frequently accompany an acute myocardial infarction.

4. Weakness may be profound.

5. Dizziness.

6. Palpitations are sometimes experienced by victims with irregular heart rhythms as a sensation that the heart is "skipping a beat."

Emergency Care

If warning signs make you suspect a heart attack, immediate care and action may mean the difference between life and death. The importance of what happens in the first few hours after an attack is emphasized by the fact that about 40% of all people with a heart attack die during this time outside the hospital because they do not receive emergency medical care at once. This is by far the most dangerous period after a heart attack has occurred.

Emergency care should be designed to create as little stress on the victim as possible. Medical care should be obtained at once. The sooner the victim can be placed in a coronary care unit and supervised by trained personnel, without endangering the victim in transit, the better.

For victims suspected of having a heart attack, the Metropolitan Insurance Company has developed these useful guidelines:

You can best help—possibly save a life—if you know in advance:

1. The nearest hospital equipped to handle heart attack emergencies.

2. How to do cardiopulmonary resuscitation (CPR).

TABLE 11-1. Chest Pain—Differences Between Angina and Heart Attack

Signs and Symptoms	Angina Pectoris	Acute Myocardial Infarction
Pain intensity	Mild to moderate	Very severe, intense.
Duration	3 to 5 minutes	30 minutes to several hours.
Precipitating factors	Physical or emotional stress	None.
Relieving factors	Rest Nitroglycerin	None.
Associated symptoms	May be none	Profuse perspiration; nausea and vomiting; fear of impending doom

Adapted from National Highway Traffic Safety Administration, *Emergency Medical Care* (Washington, D.C.: U.S. Government Printing Office).

3. How quickly to call a doctor, the hospital and/or an ambulance.
4. The fastest route to the hospital.

Knowing these things, you should:
1. Help the victim to the least painful position—usually sitting with legs up and bent at knees. Loosen clothing around the neck and midriff. Be calm and reassuring.
2. Quickly call an ambulance to get the victim to the hospital via local rescue squad, police, fire, or other available service. Once the ambulance is on the way, notify the family physician, if you have one.
3. If the ambulance is coming, comfort the victim while waiting. Otherwise, help the victim to a car, trying to keep the victim's exertion to a minimum. If possible, take another CPR-trained person with you. The victim should sit up.
4. Drive cautiously to the hospital. Watch the victim closely (or have other passenger do so). If he or she loses consciousness, check for breathing and feel for neck pulse under the side angle of the lower jaw to check for circulation. If there is no pulse, start CPR. Continue CPR until trained help arrives to take over.
5. If the victim retains consciousness to the hospital, make sure he or she is carried, not walked, to the emergency room.

Obviously, for cardiac arrest cardiopulmonary resuscitation (CPR) is performed.

STROKE

Stroke is the third most common cause of death, and in the middle-aged and older Americans it is a frequent cause of disability. Each year 500,000 adults suffer stroke and more than 250,000 die.

A stroke in medical terms is known as a cerebrovascular accident (CVA). The person who has a stroke may die shortly after the onset. However, in many cases the person survives the initial stroke to be left with a neurologic deficit or may even recover completely.

Causes of Stroke

Strokes can be divided into two broad categories. One category of stroke is the result of *infarction*, which occurs when the blood supply to a limited portion of the brain is inadequate and death of nervous tissue follows. Infarction may be caused by embolism or by blood vessel occlusion due to atherosclerosis. Emboli are usually small blood clots arising from diseased blood vessels (carotid) in the neck or from clots or material arising from the heart. Other types of emboli that may cause occlusion of cerebral blood vessels are air, tumor tissue, and fat. An infarction can also occur when there is marked narrowing of the blood vessels in the neck or within the skull due to atherosclerosis.

The second category is *hemorrhages*. The development of the hemorrhage is usually sudden and marked by a severe headache and stiff neck.

In infarction, the tissue that has died swells. This swelling may cause further damage to nearby tissue that has only a marginal blood supply. The brain cells that depend on the blood flow by a particular vessel quickly become anoxic and begin to die in less than four minutes. Furthermore, all body functions controlled or influenced by the affected area are impaired or lost. For example, if the speech area is involved, the individual may be unable to talk; if visual centers are involved, blindness may result.

Signs and Symptoms

The signs and symptoms of a stroke depend, of course, on the area of the brain involved. Among the most common are:

- Impaired speech
- Confusion and/or dizziness
- Paralysis of one side of the body
- Unequal pupil size
- Seizures
- Temporary loss of speech or trouble in speaking or understanding speech
- Temporary dimness or loss of vision, particularly in one eye
- Mouth drawn to one side of the face or drooping on one side; paralysis of facial muscles, resulting in loss of expression. (Eyelid droops on affected side.)
- Loss of bladder or bowel control
- Sudden severe headache
- Nausea and/or vomiting

It is interesting to understand that if there is a stroke on the left side of the brain, the right side of the body will be affected below the head level. This is because the motor fibers pass through at the level of the medulla and then cross over to the opposite side of the body on the lower level of the spinal cord.

Occasionally, people may have small emboli that produce transient stroke-like symptoms that are known as transient ischemic attacks (TIAs) or "mini-strokes" before they experience a typical stroke. A TIA is indicative of a transient interruption of blood supply and oxygenation to a localized area of the brain. Since the effect is brief and localized, recovery usually occurs in twelve to twenty-four hours without any damage. A TIA is thought to result from the closing of small intracranial arteries by blood clots or plaques, a sudden drop in blood pressure, or from the compression of a vertebral artery by head-turning.

Signs and symptoms are headache, light-headedness, dizziness and fainting. Though temporary in nature, these signs and symptoms are warnings that a major stroke may occur. Care of the TIA victim includes being sure that:

- The victim takes medication given by a physician.
- If another attack occurs, the victim sees a physician or goes to the emergency department.
- If a person has TIAs, he or she is under the care of a physician.
- The victim does not drive without a physician's approval.

Emergency Care

The initial care of the stroke victim should include careful attention to the victim's airway. If the victim is semiconscious or unconscious, he or she should be placed on one side, preferably with the paralyzed side down. This position frees the victim's useful extremities. The paralyzed side should be adequately cushioned. Positioning on the side will permit the pooling of secretions in the cheek rather than the throat.

Because of the impairment of blood flow to the brain, keep the victim's head propped up about fifteen degrees to allow for adequate venous drainage.

Remove dentures. Also remove any mucus and food debris from the mouth in a swabbing motion with a piece of cloth wrapped around a finger. Do not give any liquids—the throat may be paralyzed.

The first aider must often rely on the family to obtain an accurate history of the problem because the victim may be unable to provide meaningful input.

The victim may have unusual behavior. This may be manifested in being combative and using abusive and profane language.

If an eye has been affected by the stroke, consider protecting the eye by closing the lid and taping the eyelid down to prevent drying, which can result in loss of vision.

Avoid doing or saying anything that will increase the victim's anxiety. Do not overly handle the victim because it may aggravate the stroke. Calm reassurance of the victim and the family is one of the best things a first aider can do. Transportation to the medical facility must be as gentle and prompt as possible.

The first few minutes of care are critical in avoiding further injury, and the care is reassuring to the victim. Learning to recognize the signs and symptoms of stroke and providing proper emergency care until medical help arrives can help cope with this major killer and disabler.

DIABETIC EMERGENCIES*

With nearly 11 million Americans having diabetes, most of us have a friend or relative who has diabetes.

Diabetes is the inability of the body to appropriately metabolize carbohydrates. The islets of Langerhans of the pancreas fail to produce enough of a hormone called insulin. The function of insulin is to take glucose (sugar) from the blood and carry it into the cells to be used. The excess glucose remains in the blood, and the body cells must rely on fat as fuel. Since glucose is a major body fuel, when it cannot be metabolized, serious consequences can develop.

Each year about 8,000 deaths occur from diabetic emergencies in which the glucose level has become unbalanced. When the glucose level becomes too high, diabetic coma, or ketoacidosis, may occur; and the body tries to eliminate the excess urine, which can result in dehydration. Meanwhile, the cells, deprived of glucose, begin to metabolize fats for fuel. Metabolism of fat results in the production of acids and ketones as wastes. The ketones cause the victims' breath to have a fruity odor. As dehydration increases and the body is robbed of fuel, the person comes closer and closer to coma.

The opposite condition, insulin shock, can result when a person with diabetes has taken too much insulin or not eaten. The glucose level in the blood drops dangerously low and the victim becomes weak and disoriented, or unconscious.

Both of these conditions can be fatal unless something is not done to reverse them.

Diabetic Coma (Ketoacidosis or Hyperglycemia)

Diabetic coma can develop for four basic reasons. The person has undiagnosed diabetes; the diabetic has not taken insulin; the diabetic has overeaten and produced more sugar than the insulin can convert; the diabetic has an illness, injury, or stress that is affecting the insulin level.

Victims of diabetic coma often behave similarly to people who are intoxicated. The victim is in need of insulin to restore the sugar balance, but a first aider should not administer it. You can give the victim water if it can be kept down, but you should seek medical care immediately. If the victim is unconscious, maintain an open airway and be alert for vomiting. Turn the victim on his side to prevent choking. Look for a medic alert tag on the victim's wrist or neck that will indicate that the victim is diabetic. Take the victim to the hospital.

---

*Copyright by the American Diabetes Association. Reprinted with permission from the Emergency Personnel Program manual.

In an emergency

THINK

LOW Blood Sugar
(Insulin reaction or Hypoglycemia)

Symptoms
Sudden Onset
Staggering, poor coordination
Anger, bad temper
Pale color
Confusion, disorientation
Sudden hunger
Sweating
Eventual stupor or unconsciousness

Action to take:

Provide sugar! If the person can swallow without choking, offer any food or drink containing sugar, such as soft drinks, fruit juice, or candy. Do not use diet drinks when blood sugar is low.

If the person does not respond in 10 to 15 minutes, take him/her to the hospital.

HIGH Blood Sugar
(Hyperglycemia or Acidosis)

Symptoms
Gradual Onset
Drowsiness
Extreme thirst
Very frequent urination
Flushed skin
Vomiting
Fruity or wine-like breath odor
Heavy breathing
Eventual stupor or unconsciousness

Action to take:

Take this person to the hospital. If you are uncertain whether the person is suffering from high or low blood sugar, give some sugar-containing food or drink. If there is no response in 10–15 minutes, this person needs immediate medical attention.

DIABETES!

Warning: A diabetic emergency may resemble alcohol or drug intoxication. Know the symptoms of low and high blood sugar. **THINK DIABETES!**

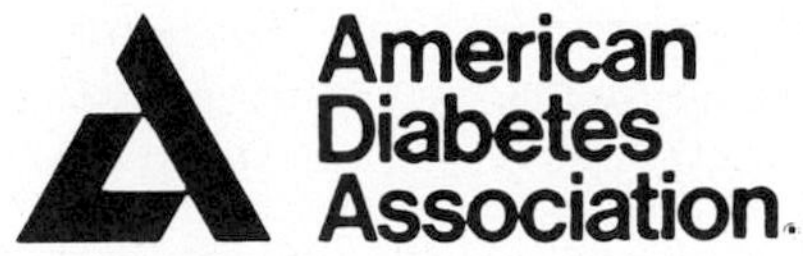

Insulin Shock (Hypoglycemia)

This condition can develop because the victim has taken too much insulin, too little food, or both. Skipping meals is dangerous for diabetics because the brain depends on glucose for its metabolism. If insulin is given and sugar is removed from the blood and there is no food to replace it, the blood sugar level drops drastically low. The brain is then unable to function. Unlike diabetic coma, insulin shock develops very rapidly and can cause bizarre behavior, which may be mistaken for mental illness.

First aid for insulin shock includes giving the victim something containing sugar, such as a soft drink, candy, or fruit juice. Do not use diet drink when blood sugar is low. Often, the victim will recover amazingly fast. If the person does not feel better in ten to fifteen minutes, take him or her to the hospital. For an unconscious victim, a cube of sugar or loose sugar may be placed under the tongue of the victim because some sugar is absorbed through the lining of the mouth.

Telling the difference between the two conditions, diabetic coma and insulin shock, can be difficult. If the victim is awake, the victim can often direct the first aider as to what to do. If the victim has eaten but not taken insulin, the problem is most likely diabetic coma. If the victim has not eaten but has taken insulin, the problem is most likely insulin shock.

If the first aider cannot distinguish between the two conditions and sugar is available, have the victim take it. If the condition is insulin shock, there will be noticeable improvement. If it is diabetic coma, there is little danger that a small amount of sugar will worsen the victim's condition. Do not give liquids to an unconscious victim. These procedures may save the life of a victim or avoid brain damage.

EPILEPSY*

More than two million Americans have epilepsy. People with epilepsy look just like everyone else, except when they have a seizure.

Epilepsy is a common neurological condition. It is sometimes called a seizure disorder. It takes the form of brief, temporary changes in the normal functioning of the brain's electrical system. These brief malfunctions occur when more than the usual amount of electrical energy passes between cells. This sudden overload may stay in just one small area of the brain, or it may swamp the whole system.

You cannot see what is happening inside a person's brain. But you can see the unusual body movements, the effects on consciousness, and the changed behavior that the malfunctioning cells are producing. These changes are what we call epileptic seizures.

Recognition of epilepsy and knowledge of first aid is important because it is very easy to mistake epilepsy for some other condition. For example, since a convulsive seizure may look like a heart attack, a first aider might apply CPR techniques when they are not necessary. A period of automatic behavior may be interpreted as public drunkenness, being drunk and disorderly, or being high on drugs. The fact that people who undergo this kind of seizure often carry phenobarbital (an anti-epileptic drug) with them adds to the confusion.

About one person in one hundred has epilepsy, and three out of four new cases begin in childhood. Epilepsy in adults may be the result of head injury—often from automobile accidents—or may date from their childhood years. Epilepsy is not contagious at any age.

Types of Seizures

Epileptic seizures may be convulsive or nonconvulsive in nature, depending on where in the brain the malfunction takes place and on how much of the total brain area is involved.

Convulsive seizures are the ones that most people generally think of when they hear the word "epilepsy." In this type of seizure the person undergoes convulsions that usually last from two to five minutes, with complete loss of consciousness and muscle spasms.

Nonconvulsive seizures may take the form of a blank stare lasting only a few seconds, an involuntary movement of arm or leg, or a period of automatic movement in which awareness of one's surroundings is blurred or completely absent.

Since these seizure types are so different, they require different kinds of action from the public, and some require no action at all. Table 11-2 describes seizures in detail and how to handle each type.

Should Medical Attention Be Called?

An uncomplicated convulsive seizure due to epilepsy is not a medical emergency, even though it looks like one. It stops naturally after a few minutes without ill effects. The average victim is able to resume normal activity after a rest period and may need only limited assistance, or no assistance at all, in getting home.

However, several medical conditions other than epilepsy can cause seizures. These require immediate medical attention and include:

encephalitis	poisoning	hypoglycemia
meningitis	pregnancy	high fever
heat stroke		head injury

**Source:* Epilepsy Foundation of America. Reprinted with permission.

TABLE 11-2. Epilepsy: Recognition and First Aid

Seizure Type	What It Looks Like	Often Mistaken For	What To Do	What Not To Do
CONVULSIVE **Generalized Tonic-Clonic** (Also called Grand Mal)	Sudden cry, fall, rigidity, followed by muscle jerks, frothy saliva or lips, shallow breathing or temporarily suspended breathing, bluish skin, possible loss of bladder or bowel control, usually lasts 2-5 minutes. Normal breathing then starts again. There may be some confusion and/or fatigue, followed by return to full consciousness.	Heart attack. Stroke. Unknown but life threatening emergency.	Look for medical identification. Protect from nearby hazards. Loosen tie or shirt collars. Place folded jacket under head. Turn on side to keep airway clear. Reassure when consciousness returns. If single seizure lasted less than 10 minutes, ask if hospital evaluation wanted. If multiple seizures, or if one seizure lasts longer than 10 minutes, take to emergency room.	Don't put any hard implement in the mouth. Don't try to hold tongue. It can't be swallowed. Don't try to give liquids during or just after seizure. Don't use oxygen unless there are symptoms of heart attack. Don't use artificial respiration unless breathing is absent after muscle jerks subside, or unless water has been inhaled. Don't restrain.
NON-CONVULSIVE **Absence** (Also called Petit Mal)	A blank stare, lasting only a few seconds, most common in children. May be accompanied by rapid blinking, some chewing movements of the mouth. Child having the seizure is unaware of what's going on during the seizure, but quickly returns to full awareness once it has stopped. May result in learning difficulties if not recognized and treated.	Daydreaming. Lack of attention. Deliberate ignoring of adult instructions.	No first aid necessary, but medical evaluation should be recommended.	
Simple Partial (Also called Jacksonian)	Jerking begins in fingers or toes, can't be stopped by patient, but patient stays awake and aware. Jerking may proceed to involve hand, then arm, and sometimes spreads to whole body and becomes a convulsive seizure.	Acting out, bizarre behavior.	No first aid necessary unless seizure becomes convulsive, then first aid as above.	
Simple Partial (Also called Sensory)	May not be obvious to onlooker, other than patient's preoccupied or blank expression. Patient experiences a distorted environment. May see or hear things that aren't there, may feel unexplained fear, sadness, anger, or joy. May have nausea, experience odd smells, and have a generally "funny" feeling in the stomach.	Hysteria. Mental Illness. Psychosomatic illness. Parapsychological or mystical experience.	No action needed other than reassurance and emotional support	
Complex Partial (Also called Psychomotor or Temporal Lobe)	Usually starts with blank stare, followed by chewing, followed by random activity. Person appears unaware of surroundings, may seem dazed and mumble. Unresponsive. Actions clumsy, not directed. May pick at clothing, pick up objects, try to take clothes off. May run, appear to be afraid. May struggle or flail at restraint. Once pattern established, same set of actions usually occur with each seizure. Lasts a few minutes, but post-seizure confusion can last substantially longer. No memory of what happened during seizure period.	Drunkenness. Intoxication on drugs. Mental Illness. Indecent exposure. Disorderly conduct. Shoplifting.	Speak calmly and reassuringly to patient and others. Guide gently away from obvious hazards. Stay with person until completely aware of environment. Offer to help getting home.	Don't grab hold unless sudden danger (such as a cliff edge or an approaching car) threatens. Don't try to restrain. Don't shout. Don't expect verbal instructions to be obeyed.
Atonic Seizures (Also called Drop Attacks)	The legs of a child between 2-5 years of age suddenly collapse under him and he falls. After 10 seconds to a minute he recovers consciousness, and can stand and walk again.	Clumsiness. Lack of good walking skills. Normal childhood "stage."	No first aid needed (unless he hurt himself as he fell), but the child should be given a thorough medical evaluation.	
Myoclonic Seizures	Sudden brief, massive muscle jerks that may involve the whole body or parts of body. May cause person to spill what they were holding or fall off a chair.	Clumsiness. Poor coordination.	No first aid needed, but should be given a thorough medical evaluation.	
Infantile Spasms	Starts between 3 months and two years. If a child is sitting up, the head will fall forward, and the arms will flex forward. If lying down, the knees will be drawn up, with arms and head flexed forward as if the baby is reaching for support.	Normal movements of the baby, especially if they happen when the baby is lying down.	No first aid, but prompt medical evaluation is needed.	

Source: Epilepsy Foundation of America. Reprinted with permission.

The following guidelines are designed to help people with epilepsy avoid unnecessary and expensive trips to the emergency room and to help you decide whether or not to call an ambulance when someone has a convulsive seizure.

Do not call an ambulance if:

1. Medical I.D. jewelry or card identified the person as epileptic, *and*

2. The seizure ends in under *ten minutes, and*

3. Consciousness returns without further incident, *and*

4. There are no signs of injury, physical distress, or pregnancy.

Call an ambulance if:

1. The seizure has happened in water.

2. There is no medical I.D. and no way of knowing whether the seizure is caused by epilepsy, *and*

3. The seizure continues for more than *five* minutes. Setting a five-minute limit on a seizure of unknown origin before calling for emergency assistance (against ten minutes if medical I.D. is worn) is a precaution based on the possibility that a serious condition other than epilepsy may be causing the convulsion.

If an ambulance arrives after the person has regained consciousness, you should ask the person whether the seizure was associated with epilepsy and whether emergency room care is wanted. The same questions should be asked of a person without medical I.D. whose seizure lasts less than five minutes and for whom an ambulance has not yet been called.

Could It Be Epilepsy?

Only a physician can say for certain whether or not a person has epilepsy. But many people miss the more subtle signs of the condition and therefore also miss the opportunity for early diagnosis and treatment. The following symptoms are not necessarily indicators of epilepsy and may be caused by some other, unrelated condition. However, if one or more is present, a medical check-up is recommended.

- Periods of blackout or confused memory
- Odd sounds, distorted vision, episodes of fear, or short-lived feelings of impending disaster
- Occasional "fainting spells" in which bladder or bowel control is lost, followed by extreme fatigue
- Excessive thrashing around while asleep, or waking with a bitten tongue or unexplained bruises
- Episodes of staring in children; brief periods when there is no response to questions or instructions
- Sudden falls in a child for no apparent reason
- Episodes of blinking or chewing at inappropriate times
- Involuntary movements
- A convulsion, with or without fever

ASTHMA

The sight of a person suffering an acute asthmatic attack is most distressing and, to first aiders inexperienced with this form of illness, very frightening.

There are about ten million asthmatics in the United States, over half of them children. At some time in their lives, 5% to 10% of the population are believed to be affected. Because it is a chronic disease, asthma accounts for many absences from school and work. Asthma kills 4,000 to 5,000 of its victims each year. It is a common cause of emergency department visits.

All asthmatics have hyperirritable airways, making the bronchial tree sensitive and overreactive to substances and conditions that do no normally adversely affect other people.

Although asthma is precipitated by various "triggers," the result is the same—an airway obstruction due to:

- Bronchospasm
- Swelling of mucous membranes in the bronchial walls
- Plugging of bronchi by thick, mucous secretions

Status asthmaticus is a severe, prolonged asthmatic attack that even a physician using epinephrine cannot break; it is a true emergency. The chest is greatly distended and the victim has great difficulty in moving air. There may be inaudible breath sounds and wheezes because of the little air movement. The victim is usually exhausted and dehydrated.

Signs and Symptoms

Asthma is characterized by a sudden narrowing of the smaller air passageways in the lungs. The victim becomes acutely short of breath and a wheezing will be heard during exhalation.

Wheezing is the most obvious sign of this condition. It is a whistling, high-pitched sound produced by air being forced through a constricted airway. The wheezing is usually quite audible, but it may be absent if the attack is very severe and there is very little movement of air. Not all wheezes are asthma. Other causes of wheezing include heart failure, smoke inhalation, and chronic bronchitis.

Other important signs leading to suspicion of asthma include:

- A known history of severe allergies or a family history of allergies
- Previous attacks of shortness of breath
- A recent respiratory infection
- Prescription medications in the form of pills and/or inhaler
- An unproductive cough
- Rapid respiration rate

During an acute attack, the victim has relatively more obstruction during exhalation than during inhalation. The result is a trapping of air in the lungs with consequent hyperinflation of the chest.

Emergency Care

The first aider may be called on to assist a person who is suffering from an acute asthmatic attack. In most cases, the first aider can do little other than recognize the nature of the ailment and, if needed, obtain medical assistance. Considerations during an emergency may include:

- The keystone of asthma care is adequate fluid intake. Doubling the intake of liquids will benefit the victim. Water given orally, if possible, is warranted.
- Often steam or vaporizer inhalations are beneficial.
- Inhalation of nebulized medication should not be done more than every one or two hours and rarely used for more than one day. Many asthmatics carry a nebulizer or inhaler or at least know which one is effective.
- Help the victim into a comfortable breathing position that he or she chooses. Do not make the victim assume a position you think will be comfortable. The best position is usually sitting straight up. The victim probably won't let you position him or her in any other way. He or she knows better than you what position enables him to breathe most comfortably.
- Place the victim in a room that is as free as possible of common allergens (e.g., dust, feathers, animals). It should also be free of odors (e.g., tobacco smoke, paint).
- Panic is often present in the acute asthmatic attack. A calm and caring attitude and a comforting voice can prevent panic from escalating.
- Keep all questions to the victim as brief and essential as possible. The victim may be struggling merely to breathe. Attempt to find out when the onset of the attack began and if previous attacks have occurred.
- Observe skin and nail bed color for cyanosis and note wheezing patterns.
- Home therapy may not be sufficient if the asthma has been present for several hours or if there have been recurrent attacks within a few days. Therefore, medical advice should be obtained.

ABDOMEN PAIN

This section deals with a variety of disorders that cause abdominal pain. It will not be either feasible or useful to distinguish among the many causes of abdominal pain because, in general, first aid and emergency care will be similar regardless of the cause.

To assess the implications of the abdominal pain, the first aider should determine the following:

- Location of the pain
- Quality of the pain. Constant abdominal pain is suggestive of inflammatory or destructive involvement of an organ, whereas cramping, intermittent pain suggests obstruction of a hollow organ (e.g., bowel obstruction, kidney stone).
- Duration of the pain. This information can be used to determine whether the problem is of recent origin or whether it has been present for a long time.
- Intensity of the pain
- Nature of onset (Sudden and abrupt or gradual onset of pain can indicate different injuries.)
- Presence of associated vomiting
- Change in bowel habits

The victim will tell you where the pain is. First examine the other three quadrants, so that any pain you elicit from the trouble spot does not tighten the rest of the abdominal muscles. Except for examining the painful area last, the order in which the quadrants are examined is not important. (*See* Figure 11-1.)

Try to make the victim relax by explaining what you are doing. If he can, have him empty his bladder before you examine him. Ask him to remove all clothing from his abdomen. Then place him comfortably on his back, knees bent and arms at his sides to keep his abdominal muscles from tensing. Your hands must be warm; keep the victim covered and warm except for the part you are examining.

Use light pressing or palpation. In light palpation, use the fingertips to depress the abdominal wall a little more than a half inch. Light palpation will reveal large masses and tender areas. This type of palpation will elicit any guarding of the abdominal wall when a sensitive area is reached. Most victims will guard (hold the abdominal muscles tight) to protect the abdomen from the pressure of the examiner's hand. First aiders should perform only light palpations.

Do not evaluate the abdomen extensively. Extensive palpation is of little value and will delay transportation and may cause unnecessary pain, which will be repeated in the emergency department.

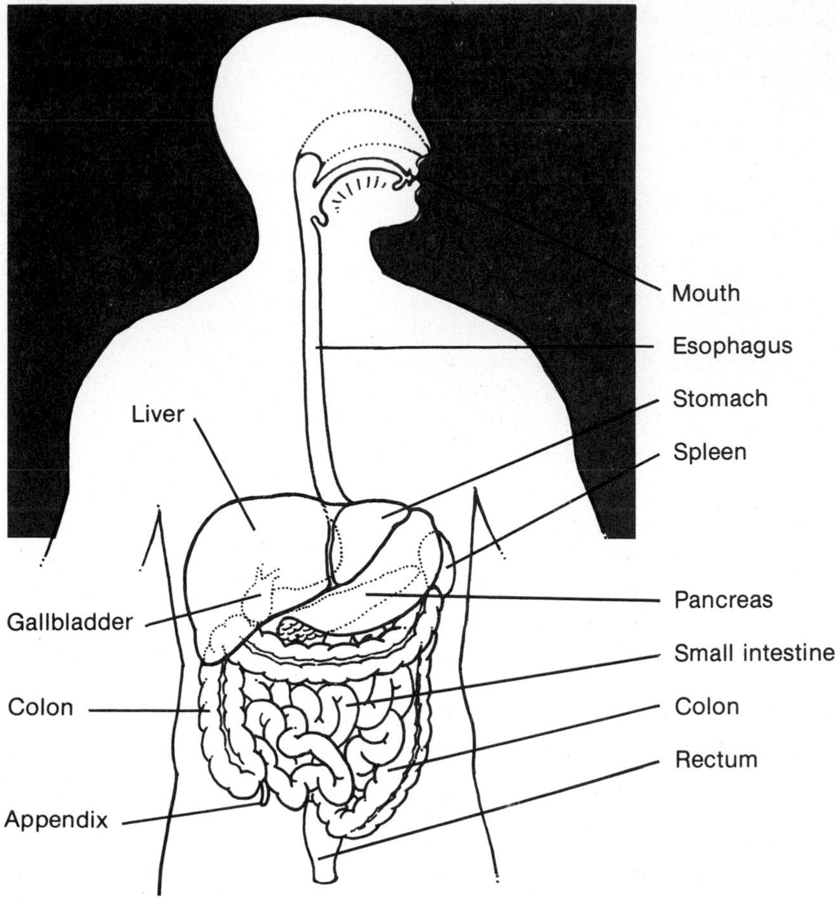

11-1. The abdominal organs

Emergency Care

The acute abdomen may require surgery, although some acute abdomens may be treated medically. In either case, immediate care by a physician is mandatory because this is a medical emergency.

Emergency care is limited; most assistance is supportive. The first aider should proceed as follows:

- Do not give anything to eat or drink. Food or fluid can aggravate many of the symptoms. If emergency surgery is needed, food in the stomach will make the surgery much more dangerous. In some cases, food will not pass out of the stomach and will only increase distention and vomiting.
- Do not give any pain medication. Pain medication will mask the symptoms and delay the diagnosis at the hospital.
- Do not give an enema or a laxative; they may cause the appendix to rupture.
- Recognize the possibility of vomiting and be prepared for it by transporting the victim on his side so that any vomitus can quickly drain out of or be cleansed from the mouth.
- Maintain the victim in a position of comfort, usually with knees bent.
- Do not waste time palpating the abdomen extensively.
- Save any stool, urine, or vomitus so it can be tested in the hospital for the presence of blood.
- Do not attempt to diagnose the victim's condition. However, do obtain a description of the pain and tenderness and other signs and symptoms so the physician may know what these were when the victim was first seen.
- Treat for shock by making the victim as comfortable as possible, conserving body heat with blankets and transporting the victim gently and quickly to the medical care.

CONSTIPATION

Constipation is the passage of hard, dry stools. The need for a daily bowel movement is a misconception.

A main cause of constipation is not taking the time to go to the bathroom. If this is the case, water from the stools eventually becomes dry as water is drawn from the stool by the large intestine.

Constipation is usually not a serious condition although it may be very painful. Most cases respond to diet changes or bowel movement habits.

Treatment consists of the following:

- Drink extra glasses of water, especially in the morning.
- Avoid laxatives, if possible.

Seek medical attention if:

- Condition persists after treatment for three days (infants), seven days (adults).
- Dark blood is seen in stools.

COUGH

Coughing is a vital reflex action—nature's way of clearing the airways of some irritating substance. Coughing can occur in perfectly healthy people and be nothing more than the body's response to a tickle in the throat. It also is a symptom of a variety of diseases, and in some cases, a person's inability to cough can be a threat to life.

There are two general types of cough. One is the dry, irritative, nonproductive cough, so called because there is no mucus or phlegm to spit out. The other is the loose, productive cough that gets its name from the fact that it is triggered by large amounts of secretions in the bronchial passages. Coughs can be transient and self-limiting—that is, they will disappear in a short time, usually without help from medication. On the other hand, coughs can hang on for a long time and become persistent and chronic.

A dry nonproductive cough can develop from breathing the dry air of overheated rooms as well as from inhaling irritating gases, dusts, or other foreign substances that sneak past the body's primary defenses in the nose and mouth. This type of cough is generally not long lasting, but it can be prolonged because the rapid expulsion of air during the act of coughing continually irritates the throat.

The common cold is probably the most frequent cause of short-term coughs, which can be either nonproductive or productive. Smoking is considered the most common cause of the persistent, chronic cough that can come from direct irritation of the bronchial passages or from damage to the lung's cleaning mechanism. Thus, the smoker is more likely to get upper respiratory infections that pave the way for more serious respiratory disease. Nonsmokers also can develop a chronic cough if they have postnasal drip from sinus and allergy difficulties or from enlarged adenoids. A cough also may be a symptom of a number of serious illnesses.

Treatment

What to do about a cough depends on what causes it. A smoker's cough, for instance, usually stops when the smoking habit is kicked. An antihistamine puts an end to postnasal drip. The dry, nonproductive cough that goes along with the common cold should disappear when the cold gets better and in many cases can be controlled without any drugs at all.

Nonmedical cough remedies that many experts recommend include sucking on a hard candy or lozenge to increase the flow of saliva and drinking liquids to keep the throat lubricated. Steam from a vaporizer, hot shower, or a tea kettle helps loosen secretions in the bronchial passages and makes them easier to cough up. Keeping moisture in the air indoors with various humidifying devices can help keep throats form becoming dry.

When the dry, nonproductive cough becomes too annoying, exhausts the cougher, or robs him and his family of much needed sleep, relief may be obtained from nonprescription medicines, called antitussives (from the Latin word *tussis*, meaning cough).

An antitussive works by depressing the cough center in the brain. Codeine is one of the most commonly used antitussives. Although it is a narcotic, there is no danger of psychological and physical dependence when codeine is used in the recommended dose for cough control. Stringent controls have been put on the sale of codeine in nonprescription cough medicines to assure that it is not misused.

A nonnarcotic antitussive considered safe and effective is dextromethorphan which—like codeine—acts on the cough center in the brain. Taken at the recommended dose, dextromethorphan produces few adverse reactions and these are usually mild and limited to drowsiness and upset stomach.

Although antitussives are useful in stilling the dry, nagging kind of cough, they should never be used to control a loose, productive cough, such as that associated with asthma, chronic bronchitis, or emphysema. In these diseases it is important to keep the airways clear. Suppressing the cough reflex only makes matters worse by slowing down or preventing the natural clearing process.

Another type of cough medicine is the expectorant, used to encourage removal of secretions from the bronchial airways by reducing their thickness or by increasing the amount of respiratory tract secretion. Many ingredients in cough remedies claim to be expectorants, but none is really effective.

Many over-the-counter (OTC) cold remedies are combinations of several ingredients. They may contain an antitussive, an expectorant, a nasal decongestant, and an antihistamine. Sometimes a bronchodilator for clearing the bronchial tubes or a fever reducer is included. Generally these products are intended to treat the various symptoms associated with the common cold—sore throat, runny nose, stuffed-up nose, headache—and should not be taken for a cough alone.

Many OTC cold remedies contain alcohol, suggesting that parents would be wise to read the label carefully before giving cough medicines to young children. Cough and cold preparations containing alcohol in excess of 10% by weight should not be used by children under six years of age except under the advice and supervision of a physician.

When To Seek Medical Attention

The average self-limiting cough usually lasts about a week. Anything longer can be a sign of more serious problems. A persistent cough may be a sign of a serious condition. If coughing persists for more than one week, tends to recur, or is accompanied by high fever, rash, or persistent headache, consult a physician.

According to the National Heart and Lung Institute and the National Tuberculosis Association, a cough that lasts more than a month is a chronic cough that could be a symptom of a chronic lung disease. A person who buys a lot of cough medicine and is constantly "popping" cough drops, or who seems to cough a lot at bedtime or when waking up in the morning may have a chronic cough. If this is the case, the cougher should not undertake self-treatment but should be checked by a physician.

DIARRHEA

Diarrhea is frequent elimination of loose, watery stools. Most diarrhea is caused by a stomach virus that overstimulates the intestines to empty themselves and push the stools through before water can be reabsorbed by the body. Dehydration is the most common complication and results from the loss of large amounts of fluid lost and are not replaced. Adult diarrhea is often caused by stress or emotional problems.

Treatment

The treatment for diarrhea includes the following:

- Avoid solid foods for one day.
- Mild foods can be added the next day. The BRAT diet—B = bananas, R = rice, A = applesauce, T = toast—is recommended.

Most things done for viral diarrhea make it worse. Although almost everyone has taken white, pink, or clear-brown stuff to stop diarrhea, *DON'T!* It is better to get rid of the infected diarrhea fluid than to keep it in to churn around in one's intestines.

Another mistake most people make in managing diarrhea is to encourage liquids like soft drinks, flavored gelatin water, apple juice and the canned electrolyte solution athletes drink. Drinking plain water is *not* a good way to replace lost fluids from diarrhea and vomiting because plain water does not contain sodium and potassium which are lost in the diarrhea along with water.

Most ordinary foods entering an inflamed intestinal tract are irritating—but many people with diarrhea go right on eating as usual, which increases bowel motility. Even milk is usually not well tolerated. So what can be done when someone has a virus causing diarrhea and vomiting?

The most important thing is to replace the lost fluid and electrolytes in the proper balance. Several products are available, such as Pedialyte™ and Infalyte™. Pedialyte™ comes as a ready to use solution in bottles for infants and in cans with a mild fruit flavor for children and adults. (The fruit flavor is merely an aroma because stronger flavors or sweetening increases diarrhea.) Infalyte™ comes as a powder which is mixed with plain water. Follow the instructions for Pedialyte™ or Infalyte™ carefully, never mixing these solutions with juices or other liquids. And remember, these solutions should be used *exclusively* until their need is over. In other words, it defeats the purpose to alternative drinking Pedialyte™ or Infalyte™ with water, juice, or something else.

Large amounts of Pedialyte™ or Infalyte™ are needed to replace lost fluids plus maintenance requirements. When an infant or young child has diarrhea and/or vomiting, a pediatrician should help guide the amounts of fluid needed, while monitoring signs of dehydration such as dry lips and skin, dull eyes, listlessness, a sunken soft spot, decreased urination, and poor skin elasticity—because dehydration can be a killer.

After the vomiting and cramping have stopped in older children and adults with viral gastroenteritis, you may try banana, broth, rice, and cooked carrots cautiously. When these are tolerated, substitute plain water for the electrolyte solution. Then slowly add other mild foods like potatoes, yogurt, and skinless chicken or white fish.

When To Seek Medical Attention

The victim of diarrhea should seek medical attention if any of the following occurs:

- Tarry or bloody diarrhea
- No improvement after twenty-four hours
- Continues for over one week
- No urine for more than eight hours
- Accompanied by vomiting
- Fever of more than 101°F for more than twenty-four hours

EARACHE

Earache or inflammation of the middle ear is common in children and youth, but it may happen in people of all ages. Though usually caused by a bacterial infection behind the eardrum, earaches can be caused by viruses or allergies. Bacterial infections require an antibiotic.

Treatment

Earaches can be treated as follows:

- Apply heat with a warm wash cloth or a heating pad to the ear.
- Take oral nasal decongestant (tablet, liquid, or capsule form).
- Use nasal decongestants (nose drops or spray four times daily) for some relief. Do not use for more than three continuous days.
- Take aspirin or acetaminophen to help relieve the pain, though some experts do not recommend them because the pain may be mocked.
- Increase humidity through the use of a vaporizer.
- Chew gum to try to relieve pain.

When To Seek Medical Attention

A person who is suffering from an earache should seek medical attention if:

- The earache is severe and lasts for one hour—even if it then stops.
- Pain increases despite treatment.
- Temperature is over 102°F.
- Person cannot touch chin to chest without pain (may be a sign of meningitis).
- Eardrum ruptures.

FEVER

"Fever" can be a frightening word, particularly when it is part of the name of a disease, as in "yellow fever," "typhoid fever," "scarlet fever," and so on.

Unless it is very high, a fever is not to be feared. It is not a disease, simply a sign, a warning sign, that something is wrong with the body that needs investigation. A fever may even serve a useful purpose. Fever usually occurs with a bacterial or viral infection or inflammation.

Treatment

There are some very good reasons for not treating a fever. For one, there is some evidence that a fever may play a role in stimulating the body's natural defenses. The ups and downs of a fever also help in diagnosing an illness and following its course. And fever is often the only way to determine whether a particular treatment is working. If a person is on an antibiotic, for instance, a persistent fever would indicate that the drug is probably not effective and that an alternative should be used.

In general, the studies reveal that parents worry a lot about fever and its possible harmful effects. They do not understand what constitutes a "high fever," they fear that if the fever is not treated it will continue to rise to dangerous levels, and they believe that even moderately high temperatures could cause permanent harm, such as "brain damage."

Many of the parents interviewed in these studies thought that temperatures as low as 100°F were serious and said they would start giving their children medication as soon as the fever thermometer reached that point.

Some parents tend to check their children's temperatures frequently—from five to eight times a day, sometimes even hourly. Quite a number of parents worry so much about fever that they wake the child to give additional medication to lower the temperature. Such aggressive treatment of childhood fevers is not always necessary, according to pediatricians.

Fever is one of the most common reasons parents bring their children to see a doctor. About 90% of these fevers are minor and self-limiting, caused by some common infectious agent such as an influenza virus. Truly high fevers—105°F or higher—are rare and may be the result of a serious infection or other condition that has upset the body's temperature regulation.

Unless the fever is very high, the temperature of a feverish child who feels reasonably well otherwise (which is often the case) does not have to be reduced, experts say. There are exceptions, of course. Persistent fevers over 103°F and fevers in infants and very young child and in those who have a history of convulsions require prompt medical attention.

Even though professional health care is not needed for all feverish children, tender, loving care is still in order. Parents can take a number of measures to make the young victim more comfortable.

- Help the body maintain its own temperature regulation. Many well-meaning parents bundle up a sick child, thus preventing natural heat loss. Keep the sick room at a moderate temperature and the bed coverings to a minimum.
- Sponging with lukewarm water can also make the victim more comfortable. This increases heat loss by evaporation. Enemas should *not* be used.
- Be sure that the child gets plenty of fluids.
- If treatment with antipyretic drugs is recommended, among the most effective are aspirin and acetaminophen (known by several brand names, such as Tylenol™, Datril™, and Panadol™, and also sold generically).

Both drugs work equally well in reducing fever, but each has other advantages of its own. Acetaminophen

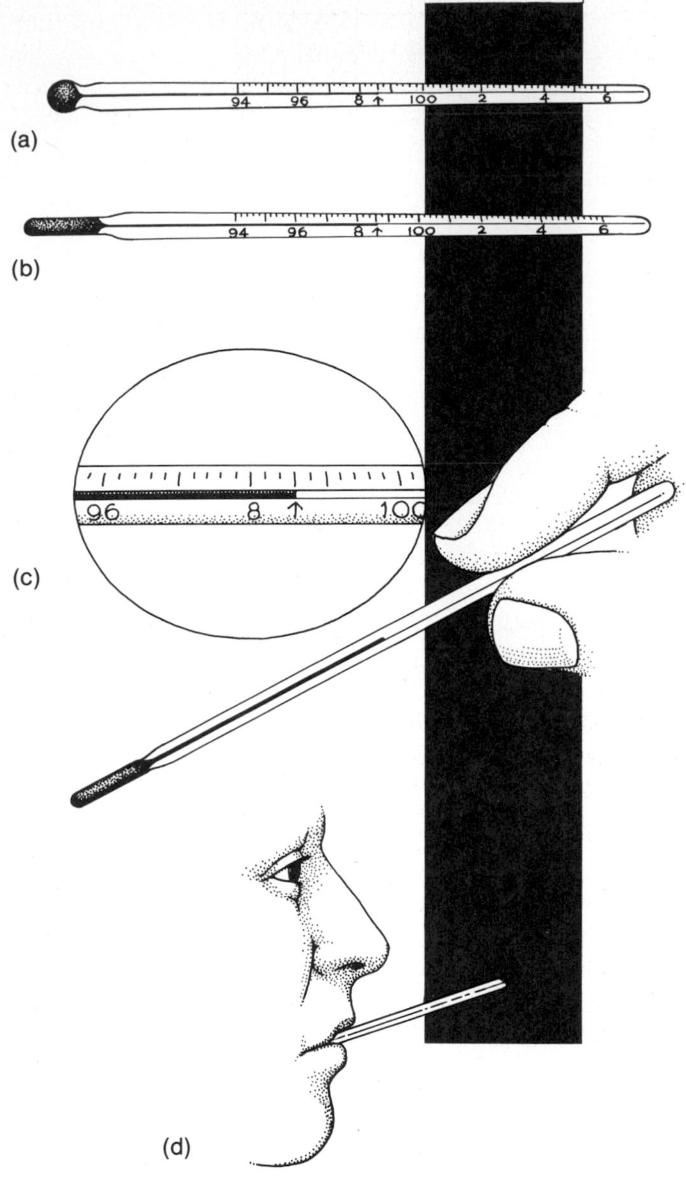

11-2. Using a thermometer
(a) Rectal thermometer
(b) Oral thermometer
(c) Reading a thermometer. An arrow usually points to 98.6°F—normal oral temperature (even if it is a rectal thermometer)
(d) To take an oral temperature, place the bulb of the thermometer under the tongue for at least three minutes.

is available in liquid form—a plus if a small child is being treated—but it is not effective in reducing inflammation. Aspirin does fight inflammation, but it can have serious side effects, including gastrointestinal bleeding and interference with blood clotting if given for prolonged periods or in excessive amounts. Both drugs can be toxic if taken in large amounts. Therefore, care should always be taken to keep the bottle out of the reach of the toddler or young child.

In addition, parents should be particularly aware that they should consult a physician before giving aspirin to children and teenagers with flu or chicken pox. Some studies have shown a possible association between such use of aspirin and the development of a rare but often fatal condition called Reyes disease.

Symptoms of Reyes disease include violent headache, persistent vomiting, lethargy, sleepiness, belligerence, disorientation, and delirium. These symptoms are very serious and can develop quickly, sometimes within half a day after the child has apparently recovered from the original flu or chicken pox. Unless emergency medical treatment is initiated promptly in a hospital setting, Reyes disease can cause brain damage and even death.

In most cases, a fever is not serious, but still, it can be a sign that something is seriously wrong. That is why it is important to follow the general rule that if the temperature goes above 103°F in an older child or adult or the fever persists for more than three days (seventy-two hours), or recurs, it is time to call the doctor. Fever in infants is potentially more serious, and if it persists or recurs, the doctor should be contacted within twenty-four hours.

Taking Temperatures

Fever thermometers come in two styles—oral and rectal. You can tell them apart because the rectal thermometer is larger is diameter. Both contain mercury in a bulb at one end. When warmed, the mercury expands and rises up the narrow tube inside the shaft.

The degrees of temperature are marked on the shaft of the thermometer. Each little space between the numerals is equal to 0.2°F. The normal temperature is marked with an arrow.

Temperatures should not be taken orally just after the person has had a cold drink or brushed his or her teeth. Wait fifteen or thirty minutes. Then follow these basic steps (*see* Figure 11-2):

1. Wash your hands and rinse the thermometer in cool water.

2. Holding the thermometer by the top (not the bulb end), shake it with a quick snap of the wrist until the mercury goes to 96°F or lower.

3. Place the bulb end of the thermometer well under the victim's tongue with the instruction to keep the mouth closed without biting for at least three minutes. Young children and infirm elderly persons should not be left alone with a fever thermometer in place.

4. Remove the thermometer and rotate it until you can see the mercury level. A good light helps, but do not hold the thermometer close to a lamp. The heat could affect the reading.

When a person cannot hold an oral thermometer in the mouth—as with an infant, for example—the temperature can be taken rectally (*see* Figure 11-3).

To do so, follow steps 1 and 2, and then:

3. Lubricate the thermometer with a lubricant such as Vaseline™.

4. Have the person lie on one side and breathe through the mouth. Infants and small children may be on their sides, backs or tummies. Gently separate the person's buttocks with your free hand and gently insert the thermometer almost half an inch (the length of the bulb) into the rectum. Leave it or hold it in place, especially in infants and toddlers, about four minutes.

5. Remove, wipe off the lubricant, and read it like an oral thermometer. Rectal temperatures are about one degree higher than oral readings.

6. After use, wash the thermometer in cool, soapy water. Never wash it in warm or hot water, and do not store it near heat.

A less reliable device for measuring body temperature is a strip of blackened plastic in which liquid crystals are embedded. When pressed against the forehead for 15 to 60 seconds, these "fever strips" register rises in skin temperature by markings such as letters (N for normal, F for fever) or numbers. They also may turn various colors—tan (warm), green (warmer), and blue (warmest).

One problem with fever strips is that normal, nonfeverish forehead surface temperatures can vary two to eight degrees among individuals. In addition, the skin temperature can be affected by air temperature, artificial light, and even flushing of the face caused by an emotional state—factors that do not affect the internal body temperature.

If you use fever strips, read the product directions carefully and double check with a clinical thermometer when a high reading is registered by the fever strip or anytime you suspect a fever even though the strip registers normal.

HEADACHE

Many things can cause headaches. Most are minor and will go away in time. Most occur when the muscles of the head or neck become tense resulting in the blood vessels of the head to go into spasm. These headaches can be very painful and last for hours or even days.

Treatment

Headaches can be treated as follows:

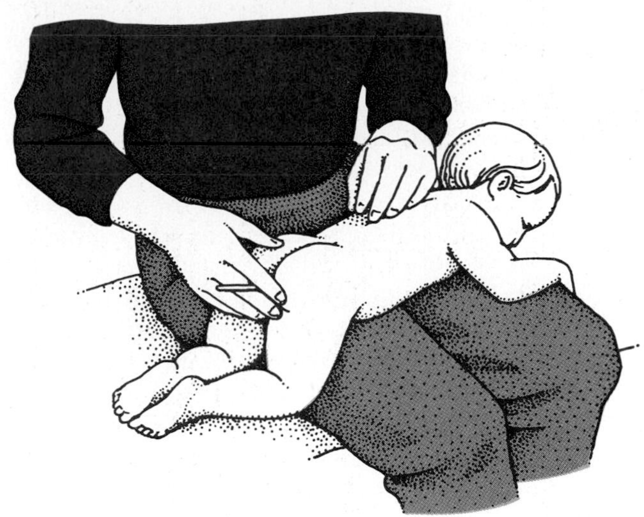

11-3. Taking a baby's rectal temperature

- Use aspirin or acetaminophen as needed.
- Give decongestants with antihistamines for allergic or cold symptoms.
- Attempt to relax by placing your head on a pillow so that your muscles can relax. Move head slowly around in a circle and massaging the neck and scalp can relieve pain.
- Some people find that placing a washcloth dipped in cold water on the forehead relieves the pain.

Seek Medical Attention

Rarely will a headache be a sign of a serious illness, but you should seek medical attention if any of the following occurs:

- Sudden onset of pain happens without a specific cause.
- Pain wakes you in the middle of the night.
- Accompanied by high fever of 103°F and headache with no other symptoms.
- A stiff neck; victim cannot touch chin to chest without pain.
- Recurring headaches in children.
- Headaches increasing in frequency and severity.
- Accompanied by loss of coordination or double vision.
- Severe and after a blow to the head.

SORE THROAT

Most (about 80%) sore throats are caused by viral infections or irritations from smoking, yelling, and postnasal drainage. Some are caused by bacteria and are known as "strep" throat, which should be treated medically with penicillin or erythromycin. The only way to diagnose a strep throat accurately is by a throat culture. Viral sore throats cannot be successfully treated with antibiotics.

Most sore throats are minor. Strep throat is a serious problem and is less frequent in adults than in children.

Telling the difference between a sore throat caused by strep and one caused by virus germs is not always easy. Sometimes the clinical picture of strep is classic, with high fevers, a very red throat, pus on the tonsils (or where they were), weakness, aches and pains all over—especially in the joints, and sometimes a diffuse, fine, sandpaper-like rash. But all these symptoms are not always present. Sometimes a strep infection will look just like a virus-caused sore throat—and sometimes a virus infection will mimic a strep infection.

If a strep infection is not properly treated (with antibiotics for ten days), rheumatic fever or kidney inflammation may be a complication. Rheumatic fever is a complex illness that may occur weeks after a strep throat has come, gone, and is all but forgotten. Besides fever and weakness, the symptoms of rheumatic fever may include various combinations of other things like swollen joints, a strange looking rash, damage to a valve of the heart, as well as heart failure. An inflammatory process in the kidney that causes the loss of protein and red blood cells in the urine can also occur.

Strep infections are miserable. Treating them with adequate penicillin or another appropriate antibiotic helps a person get well much more quickly. But of even more importance, treating a strep infection for ten days with the right antibiotic can prevent rheumatic fever and kidney inflammation. You do not want anyone in your family to have either of these long-term problems.

Children and adults with sore throats can now be tested for strep with an excellent antibody test that takes only ten minutes without having to wait overnight for a throat culture.

Treatment

Treatment of sore throats includes the following procedures:

- Humidify the home, especially the bedroom.
- Gargle with hot salt water (1 teaspoonful in 8 ounces of water) or with commercial mouthwash every two hours.
- Suck cough drops or hard candy or honey.
- Drink more fluids and juices or lemonade.
- Stop smoking and avoid smoke.
- Give pain reliever (aspirin or acetaminophen) for severe discomfort.
- Check temperature three times daily.

When To Seek Medical Attention

Medical attention should be sought if the victim has any of the following:

- A skin rash
- Severe difficulty with breathing
- Exposure to strep throat
- History of frequent strep throats
- Sore throat accompanied by fever of 101°F several times daily.
- Cannot trace cause to a cold, low humidity, excessive yelling, etc.
- Lasts more than three days or after treatment began (four days in adult)
- Very bright red throat or throat with white spots or pus on it
- Foul mouth odor
- Cannot touch chin to chest without pain
- Earache.

VOMITING

Vomiting is usually a sign of a viral infection of the stomach and intestine, excessive drinking of alcohol, or emotional upsets. Antibiotics do not help.

Dehydration is a threat. Signs of dehydration include thirst, dark yellow urine, dry mouth, sunken eyes, and skin that has lost its elasticity (pinch skin which should spring back immediately afterwards—compare with healthy person).

Treatment

Vomiting should be treated as follows:

- Nothing by mouth for four hours.
- Clear liquids (apple or grape juice, flat soda, clear soup) only for twenty-four hours.
- Bed rest.
- Replace lost fluids with soups, mild foods, and liquids only on second day and until all symptoms are gone for forty-eight hours.
- Avoid giving aspirin to children.

When to Seek Medical Attention

Seek medical attention if any of the following occurs:

- Severe vomiting (shoots out in large quantities)
- Does not stop after twelve hours of treatment (two to six hours for small children)
- Blood or dark, coffee-ground material appears in the vomit
- Signs of dehydration

- Severe or constant abdominal pain
- Yellow or green vomit on several occasions
- Combined with a severe persistent headache
- Accompanied by fever, dizziness, or pain (especially abdominal)
- Occurs after a recent head injury

HYPERVENTILATION

Hyperventilation syndrome is common. One in ten people will experience at least one episode of hyperventilation in their lives. Most cases will be temporary in duration.

There is a lack of medical literature and instruction about hyperventilation. Most victims neither are aware of overbreathing nor appear overly short of breath. Hyperventilation occurs more often in female than male adolescents; but by early adulthood, its incidence in women and men is almost equal.

Almost any sudden shock can trigger hyperventilation: a broken romance, death of a loved one, or anticipated stress, such as having to give a speech or go to a job interview. Often at rock concerts, teenaged girls have hyperventilated during the excitement of seeing and hearing their favorite singers. The person experiencing hyperventilation does not do it on purpose.

Hyperventilation is described as overbreathing to the extent that arterial carbon dioxide is abnormally lowered. When overbreathing blows off too much carbon dioxide, the blood pH (a measure of blood acidity) will be raised above normal and alkalosis, which is the cause of many of the symptoms associated with hyperventilation, develops.

Rarely do victims exhibit the textbook picture of overt hyperventilation. In fact, it has a vast number of symptoms:

- Chest pain, rapid pulse
- Dizziness, faintness, "blackouts," lightheadedness
- Dry mouth
- Dyspnea (labored breathing)
- Numbness, tingling, coolness of extremities
- Stiffness, cramping, tremors

Memorization of a long list of symptoms is a waste of time.

The human body's reaction to anxiety is sympathetic arousal (i.e., fight-or-flight response). Thus, hyperventilation is an expected result of anxiety. Although unusual, there are organic causes of hyperventilation.

Unless the person says that hyperventilation problems have happened before, the first aider may be fooled into believing the victim is having a heart attack. Some hyperventilating victims will have not only sharp chest pains but also many of the other signs of a heart attack.

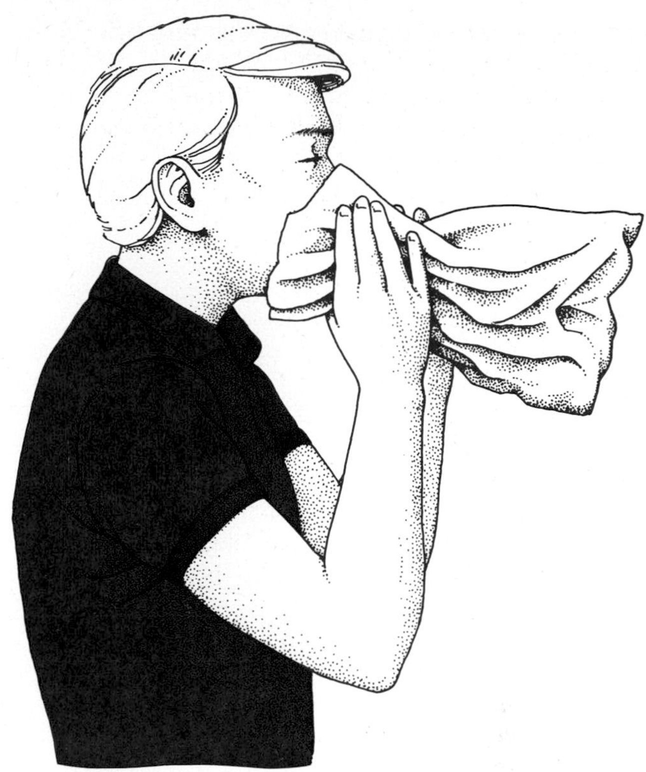

11-4. Breathe into a paper bag in case of hyperventilation

Treatment

Hyperventilation can be treated as follows:

- Avoid frequent sighing.
- Avoid temptation to "clear lungs" with deep breath.
- Hold breath for brief periods.
- Lie down in quiet place for fifteen to thirty minutes.
- Use a paper bag to "rebreathe" for three to five minutes. Breathing into a paper bag has long been thought to be the solution for hyperventilation. The paper bag remedy probably works because the technique may slow the victim's rate and depth of respiration. (*See* Figure 11-4.)

BLEEDING (RESPIRATORY AND DIGESTIVE TRACTS)

It is sometimes difficult to differentiate between bleeding from the respiratory tract and bleeding from the digestive tract. Blood from the nose, throat, or lungs may be swallowed. Thereafter it will have the same appearance in the stool as blood from the

TABLE 11-3. Bleeding from the Mouth

Color and Appearance	Amount and Method	Most Likely Source	Cause	Remarks on Treatment
Bright red	Blood-streaked sputum	Local: From mouth tissues, gums, throat, back of nose	Pyorrhea, cold in head, laryngitis, pharyngitis	Mouthwash or other symptomatic treatment. See dentist.
Bright red	Coughed up (teaspoonful or more)*	Lungs	Tuberculosis of lung, cancer	Symptomatic treatment (see below). See doctor.
Bright red	In sputum or phlegm: Coughed up, frothy, bubbly, pink or red	Lungs	Heart disease	Symptomatic treatment (see Heart Disease). See doctor.
Brown (like prune juice)	In phlegm: Coughed up (½ to 1 teaspoonful)	Lungs	Pneumonia	See doctor.
Bright red	Vomited (cupful or more)	Stomach	Hemorrhage from ulcer, cancer, ruptured vessel. Probably very recent or still continuing	Symptomatic. Use icebag.
Dark brown (like coffee-grounds)	Vomited (usually considerable in amount; one pint or more)	Stomach (old blood, mixed with partly digested food)	Stomach or duodenal disease, or blood swallowed after extraction of tooth. Bleeding probably occurred 2 or 3 hours previously, and has stopped or lessened in amount.	Ulcer, cancer.

Source: U.S. Public Health Service, *The Ship's Medicine Chest and Medical Aid at Sea,* U.S. Department of Health, Education, and Welfare.

*Coughed-up blood may result from a paroxysm of coughing or it may come from the back of the throat without any great amount of coughing, until the blood actually is in the mouth.

TABLE 11-4. Blood in Stools

Color and Appearance	Amount and Method	Most Likely Source	Cause	Remarks on Treatment
Bright red	Streaked feces	Lower end of digestive tract: hemorrhoids, anal fissure	Constipation (hard fecal matter that injures mucous membrane), local injuries, fissures, piles, cancer	If present with every stool and not reduced by cathartics which soften stools, see docor.
Bright red	Teaspoonful or more	Lower end of digestive tract	Ulcer or tumor of rectum, ulcerative colitis, dysentery, typhoid	See doctor.
Tarry	Abundant	Upper part of digestive tract	Stomach or duodenal ulcer; gastritis; liver; kidney or heart disease; typhoid; dysentery; tumor; cancer	Symptomatic treatment. See doctor.

Source: U.S. Public Health Service, *The Ship's Medicine Chest and Medical Aid at Sea,* U.S. Department of Health, Education, and Welfare.

digestive tract. To find the source of blood discharged from either the mouth or rectum, the factors that follow must be considered.

The blood may be bright red, leaving no doubt that it is blood; or it may not look like ordinary blood. If vomited and partly digested, the blood will appear dark and granular like coffee grounds. The vomitus mixed with partly digested food and other stomach contents makes for further confusion. Also, blood may give a stool a black appearance like tar.

There may be much or only a little bleeding. Sputum may be only blood-streaked, as in some mouth diseases. A teaspoonful or more of bright blood may be coughed up or vomited if the trouble is farther down the throat, in the lungs, or in the stomach. A pint or more of partly digested material like coffee grounds may be vomited. Or there may be smaller or larger amounts of bright red blood usually from a local disease of the anus or rectum, such as piles or a tumor. Digested blood in tarry stools usually occurs in large amounts.

Bleeding from the digestive or respiratory tract usually does not produce pain or other obvious signs or symptoms, except those associated with considerable loss of blood, such as faintness, weakness, dizziness, pale moist skin, and rapid pulse.

Tables 11-3 and 11-4 list some of the usual characteristics of respiratory and digestive tract bleeding.

The cause of the bleeding will determine treatment. In all cases of bleeding from the lungs or the gastrointestinal tract, the victim should see a physician.

Heart Attack

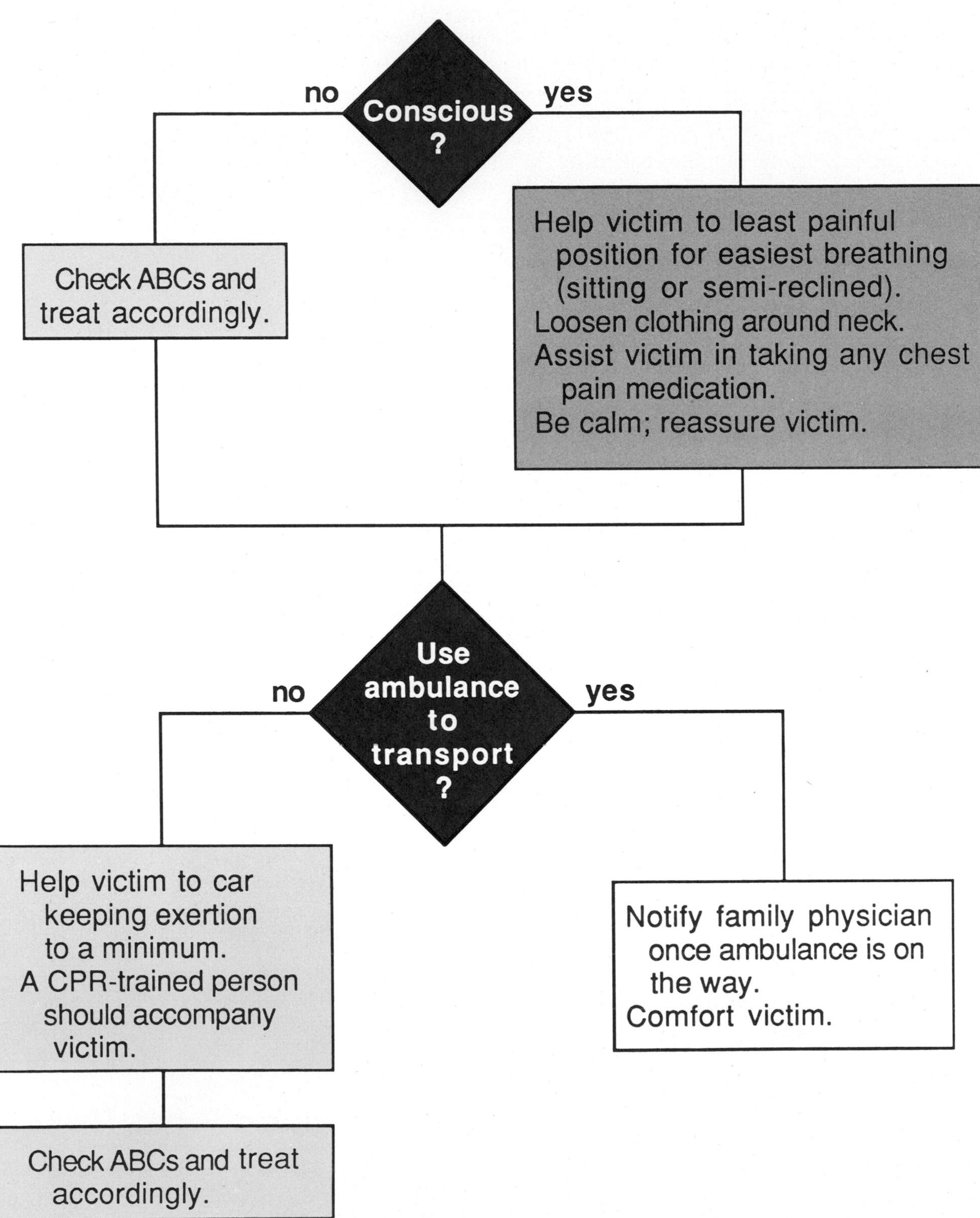

Stroke

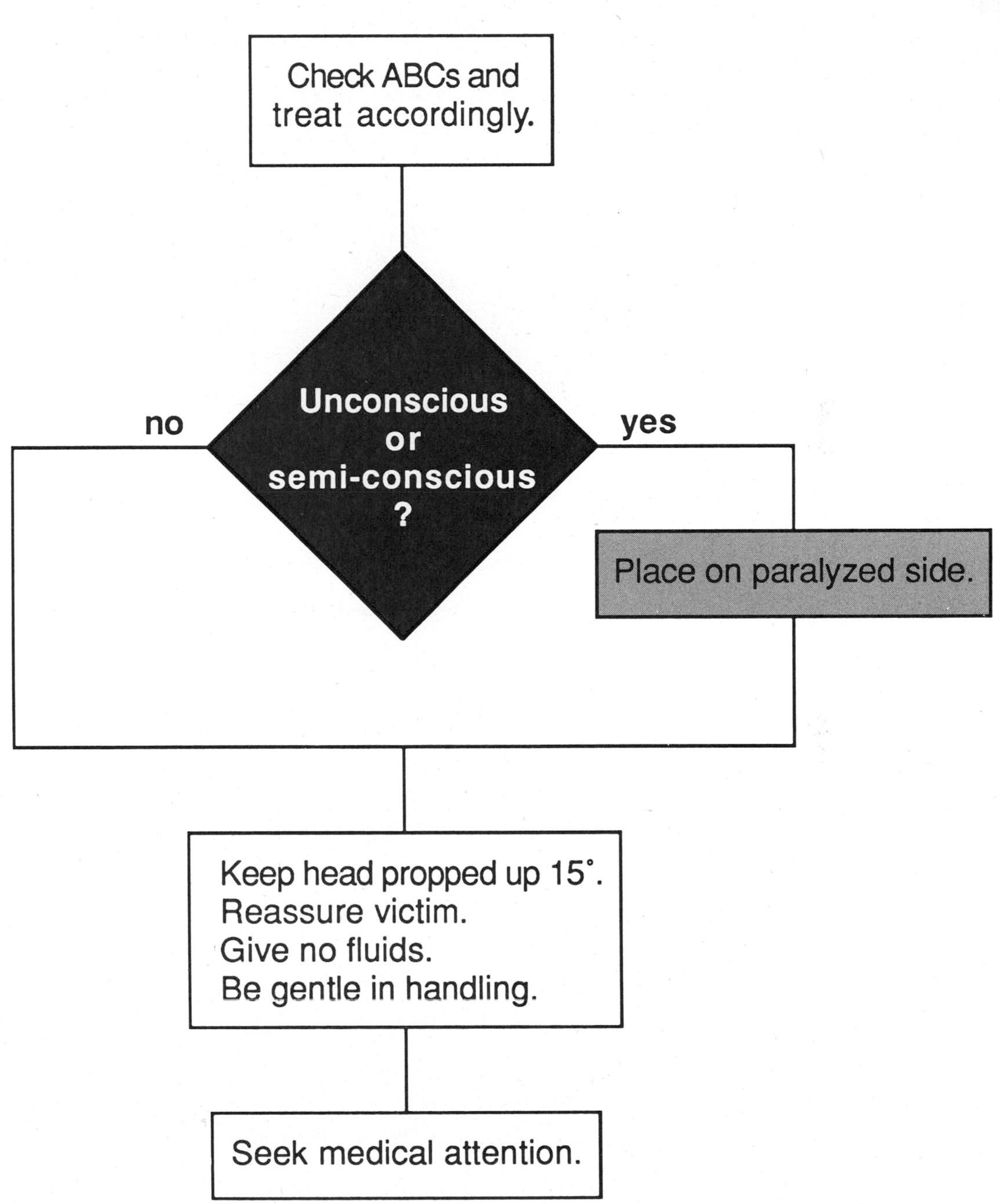

Check ABCs and treat accordingly.
Unconscious or semi-conscious ?
no
yes
Place on paralyzed side.
Keep head propped up 15°.
Reassure victim.
Give no fluids.
Be gentle in handling.
Seek medical attention.

Diabetic Emergencies

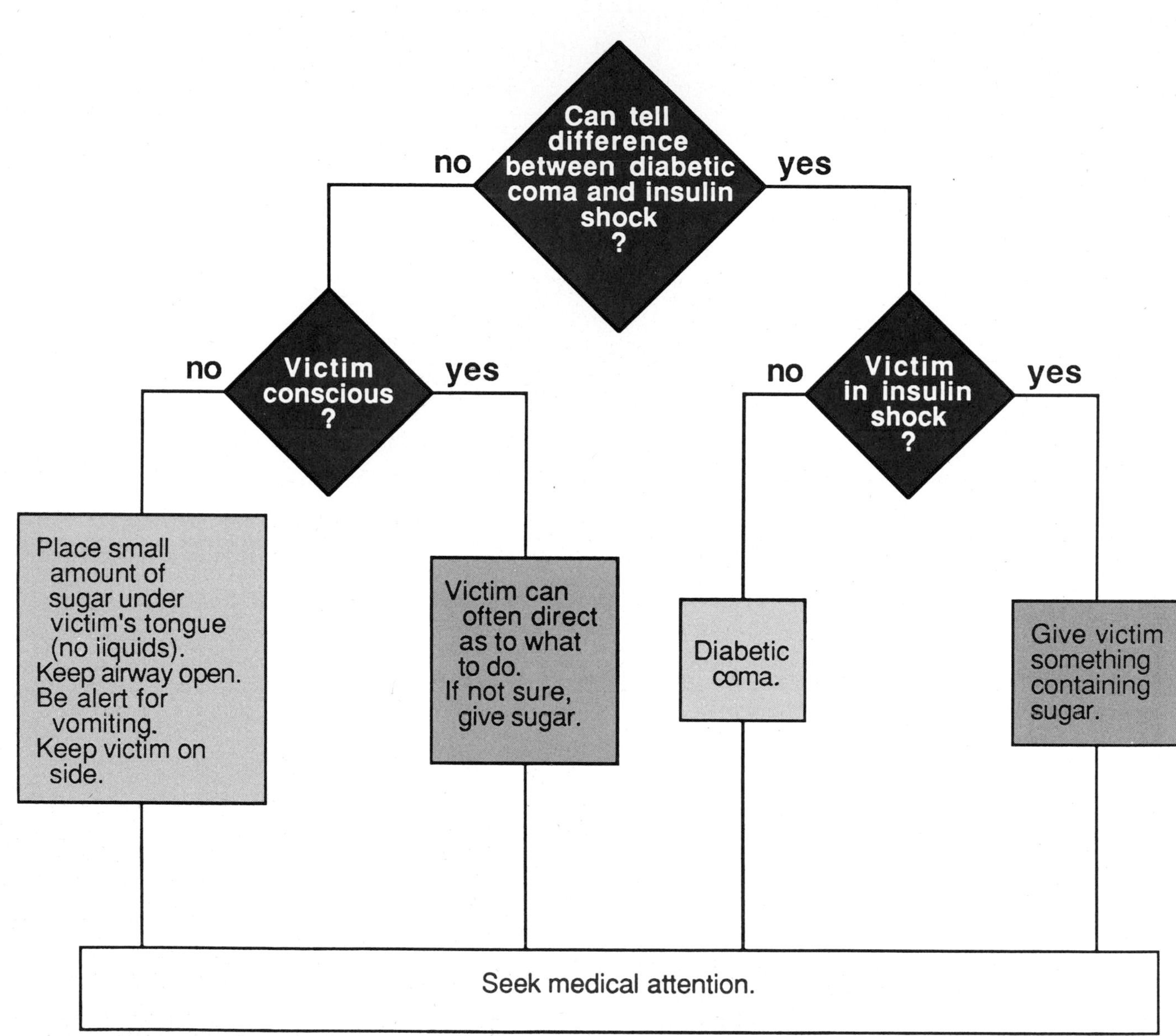

Seizures

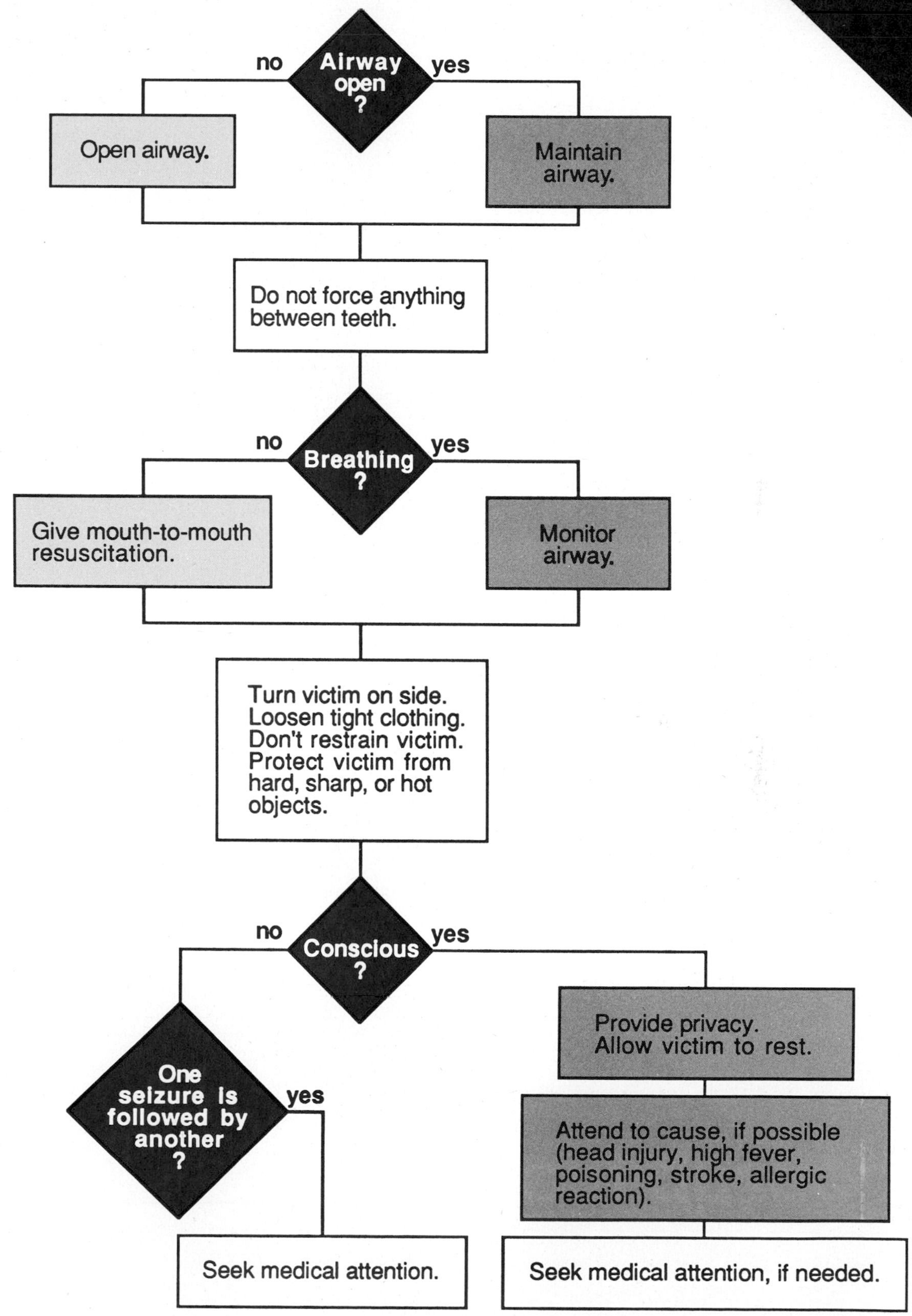

Airway open ?
no
yes
Open airway.
Maintain airway.
Do not force anything between teeth.
Breathing ?
no
yes
Give mouth-to-mouth resuscitation.
Monitor airway.
Turn victim on side.
Loosen tight clothing.
Don't restrain victim.
Protect victim from hard, sharp, or hot objects.
Conscious ?
no
yes
One seizure is followed by another ?
yes
Provide privacy.
Allow victim to rest.
Attend to cause, if possible (head injury, high fever, poisoning, stroke, allergic reaction).
Seek medical attention.
Seek medical attention, if needed.

Asthma

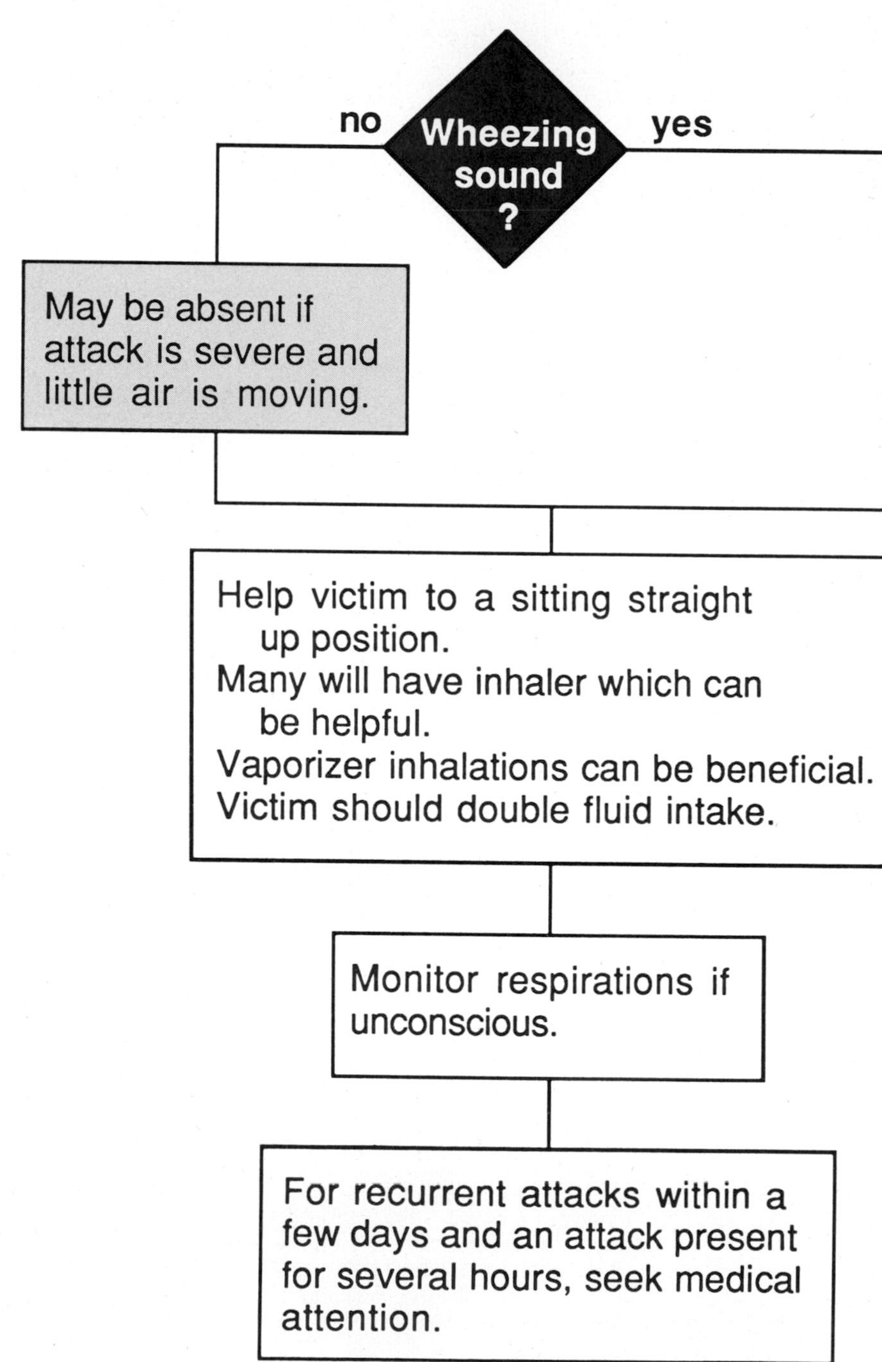

no
Wheezing sound ?
yes
May be absent if attack is severe and little air is moving.
Help victim to a sitting straight up position.
Many will have inhaler which can be helpful.
Vaporizer inhalations can be beneficial.
Victim should double fluid intake.
Monitor respirations if unconscious.
For recurrent attacks within a few days and an attack present for several hours, seek medical attention.

Abdominal Pain

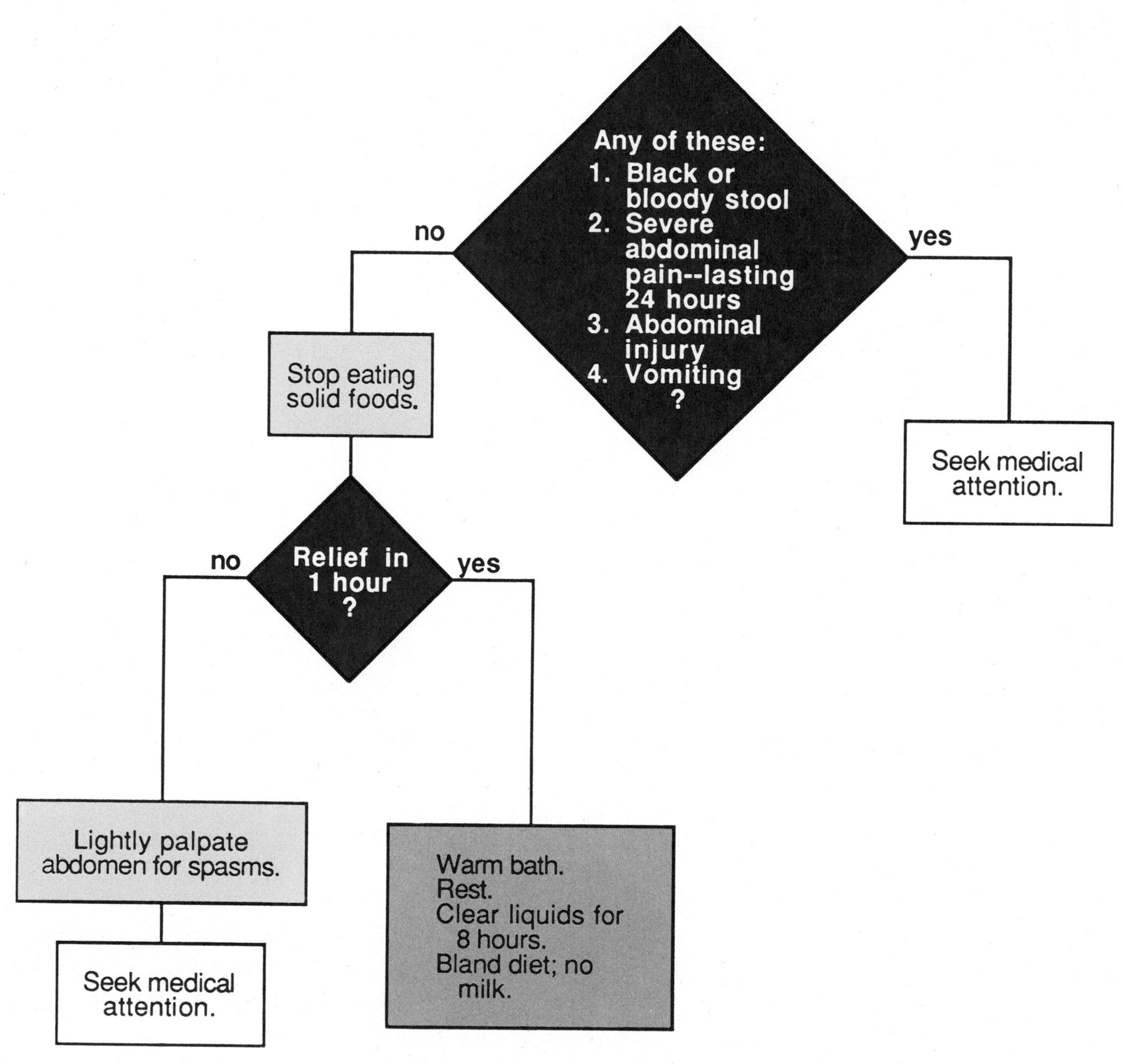

Constipation

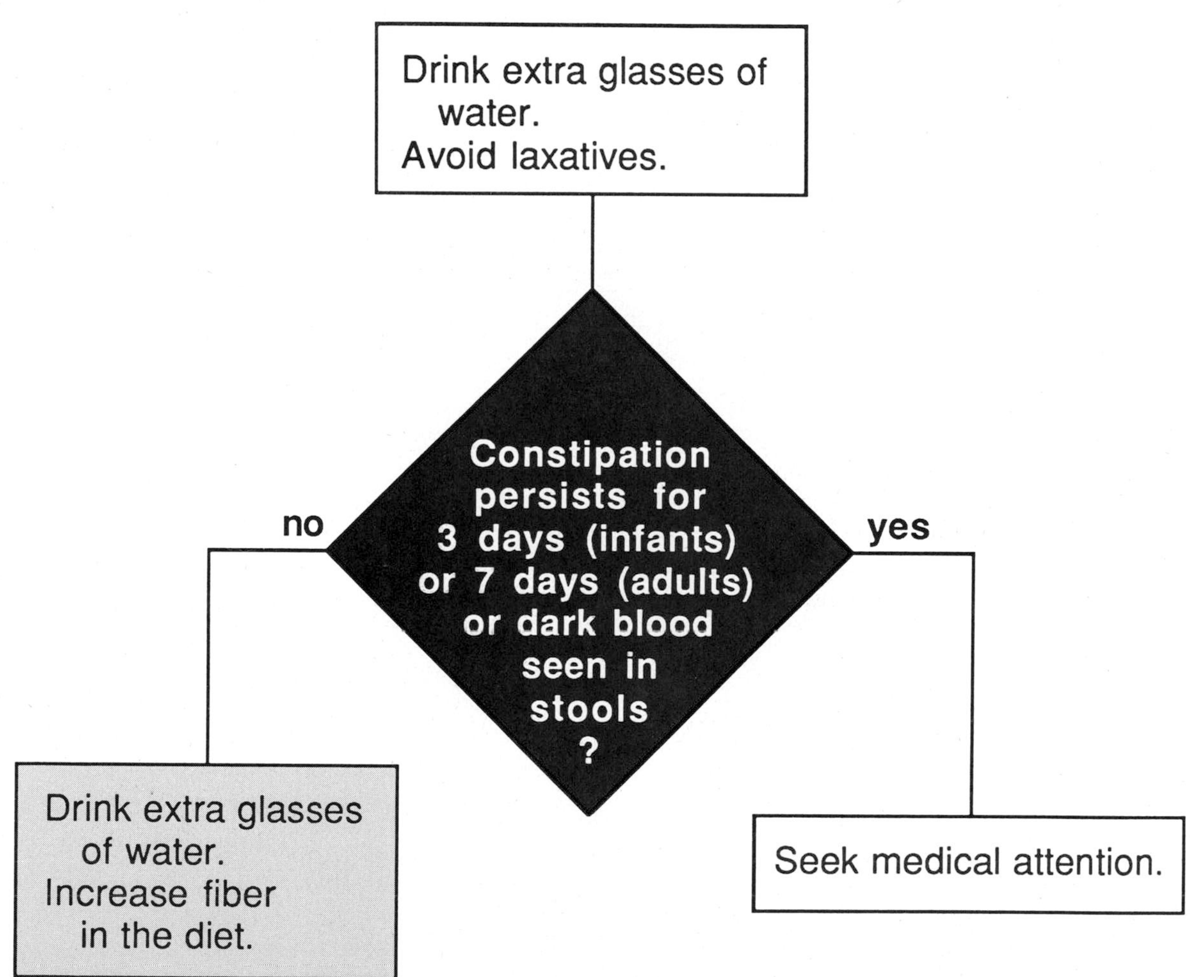

Coughing

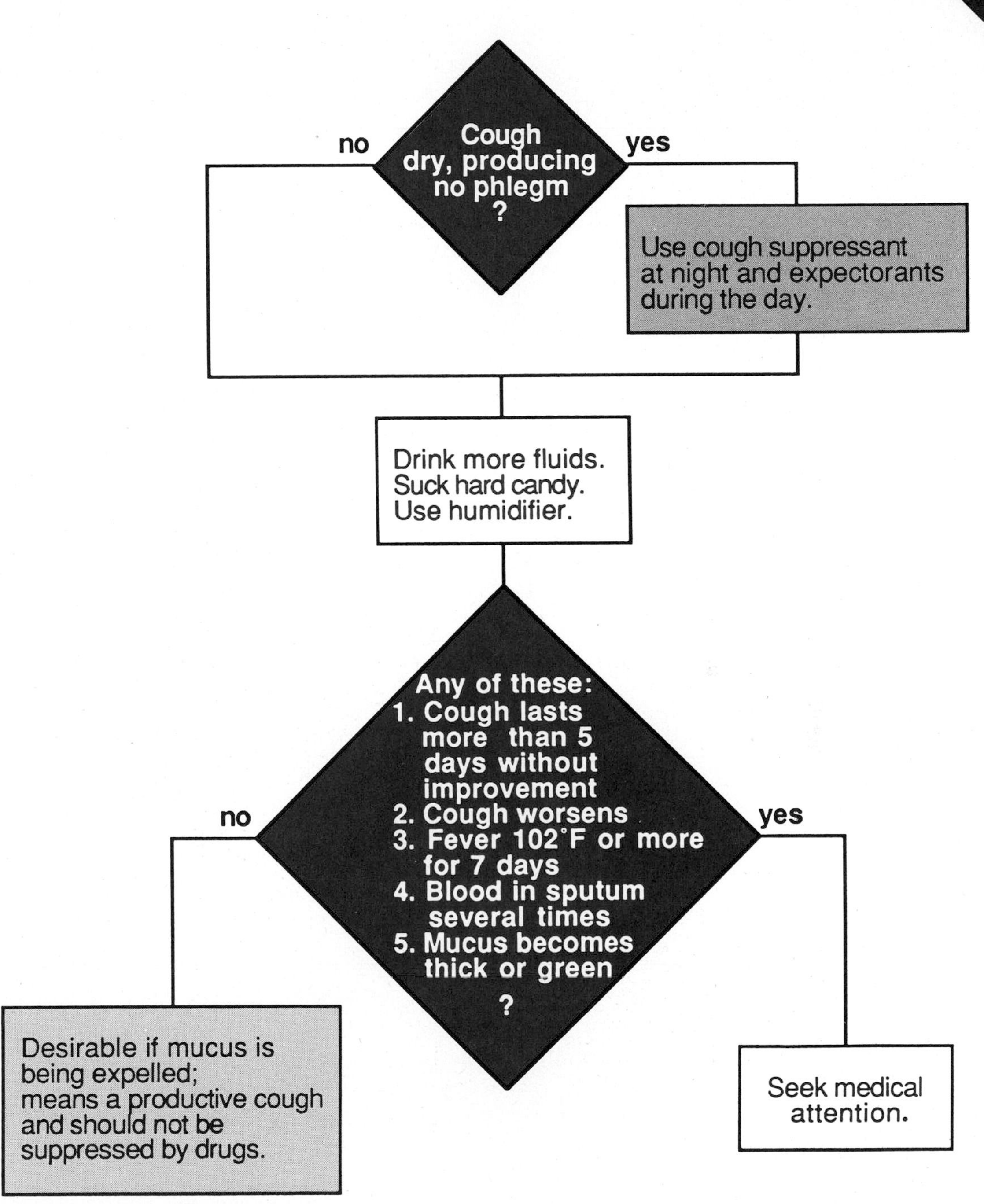

no
Cough dry, producing no phlegm ?
yes
Use cough suppressant at night and expectorants during the day.
Drink more fluids.
Suck hard candy.
Use humidifier.
Any of these:
1. Cough lasts more than 5 days without improvement
2. Cough worsens
3. Fever 102°F or more for 7 days
4. Blood in sputum several times
5. Mucus becomes thick or green
?
no
yes
Desirable if mucus is being expelled; means a productive cough and should not be suppressed by drugs.
Seek medical attention.

Diarrhea

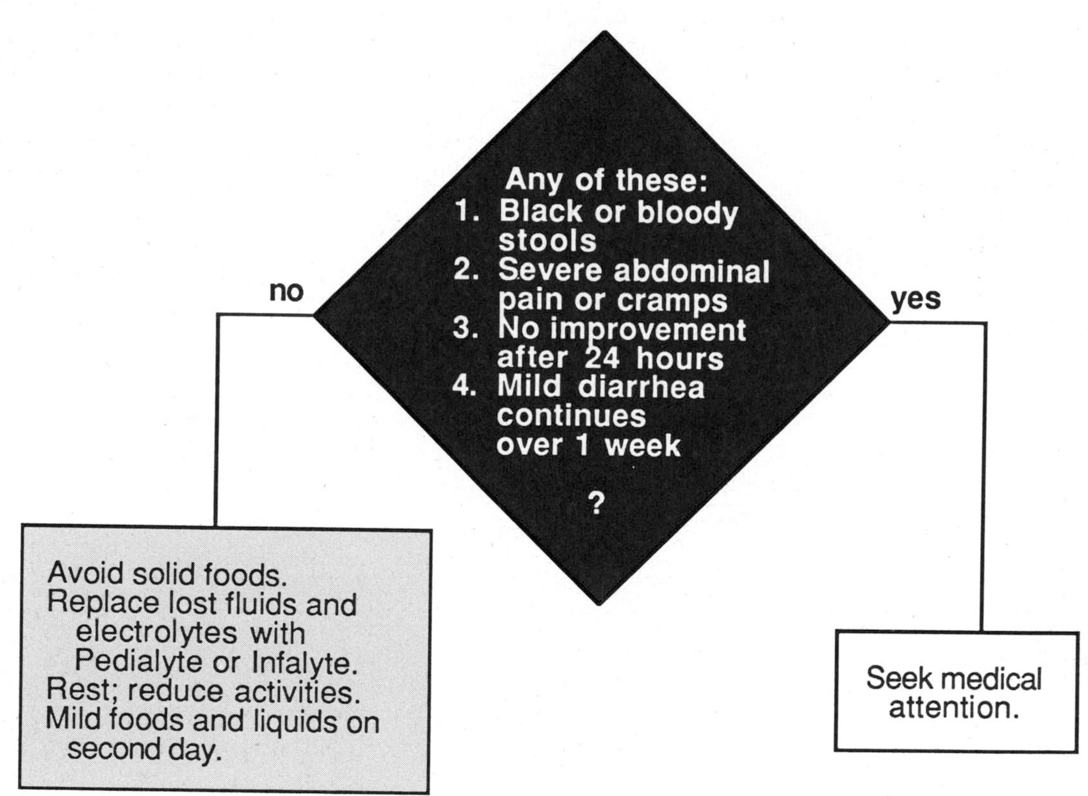

Any of these:
1. Black or bloody stools
2. Severe abdominal pain or cramps
3. No improvement after 24 hours
4. Mild diarrhea continues over 1 week
?
no
yes
Avoid solid foods.
Replace lost fluids and electrolytes with Pedialyte or Infalyte.
Rest; reduce activities.
Mild foods and liquids on second day.
Seek medical attention.

Earache

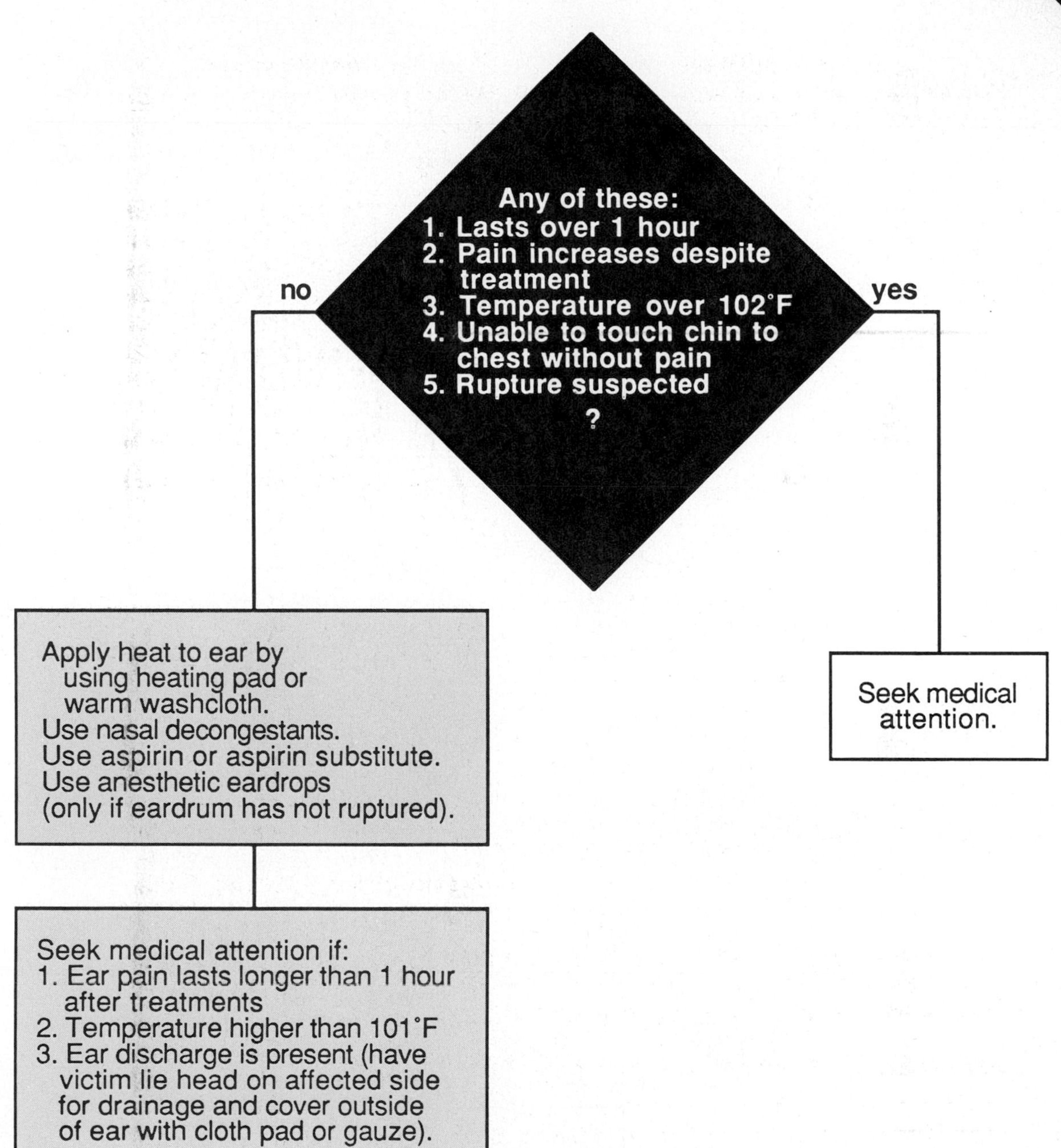
Any of these:
1. Lasts over 1 hour
2. Pain increases despite treatment
3. Temperature over 102°F
4. Unable to touch chin to chest without pain
5. Rupture suspected
?
no
yes
Apply heat to ear by using heating pad or warm washcloth.
Use nasal decongestants.
Use aspirin or aspirin substitute.
Use anesthetic eardrops (only if eardrum has not ruptured).
Seek medical attention.
Seek medical attention if:
1. Ear pain lasts longer than 1 hour after treatments
2. Temperature higher than 101°F
3. Ear discharge is present (have victim lie head on affected side for drainage and cover outside of ear with cloth pad or gauze).

Fever

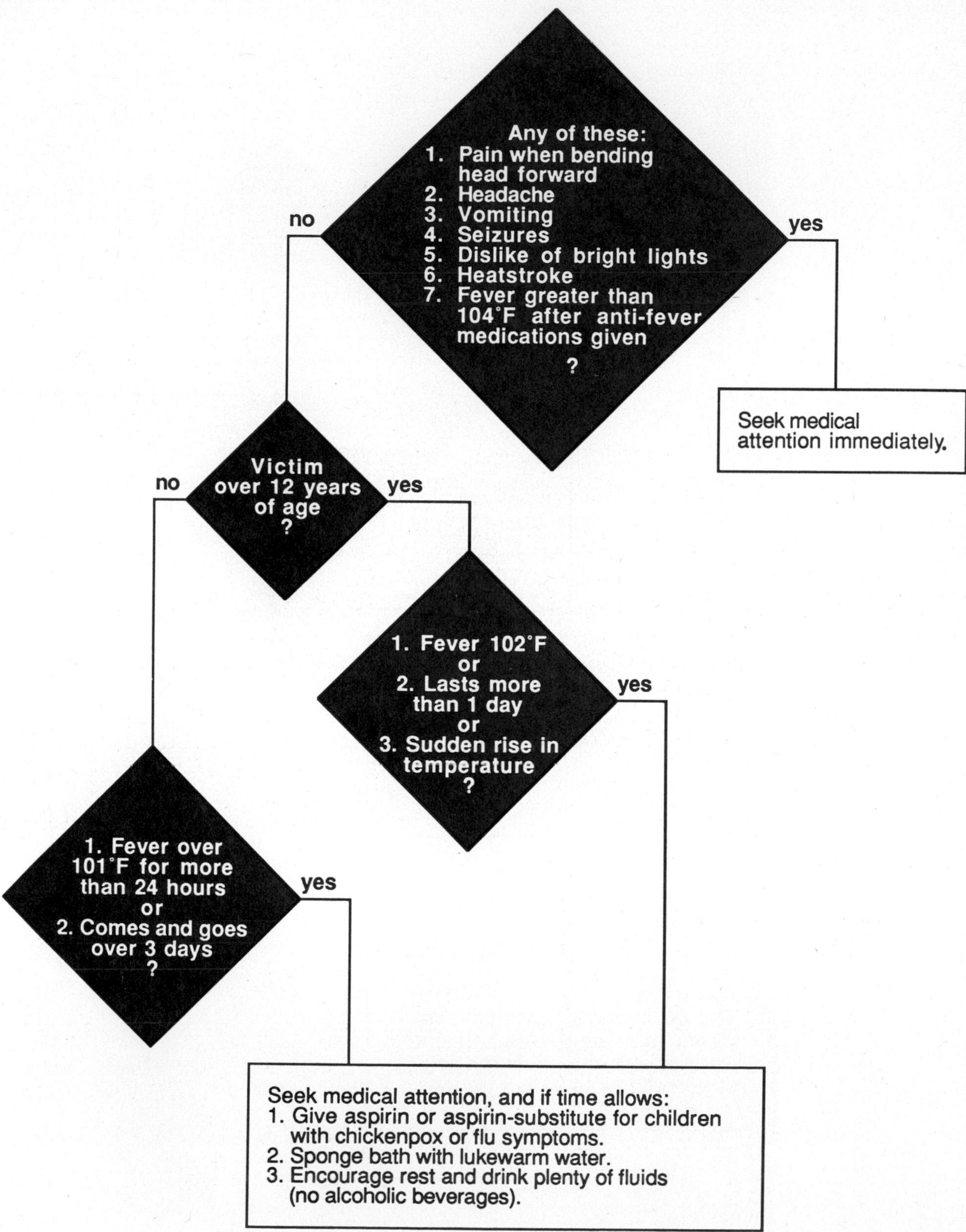

Any of these:
1. Pain when bending head forward
2. Headache
3. Vomiting
4. Seizures
5. Dislike of bright lights
6. Heatstroke
7. Fever greater than 104˚F after anti-fever medications given
?
no
yes
Seek medical attention immediately.
Victim over 12 years of age ?
no
yes
1. Fever 102˚F or 2. Lasts more than 1 day or 3. Sudden rise in temperature ?
yes
1. Fever over 101˚F for more than 24 hours or 2. Comes and goes over 3 days ?
yes
Seek medical attention, and if time allows:
1. Give aspirin or aspirin-substitute for children with chickenpox or flu symptoms.
2. Sponge bath with lukewarm water.
3. Encourage rest and drink plenty of fluids (no alcoholic beverages).

Headache

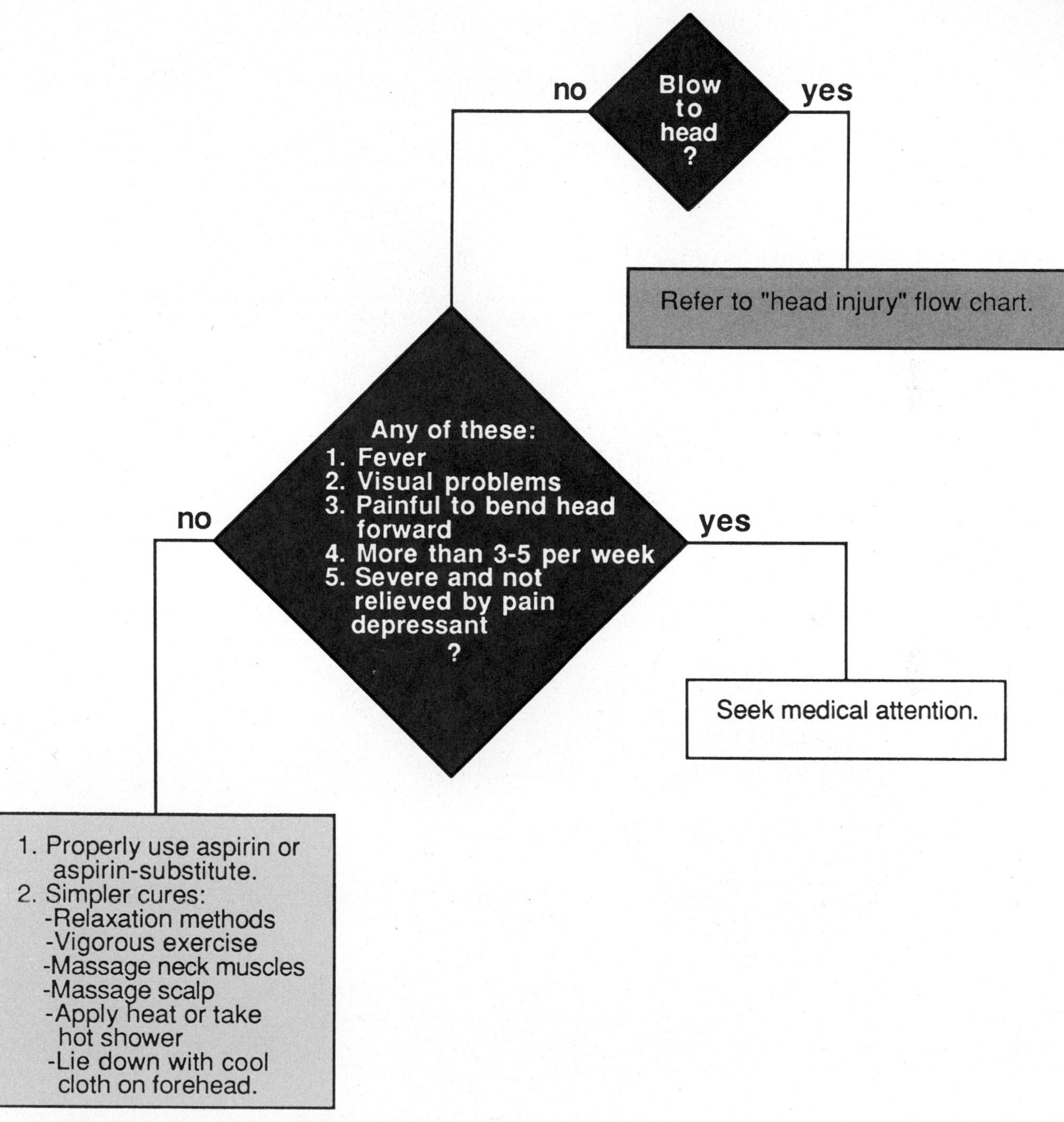

Blow to head ?
no
yes
Refer to "head injury" flow chart.
Any of these:
1. Fever
2. Visual problems
3. Painful to bend head forward
4. More than 3-5 per week
5. Severe and not relieved by pain depressant
?
no
yes
Seek medical attention.
1. Properly use aspirin or aspirin-substitute.
2. Simpler cures:
-Relaxation methods
-Vigorous exercise
-Massage neck muscles
-Massage scalp
-Apply heat or take hot shower
-Lie down with cool cloth on forehead.

Sore Throat

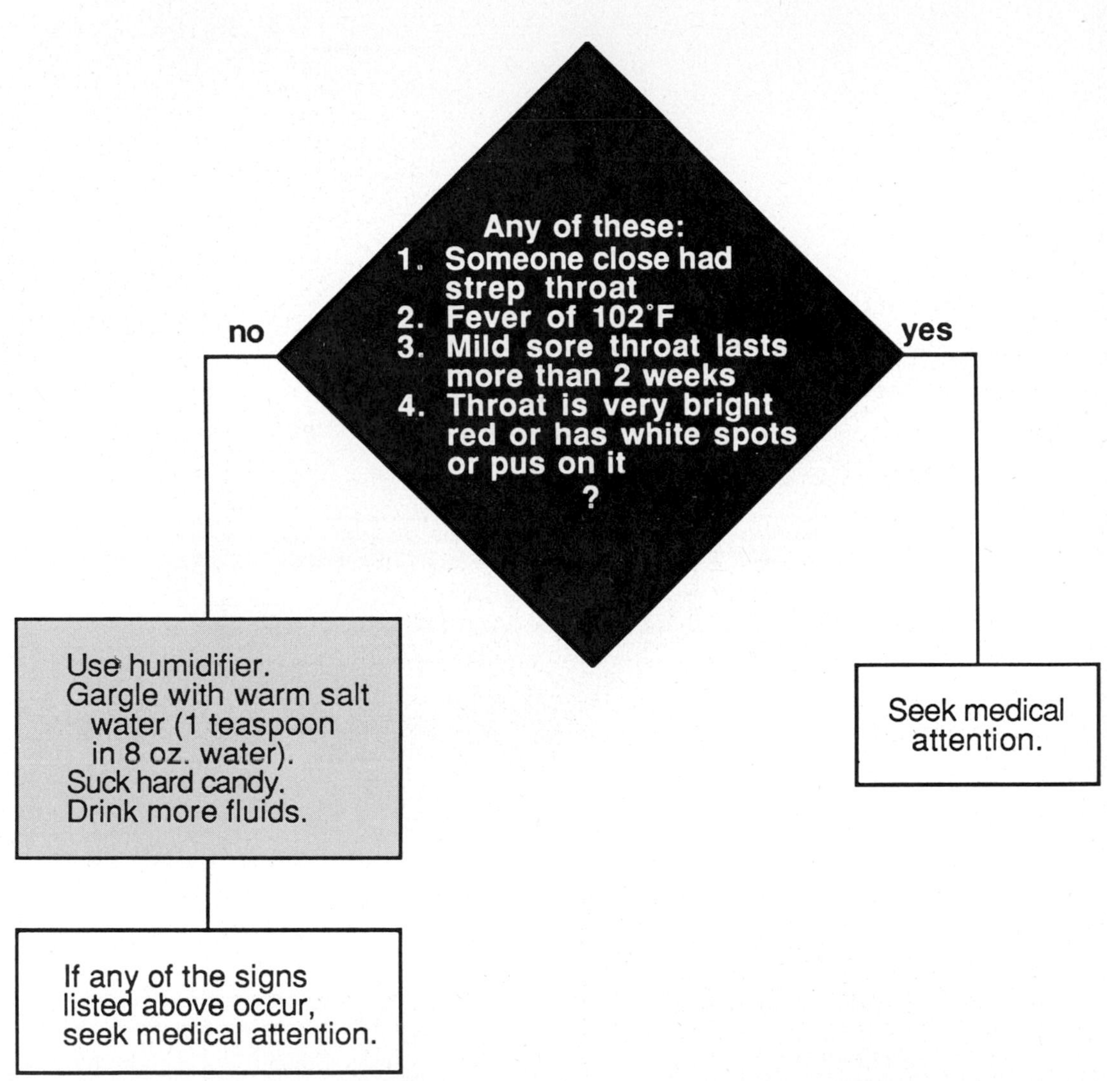

Any of these:
1. Someone close had strep throat
2. Fever of 102°F
3. Mild sore throat lasts more than 2 weeks
4. Throat is very bright red or has white spots or pus on it
?
no
yes
Use humidifier.
Gargle with warm salt water (1 teaspoon in 8 oz. water).
Suck hard candy.
Drink more fluids.
If any of the signs listed above occur, seek medical attention.
Seek medical attention.

Vomiting

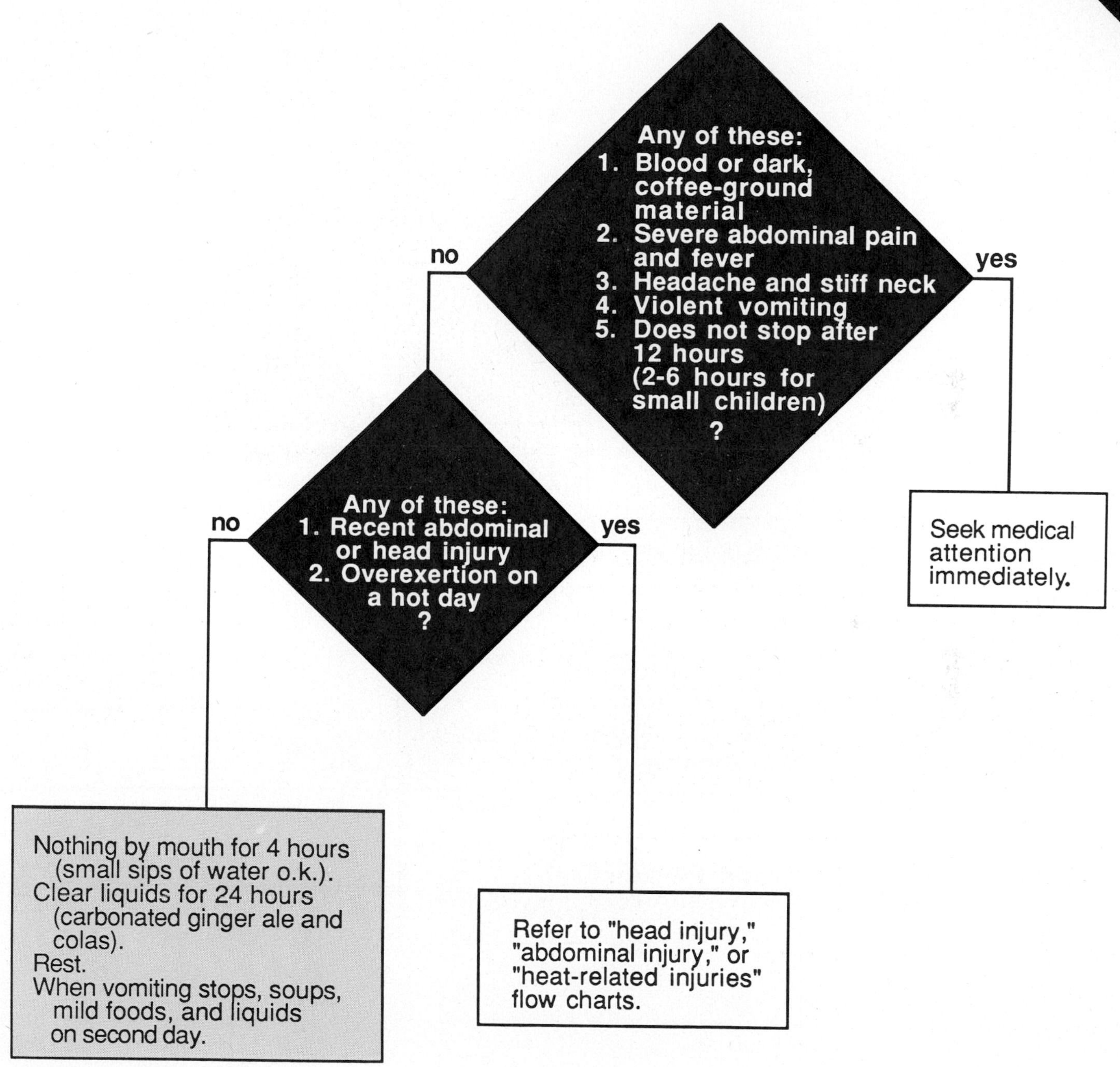

Any of these:
1. Blood or dark, coffee-ground material
2. Severe abdominal pain and fever
3. Headache and stiff neck
4. Violent vomiting
5. Does not stop after 12 hours (2-6 hours for small children)
?
no
yes
Seek medical attention immediately.
Any of these:
1. Recent abdominal or head injury
2. Overexertion on a hot day
?
no
yes
Nothing by mouth for 4 hours (small sips of water o.k.).
Clear liquids for 24 hours (carbonated ginger ale and colas).
Rest.
When vomiting stops, soups, mild foods, and liquids on second day.
Refer to "head injury," "abdominal injury," or "heat-related injuries" flow charts.

Hyperventilation

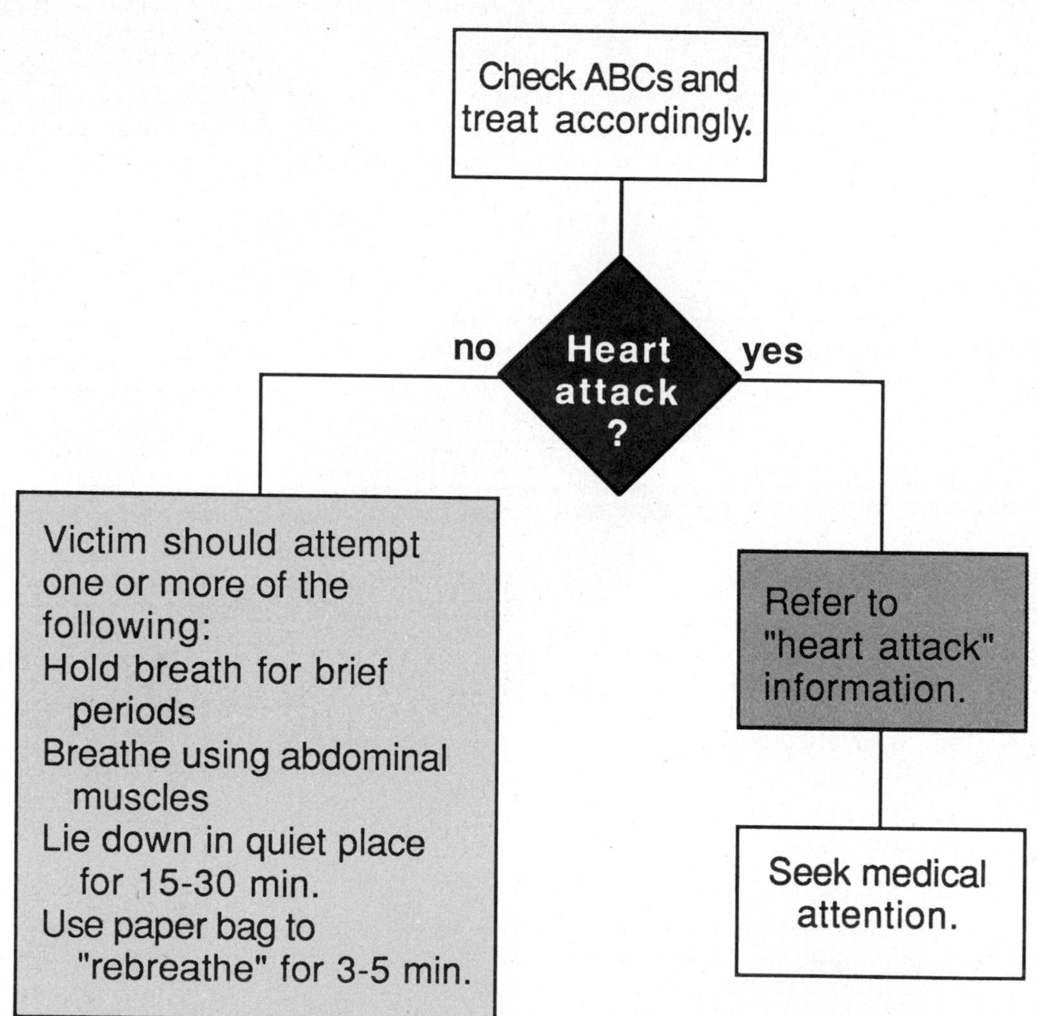

Heart Attack

LEARNING ACTIVITIES

T F 1. When an artery in the heart becomes blocked, the part of the heart muscle it serves dies.
T F 2. If a small part of the heart muscle dies, the heart ceases to pump.
T F 3. A feeling of crushing pressure in the chest is one sign of a heart attack.
T F 4. Heart attack victims can breathe more easily and there is less pain if they are lying flat on their backs.
T F 5. Angina is a narrowing of an artery in the heart.
T F 6. The greater the pain during a heart attack, the greater the damage to the heart.
T F 7. "Heart attack" is only one of several names for the same condition.
T F 8. There are three main coronary arteries on the heart.
T F 9. The dead heart muscle resulting from a heart attack is called a myocardial infarction.
T F 10. It is often difficult to determine if a person is having a heart attack.
T F 11. The main difference between pain of angina and the pain of myocardial infarction is its duration.
T F 12. All heart attack victims need CPR.

Case 1: A 54-year-old male awakens in the morning after a restless night. He has experienced a mild "tightness" in his chest.

1. Which of the following symptoms would a victim suffering a classic acute myocardial infarction (heart attack) describe?

A. ______ Profuse perspiration
B. ______ Pain in the jaw radiating to the shoulders, arm, and back
C. ______ Nausea and vomiting
D. ______ Shortness of breath
E. ______ "Heartburn" or "indigestion"
F. ______ Anxiety and restlessness
G. ______ All of the above

2. List the appropriate emergency care for a person who has the symptoms and signs of an acute myocardial infarction (heart attack).

A. ______________________________

B. ______________________________

C. ______________________________

3. List the emergency care you would provide to an unconscious victim who appeared to have an acute myocardial infarction.

A. ______________________________

B. ______________________________

C. ______________________________

4. List some of the most common major contributing risk factors in heart disease.

A. ______________________________

B. ______________________________

C. ______________________________

D. ______________________________

E. ______________________________

F. ______________________________

G. ______________________________

H. ______________________________

Case 2: You find an extremely overweight male who complains of a crushing pain in his chest. He is sweating profusely and has trouble catching his breath. He indicates that the pain has lasted about one hour, and he has taken three nitroglycerin tablets without relief. He reports that he is 67 years old.

1. What condition is this victim most likely experiencing?

____

2. What are the major symptoms of angina pectoris, myocardial infarction, and congestive heart failure? From the following list of symptoms, write A if symptomatic of angina pectoris, and write M if symptomatic of myocardial infarction. (Each symptom may be associated with more than one condition.)

A. ______ Severe pain
B. ______ Shortness of breath
C. ______ Fear
D. ______ Sweating and nausea

3. What are two major differences in pain that are associated with angina pectoris and myocardial infarction?

A. ______________________________
____

B. ______________________________
____

Case 3: You answer a call from an elderly female neighbor. At her home you find a woman who complains of severe chest pain. She has just completed some strenuous housework. She reports a history of having a "bad heart." She further reports that the pain lasted ten minutes and was promptly relieved with her medication.

1. This victim is most likely suffering from which problem?

A. ______ Cerebrovascular accident
B. ______ Myocardial infarction (heart attack)
C ______ Angina pectoris

2. Match the heart problems with the appropriate descriptions.

A. ______ Myocardial infarction
B. ______ Angina pectoris
1. Occurs when the heart temporarily does not have enough oxygen for its own needs.
2. Occurs when a coronary vessel becomes occluded.

3. Match the symptoms(s) with the appropriate heart conditions.

A. ______ Difficulty in breathing
B. ______ Chest pain greater than twenty minutes
C. ______ Pressure or squeezing sensation of chest
1. Angina pectoris
2. Myocardial infarction
3. All of the above

4. What emergency care should be provided to the person suffering from angina pectoris?

A. ______________________________
____

B. ______________________________
____

C. ______________________________
____

5. What emergency care should be provided to the person suffering an acute myocardial infarction?

A. ______________________________
____

B. ______________________________
____

C. ______________________________
____

D. ______________________________
____

Stroke

T F 1. A stroke is caused by a blood clot in an artery in the heart.
T F 2. Numbness or paralysis of the extremities is one sign of a stroke.
T F 3. Because of paralysis of the facial muscles, tongue, and throat, a stroke victim may not be able to speak.
T F 4. Strokes usually occur in older people with hardening of the arteries.
T F 5. Stroke victims may have difficulty with speech.
T F 6. Stroke victims should be transported on their backs.

Case: A 76-year-old woman was found by her daughter after she blacked out and fell. On your arrival at the scene, the victim has complete loss of movement to her left side and is unable to speak.

1. From the following list, check all the signs and symptoms of a cerebrovascular accident (CVA or stroke).

A. ______ Weakness or paralysis of one or both sides of the body
B. ______ Confusion, dizziness
C. ______ Unequal pupil size
D. ______ Rapid pulse
E. ______ Shortness of breath
F. ______ Nausea, vomiting
G. ______ Headache, unconsciousness
H. ______ All of these

2. List the proper emergency care for a person whom you suspect has suffered a cerebrovascular accident.

A. ______________________________

B. ______________________________

C. ______________________________

D. ______________________________

E. ______________________________

F. ______________________________

3. List and describe two main causes of a cerebrovascular accident:

A. ______________________________

B. ______________________________

4. What is a common result from all causes of cerebrovascular accidents? What is a main danger to the victim?

____

Diabetic Emergencies

T F 1. Diabetes is a condition in which the body is unable to use sugar normally.
T F 2. The brain needs a constant supply of sugar and oxygen.
T F 3. Insulin permits sugar to pass from the body cells into the bloodstream.
T F 4. If there is too much insulin in the body, there will be too much sugar in the bloodstream and not enough in the body cells.
T F 5. If there is too much sugar in a person's bloodstream and not enough in his body cells, he may go into a diabetic coma.
T F 6. The onset of diabetic coma occurs within minutes.
T F 7. It is often difficult to distinguish between the signs of insulin shock and those of diabetic coma.
T F 8. Sugar may save the life of a person in a diabetic coma.
T F 9. A first aider can only provide immediate transportation to a medical facility for a person in a diabetic coma.
T F 10. Insulin shock is the same thing as diabetic coma.
T F 11. In diabetic coma, there is too much sugar in the blood.
T F 12. In insulin shock, there is insufficient sugar in the blood.
T F 13. The main visible difference between diabetic coma and insulin shock is the victim's breathing.
T F 14. First aid treatment for diabetic coma is to increase the victim's blood sugar concentration.
T F 15. The onset of diabetic coma generally occurs in ten to twenty minutes.

Case 1: A 45-year-old man is found lying under a bridge. He appears drowsy and confused; his speech is incoherent. An unusual sweet odor is noted on his breath. Pulse and respiration rates are rapid. His skin is very dry. No other history is available.

1. What is the most likely diagnosis in this case?

____

____

2. What emergency care should be initiated?

A. ______________________________

____

____

____

B. ______________________________

____

____

____

C. ______________________________

____

____

____

3. What mistake must be avoided when attempting to make a diagnosis on the basis of breath odor?

____

____

____

____

____

Case 2: During a tennis tournament, a 14-year-old female suddenly appears to lose her concentration. Her game, which has been very good until this time, falls apart. Becoming irritable and excited, she yells frequently at her opponent. Between sets she complains of tingling and numbness in her hands and feet and she is too weak to continue play. She is wearing a tag indicating that she is a diabetic.

1. To determine the emergency care necessary in this case, what two questions should be asked of the young woman?

A. ______________________________

____

B. ______________________________

____

2. The young woman indicates she has not yet eaten that day. From which diabetic reaction is she most likely suffering?

A. ______ Diabetic coma
B. ______ Insulin shock
C. ______ Neither

3. What is the most immediate emergency care for this situation?

A. ______ Transport to a medical facility
B. ______ Administer food or drink containing sugar
C. ______ Neither

Match the following diabetic reactions with their associated symptoms in questions 4 to 15. For each symptom, mark:

A—if the symptom is associated with diabetic coma *only*
B—if the symptom is associated with insulin shock *only*
C—if the symptom is associated with *both* A and B
D—if the symptom is associated with *neither* A nor B

4. ______ Skin—flushed, dry
5. ______ Skin—pale, moist
6. ______ Ill, weak appearance
7. ______ Sudden onset
8. ______ Gradual onset
9. ______ Breath—normal odor
10. ______ Breath—fruity odor
11. ______ Hallucinations
12. ______ Need to urinate
13. ______ Tingling sensation in extremities
14. ______ Respiration—normal, shallow
15. ______ Respiration—rapid, deep
16. If you are at all uncertain about the specific diabetic reaction, what is the *best* emergency care to provide?

____

Case 3: You find a teenage boy sprawled out in a hallway. He is unconscious but has a slow, steady pulse. Pupil response is slow but regular. A fruity odor is detected on his breath. His mother informs you that he was recently given a clean bill of health from a physician and is a "good boy" who does not drink or take drugs.

1. What emergency conditions(s) should you consider? (Check all that apply.)

A. ______ Insulin shock
B. ______ Diabetic coma
C. ______ Alcohol intoxication
D. ______ Drug overdose
E. ______ None of the above

2. What is the appropriate emergency care for this young man?

A. ______ Induce vomiting and transport to a medical facility.
B. ______ Give sugar and transport to a medical facility.
C. ______ Maintain observation of victim and transport to a medical facility.

3. Match the following medical emergencies with their recognized signs or symptoms. Match each sign or symptom with *one or more* medical emergencies. Write the corresponding number for each medical emergency in the space provided.

A. ______ Confusion	1. Insulin shock
B. ______ Weak, dizzy	2. Diabetic coma
C. ______ Nausea, vomiting	3. Alcohol intoxication
D. ______ Dry, flushed skin	
E. ______ Sweetish breath	
F. ______ Profuse sweating	
G. ______ Urinary frequency	
H. ______ Unconsciousness	

Case 4: A 68-year-old widow with adult onset diabetes mellitus has not taken her insulin for seven days. You find her confused and her face flushed. Her skin is warm to touch, her breath smells like "nail polish remover," and her respirations are deep, rapid, and sighing.

1. This woman is in ________________________ .

2. From the following list of signs and symptoms, choose those that are associated with sudden onset of insulin shock.

A. ______ Cool, clammy skin
B. ______ Normal blood pressure, normal respiration
C. ______ Hot, dry skin
D. ______ Bounding, full pulse
E. ______ Steady pulse
F. ______ Elevated blood pressure, shallow respiration
G. ______ Dizziness, headache, irritability

3. Which diabetic-related emergency is frequently mistaken for drunkenness?

____

____

4. From the following list, identify the proper emergency care for a victim in diabetic coma or insulin shock. The care may be the same for both medical emergencies. Use a D for diabetic coma and an S for insulin shock.

A. ______ For a conscious victim, find out if he has eaten or taken insulin that day.
B. ______ If the victim is fully conscious, give sugar in a concentrated form (e.g., granulated sugar, hard candy, sweetened fruit juice).
C. ______ For an unconscious victim, look for a medical alert identification bracelet, necklace or card, and observe the victim's respiratory rate.
D. ______ Transport to the nearest hospital as soon as possible for evaluation and treatment.
E. ______ Monitor vital signs and give psychological support.

Epilepsy

T F 1. Epileptics are usually unconscious during convulsions and remain so for about five minutes or so.
T F 2. Epileptics should be encouraged to rest after a seizure because any activity could precipitate another attack.
T F 3. An ambulance should be called for all victims of seizures because they are true emergencies.
T F 4. Epilepsy is the only cause for seizures.
T F 5. A padded object should be placed between a victim's teeth in order to prevent the tongue from being bitten.
T F 6. Petit mal seizures are characterized by unconsciousness and uncontrollable muscular contractions.
T F 7. Grand mal seizures do not cause unconsciousness and may be hard to detect.
T F 8. Victims of an epileptic seizure should be restrained.
T F 9. The first aid care for epilepsy and other types of seizures is similar.

Case: At a playground area you find a young child lying on the ground with his extremities in spasmodic contractions. The facial area is cyanotic, and there is a slight frothing at the mouth.

1. From what is this child most likely suffering?

   A. ______ Poisoning
   B. ______ Aspiration
   C. ______ Epilepsy
   D. ______ Heat exhaustion

2. What are the two most common types of epileptic seizures?

   A. ______________________________

   B. ______________________________

3. Describe the emergency care for this child.

   A. ______________________________

   B. ______________________________

   C. ______________________________

   D. ______________________________

   E. ______________________________

Asthma

T F 1. Status asthmaticus is a true emergency.
T F 2. Wheezing is the most obvious sign of asthma.
T F 3. In most asthma cases there is little the first aider can do except obtain medical assistance if needed.
T F 4. Vaporizer inhalations are detrimental.
T F 5. Unconscious victims of asthma need to be resuscitated.

Case: A middle-aged woman complains of being short of breath and reports that she has had previous such episodes of asthma. You can hear a "wheezing" sound as she breathes.

1. What do many asthmatics carry with them for their asthma?

   ____

2. What position is usually the most comfortable?

   ____

3. What type of communication is an asthmatic limited to during an attack?

   ____

4. What two other procedures might be helpful?

   A. ______________________________

   B. ______________________________

Abdomen Pain

T F 1. Vomiting of bright red blood indicates bleeding in the large intestines.
T F 2. Dark, coffee ground colored vomit suggests bleeding in the stomach such as from a peptic ulcer.
T F 3. The first aider should not press any deeper than a half inch when palpating the abdominal area.
T F 4. Food and/or fluid can be given to a victim in order to alleviate the stomach distress.
T F 5. A laxative and/or enema may cause the appendix to rupture.

T F 6. A laxative may provide abdominal pain relief and should be given.
T F 7. Extensive pressing or palpating will be needed to identify the location of an abdominal problem.
T F 8. Emergency care for abdominal pain is generally the same regardless of the cause.
T F 9. Food and fluids should *not* be given to those with acute abdominal pain.
T F 10. The color of blood in vomit can provide a clue as to the source of the blood.

Case: A teenage girl complains of a severe stomach ache. She is also experiencing chills.

1. Pain from hollow organs tends to be ______ .
2. Pain from solid organs tends to be ______ .
3. Palpation (pressing) should never be more than ______ inch.
4. ______ color can indicate the location of an internal problem.
5. Do not try to ______ the victim's problem.

Cough

T F 1. Coughs can sometimes be useful and should not be stopped.
T F 2. Cough suppressants can be helpful when sleep is needed.
T F 3. Sucking hard candy can help some coughs.
T F 4. Adding humidity to the air can keep throats from becoming dry.
T F 5. An antitussive works by depressing the cough center in the brain.

1. What are the two types of cough?
   A. ______
   B. ______
2. Nonmedical cough remedies include:
   A. ______
   B. ______
   C. ______
3. How do antitussives work?
   ______
4. Cite two examples of antitussives.
   A. ______
   B. ______
5. What should be done for a cough that lasts more than a month?
   ______

Diarrhea

T F 1. Stomach bacteria causes most diarrhea.
T F 2. Plain water, soft drinks, and apple juice are suggested drinks to avoid dehydration in cases of diarrhea.
T F 3. Most things done for viral diarrhea make it worse.
T F 4. The victim with fever accompanying diarrhea should seek medical attention.

1. What is the most common complication of diarrhea?

____

____

2. The initials BRAT represent:

B = ______
R = ______
A = ______
T = ______

3. Give the best recommendation for diarrhea.

____

____

4. Cite when a physician should be consulted.

____

____

Earache

T F 1. Earaches are limited to children.
T F 2. Ruptured eardrums should be seen by a physician.
T F 3. Decongestants can help relieve an earache.

Case: A child complains of a severe earache. Before seeking medical advice, you decide to alleviate the earache.

1. Which are ways of reducing the pain?

A. ______ Use nasal decongestants
B. ______ Apply heat with a heating pad
C. ______ Puncture the eardrum to allow drainage
D. ______ Blow the nose
E. ______ Use a vaporizer to increase the humidity

2. What usually causes most earaches?

____

____

Fever

T F 1. All fevers should be reduced.
T F 2. Truly high fevers (105°F) are rare.
T F 3. Ice water can be effectively used to reduce a fever.
T F 4. Before giving aspirin to a child with a high fever, a physician should be consulted.
T F 5. Persistent fevers over 103°F and those with a history of convulsions require prompt medical attention.

Case: An infant has a high fever. Before seeking medical attention, you decide to provide emergency care.

1. What is the best solution to use in reducing a fever?

   A. ______ Rubbing alcohol
   B. ______ Ice water
   C. ______ Lukewarm water
   D. ______ Tap water
   E. ______ Rubbing alcohol and ice water

2. What condition may be associated with high fever?

   ____
   ____

3. To what condition can a prolonged high fever lead?

   A. ______ Loss of senses
   B. ______ Loss of bodily functions
   C. ______ Dehydration
   D. ______ Heart damage

4. Describe the emergency care for this particular case.

   ____
   ____
   ____
   ____
   ____
   ____
   ____

Headache

T F 1. Most headaches are of a serious nature.
T F 2. Seek medical attention if headache pain wakens you in the middle of the night.
T F 3. Massaging the neck and scalp may relieve a headache.
T F 4. Acetaminophen is ineffective against headaches.

Case: After a difficult and stressful day, a headache occurs.

Before trying pain medication or other medications, attempt to alleviate the headache by:

A. ______________________________
____
B. ______________________________
____
C. ______________________________
____

Sore Throat

T F 1. Bacteria causes most sore throats.
T F 2. Antibiotics should be used for viral sore throats.
T F 3. A throat culture is the only way to diagnose a strep throat accurately.
T F 4. A strep throat is caused by bacteria.
T F 5. Sucking hard candy can sometimes provide relief from a sore throat.
T F 6. A sore throat accompanied by a fever of 101°F should be seen by a physician.

Case: Your 6-year-old son complains about a sore throat and does not want to go to school. Realizing that most sore throats are minor, you suspect his reason for not wanting to attend school.

1. The classic signs of a strep throat are:

   A. ______________________________
   ____
   B. ______________________________
   ____
   C. ______________________________
   ____
   D. ______________________________
   ____

2. A sore throat can be tested for strep with a ______________________________.

3. The best treatment for a strep throat is a ____
____.

4. Cite three home treatments for a sore throat.
____
____

5. When should a physician be consulted?
____
____
____
____

Vomiting

T F 1. Dehydration can result from excessive vomiting.
T F 2. Dark yellow urine can be an indication of dehydration.
T F 3. Seek medical attention if blood appears in vomit.
T F 4. Antibiotics is helpful in cases of vomiting.

Case: A child has had several bouts of vomiting during the past several hours.

Which procedures could be done?

A. ______ Give milk to settle the stomach.
B. ______ Give nothing by mouth for several hours.
C. ______ Give aspirin to reduce pain.
D. ______ Replace lost fluids after twenty-four hours.

Hyperventilation

T F 1. Hyperventilation can be confused with a heart attack.
T F 2. Hyperventilation is a reaction to stress.
T F 3. Hyperventilation results in too little carbon dioxide in the blood.
T F 4. The "paper bag" remedy works for hyperventilation because it may slow the victim's respiration rate and depth.
T F 5. Holding one's breath can help the hyperventilation victim.

Case: At a rock concert, a teenager suddenly collapses. She is carried out to the foyer where she regains consciousness.

1. What is her condition?
____
____

2. How prevalent is it?
____
____

3. With what other condition can it be confused?
____
____

4. What is the traditional care for this condition?
____
____
____
____
____
____
____

5. Name other methods that could be tried?

A. ____
____

B. ____
____

Internal Bleeding

Identify the source (organ) of internal bleeding if the following signs are manifested:

Signs
1. Coughed-up blood (bright and frothy)
2. Coughed-up blood (bright red)
3. Coughed-up blood (coffee ground-like)
4. Jet black stools
5. Blood streaked stools
6. Bright red stools (teaspoon or more)

Source
1. ______________________________
2. ______________________________
3. ______________________________
4. ______________________________
5. ______________________________
6. ______________________________

12 Emergency Childbirth*

- **Emergency Childbirth Procedures from the popular nursing journal RN.**

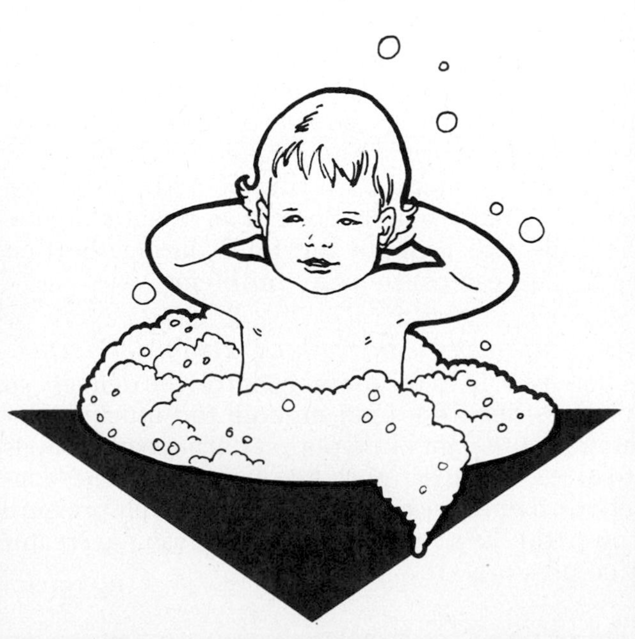

It could happen when you are on vacation, on a bus, in a store, on the street, or anywhere. Suddenly you are faced with a woman about to give birth and you are the only one around who can help. What should you do? How should you go about helping her deliver the baby? What if the cord is around the baby's neck? What if the mother bleeds excessively?

Stages of Labor

Labor is the process in which the uterus repeatedly contracts to push the fetus and placenta out of the mother's body. Delivery is the actual birth of the baby at the end of the second stage of labor.

At the beginning of labor, contractions are far apart. As labor progresses, contractions occur closer together. During the most active stage of labor, contractions occur every two to three minutes and last thirty to forty-five seconds.

There are three stages of labor. The first stage begins with the first uterine contraction and lasts until the cervix is completely open (dilated). The first stage lasts about twelve hours in a woman who has previously borne a child. The amniotic sac frequently ruptures when the cervix is completely expanded.

The second stage of labor begins when the fetus starts descending into the vagina. Normally, the head descends first. If the buttock descends first, it is called a breech delivery. During the second stage of labor, the woman will bear down with each contraction. When the first part (usually the head) appears and remains visible between contractions, it is called crowning. In a normal delivery, the head will appear first and the shoulders and trunk soon after. The second stage of labor lasts about an hour in a woman having a first baby and from fifteen to

*Published in *RN*, the full-service nursing journal. Copyright 1981, Medical Economics Company, Inc., Oradell, N.J. Reprinted with permission.

twenty minutes in a woman who has previously borne a child.

In the third stage of labor, uterine contractions expel the placenta. When the placenta separates from the uterine wall, a small amount of blood gushes out through the vagina. The placenta is then pushed out of the uterus and through the vagina. The third stage of labor usually lasts about fifteen minutes.

Unplanned delivery outside of a hospital is a nerve wracking, challenging, and exciting experience. By following the simple but essential steps, you will be able to deliver a new mother safely.

Is There Time to Get to the Hospital?

To decide, you will need the answers to a few questions:

What are the woman's symptoms?

Delivery is usually imminent if:

- The perineum is bulging.
- The baby's head is at the opening of the vagina (known as crowning).
- Strong uterine contractions occur two minutes apart or less and last forty-five to sixty seconds.
- The woman is straining or pushing during contractions.

How many deliveries has she had?

First deliveries are usually slower than subsequent ones. First babies generally take about one hour to push out after the mother becomes completely dilated. So, if this is the woman's first delivery, you *may* be able to get her to the hospital if it is no more than fifteen to twenty minutes away, even though a nickel's size of the baby's head is already visible at the opening of the vagina.

If this is a second or subsequent delivery, do not try to make it to the hospital if the woman is pushing and the perineum is bulging. Bulging is a sign that delivery is less than ten minutes away. Even if the baby's head is not visible, you do not have much time. Once a mother has the urge to push, the delivery will usually take place within half an hour.

How far away is the hospital?

Once you have estimated how much time you are likely to have, find out where the hospital is and the fastest way to get there. If you do not think you will make it, prepare yourself and the woman for the delivery. If possible, ask a bystander to contact the woman's doctor and hospital, or do it yourself, so they will be prepared for the woman's arrival after the delivery.

If Deliver You Must, Here Is What To Do (see Figure 12–1)

Be reassuring while you prepare the delivery area.

You want the woman to stay as calm as possible so she can follow your instructions. If you have the facilities and time allows, move the woman to an area with as much privacy as possible and have her lie down on her back with her knees bent and separated. Remove any hampering clothing. Wash your hands, if possible, and place the cleanest available material under her buttocks. One suggestion is the inside of an unused newspaper, which is very clean when it comes off the press.

Most films of deliveries depict the mother lying flat on her back with her legs up. This position gives you the best view, but may be harder for the mother. Remember, she is the one doing the work. If she prefers to sit up, with someone behind her to support her back, or even to squat, you should allow her to do so. These positions allow her to use the force of gravity to her benefit. In addition, less tension is placed on her vaginal tissues, reducing the likelihood of a tear. Another position commonly used for comfort is side-lying. Position the woman on her left side, to improve blood return to her heart. Have someone hold her right leg up out of the way, so you can see the mother's vaginal opening.

Do not place your hands inside the vagina.

Remind yourself that a woman is very vulnerable to infection during childbirth because of the exposed blood vessels in her uterus.

Tear the amniotic membrane (bag of waters), if it is still intact and visible outside the vagina.

To do this, snag the membrane with your fingernail and pull or pinch it. If this does not work, pierce it with the sharp point of a pocket knife, scissor, pen, or other available object. The cleaner, the better.

Make sure to tear the membrane *before* the head emerges. A baby who is born in an intact amniotic membrane will aspirate the fluid during the first breath. This can cause many problems.

Do not attempt to restrain or delay delivery.

Do, however, help the mother control the delivery so the baby's head does not emerge too quickly. Encourage her to pant like a puppy during contractions instead of trying to push the baby out. The contractions themselves should create enough pressure to push the head out. Deliberate pushing creates undue pressure.

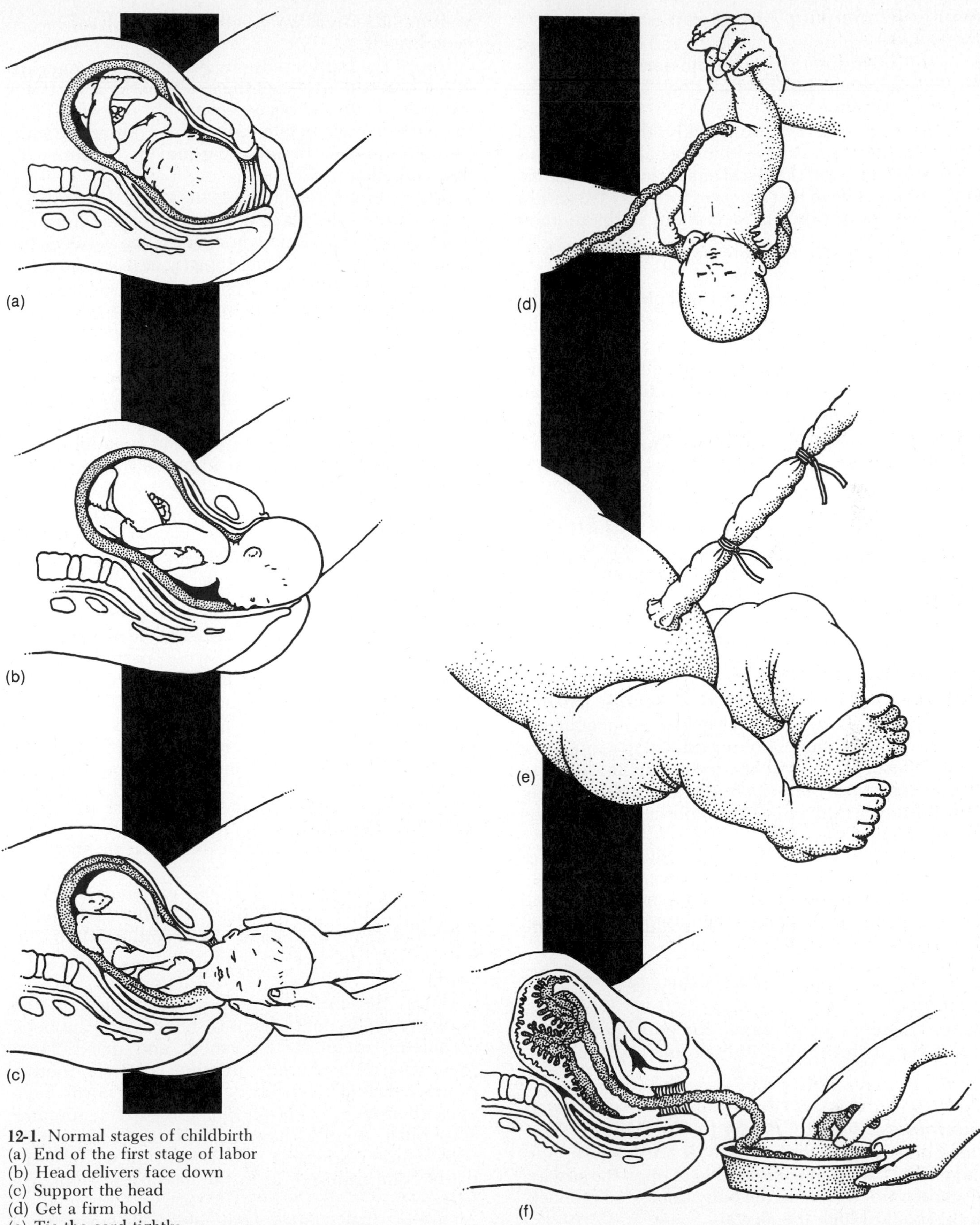

12-1. Normal stages of childbirth
(a) End of the first stage of labor
(b) Head delivers face down
(c) Support the head
(d) Get a firm hold
(e) Tie the cord tightly
(f) Placenta is expelled in five to twenty minutes

Do not let the baby's head pop out.
As the head emerges, place one hand over it and apply gentle pressure to keep it from emerging suddenly. This action controls—but does not delay—the speed of delivery.

If the head emerges too quickly, there may be a rapid change in pressure within the baby's skull. This can cause tearing in the dural or subdural membrane of the brain. A head that emerges too quickly can also cause vaginal or perineal lacerations in the mother.

Check for presence of the cord as the head emerges.
Feel for a loop of cord around the infant's neck. If the cord is present and wrapped loosely around the baby's neck, slip it over the baby's head. You can probably do this without much difficulty. Make sure you do not restrict the movement of the baby's head as it is coming out.

Wipe out the baby's mouth and nose.
Do this as soon as the head emerges and the cord is checked.

As the shoulders emerge, support and lift the baby's head and neck slightly.
The rest of the baby's body will slip out very quickly. Support the body as it emerges.

Get a firm hold on the baby.
Newborns are very slippery.

Dry the baby immediately and keep it warm.
Keeping a newborn warm will help prevent unnecessary stress. A cold newborn may develop respiratory problems because it will have to use up its energy to keep warm. Newborns have difficulty maintaining their body warmth and wet newborns get hypothermic very rapidly.

The action of drying the baby will help to stimulate its breathing. Rubbing the back and flicking the feet should also stimulate breathing. Most newborns cry and breathe spontaneously within one minute after birth.

Make sure nothing obstructs the baby's breathing.
Wipe the baby's mouth again. Keep its head slightly lower than its feet to facilitate drainage of fluid and mucus.

If the baby does not begin to breathe within one minute, begin CPR (refer to Chapter 3).
Place one hand under the baby's back for support and extend the head back slightly to open the airway. Be careful not to extend the baby's neck too far back, as this could block the airway.

Make a tight seal on infant's mouth and nose with your mouth. Give two breaths, with a pause between each breath.

Check the baby's pulse by placing your fingertips at the brachial artery on the inside of the arm. If it is adequate (110–130 beats per minute is normal) and the baby has not begun to breathe, continue mouth-to-mouth-to-nose breathing, using one breath every three seconds.

If you do not feel a pulse, start cardiac compressions. To do this, place two fingers on the sternum, one finger's width below imaginary line between the nipples. Push smoothly and gently at least 100 times per minute and continue the respiratory efforts. You should be giving five compressions to every one breath. Be sure the baby's head is on the same level as its heart or slightly lower; otherwise, chest compressions will not pump enough blood up to the brain. Continue CPR until the baby responds or help arrives.

Check periodically for pulse and breathing. The baby's color will begin to improve if the CPR is working.

Keep the newborn level with the mother's vagina.
Never place the infant above or below the vaginal opening before the cord is clamped or tied. Lowering the baby can cause circulatory overload if the placental blood drains quickly from the placenta into the baby. This could be disastrous, particularly in a premature baby. Elevating the baby above the opening can drain the infant's blood through the cord and back into the placenta, causing anemia or circulatory problems. For the same reason, do not place the baby on the mother's abdomen before you clamp the cord.

Tie the cord tightly.
Using the cleanest available material, tie the cord tightly enough to prevent leakage. A square knot works best. One of the best tying materials is a clean shoelace. Other possibilities are strips of material torn from a shirt or other article of clothing. Remember, do not use wire because it will cut through the cord.

Unless the cord is wrapped tightly around the baby's neck, do not tie it until after the baby has been completely delivered, warmed, and dried. How soon after delivery the cord should be clamped is somewhat controversial. Babies whose cords have been clamped quickly—within three to five minutes after birth—tend to have complications later. This could cause respiratory problems if the infant is already compromised, as in the case of a premature baby.

On the other hand, infants whose cords have not been clamped as quickly tend to fare better. They do, however, risk circulatory problems if they are not kept level with the mother's vagina.

Wait to cut the cord.

The cord can stay uncut until the mother and baby reach the hospital if you do not have a sterile knife or scissors.

If you have facilities for sterilization (a pot of boiling water will do), cut the cord by following this procedure:

- Make sure the cord is tied four to six inches from the infant's body and that the knot is tight enough to prevent leakage. If not, retie it.
- Make a second knot about four inches from the first one.
- Make a sharp cut between the two knots.
- If there is more than momentary bleeding, recheck the knots for tightness. If necessary, make another knot, but do not open the one already in place.

Never pull on the placenta.

The placenta will usually expel itself within twenty or thirty minutes after the birth of the baby. If not, seek immediate medical help. You will know that the placenta has separated when there is a lengthening of the cord and a gush of bloody discharge from the vagina. To help the mother deliver the placenta, instruct her to push or bear down as if to have a bowel movement.

If the perineum is torn and bleeding, apply pressure.

Treat it like an open wound by applying direct pressure with gauze or the cleanest material available. Sanitary pads work very well. Place the pad on the perineum and tell the mother to press her thighs together tightly.

Be on the alert for excessive bleeding.

If this occurs, seek immediate medical attention because the mother may be hemorrhaging and at risk of shock. Remember, there is a big difference between blood mixed with uterine and vaginal secretions and bleeding.

Save the placenta.

After the placenta is delivered, inspect it to make sure it is intact. Take it to the hospital with the mother and baby. You can place the baby on the shiny side of the placenta and wrap them together for warmth.

Massage the mother's uterus until it is firm.

Massage will stimulate the uterus to contract and become firm. This helps to minimize the discharge and may prevent hemorrhaging. To massage the uterus, hold it just above the pubic bone with one hand. With the other hand, apply gentle downward pressure on the uterus area. Check every five minutes for firmness and massage as necessary.

If the uterus does not stay firm with massage, try putting the baby to the mother's breast. Suckling helps to contract the uterus and keep it firm.

Offer liquids to the mother.

This is especially important if transportation to the hospital is delayed.

Write down important information.

Record pertinent data, including the following:

- Time of delivery
- Exact position of the cord if it was around the neck
- Appearance of the amniotic fluid, especially if it was green or brown
- Time the placenta was expelled and its condition
- Condition of mother and baby
- Mother's blood type and Rh factor, if she knows it.

Seek medical attention for mother and baby.

What To Do If Complications Occur

If the cord is wrapped tightly around the baby's neck, immediately tie it in two places and then cut it.

This is the only way to prevent the baby from strangling. Tie the cord tightly in two places several inches apart from each other and cut between the ties. It is more important to concentrate on getting the job done quickly than on preventing infection, so use anything at hand to tie the cord, as long as it is not wire, which will cut right through. If you do not have anything to tie the cord with, cut it and hold the ends tightly closed (or ask someone nearby to do this) until you can tie them.

If the baby's buttocks emerge first (breech birth), simply support them and the baby's trunk as they come out.

Never attempt to pull the baby from the vagina by his legs or trunk.

As soon as the legs are delivered, support the baby's body in the palm of your hand. After the shoulders emerge, the baby's body should naturally rotate so that its chest is facing downward as the head emerges. If the head is not delivered within about thirty seconds, support the baby's body with one arm and reach two fingers into the vagina to locate the baby's mouth. Use the two fingers to pull down slightly on its mouth. With your other hand, apply constant pressure on the mother's uterus. This will almost always cause the baby's head to be delivered. If it does not emerge within two minutes, keep your hands in position and transport the mother and baby to the nearest hospital as quickly as possible.

When an arm, leg, or shoulder emerges first, do not pull it out.
Transport the woman to the hospital immediately. Normal delivery is risky and special obstetrical procedures should be employed.

If the cord emerges before the baby (prolapsed cord), do not push the cord back into the vagina.
Put your hand into the vagina and push the baby's head away from the cervix so its circulation is not compromised. Elevate the mother's hips with a pillow, blanket, or rolled-up newspaper and place her in a knee-chest position. Keep the exposed cord moist and cover it with the cleanest available material. Get the woman to a hospital immediately. Breech presentation and prolapsed cord are the only two cases in which a first aider should place his or her hand in the mother's vagina.

If the baby's shoulders become wedged in place after the head has been delivered, do not attempt to pull the baby out.
Suction the baby's mouth and nose, and carefully and quickly transport the woman to a hospital.

Suspect multiple birth:
If you see distended abdomen, strong uterine contractions, or baby's size out of proportion to mother's abdomen, suspect multiple deliveries. Tie the cord of the first baby to prevent hemorrhaging. Deliver the second and subsequent babies in the same manner as single babies and care for the cord and placentas as for a normal delivery.

If a baby is premature, use extra care.
Premature babies (under 5.5 pounds or born before 38 weeks' gestation) are extremely susceptible to respiratory distress, infection, and other problems. Wrap the baby in the cleanest and warmest material available. If you have aluminum foil, use it as outer wrapping for extra insulation. Leave the baby's face uncovered and keep the mouth and nose clear of fluid.

If there is any bleeding from the cord, reclamp or tie it in another place close to the original closure. A premature baby cannot tolerate even the slightest loss of blood.

Avoid contamination by keeping your breath from the baby's face and having other people stay back.

Assisting in the birth of a baby is one of the few situations in which a first aider will have the opportunity to participate in a happy event rather than an unpleasant one.

Emergency Childbirth

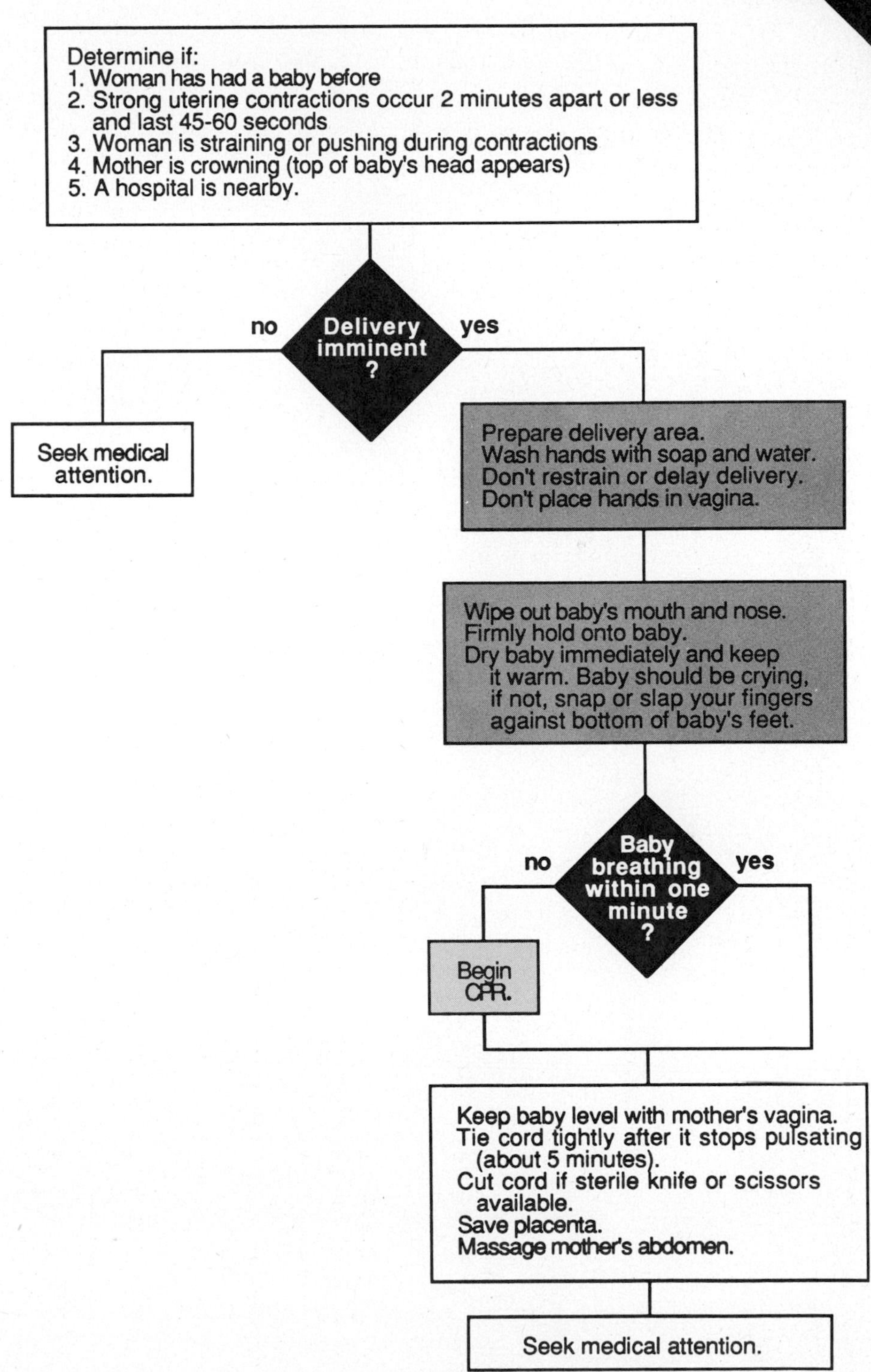

Emergency Childbirth

LEARNING ACTIVITIES

T F 1. In childbirth, the head of the baby usually emerges first.
T F 2. The baby's body is slippery and must be held firmly.
T F 3. The delivered baby should be placed on the mother's abdomen with its head down and to one side.
T F 4. A baby who does not breathe should be slapped firmly on the back.
T F 5. Blood and mucus should be wiped from the baby's mouth with a sterile gauze pad.
T F 6. Both mother and baby should be kept warm.
T F 7. The afterbirth should be preserved.
T F 8. Never tell the woman to cross her legs to delay delivery.
T F 9. Do not pull on the baby during the delivery.
T F 10. If the baby's head passes through the birth canal with the bag of waters still unbroken, tear the bag with your fingers.
T F 11. The umbilical cord should not be cut closer than four inches from the baby's navel.
T F 12. There is nothing a first aider can do except transport when only a foot or a leg is presented first.

Case 1: A woman is expecting her first child. Her amniotic sac (bag of waters) broke one hour earlier and her contractions are about ten to twelve minutes apart.

1. What stage of labor is this woman experiencing?

____

____

____

____

2. How long does the first stage of labor typically last?

A. ______ 4 hours
B. ______ 6 hours
C. ______ 8 hours
D. ______ 12 hours
E. ______ A full day

3. Describe the second stage of labor and how long it typically lasts.

____

____

____

____

The following presents an opportunity for self evaluation and review of situations surrounding emergency childbirth.

1. When is it necessary for a first aider to assist in or perform an emergency on-site delivery of a baby?

A. _______________________________________

____

B. _______________________________________

____

C. _______________________________________

____

2. What factors must be considered to determine if the mother is in advanced stages of labor?

A. _______________________________________

____

B. _______________________________________

____

C. _______________________________________

____

3. What should the first aider do when it is determined that an emergency on-site delivery is necessary?

A. _______________________________________

____

B. _______________________________________

____

C. _______________________________________

____

4. When the baby's head first appears during the normal delivery, the first aider should (check one)

A. ______ Gently pull on the head to ease delivery.
B. ______ Apply gentle pressure to the top of the head.

5. What should you do if the umbilical cord is wrapped around the baby's neck?

____

____

____

____

6. What steps should be taken to care for the normal newborn child?

   A. ______________________________

   B. ______________________________

   C. ______________________________

7. If the child is not breathing and artificial respiration must be used, how does artificial respiration in a newborn differ from artificial respiration in an adult?

   A. ______________________________

   B. ______________________________

8. What steps are involved in caring for the child's umbilical cord?

   A. ______________________________

   B. ______________________________

9. The placenta is usually delivered a few minutes after the baby is born. However, this process may take as long as ______ .

   A. 15–30 minutes
   B. 30–60 minutes
   C. 1–2 hours
   D. Over 2 hours

10. List three types of complicated deliveries.

   A. ______________________________

   B. ______________________________

   C. ______________________________

11. Describe the two conditions under which the first aider should have contact with the mother's vaginal area.

   A. ______________________________

   B. ______________________________

12. What should the first aider do after the baby and placenta have been delivered?

____

Case 2: A pregnant woman lives in a rural setting approximately twenty-five minutes from the closest medical facility. When you reach her home, she indicates she is having painful contractions three to five minutes apart and feels the urge to have a bowel movement. She informs you that she has two other children. On examination you see that the woman's vagina is bulging.

1. What would be your decision regarding moving the mother-to-be? Why?

____

2. What is the very first thing that should be done once the baby's head has been successfully delivered?

____

3. The umbilical cord is cut after the baby is delivered because the child no longer depends on it for oxygen and nourishment.

   A. ______ True
   B. ______ False

4. What occurs during the third stage of labor?

____

5. Why is it necessary to save the placenta and deliver it to the hospital with the mother and newborn? ______________________________

Case 3: A pregnant mother tells you she feels as if she has to have a bowel movement. On examination, you see that an arm is presenting.

1. What is the appropriate emergency medical treatment in this situation?

____

2. A breech delivery is when:

   A. ______ A limb is presenting first.
   B. ______ The umbilical cord emerges first.
   C. ______ The buttocks appear first.
   D. ______ Both A and C.
   E. ______ Both B and C.

3. What is appropriate treatment in a breech situation?

   A. ______________________________

   B. ______________________________

4. If the baby is not spontaneously delivered at this point, what is the appropriate intervention?

   ____

5. What specific condition indicates that delivery is imminent?

   ____

13 First Aid Skills

- Bandaging
- Splinting

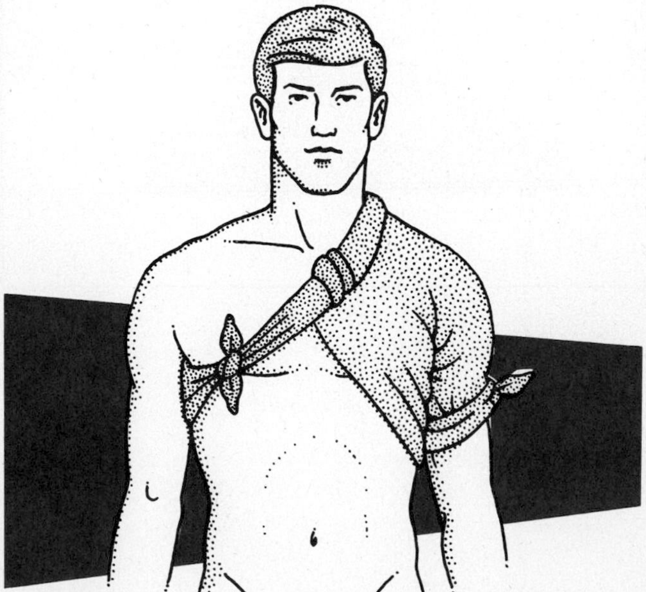

The following illustrations show suggested bandaging and splinting skills. This compilation represents the skills needed for most first aid situations likely to be encountered.

Triangular and Cravat Bandages

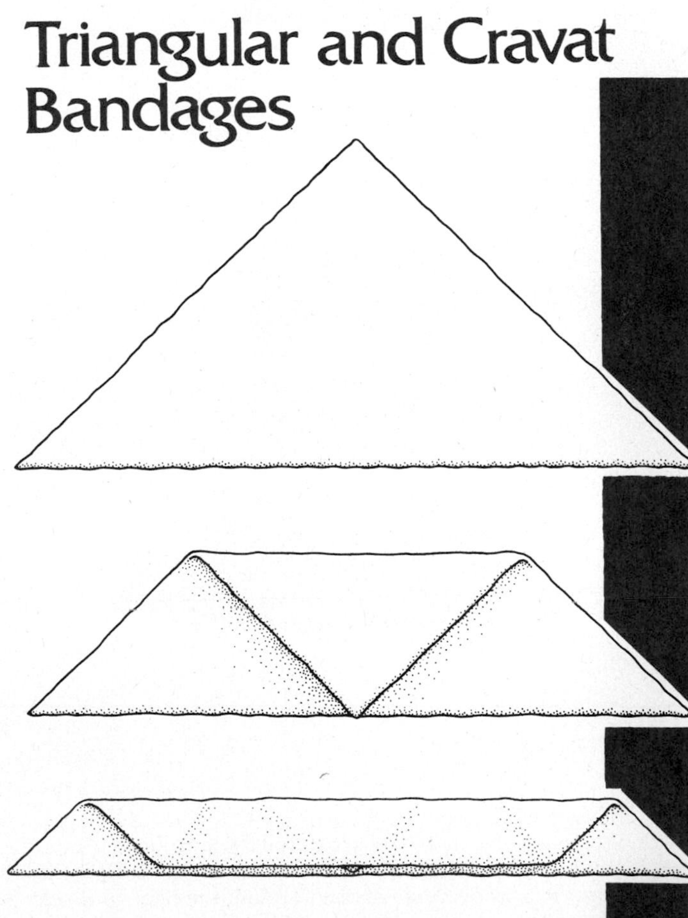

13-1. Fold the triangular bandage to make a cravat. Size of a triangular is about 55 inches at the base and from 36 to 40 inches along the sides.

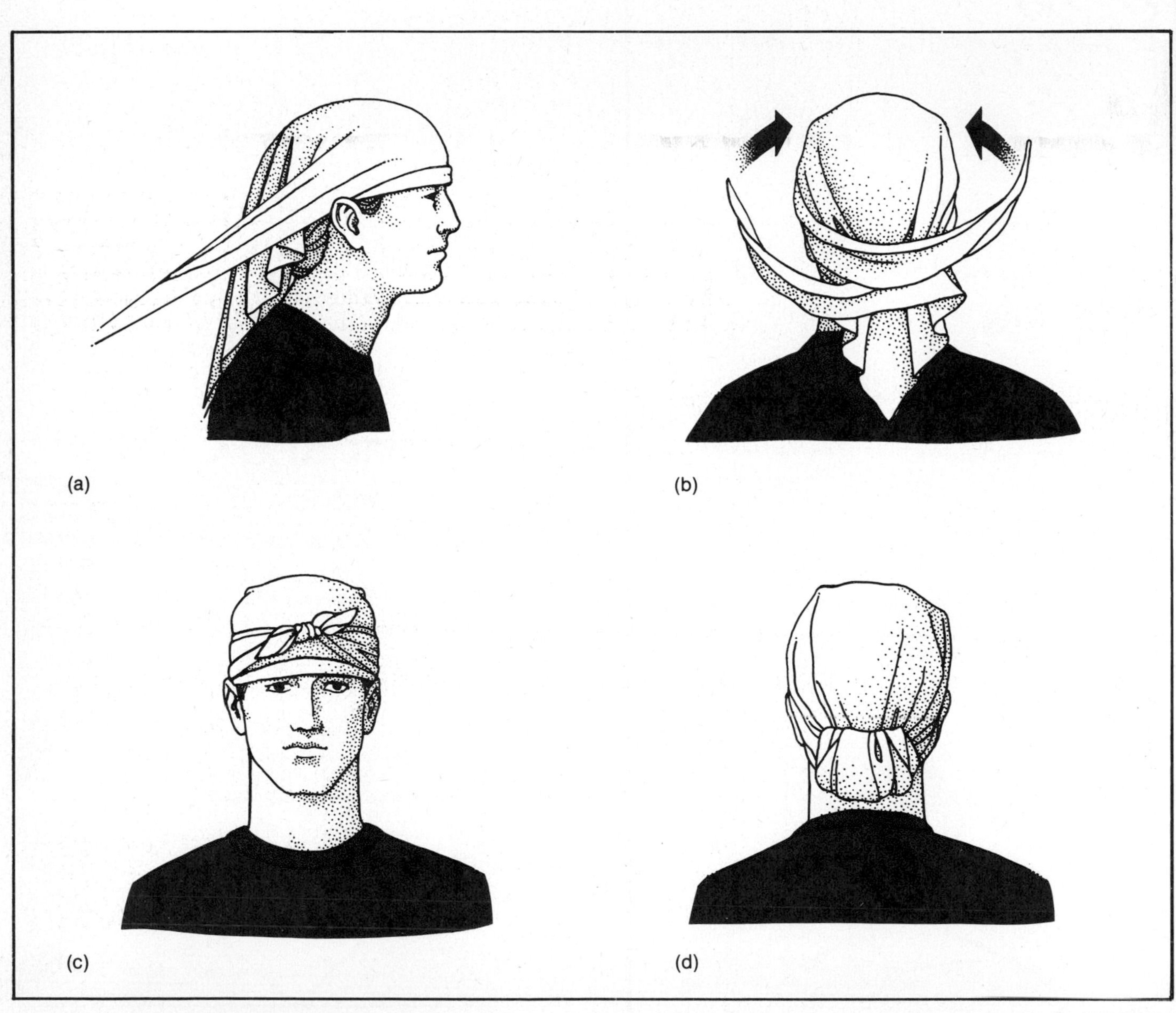

13-2. Triangular bandage for the head
(a) Place center of triangle base across the forehead so that it lies just above the eyes, with point of bandage down the back of the head. Bring ends above the ears and around the back of head.
(b) Cross the two ends snugly over each other just below the lump at the back of the head. Bring ends back around to center of forehead.
(c) Tie ends in a knot.
(d) Tuck point in fold where bandage crosses.

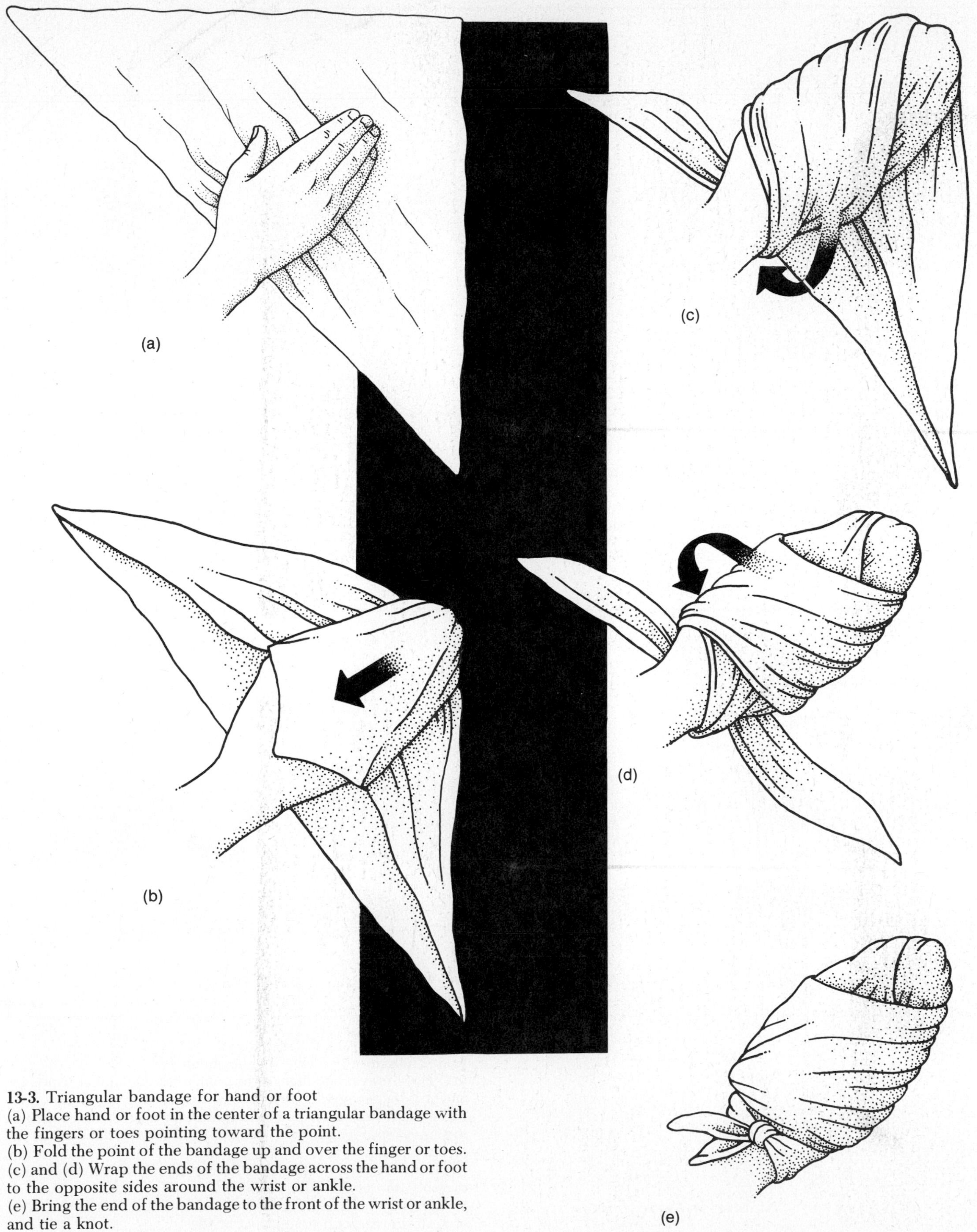

13-3. Triangular bandage for hand or foot
(a) Place hand or foot in the center of a triangular bandage with the fingers or toes pointing toward the point.
(b) Fold the point of the bandage up and over the finger or toes.
(c) and (d) Wrap the ends of the bandage across the hand or foot to the opposite sides around the wrist or ankle.
(e) Bring the end of the bandage to the front of the wrist or ankle, and tie a knot.

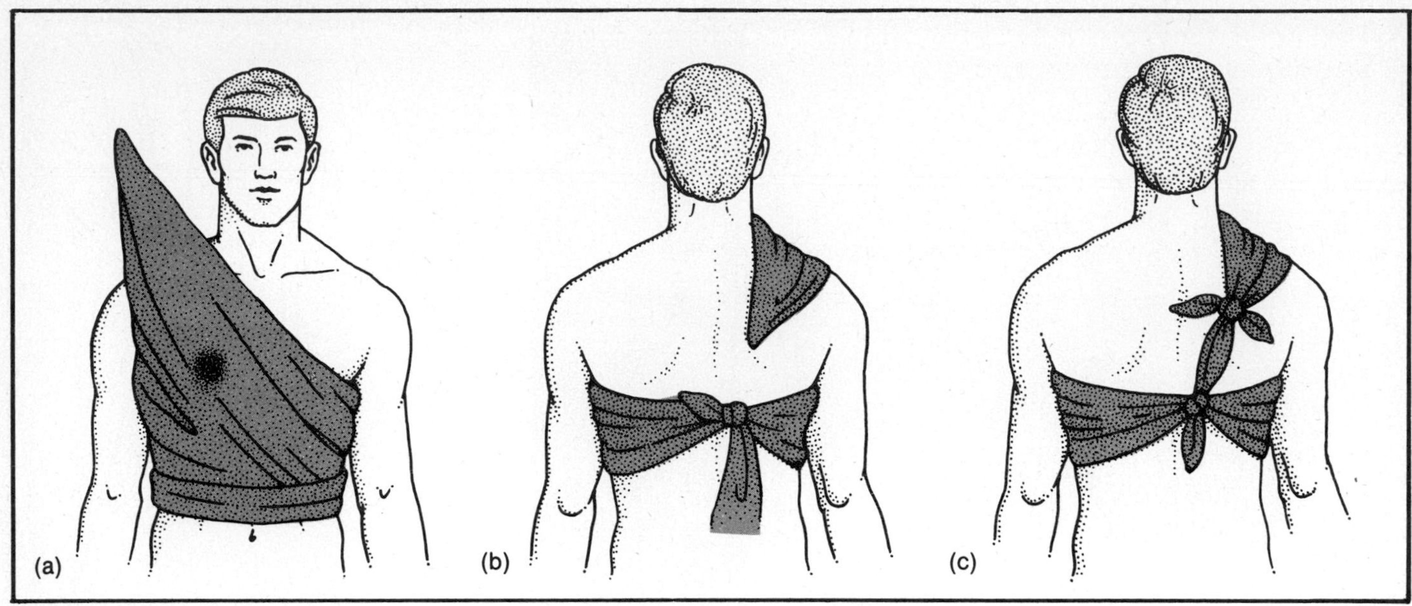

13-4. Triangular bandage for chest or back
(a) Fold the base of the bandage up far enough to secure the dressing and tie the ends around the torso. Tie so there is one long and one short and will be left.
(b) Place the point of the bandage over the shoulder.
(c) Bring the long end up to the shoulder and tie it to the point of the triangle.

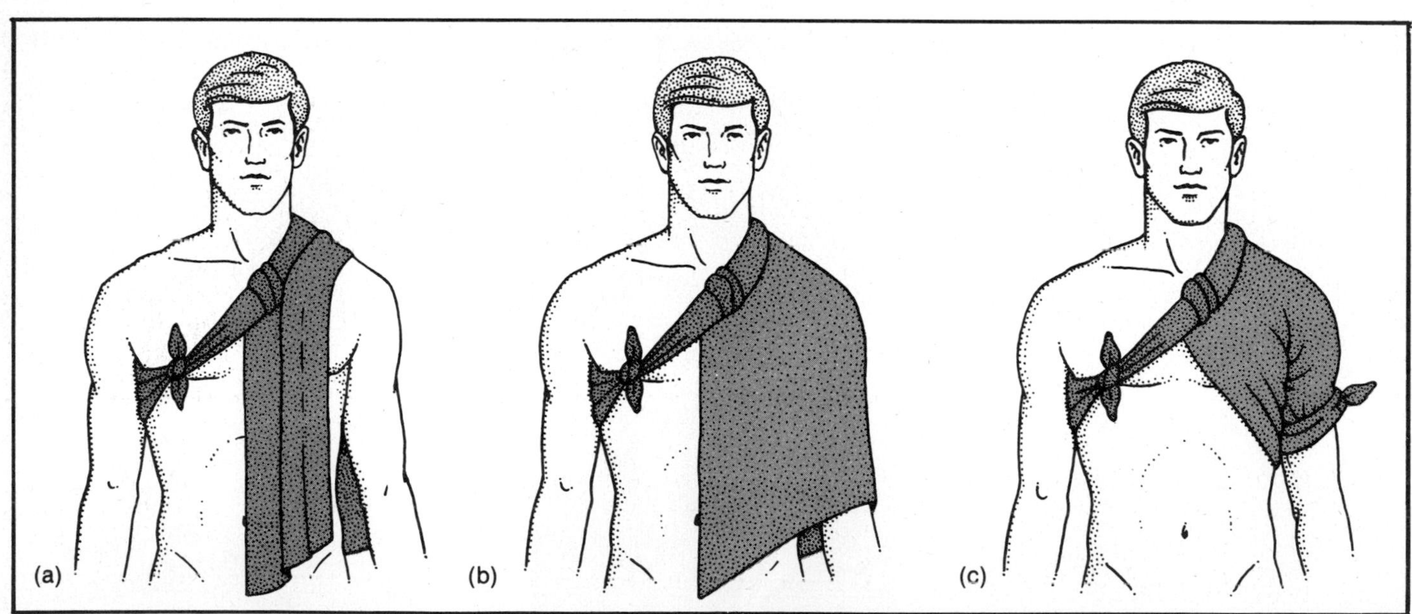

13-5. Triangular bandage for the shoulder
(a) Place a cravat bandage on the point of the triangular bandage and roll them together several times toward the triangle base. Place the cravat over the injured shoulder near the neck. Bring the cravat ends under the opposite armpit and tie slightly in front or back of it.
(b) Bring the base of the triangular bandage down and over the dressing on the shoulder.
(c) Fold up the base of the triangular bandage. Wrap the ends around the arm and tie on the outside.

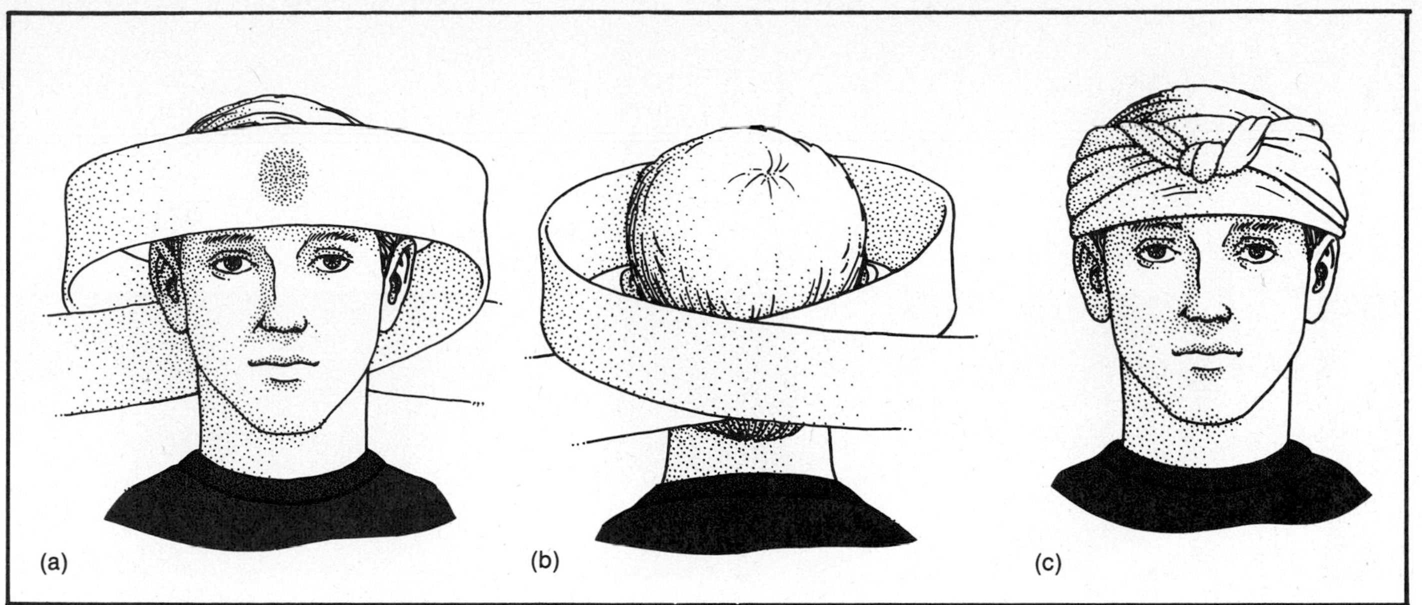

13-6. Cravat bandage for the head, ear, or eyes
(a) Place middle of bandage over the dressing covering the wound.
(b) Cross the two ends snugly over each other.
(c) Bring ends back around to where the dressing is and tie the ends in a knot.

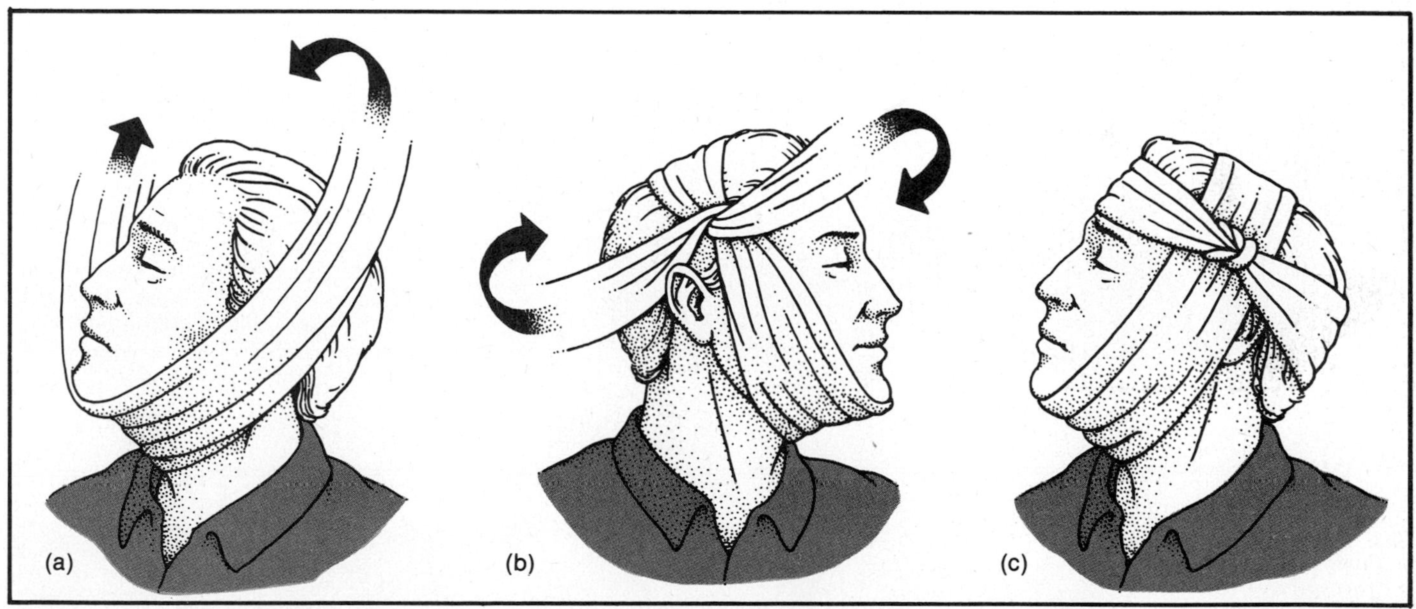

13-7. Cravat bandage for cheek, ear, or head
(a) Place bandage under chin and carry ends upward. Adjust bandage to make one end longer than the other.
(b) Take longer end over top of head to meet short end at temple. Cross ends.
(c) Take ends in opposite directions to other side of head and tie them over the part of bandage applied first.

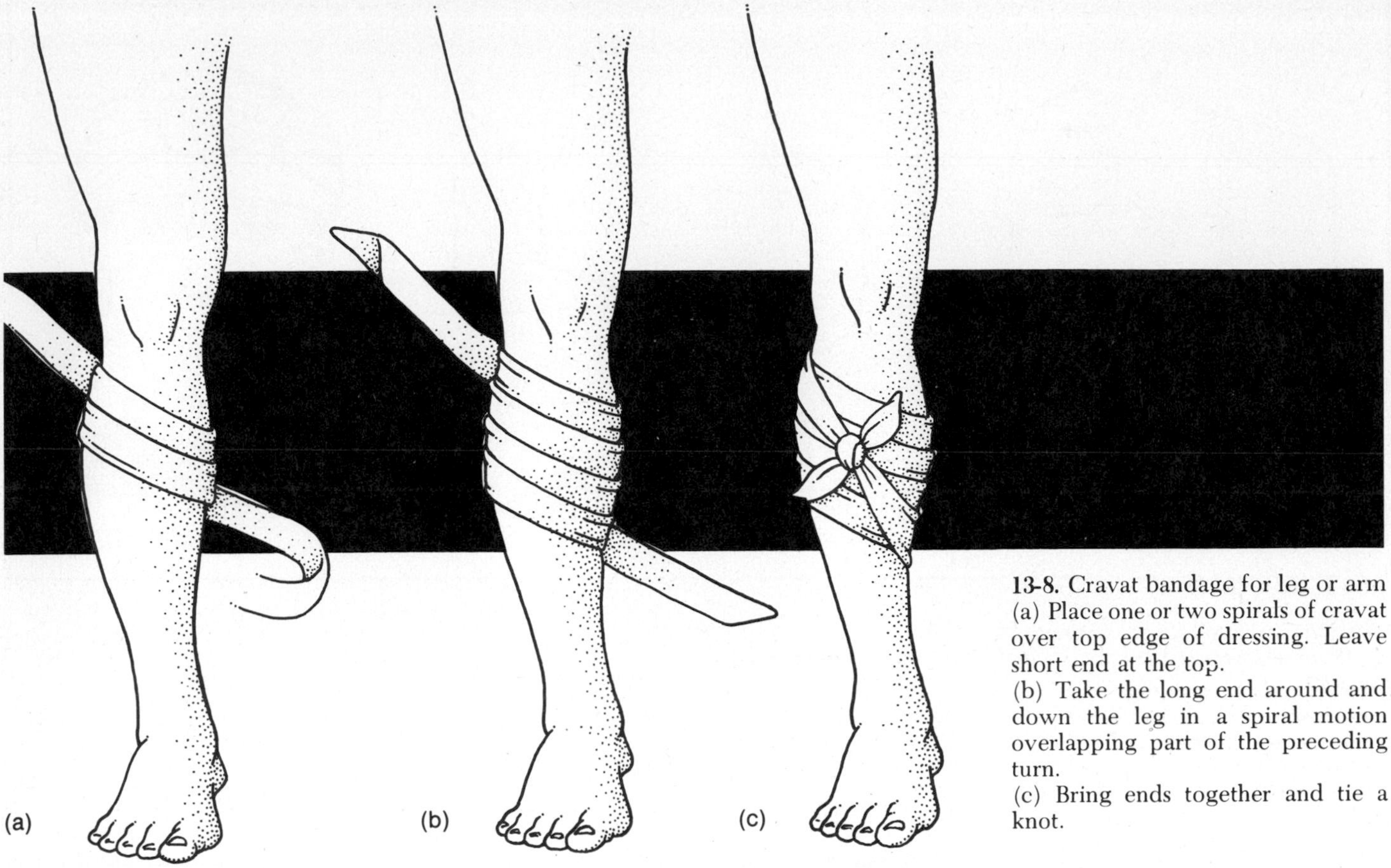

(a) (b) (c)

13-8. Cravat bandage for leg or arm
(a) Place one or two spirals of cravat over top edge of dressing. Leave short end at the top.
(b) Take the long end around and down the leg in a spiral motion overlapping part of the preceding turn.
(c) Bring ends together and tie a knot.

Roller Bandage

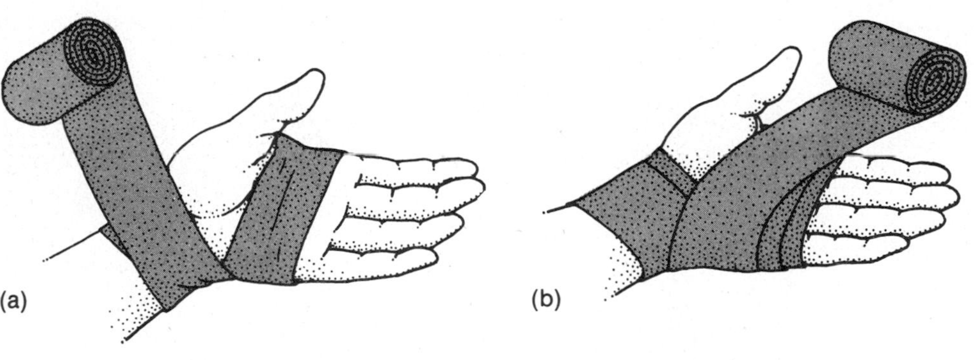

13-9. Roller bandage for hand
(a) Anchor the bandage with one or more turns around the palm of the hand. Then, carry it around the wrist.
(b) Repeat this figure-of-eight maneuver as many times as is necessary to fix the dressing properly.

13-10. Roller bandage for knee
(a) Make several anchoring turns above the knee joint, overlapping the top edge of the dressing. Proceed diagonally downward across the dressing. Circle below the joint.
(b) Proceed diagonally upward across the dressing and downward across the dressing.
(c) Repeat the figure-of-eight process until the area is sufficiently covered.

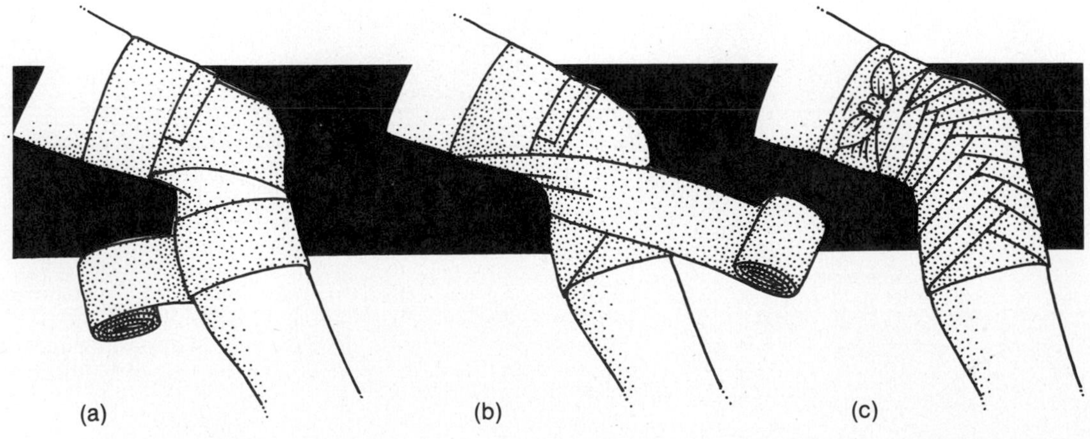

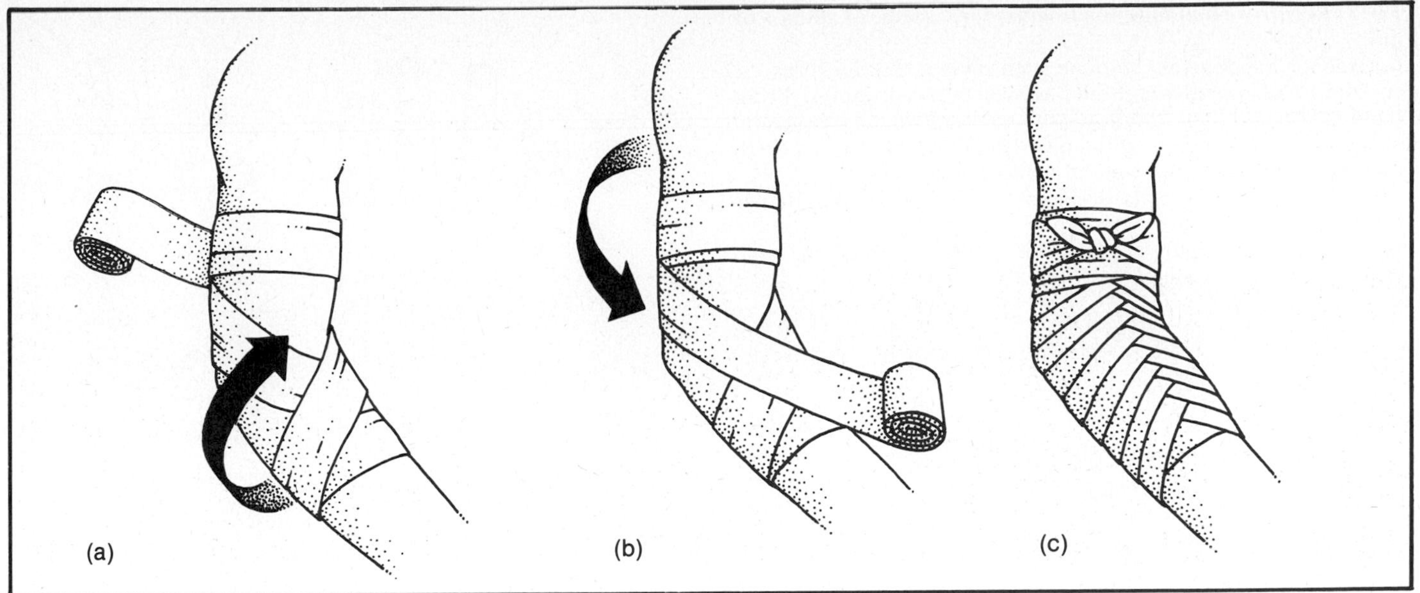

13-11. Roller bandage for elbow
(a) Make several anchoring turns above the elbow joint, overlapping the top edge of the dressing. Proceed diagonally downward across the dressing. Circle below the joint and proceed upward diagonally.
(b) Proceed downward diagonally.
(c) Repeat the figure-of-eight process until the area is sufficiently covered.

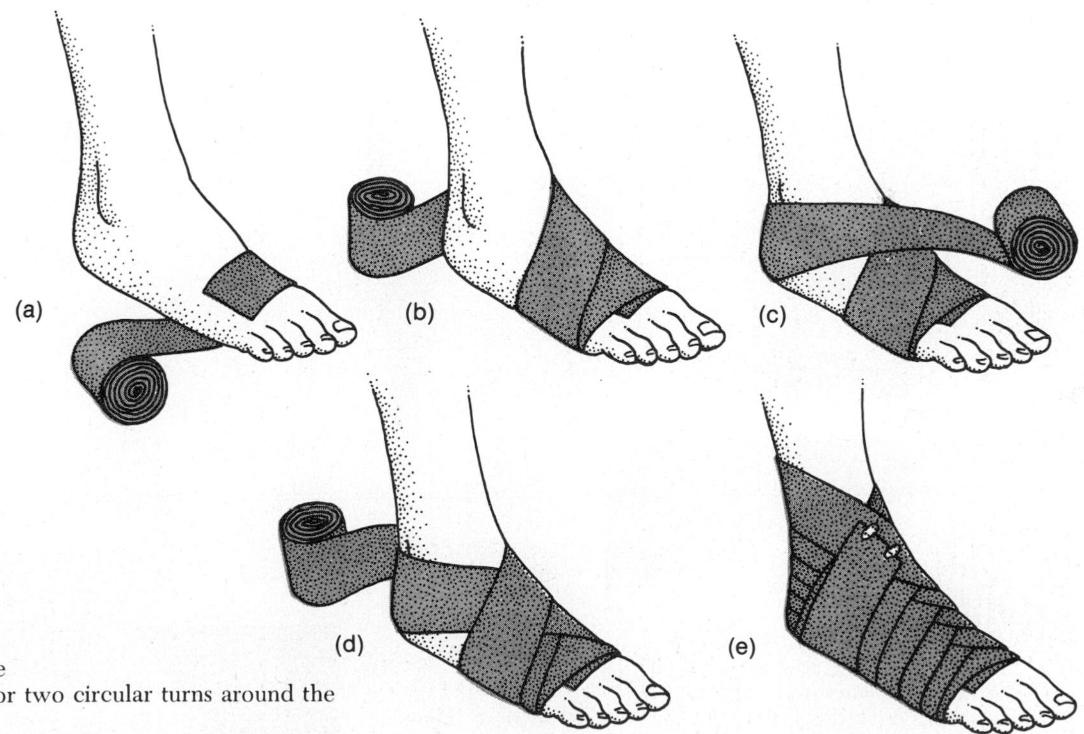

13-12. Roller bandage for ankle
(a) Anchor bandage with one or two circular turns around the foot.
(b) Bring bandage diagonally across the top of the foot and around the back of the ankle.
(c) Continue bandage down across the top of the foot and under the arch.
(d) Continue figure-of-eight turns, with each turn overlapping the last turn by about three-fourths of its width.
(e) Bandage until the foot (not toes) and lower leg are covered. Secure bandage with tape or clips.

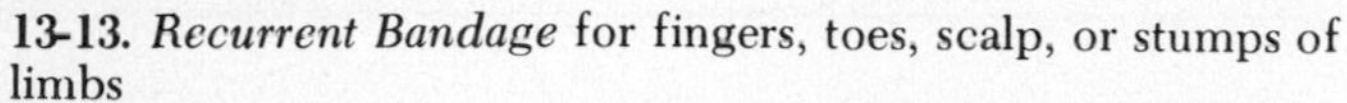

13-13. *Recurrent Bandage* for fingers, toes, scalp, or stumps of limbs
(a) Anchor bandage at the bone with several circular turns.
(b) Hold bandage down at the base where it is anchored. Bring bandage up and over and down the back side to the base again.
(c) Hold down bandage at the base. Repeat the back-and-forth bandaging process until several layers are covered.
(d) To hold bandage in place, start at the base, and make circular turns up and back to the base.
(e) To secure bandage, apply piece of tape up and then down other side.

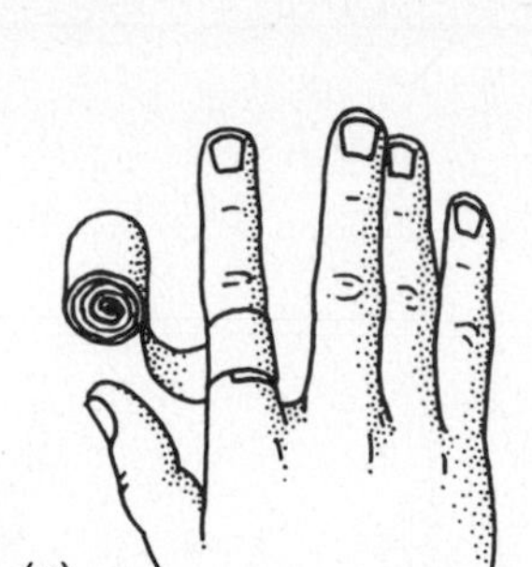

(a) 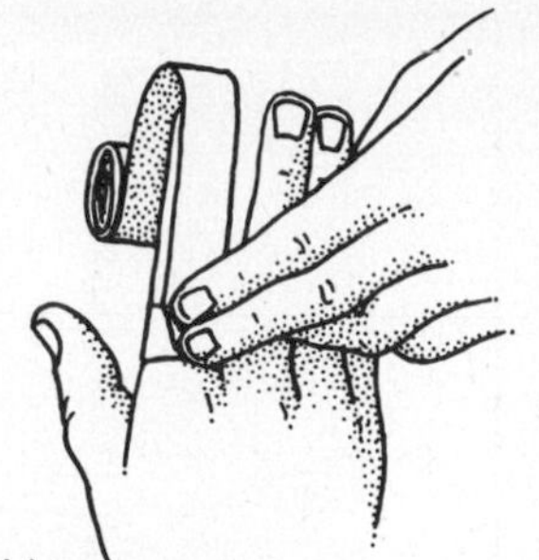 (b)

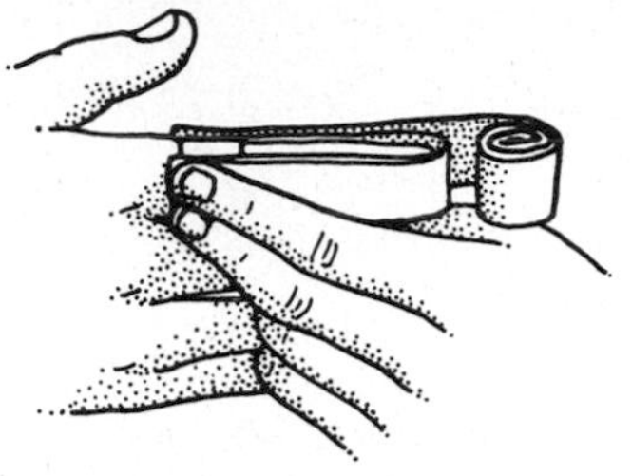

(c) 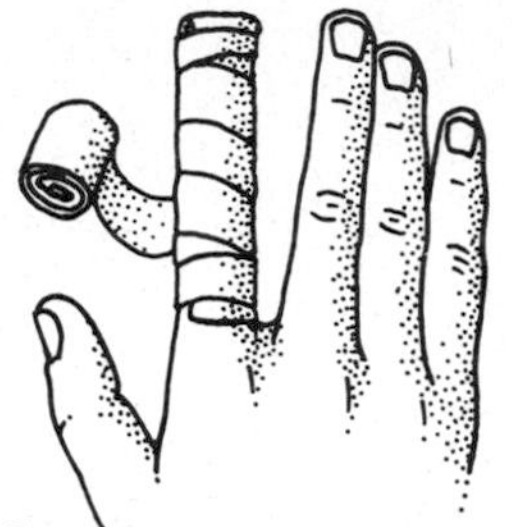 (d) 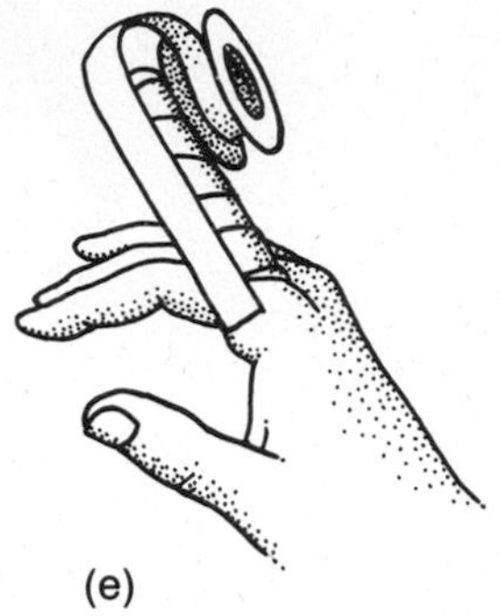 (e)

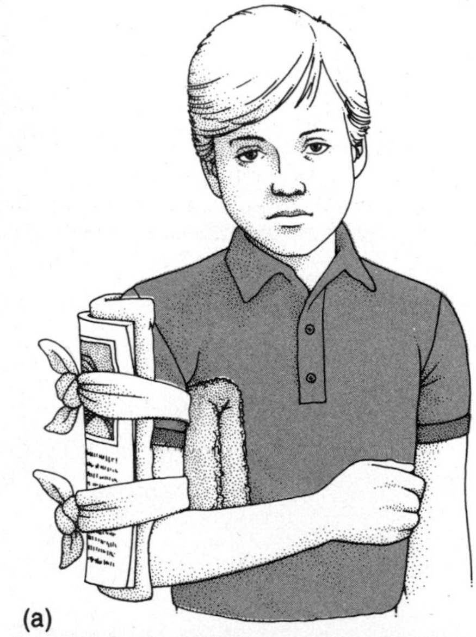

(a)

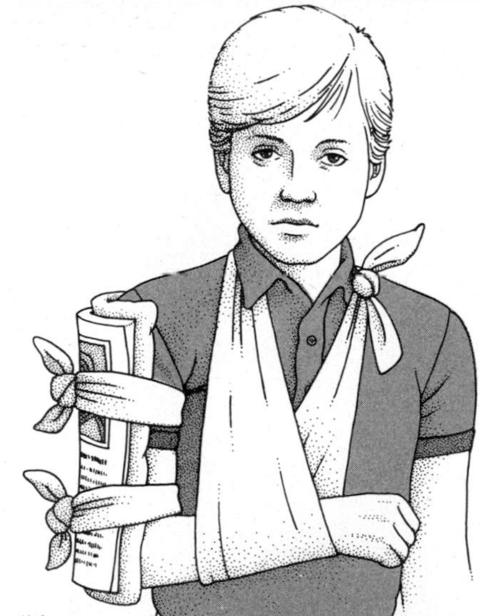

(b)

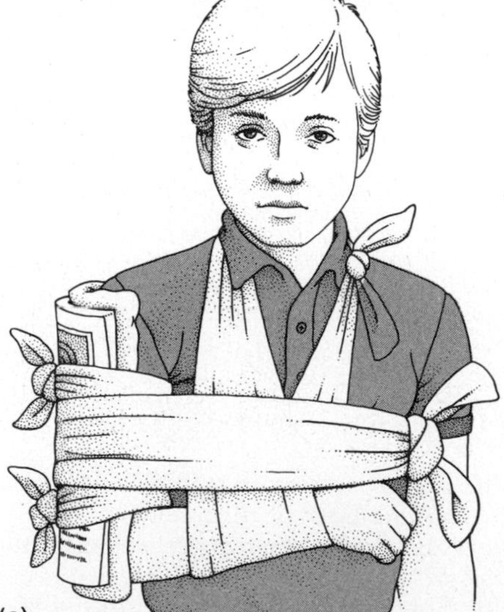

Splinting

13-14. Splinting a fractured humerus and clavicle
(a) Place a pad (i.e., towel) between the arm and the body. Place a padded splint (i.e., newspaper or board) along the outer side of the arm. Tie it to the arm.
(b) Support the arm with a wide cravat bandage. The knot should not press against the neck.
(c) Use a wide cravat bandage as a swathe to bind the arm to the chest. A broken clavicle (collarbone) can be splinted the same way except the padded splint along the outer side of the arm is not used.

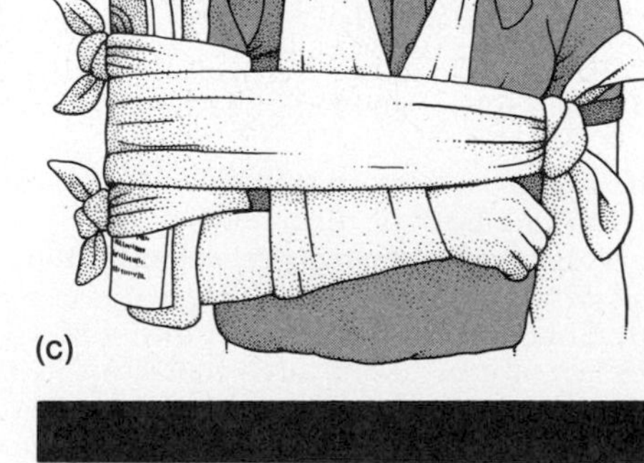

(c)

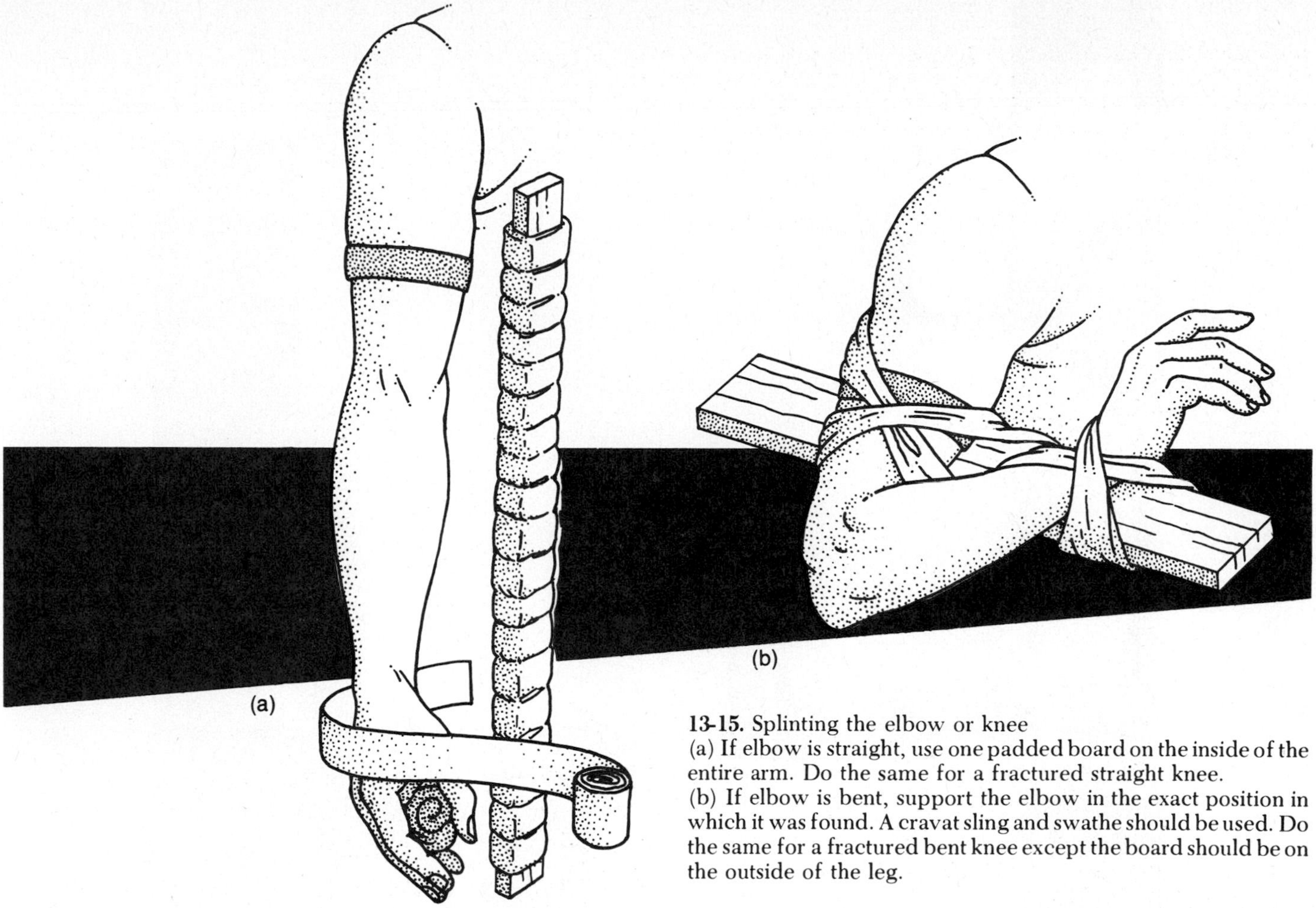

(a)

(b)

13-15. Splinting the elbow or knee
(a) If elbow is straight, use one padded board on the inside of the entire arm. Do the same for a fractured straight knee.
(b) If elbow is bent, support the elbow in the exact position in which it was found. A cravat sling and swathe should be used. Do the same for a fractured bent knee except the board should be on the outside of the leg.

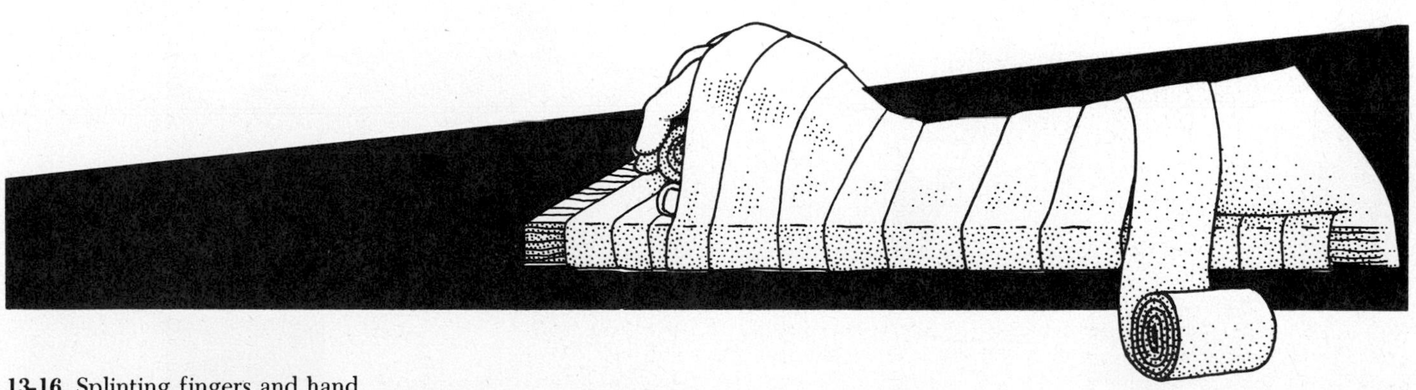

13-16. Splinting fingers and hand
Most injured fingers will be found in the position of function (cupped). Place a ball of gauze or cloth under the victim's fingers to hold them in a cupped position. Roller gauze, elastic bandage, or several cravat bandages may be used to secure the hand and fingers to the splint. Taping the injured finger to an adjacent finger or to a small piece of wood are other alternatives.

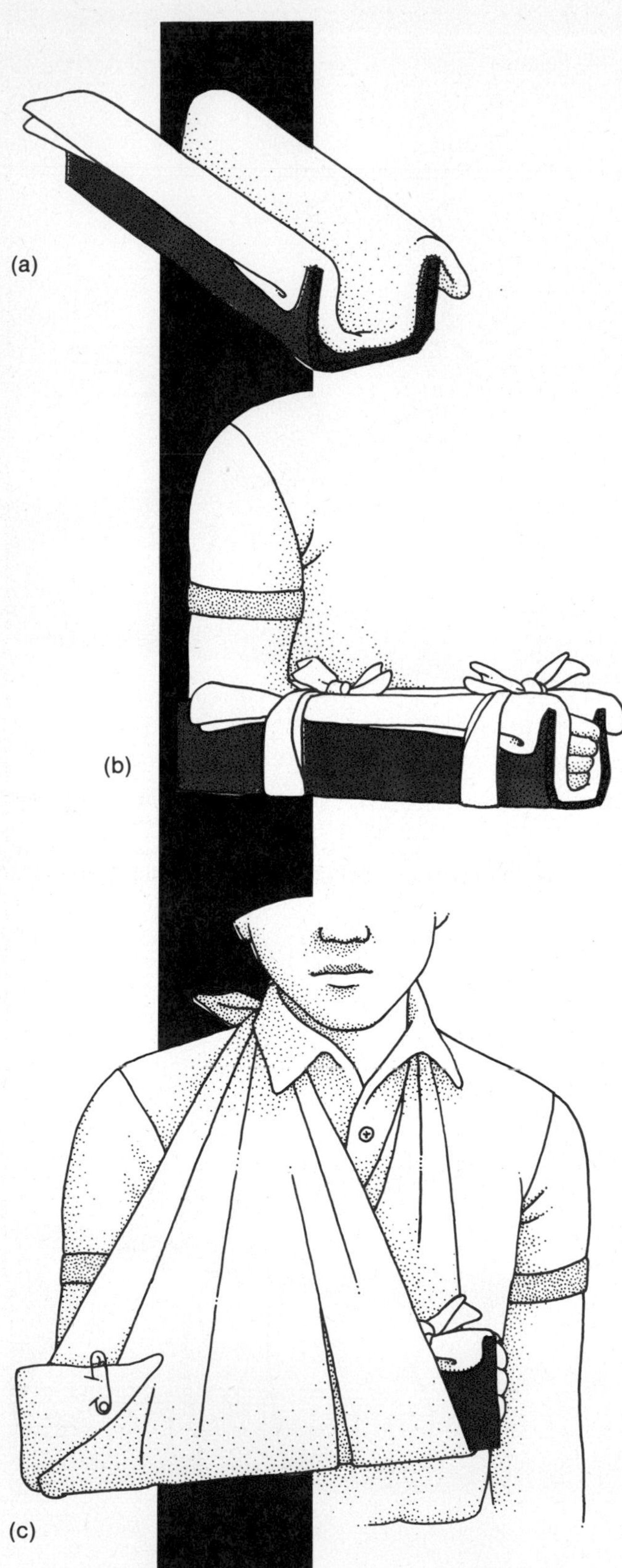

13-17. Splinting a fractured forearm
(a) Use padded splint made of cardboard, newspaper, or board.
(b) Tie the splint in place.
(c) Place the forearm in a sling. Not shown is the use of a wide cravat bandage as a swathe.

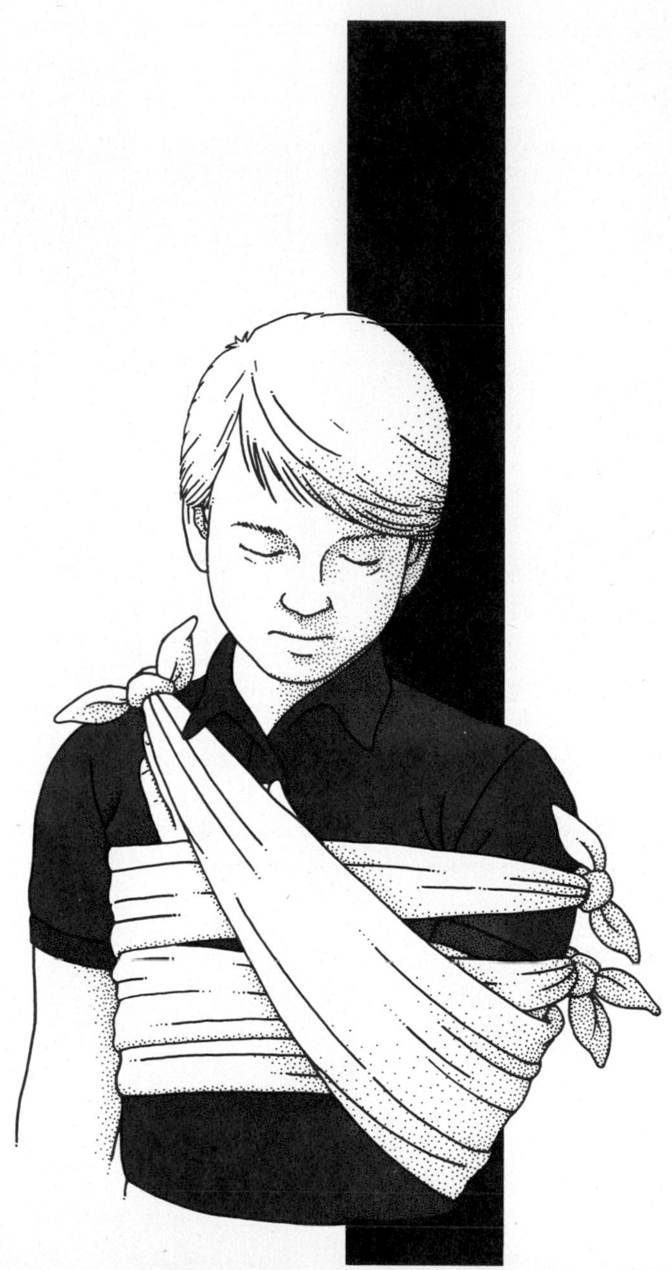

13-18. Splinting rib fractures
Place arm of injured side across chest.
Bind arm tightly to chest with cravat bandages.
Tie a cravat bandage along angle of arm for support.

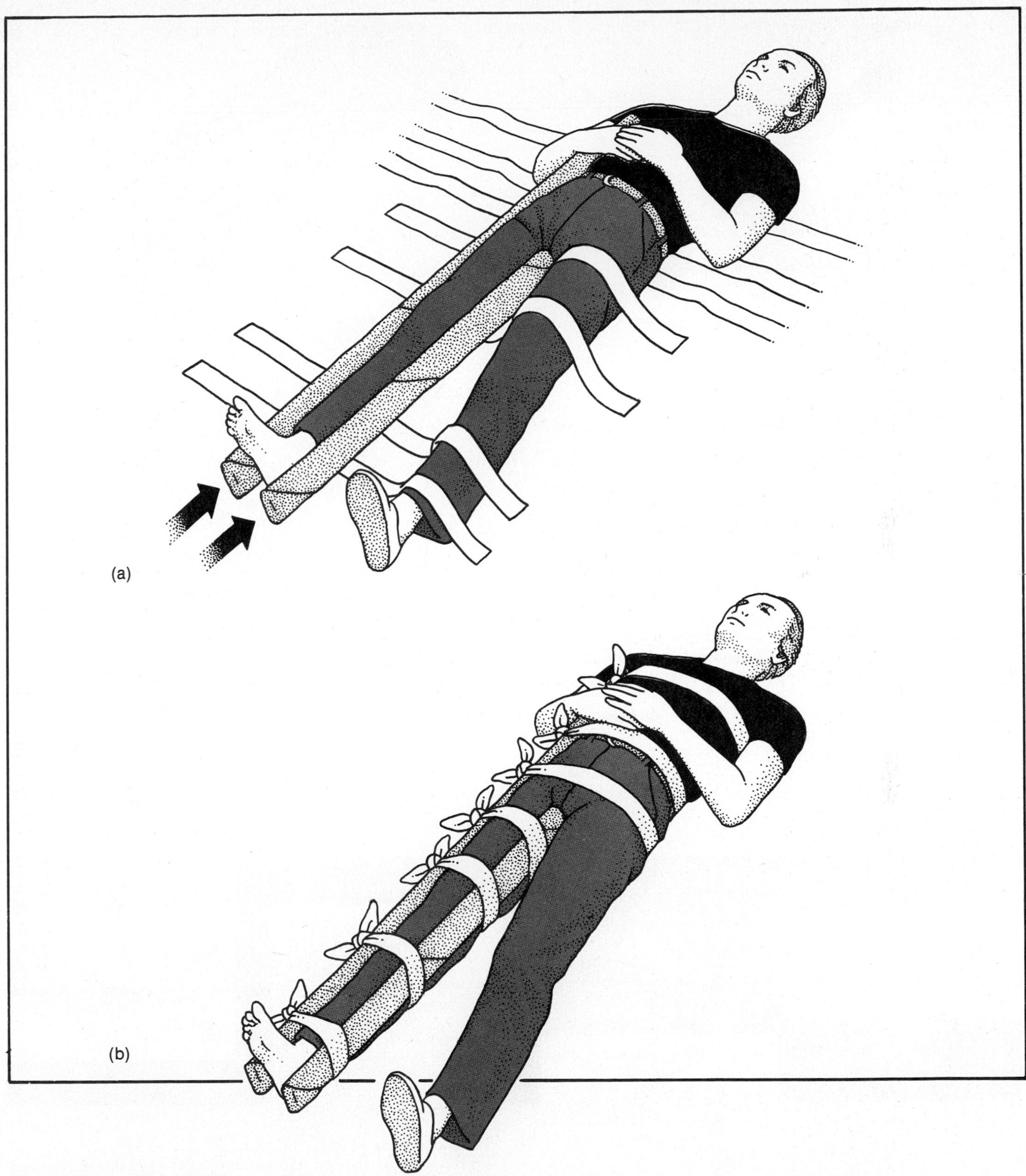

13-19. Splinting hip or femur
(a) Use a stick to slide cravat bandages or cloth strips into position. One splint should be long enough to reach from the crotch to past the heel. The other should reach from the armpit to past the heel.
(b) Tie the splints on snugly. The knots should not press the body.

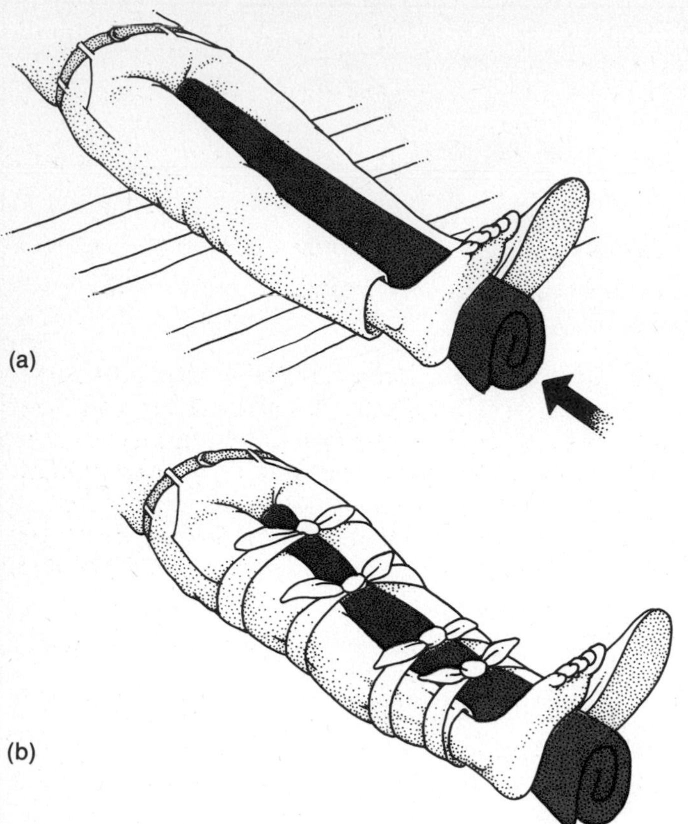

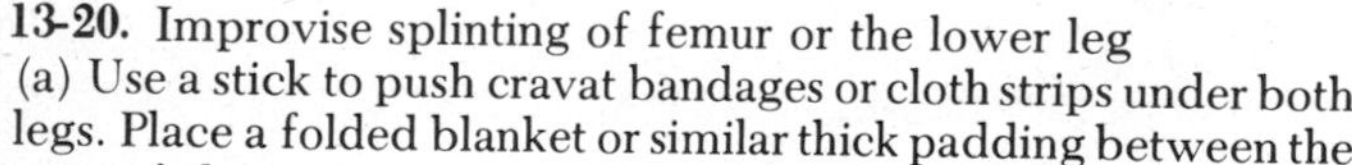

13-20. Improvise splinting of femur or the lower leg
(a) Use a stick to push cravat bandages or cloth strips under both legs. Place a folded blanket or similar thick padding between the person's legs.
(b) Tie the person's legs together so that the uninjured leg can immobilize the injured leg.

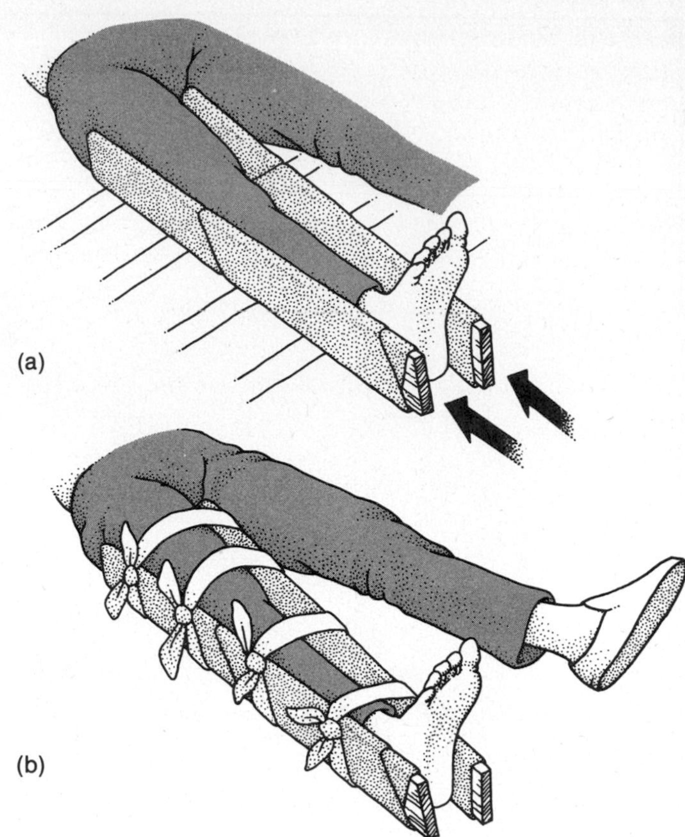

13-21. Splinting the lower leg
(a) Use a stick to push cravat bandages or cloth strips under the leg. Place padded boards or other suitable objects along the inner and outer sides and the injured leg. Both boards must reach from well above the knee to past the heel.
(b) Tie the splints in place. The knots should not press the body.

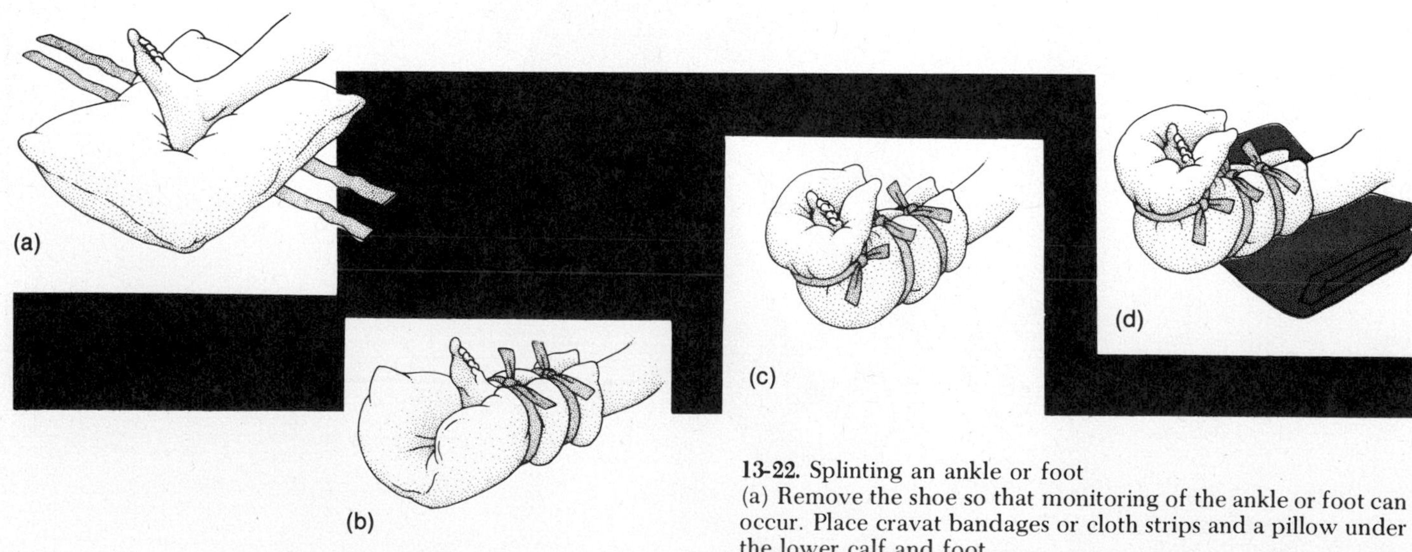

13-22. Splinting an ankle or foot
(a) Remove the shoe so that monitoring of the ankle or foot can occur. Place cravat bandages or cloth strips and a pillow under the lower calf and foot.
(b) Fold the upper part of the pillow around the ankle and tie it in place.
(c) Fold the lower part of the pillow and tie it in place, leaving the toes exposed.
(d) Elevate the foot to decrease swelling.

Traction Splints

Traction splints are used to provide constant pull on an extremity. They supply the traction that is always a part of the immobilization of a fracture, and they prevent broken bone ends from overriding due to muscle contraction. They do not reduce the fracture but simply immobilize the bone ends and prevent further injury. Traction splints are generally used for fractures of the femur or the hip.

The most commonly used traction splints are the Thomas half ring splint and the Hare traction splint. The basic principles of application are the same for both:

- Traction is applied to the injured leg by grasping the ankle and calf and gently pulling.
- While the first rescuer maintains this traction, the second rescuer slides the splint under the leg and secures the half ring splint in position, pressing firmly against the ischial tuberosity—the rounded projection of the hipbone.
- When the half ring has been fastened, the second rescuer applies and secures the ankle hitch.
- Traction is developed by tightening the winding device, or windlass, until the victim experiences relief of pain.
- The splint is then elevated so that the victim's foot is clear of the ground and the leg is secured by cravats or Velcro straps at intervals along the splint.

A Hare traction splint is applied in much the same way as the Thomas half ring splint. But with the Velcro straps between the two longitudinal rods and the traction apparatus at the foot, the application of traction becomes much simpler and much faster.

Pulses, color, and capillary refilling must be checked every five to ten minutes after applying either splint.

14 Moving and Rescuing Victims

- Emergency Moves
- Nonemergency Moves
- Water Rescue

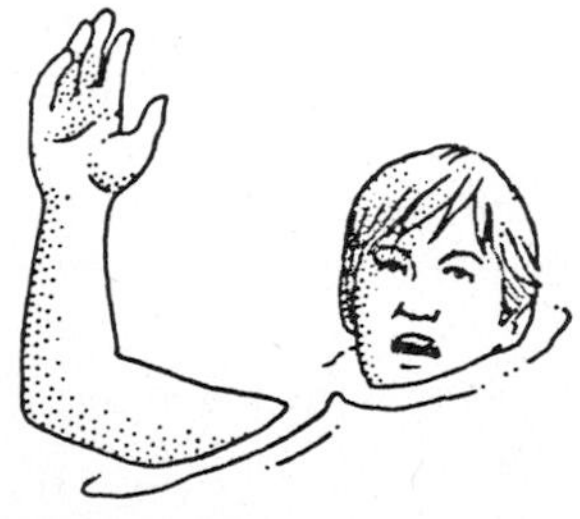

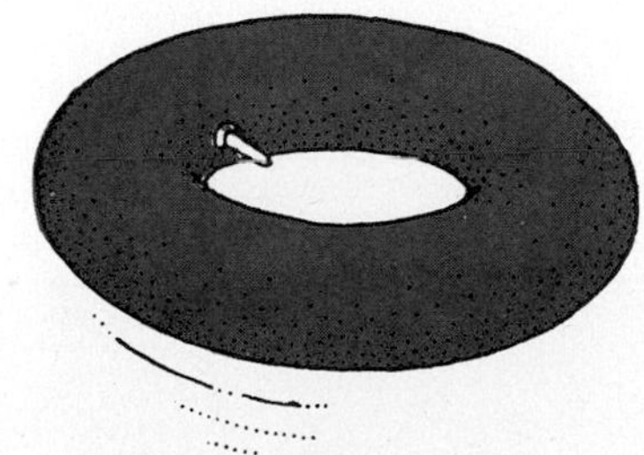

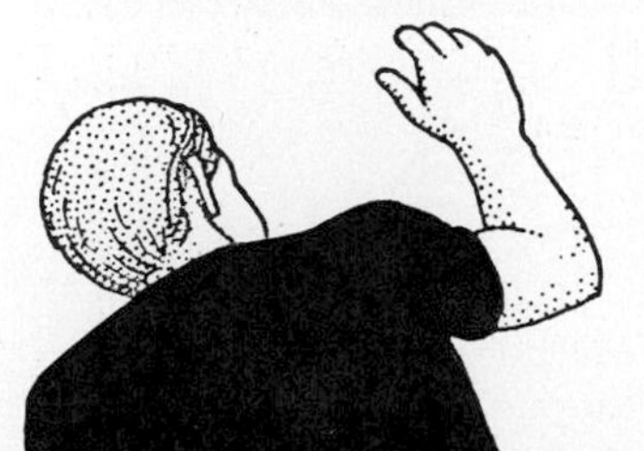

In general, a victim should not be moved until he or she is ready for transportation to a hospital, if required. All necessary first aid should be provided first. A victim should be moved only if there is an immediate danger to him or others if he is not moved, that is:

- There is a fire or danger of fire.
- Explosives or other hazardous materials are involved.
- It is impossible to protect the accident scene.
- It is impossible to gain access to other victims in a vehicle who need life-saving care.

Note that a cardiac arrest victim would typically be moved unless he is on the ground or floor because cardiopulmonary resuscitation must be performed on a firm surface.

If it is necessary to move a victim, the speed with which he is moved depends on the reason for moving him, for example:

- *Emergency move.* If there is a fire, pull the victim away from the area as quickly as possible.
- *Nonemergency move.* If the victim needs to be moved to gain access to others in a vehicle, give due consideration to his injuries before and during movement.

EMERGENCY MOVES

The major danger in moving a victim quickly is the possibility of aggravating spine injury. In an emergency, every effort should be made to pull the victim in the direction of the long axis of the body to provide as much protection to the spine as possible. If the victim is on the floor or ground, he can be dragged away from the scene by tugging on his clothing in the neck and shoulder area. It may be easier to pull the victim onto a blanket and then drag the blanket away from the scene. Such moves are emergency moves only. They do not adequately protect the spine from further injury.

NONEMERGENCY MOVES

All injured parts should be immobilized before moving and then protected during the moving. To protect yourself, the first aider should use the following principles in all nonemergency moves:

- Keep in mind physical capabilities and limitations and do not try to handle too heavy a load. When in doubt, seek help.
- Keep yourself balanced when carrying out the move.
- Maintain a firm footing.
- Maintain a constant and firm grip.
- Lift and lower by bending your legs and not your back—keep your back as straight as possible at all times; bend knees and lift with one foot ahead of the other.
- When holding or transporting, keep your back straight and rely on shoulder and leg muscles; tighten muscles of your abdomen and buttocks.
- When performing a task that requires pulling, keep your back straight and pull using your arms and shoulders.

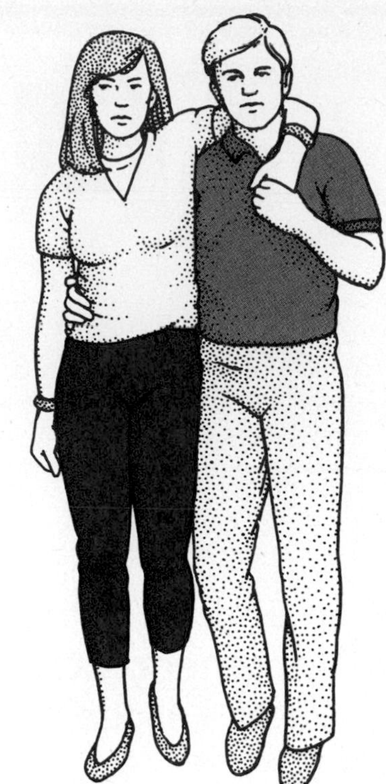

14-1. Helping the person to walk.

- Carry out all tasks slowly, smoothly, and in unison with your partner.
- Move body gradually; avoid twisting and jerking when conducting the various victim-handling tasks.
- When handling a victim, try to keep your arms as close as possible to the body in order to maintain balance.
- Do not keep muscles contracted for a long period of time.

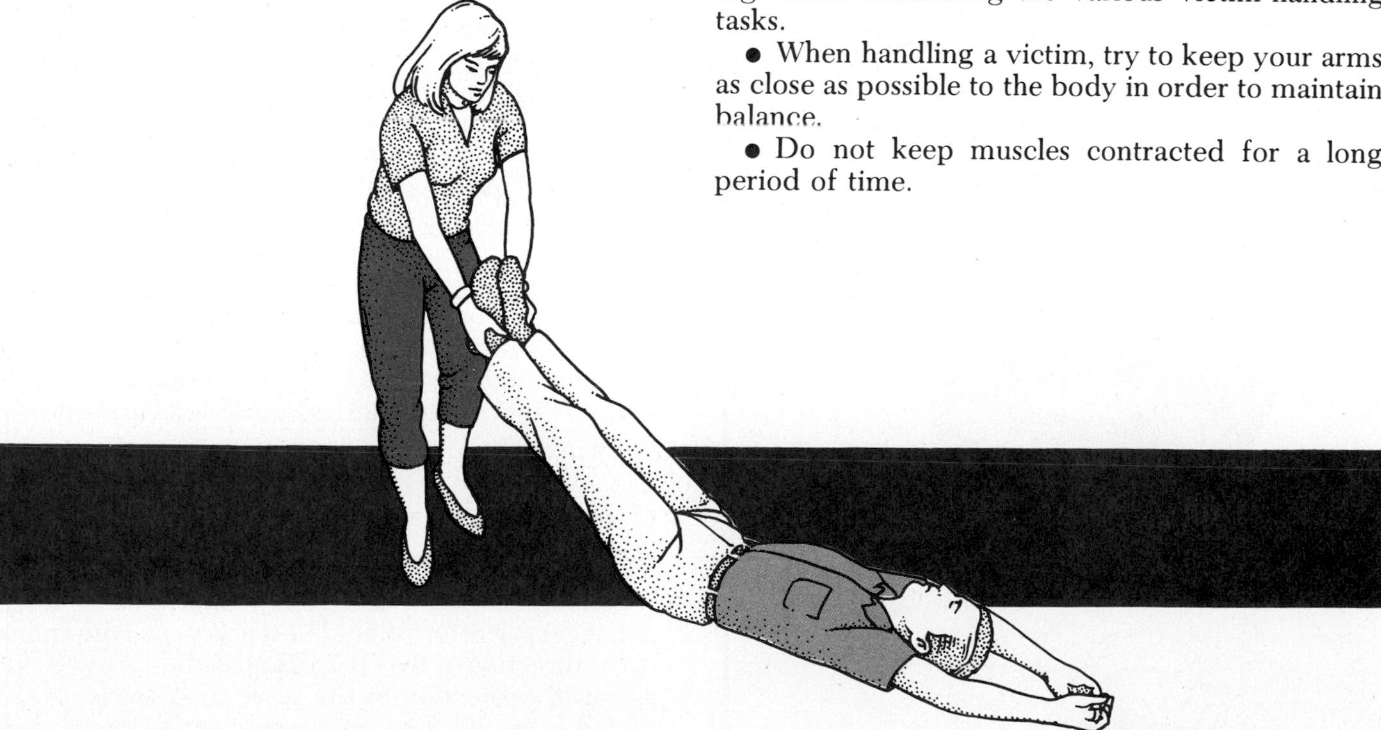

14-2. Ankle pull. The fastest method for a short distance on a smooth surface.

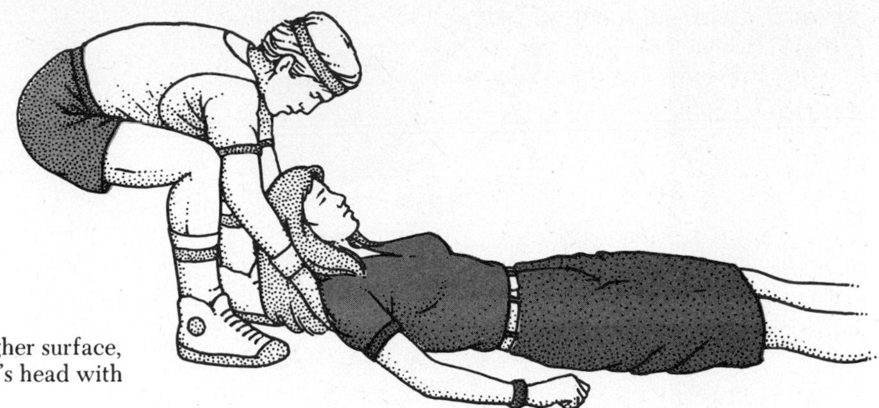

14-3. Shoulder pull. For short distances over a rougher surface, pull the person by both shoulders. Stabilize person's head with your forearms.

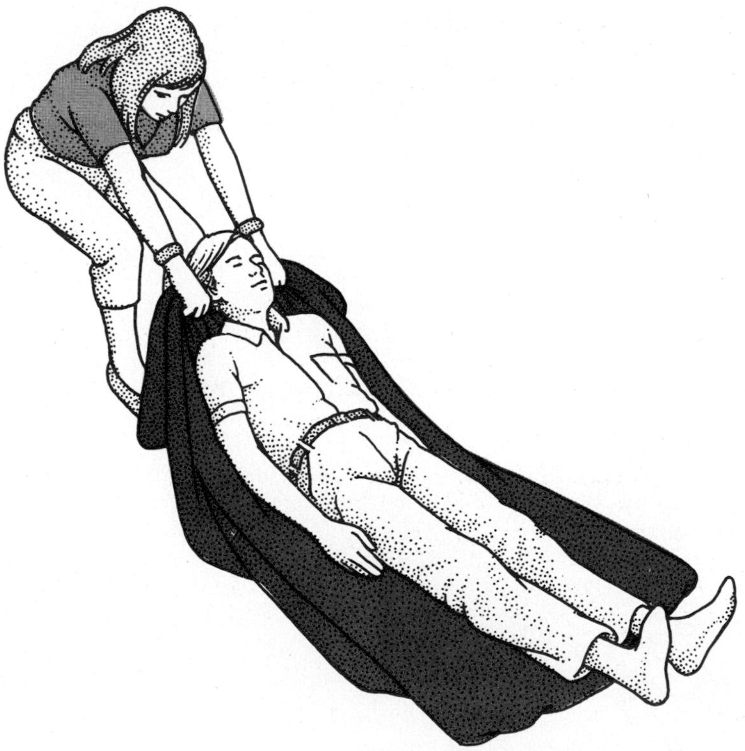

14-4. Blanket pull. Roll the person onto a blanket and pull from behind his head.

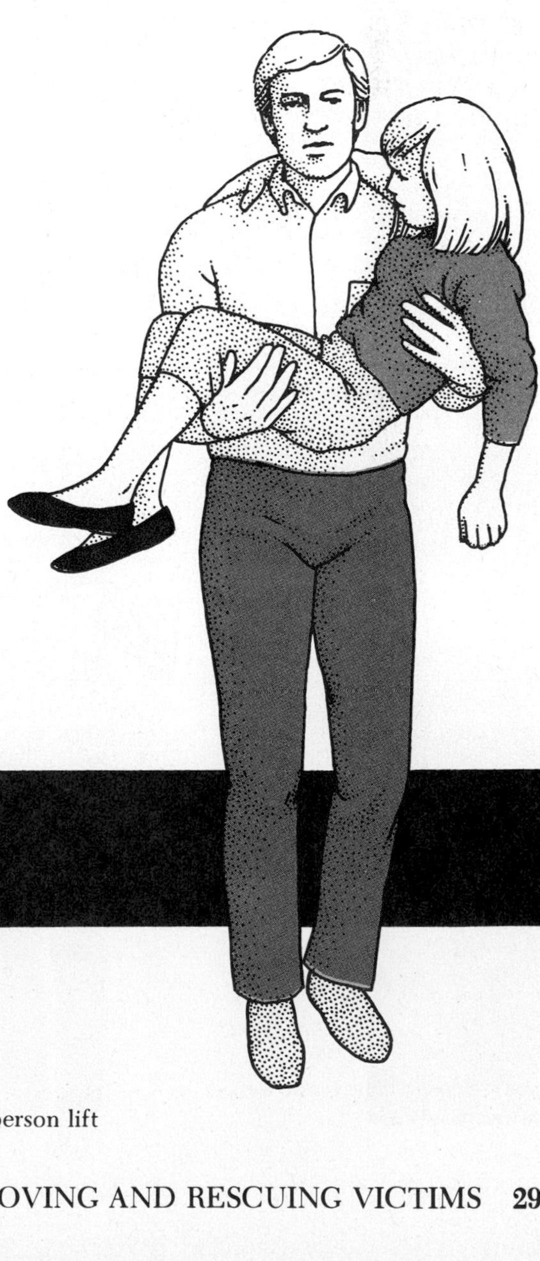

14-5. One-person lift

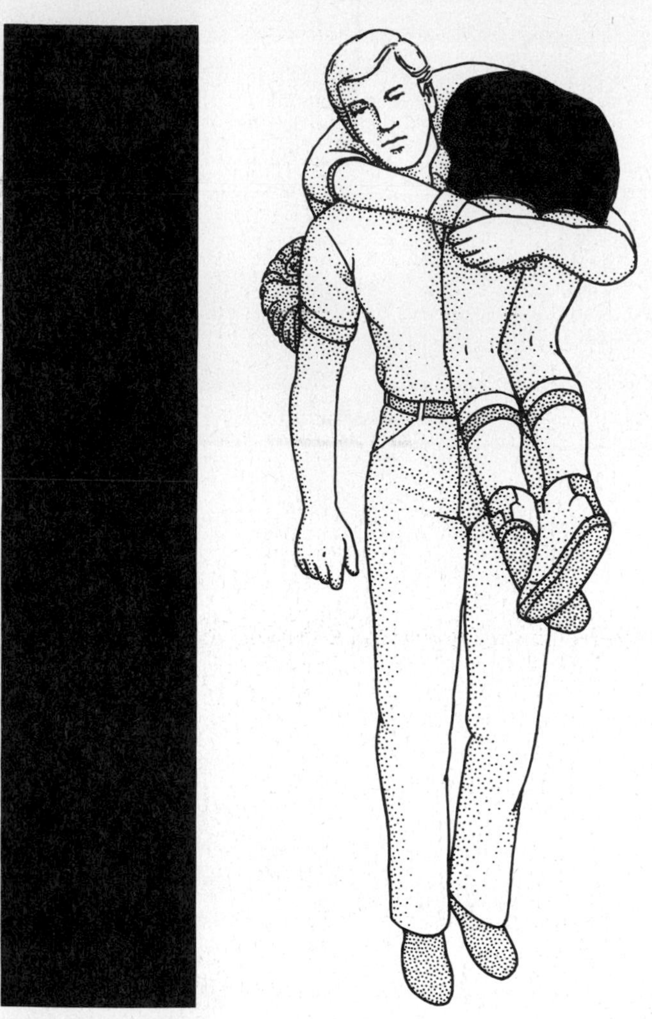

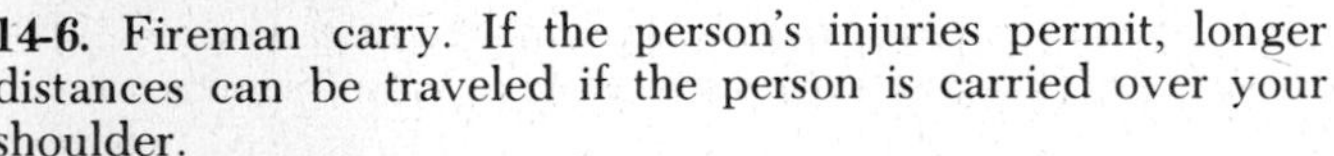

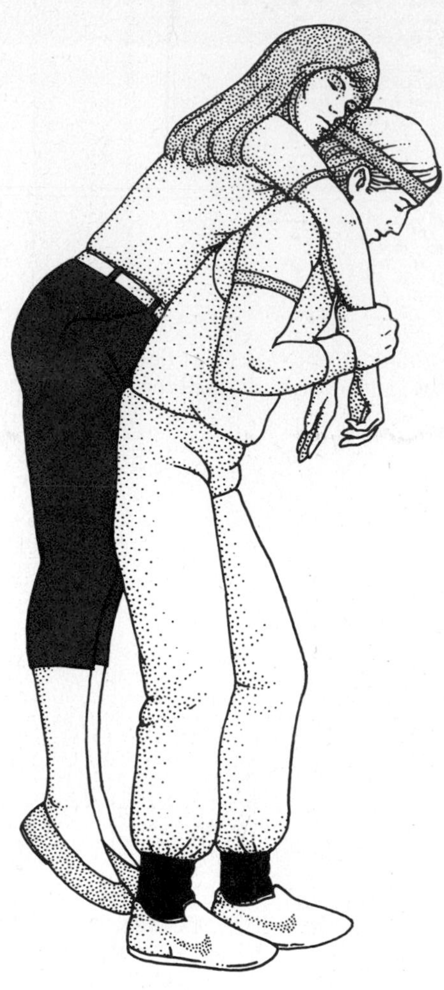

14-6. Fireman carry. If the person's injuries permit, longer distances can be traveled if the person is carried over your shoulder.

14-7. Pack-strap carry. When injuries make the fireman carry unsafe, this method is better for longer distances than the one-person lift.

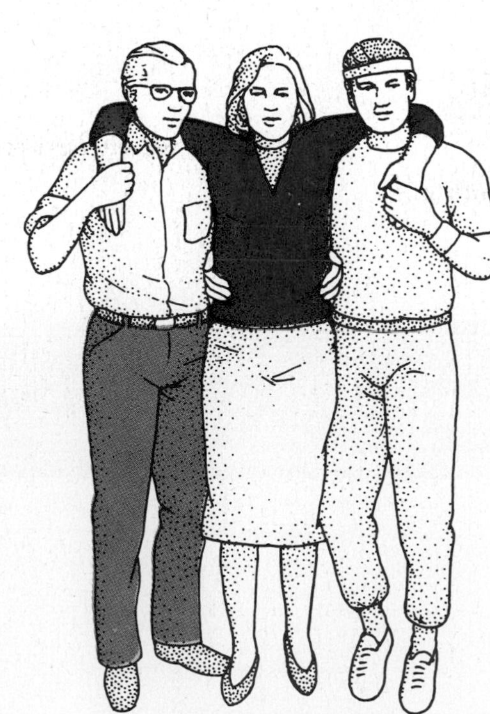

14-8. Helping the person to walk

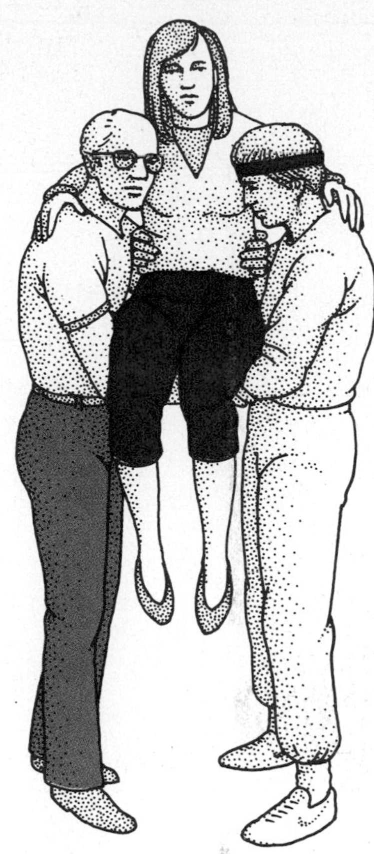

14-9. Two-handed seat carry

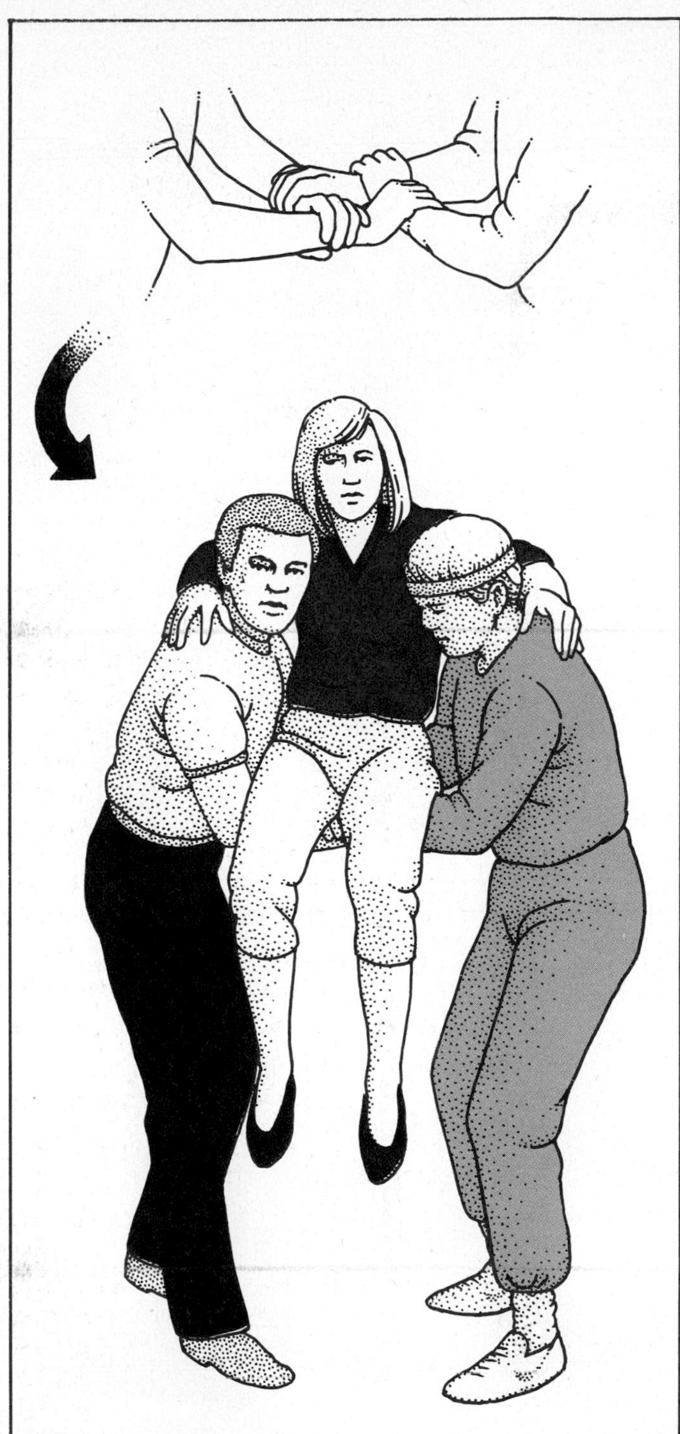

14-10. Four-handed seat carry. This is the easiest two-man carry when no equipment is available.

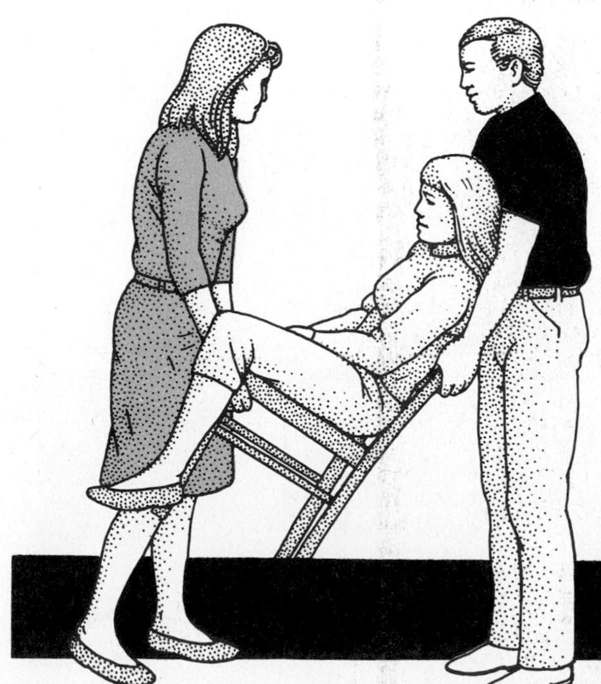

14-11. Chair carry

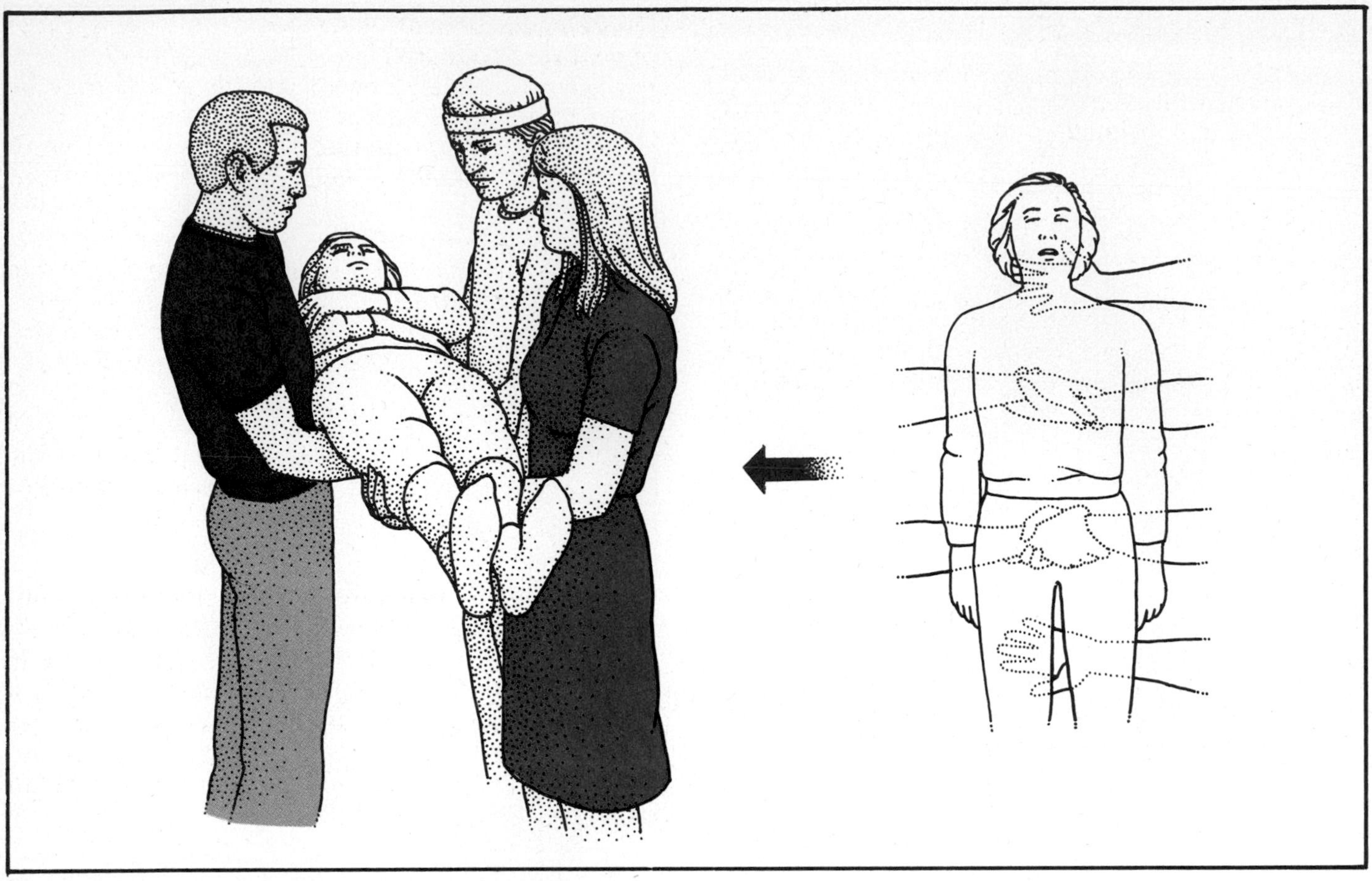

14-12. Hammock carry. Three to six people stand on alternate sides of the injured person and link hands beneath him.

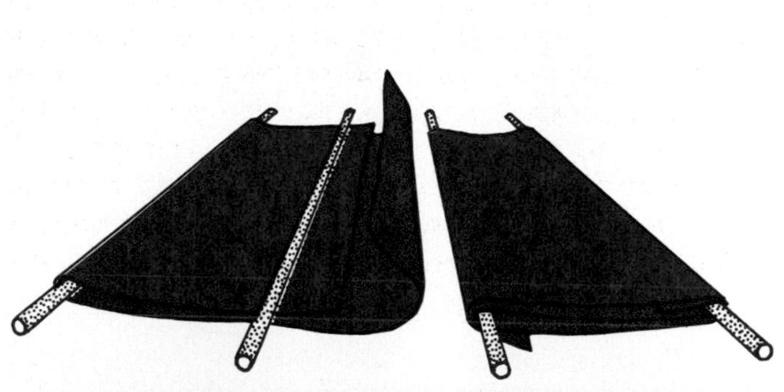

14-13. Blanket and pole improvised stretcher. If the blanket is wrapped as shown, the person's weight will keep it from unwinding.

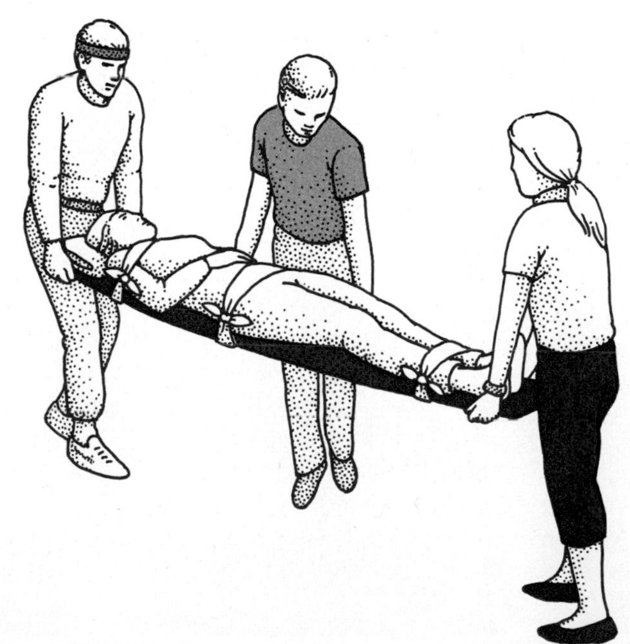

14-14. Board improvised stretcher. This is sturdier than a blanket-and-pole stretcher but heavier and less comfortable. Tie the person on to prevent rolling off.

WATER RESCUE

About 7,000 Americans die each year from drowning, making it the third leading cause of accidental death. Drowning statistics do not reflect the whole problem. An estimated 70,000 people are near-drowning victims each year. Even this figure does not give the entire picture because in many instances the victim recovers and the incident is not reported.

Since drowning situations seem to happen all the time, especially during the summer months, all adults and teenagers should be familiar with the basic rescue techniques available to poor swimmers or nonswimmers.

Reach-Throw-Row-Go

Reach-throw-row-go identifies the priority list for attempting rescue.

Reach

The first and simplest rescue technique is the reach. This method is easily mastered, but it requires the ability to judge distance accurately and a lightweight pole, ladder, long stick, or any object that can be extended to the victim. (*See* Figures 14–15(a) and 14–15(b).)

Once you have your "reacher," secure your footing. Also have a bystander grab your belt or pants for stability. Make sure you are secure before reaching down to assist the victim. Keep talking; this not only calms the victim, it helps you think through each step.

Throw

Throwing is another elementary rescue. It provides a maximum range of about fifty feet for the average untrained rescuer. You can throw anything that floats—objects such as empty fuel or paint cans, plastic containers, life jackets or floating cushions, short pieces of wood—whatever is available. If there is rope handy, tie it to the object to be thrown because you can then retrieve it in case you miss. (*See* Figure 14–15(c).)

Row

If the victim is beyond reach and you can find a nearby sailboard, boogie board, rowboat, canoe, or an outboard craft that can be started, you may attempt this form of rescue. Using these crafts requires skill only acquired through practice. In a life-or-death situation, however, even the inept use of these craft will be safer and faster than a swimming rescue. There is an element of danger for the rescuer that should be considered.

Craft powered by hand, paddle, or oar may be slower but they are safer than a motor-driven craft with which you are unfamiliar. Inexperienced hands on a throttle are more dangerous than inexperienced hands on an oar.

If rowing out to a victim, align with an object on the shoreline and in line with the victim. Fix this in your memory. Since you must row facing the opposite direction, you will need to turn your head every five or so strokes to check on the victim and your position.

Upon reaching the victim, never attempt to pull the victim in over the sides of a boat but over the stern or rear end. This has been the cause of countless double drownings. (*See* Figure 14–15(d).)

Go

If the previous "reach-throw-row" priorities are impossible to do, you must make an assessment, weighing the potential risk to yourself versus the reward to the victim. Entering even calm water to make a swimming rescue is difficult and hazardous. It takes skill, training, and excellent physical condition. All too frequently a would-be rescuer becomes a victim as well. (*See* Figure 14–15(e).)

After The Rescue

Once the victim is out of the water, protect yourself and the victim against the cold. Get into dry clothing as soon as possible. Be prepared to administer mouth-to-mouth resuscitation. All rescued victims should be seen by a physician and hospitalized because victims can die a few minutes or up to ninety-six hours or more after the incident of secondary complications. Aspiration pneumonia is a late complication of near-drowning episodes, occurring after forty-eight to seventy-two hours have elapsed.

More and more people are taking to the water in recreational activities. All adults and teenagers should be prepared to rescue those in a drowning situation.

Ice Rescue

Attempt to reach the person from shore with a long object (e.g., a branch, a rope, a board, etc.). If there is no equipment, form a human chain reaching from the shore. (*See* Figure 14–16.) Lie flat to distribute the weight. Seek medical attention immediately for someone who has fallen through broken ice.

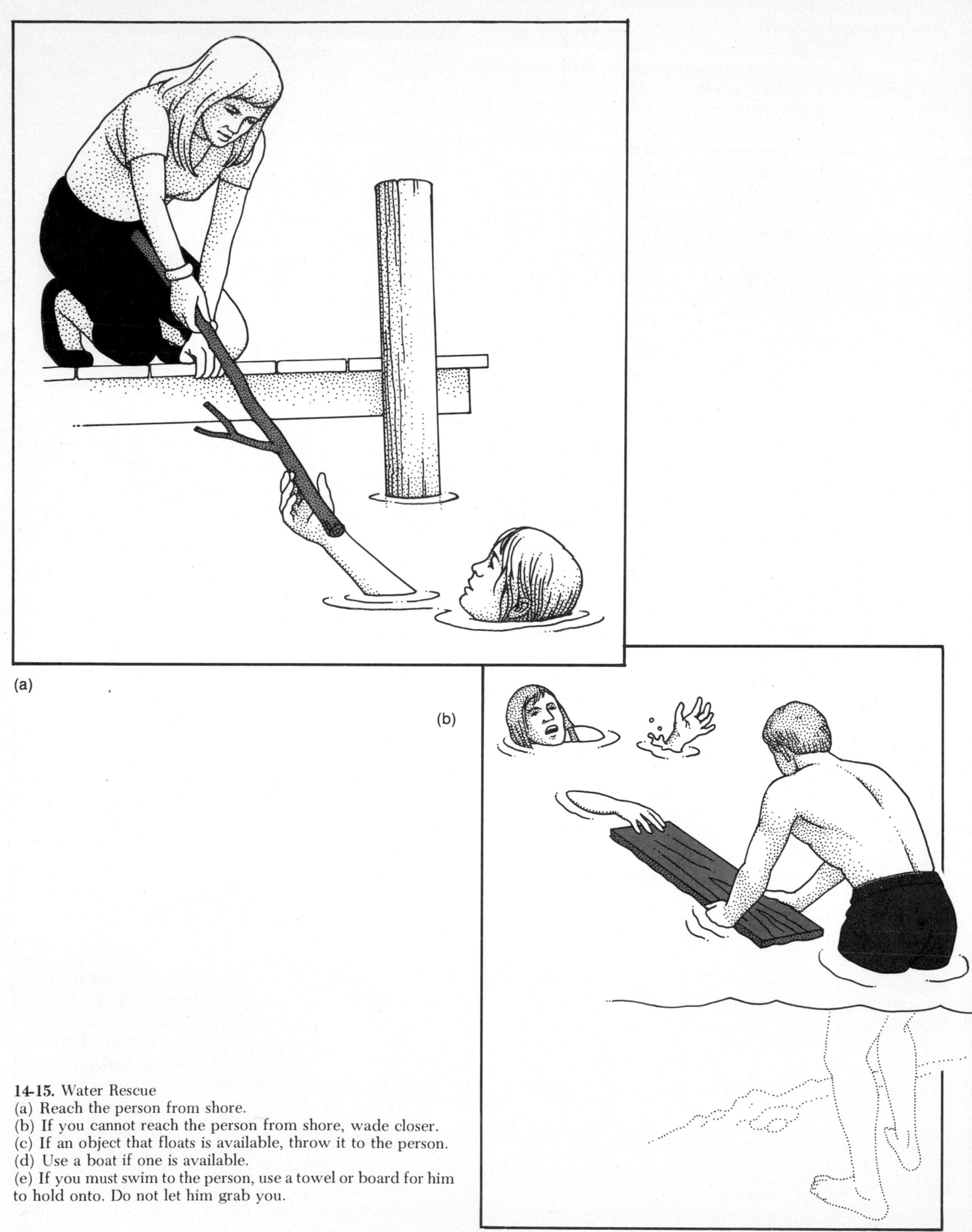

14-15. Water Rescue
(a) Reach the person from shore.
(b) If you cannot reach the person from shore, wade closer.
(c) If an object that floats is available, throw it to the person.
(d) Use a boat if one is available.
(e) If you must swim to the person, use a towel or board for him to hold onto. Do not let him grab you.

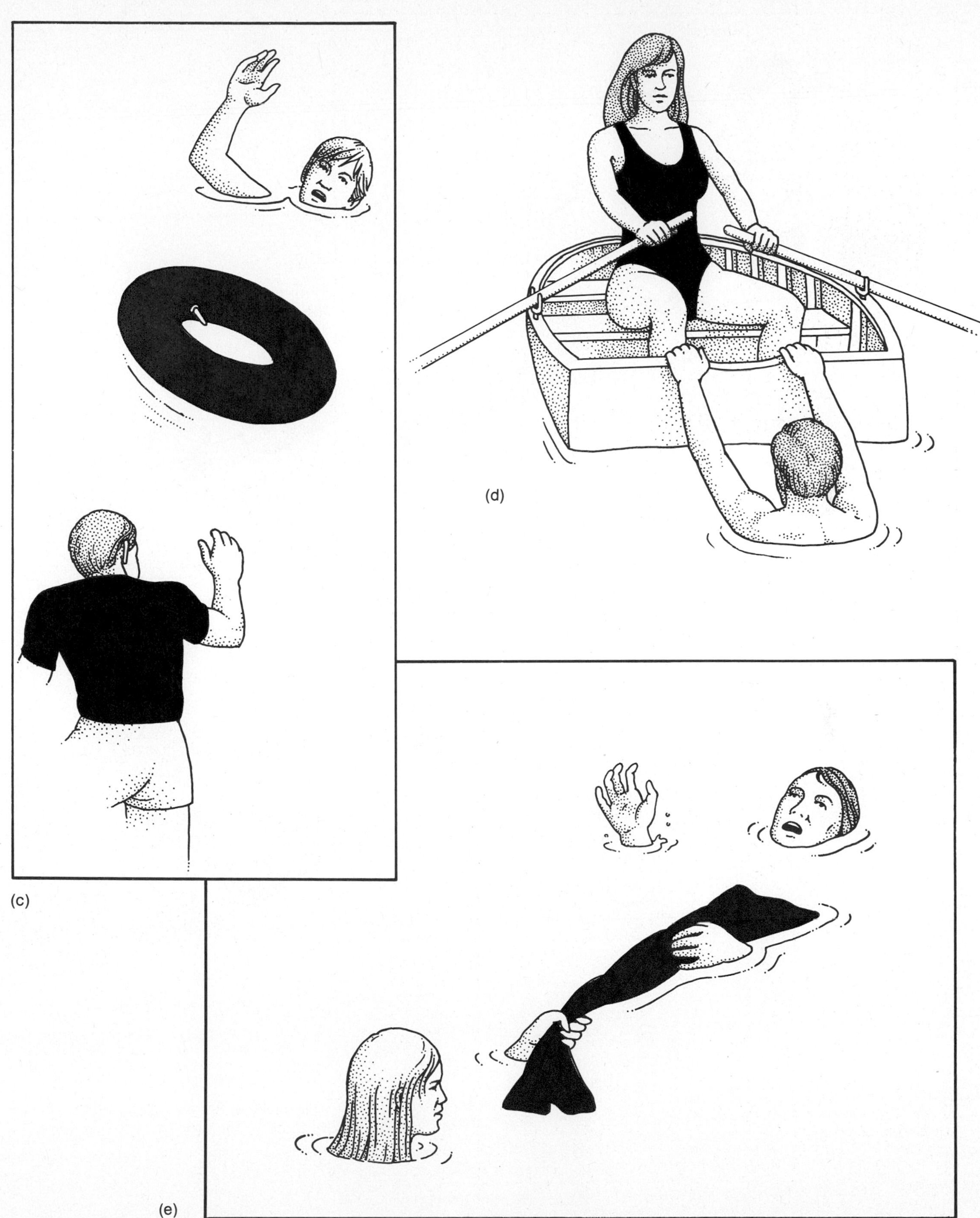
(c)
(d)
(e)

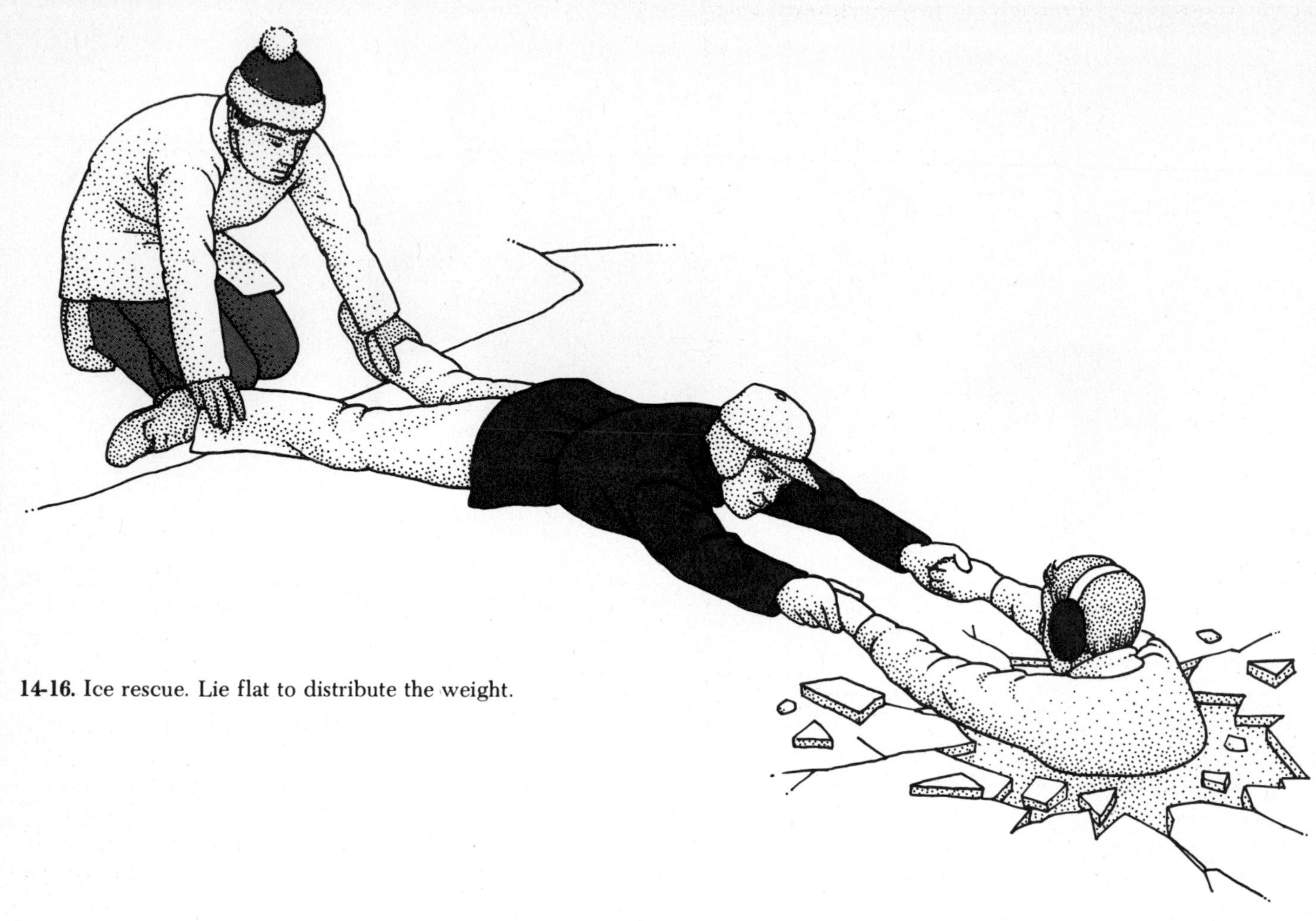

14-16. Ice rescue. Lie flat to distribute the weight.

15 Medicine Chest and First Aid Supplies

MEDICINE CHEST

It is a good idea to have useful medical supplies on hand for emergencies and to treat minor ills, but the family medicine chest does not have to be a mini-drugstore. What should be kept in the average household depends on the makeup of the family.

Generally, medicine chests should include only those health care products likely to be used on a regular basis. A person rarely bothered by constipation, for instance, would have little need for a laxative.

Some drug products lose their potency on the shelf in time, especially after they are opened. Other drugs change in consistency. Milk of magnesia, for instance, dries out if it remains on the shelf for a while after opening. Buying the large "family size" of a product not used frequently may seem like a bargain, but it is poor economy if it has to be thrown out before the contents are used up. Ideally, supplies in the medicine chest should be bought to last over a period of no more than six to twelve months.

Obviously, selecting health care items for the family medicine chest is matter of common sense. Here are some suggested items that will meet the needs of most families:

Non-Drug Products

Adhesive bandages of assorted sizes
Sterile gauze in pads and a roll
Absorbent cotton
Adhesive tape
Elastic bandage
Small blunt-end scissors
Tweezers
Fever thermometer, including rectal type for young child
Hot water bottle
Heating pad
Ice bag

Dosage spoon (common household teaspoons are rarely the correct dosage size)
Vaporizer or humidifier
First aid manual

Drug Items

Analgesic—aspirin and/or acetaminophen. Both reduce fever and relieve pain, but only aspirin can reduce inflammation.
Emetic—syrup of ipecac to induce vomiting and activated charcoal. Read the instructions on how to use these products.
Antacid
Antiseptic solution
Hydrocortisone creams for skin problems
Calamine for poison ivy and other skin irritations
Petroleum jelly as a lubricant
Antidiarrheic
Cough syrup—nonsuppressant type
Decongestant
Antibacterial topical ointment
Seasonal items, such as insect repellents and sunscreens, round out the list.

When it comes to storing these health care items, the cardinal rule is to keep all medicines out of the reach of children. In addition, be sure all medications have child-resistant caps. Elderly people who have difficulty opening such caps can ask the pharmacist for regular closure. However, they should be extra careful to see that young visitors cannot get to these drugs.

Both prescription and nonprescription drugs should be kept in a cool, dry place away from foods and other household products. Some drugs may need to be kept in the refrigerator. This should be indicated on the label. If in doubt, ask the pharmacist.

Many people keep medicines on a high shelf in a hall or bedroom closet. Some experts suggest using a locking box. A tackle box might do. A word of warning, however: Be sure all responsible adults in the family know where the key is kept.

To avoid confusion keep prescription and nonprescription drugs in separate boxes clearly labeled to distinguish one type of drug from the other. A list of what is in each box, attached to the outside if possible, will make it easier to find specific items, particularly in an emergency.

The medicine chest should be checked periodically to be sure supplies have not run low and to get rid of drugs that may have gone bad or become outdated. Many drug labels have an expiration date beyond which the product should not be used. If there is no date, put a label on the container with the date of purchase and the date it was first opened. Then, if there are any questions in the future, a pharmacist can tell whether the product is safe to use.

Tablets that have become crumbly and medicines that have changed color, odor, or consistency, or are outdated should be destroyed. Empty the bottle of medicine into the toilet, flush it down, and rinse out the bottle. Do not put leftover drugs in the trash basket where they can be dug out by inquisitive youngsters. Newly purchased drug products that do not look right should be returned to the pharmacy. Drug products that have lost their labels also should be destroyed.

Keep the telephone numbers of the local poison control center, physician, hospital, rescue squad, and fire and police departments near every phone in the house. Tape the emergency phone list inside the bathroom medicine cabinet door, and also keep it with the emergency supplies.

Each family's medicine chest is bound to contain some different items. For help in selecting appropriate health care products, check with a physician and a pharmacist.

FIRST AID SUPPLIES

Suggested First Aid Kit Contents

Activated charcoal
Adhesive strip bandages, assorted sizes
Adhesive tape, 1- and 2-inch rolls
Alcohol (70%)
Alcohol wipes
Antimicrobial skin ointment
Baking soda
Calamine lotion
Cotton balls
Elastic bandages, 2- and 3-inch widths
Epsom salts
Flashlight and extra batteries
Gauze pads, 2x2 and 4x4 inches
Hot-water bottle
Ice bag (plastic)
Matches
Measuring cup and spoons
Needles
Paper and pencil
Paper drinking cups
Roller gauze bandage, 2-inch width
Safety pins, various sizes
Salt
Scissors
Sugar
Syrup of ipecac
Thermometer—1 oral, 1 rectal
Triangular bandages, 2 or 3
Tweezers

These items can be placed in a fishing tackle box for storage and transporting.

16 Patient Education Aids

• **These are reprints of doctor-to-patient instructions for self care taken from the popular physician journal, Patient Care.**

The Patient Education Aids that follow are reproduced with the permission of Patient Care Communications, Inc., as follows:

"Understanding and treating heat disorders," reproduced with permission from *Patient Care*, May 15, 1986. Copyright © 1986, Patient Care Communications, Inc., Darien, CT. All rights reserved.

"Recognizing heart attack," reproduced with permission from *Patient Care*, November 15, 1981. Copyright © 1981, Patient Care Communications, Inc., Darien, CT. All rights reserved.

"Understanding stroke," reproduced with permission from *Patient Care*, August 15, 1982. Copyright © 1982, Patient Care Communications, Inc., Darien, CT. All rights reserved.

"Understanding diabetic emergencies," reproduced with permission from *Patient Care*, March 15, 1980. Copyright © 1980, Patient Care Communications, Inc., Darien, CT. All rights reserved.

"Questions and answers about epilepsy," reproduced with permission from *Patient Care*, October 15, 1983. Copyright © 1983, Patient Care Communications, Inc., Darien, CT. All rights reserved.

"First aid for epileptic seizures," reproduced with permission from *Patient Care*, September 15, 1983. Copyright © 1983, Patient Care Communications, Inc., Darien, CT. All rights reserved.

"Questions and answers about asthma," "Helpful hints for controlling asthma," reproduced with permission from *Patient Care*, November 15, 1981. Copyright © 1981, Patient Care Communications, Inc., Darien, CT. All rights reserved.

"Constipation," reproduced with permission from *Patient Care*, February 29, 1984. Copyright © 1984, Patient Care Communications, Inc., Darien, CT. All rights reserved.

"Home care for diarrhea," reproduced with permission from *Patient Care*, March 15, 1981. Copyright © 1981, Patient Care Communications, Inc., Darien, CT. All rights reserved.

"Tips for managing diarrhea while traveling," reproduced with permission from *Patient Care*, September 15, 1982. Copyright © 1982, Patient Care Communications, Inc., Darien, CT. All rights reserved.

"When your child has a fever," "How to take your child's temperature," reproduced with permission from *Patient Care*, September 30, 1980. Copyright © 1980, Patient Care Communications, Inc., Darien, CT. All rights reserved.

"Questions and answers about sore throat," reproduced with permission from *Patient Care*, December 15, 1980. Copyright © 1980, Patient Care Communications, Inc., Darien, CT. All rights reserved.

"Facts about the common cold," reproduced with permission from *Patient Care*, November 15, 1983. Copyright © 1983, Patient Care Communications, Inc., Darien, CT. All rights reserved.

patient care®
patient education aid

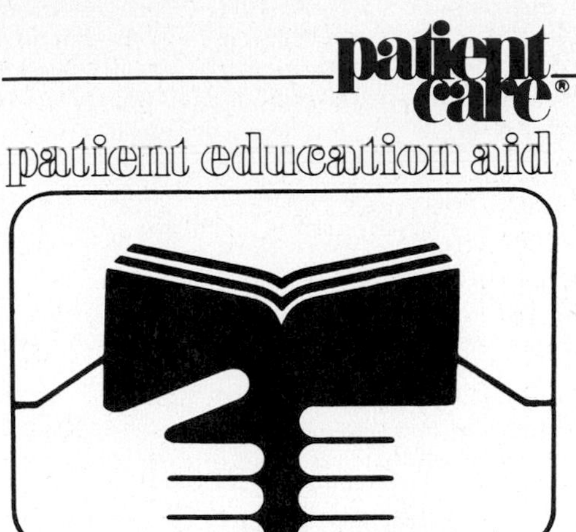

Helping your wound heal

INSTRUCTIONS

While the wound is stitched
The stitches used to close your wound will later be removed. Until then, follow these instructions to promote healing and avoid infection:
1. Keep the wound *clean* and *dry*. The doctor will tell you if you can bathe or shower.
2. If the wound has been covered with a dressing, keep the dressing clean and dry.
3. If a splint or dressing has been applied, do not remove it unless it becomes wet or dirty.
4. If the dressing becomes wet or dirty:
[ ] You can change it yourself.
[ ] Return here to have it changed for you.
If in doubt, call your doctor's office for guidance on changing the dressing.
5. Do not apply medications, lotions, ointments, or other preparations to the wound unless the doctor tells you to.
6. If you notice any of these signs of infection, call the doctor immediately:

☎ Redness, excessive swelling, tenderness, or increased warmth of the skin around the wound
☎ Red streaks in the skin near the wound
☎ Pus or watery discharge from the wound
☎ Tender bumps or swelling in your armpit or groin
☎ Foul smell from the wound
☎ Generalized body chills or fever

7. Return on ________________ at ______________
to have the wound checked and, if necessary, the dressing changed.
8. Additional instructions:
____
____
____
____

Reducing swelling
After your wound has been treated, you may have some swelling. If the wound is on your arm, hand, leg, or foot, you can help reduce swelling by keeping the injured part elevated *above the level of your heart* as much as possible. These suggestions may be useful:
≫ Elevating your hand or arm:
1. When you sleep, use three pillows—one for your head, one to elevate the injured arm, and one to bring your uninjured arm to the same level. (If you sleep on your side or your stomach, use one or both of the extra pillows to elevate your injured arm.)
2. When you are sitting, sit by a table with your elbow resting on a rolled towel, a cushion, or another soft, firm support.
3. When you are standing, rest the hand of your injured arm on top of your head. Or rest your hand on the opposite shoulder, supporting your elbow with the hand of the uninjured arm.
≫ Elevating your leg or foot:
1. When sitting, use a chair or another support that will keep your leg elevated as far as you comfortably can. If the support has a hard surface, place a soft but firm object (such as a pillow or rolled towel) on it for comfort—and added height.
2. When lying down, keep a pillow under the injured leg to elevate it.

After the stitches are out
Healing may take several weeks after the stitches are removed. Follow these guidelines until your wound is healed completely:
1. Be careful to limit your activities if your doctor advises you to. Until the wound is sufficiently healed, vigorous activity may cause it to reopen. Depending on the severity of your wound, you may have to limit certain activities for a few days to a few weeks.
2. While the wound is still red or pink, protect it from excess exposure to sunlight by applying a sunscreen. Healing wounds are more sensitive to sunlight than normal skin.
3. Do not be alarmed if the wound becomes red, slightly raised, or thickened during the first few weeks after the stitches are removed. This is normal. You may find it helpful to massage the wound gently every day. Use bland ointment such as baby oil, petrolatum (petroleum jelly), or moisturizing cream.
4. If the wound is still thickened, red, and raised or very sensitive eight weeks after your injury, consult your doctor. You may be developing excess scar, sometimes referred to as "keloid" or "hypertrophic" scar.

If you have any questions or concerns about your wound that have not been answered, feel free to call.

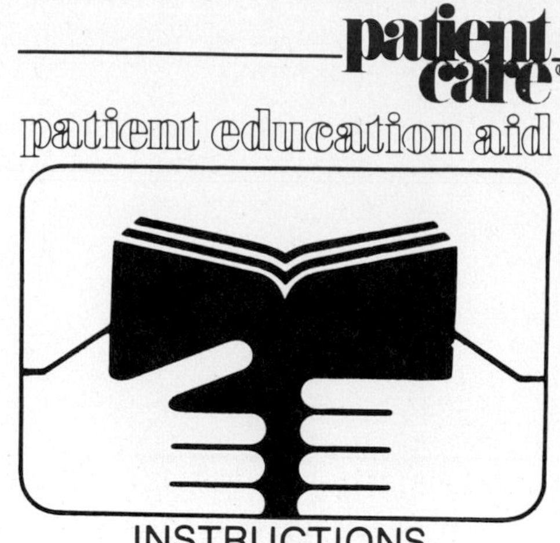

Head injury instructions

At this time, we have found no evidence that your child's head injury is serious. However, it is important that you observe him (or her) closely for the next 48 hours in case a sign of serious injury develops.

After the child goes to bed tonight, be sure to *wake him and talk to him every two hours.* Unless your doctor instructs you otherwise, you can let the child sleep through the second night.

Immediately call your doctor's office if you notice that your child has one or more of the following symptoms:

1. Unequal pupil size.

2. More than one episode of nausea or vomiting or one episode that lasts an hour or longer; mild nausea for a short time is common after a head injury.

3. Persistent trouble with vision such as blurring or double vision.

4. Severe headache after an interval of mild or no headache. Mild headache is common after head injury (see instructions on headache medication under "Further instructions," below).

5. Falling asleep easily, then being hard to arouse or appearing confused or delirious when you try to arouse.

6. Unusual awkwardness or clumsiness when walking or using hands.

7. Blood or clear fluid dripping from ears or nose.

8. Convulsions.

9. Incoherent or slurred speech.

10. Change in personality; for example, the child becomes unusually irritable.

Further instructions: Unless a doctor gives you special diet instructions, let the child eat the same food as usual. You may give acetaminophen for headache; however, give nothing else. In particular, do not give the child a sedative, tranquilizer, narcotic, or anything containing alcohol for the next 48 hours unless a physician instructs you specifically to do so.

patient care®

patient education aid

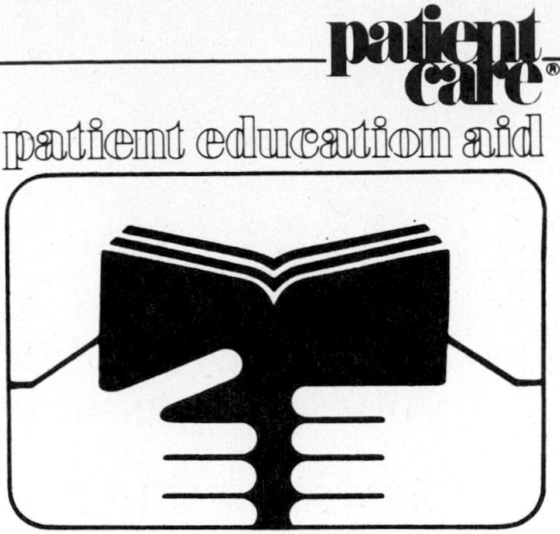

Protecting yourself against bee stings

If you've been stung by a wasp, bee, yellow jacket, or hornet, you probably want to do what you can to avoid being stung again. And if you are allergic to the venom of these insects, avoiding being stung may save your life. The following suggestions can decrease your risk of stings:

1. Wear shoes or sandals when walking outdoors.

2. Do not use after-shave lotion, perfume, cologne, or the like when you plan to spend a day or evening outdoors.

3. Whenever you can, wear slacks and a long-sleeved shirt or blouse.

4. Select summer clothing of neutral patterns and colors such as tan, white, black, or beige. Bright colors and floral patterns are attractive to bees and wasps.

5. Stay away from public picnic areas and waste cans, favorite haunts for yellow jackets.

6. After outdoor bathing, shake your towel before drying off; shake your clothing as well before putting it on.

7. Use caution when entering areas that stinging insects tend to inhabit: attics, abandoned buildings, trees and bushes, gardens, orchards, and grass.

Storing bee sting treatment kits

If you are allergic to stinging insect venom, your doctor has probably prescribed a treatment kit to use in an emergency. To get the best use from the kit:

1. Store it in a cool, dark place. If you choose the refrigerator, remember to take the kit with you when you go outdoors or on vacation.

2. Be sure to check the expiration date on the label before using the kit. If the kit includes a *glass* container of epinephrine (the drug provided with the kit), check the color of the drug. Epinephrine that is unfit for use is pinkish-brown rather than clear.

3. You might want to keep several kits in various places. For instance, you might keep one in your knapsack if you go hiking, one in your purse or the glove compartment of your car, or one at work or in your school locker in addition to one at home.

What if you do get stung?

If you are allergic to bee stings and you are stung by a bee or wasp, your treatment kit should control any allergic reaction. If you do not have a kit available, contact your doctor immediately if any of the following develop:

- ☎ Hives, flushing, or itching over large parts of your body
- ☎ Breathing difficulties, such as wheezing or hoarseness
- ☎ Tightness in your chest
- ☎ Difficulty swallowing or the feeling of a lump in your throat
- ☎ Faintness or dizziness
- ☎ Stomach cramps, vomiting, or diarrhea
- ☎ A vague feeling of illness or impending doom ☐

Additional information: ____________________

____

____

____

____

____

____

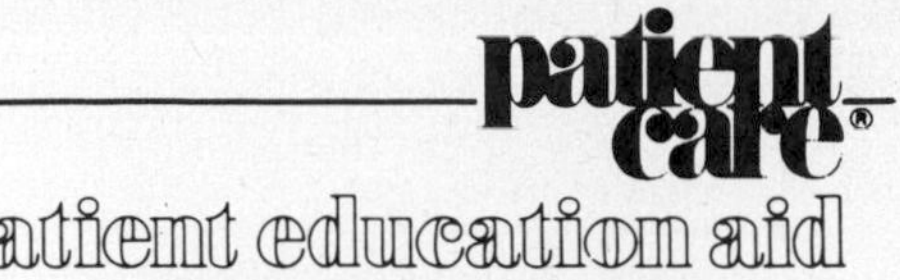

INSTRUCTIONS

Tips for protecting yourself against ticks

Most ticks are harmless. A few, however, carry infectious microorganisms that can cause serious illnesses, including Rocky Mountain spotted fever, a life-threatening disease requiring prompt treatment. If ticks are present in your area, you'll want to know how to recognize and avoid them and how to remove them, particularly if you have children or pets who roam in woods or long grass. The following information and guidelines will help protect you—and your family—against tick bite.

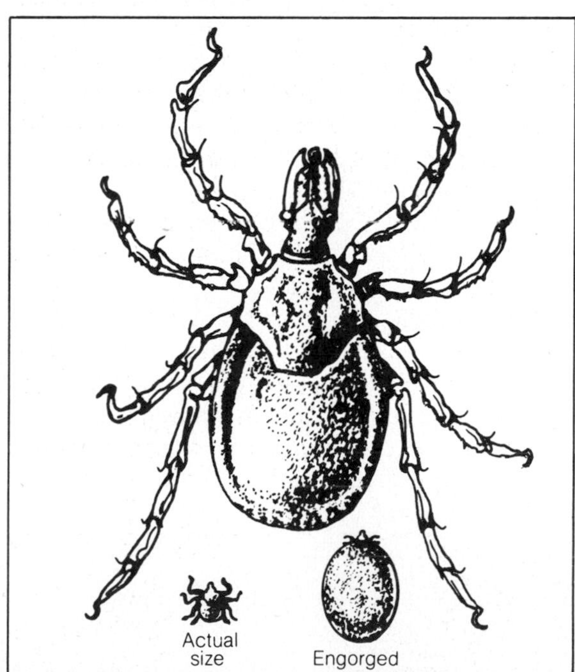

1. The tick feeds on the blood of warm-blooded animals, including man, by attaching itself to the host's skin with its mouth parts. As the tick feeds, it fills its abdomen with blood and becomes enlarged, or engorged. An engorged tick may be as large as the size of a small grape—up to almost 1 inch long.

2. When you're outdoors, be sure to wear clothing that protects your skin against ticks. Tuck the bottom of your pants inside socks or boots, and keep your blouse or shirt buttoned and your shirttails tucked in.

3. If you live in an area where ticks are prevalent, examine yourself, family members, and your pets for ticks several times a day, especially at bedtime. Part and comb through long hair to check for ticks attached to the scalp. Check clothing as soon as it is removed, before any ticks have the chance to crawl off.

4. *Remove a tick as soon as you discover it.* The longer the tick remains attached to the skin, the more likely an infection will result.

5. Use tweezers when removing a tick, or cover your fingers with a tissue; if you touch the tick, you may contaminate yourself. However, if you do not have tweezers and cannot cover your fingertips, pull the tick off right away rather than waiting and looking around for an appropriate implement.

6. To remove a tick, grasp it as close as possible to the point where it is attached to the skin. Pull firmly and steadily until the tick is dislodged, then flush it down the toilet. Avoid squashing an engorged tick during removal: Infected blood may spurt into your eyes, mouth, or into a cut on the surface of your skin.

7. Once the tick is removed, wash your hands and the bite area thoroughly with soap and water and apply an antiseptic to the area to prevent a bacterial infection.

8. If you or a member of your family develops fever with chills, headache, or muscle aches after being exposed to a tick, call your doctor right away. Such symptoms following exposure to a tick may indicate Rocky Mountain spotted fever and immediate treatment by a physician may be necessary.

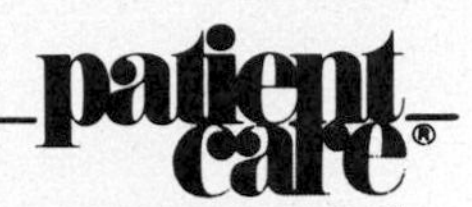

How to identify poison ivy, poison oak, and poison sumac

Being able to identify poison ivy, poison oak, and poison sumac is your best defense against the uncomfortable aftereffects of contact with these plants. The following descriptions—and the accompanying illustrations—will help you spot the offending plants before it's too late.

Poison ivy

When watching out for poison ivy, remember, "Leaflets three: Let it be!" To differentiate between poison ivy and other three-leaved plants, remember that the stem of the central leaflet of poison ivy is always longer than the stem of either of the two side leaflets. Poison ivy commonly:

≫Grows as a low plant, shrub, or climbing vine
≫Has yellow-green flowers and whitish berries
≫Produces green leaves that are shiny when they first come out, turn red and yellow toward late fall, and then drop off

Poison oak

Neither of the two poison oak varieties growing in the U.S. are actually oak plants, although their leaves are similar to those of their namesake. Western poison oak also closely resembles poison ivy. This variety is found only on the West Coast below 5,000-foot elevation levels and in low areas and wooded slopes. The more common variety also has three leaves but is found in New Jersey, Maryland, Tennessee, southern Missouri, Kansas, and south to northern Florida and Texas. It grows as a shrub, identifiable by clusters of hairy, yellowish berries. The undersides of the leaves are dense with hair.

Poison sumac

Poison sumac, another in the don't-touch category, is easy to distinguish from other harmless types of sumac:

≫Poison sumac is never found in land that is dry the year round; it prefers marshes or bogs.
≫Each leaf stalk of the poison sumac has 7-13 leaflets, while harmless sumacs may have up to 25 leaflets per stalk.
≫The leaflets of the poison sumac have smooth edges; those of its harmless relatives have saw-toothed edges.
≫Poison sumac has cream colored berries that hang from the branches in loose clusters; harmless varieties of sumac have dull red berries in tight clusters that stand upright at the twig's end.

Poison sumac is generally found east of the Mississippi River.

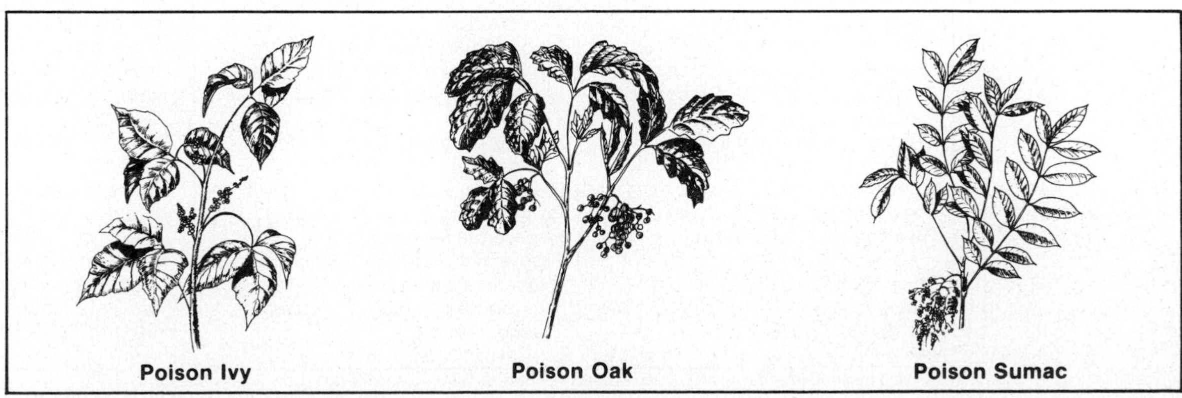

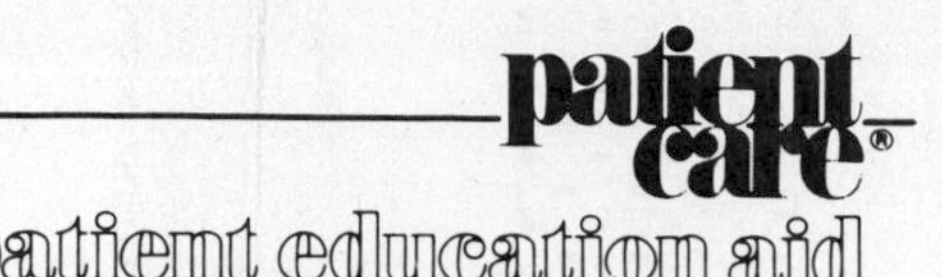

INSTRUCTIONS

Tips for safeguarding your family from plant poisoning

1. Train children not to put strange plants in their mouths; allow them to eat only plants that are given to them as food. (Check the list of poisonous or suspect berries or fruits on page 235.)

2. Keep all house plants and plant materials out of reach of very young children.

3. When you buy plants, ask about toxicity; if you have young children, buy only nontoxic plants. (A list of nontoxic plants is given below.)

4. Do not use branches of unknown plants or of plants known to be poisonous as skewers for roasting foods.

5. Do not eat any part of any plant (roots, stalks, leaves, flowers, berries, bark) unless you are absolutely certain it is edible.

6. Do not assume that a plant is safe for you to eat simply because animals have been observed eating it.

Nontoxic plants (recommended for households with young children)*

African violet *Saintpaulia ionantha*
Aluminum plant *Pilea cadierei*
Begonia *Begonia* spp.
Bloodleaf plant *Iresine* spp.
Boston fern *Nephrolepsis exaltata bostoniensis*
Chenille-plant (red-hot cattail) *Acalypha hispida*
Chinese evergreen *Aglaonema modestum*
Christmas cactus *Schlumbergera bridgesii*
Coleus *Coleus* spp.
Corn plant *Dracaena fragrans massangeana*
Creeping Charley *Pilea nummularifolia*
Crocus *Crocus* spp.
Devil's-walking-stick (Hercules' club) *Aralia spinosa*
Donkey tail (burro's tail) *Sedum morganianum*
Dusty Miller *Senecio cineraria*
Dwarf orchid cactus *Epiphyllum*
Dwarf palm (parlor palm) *Chamaedorea elegans*
False aralia *Dizygotheca elegantissima*
Gardenia *Gardenia* spp.
Geranium *Geranium* spp. or *Pelargonium* spp.
Grape hyacinth *Muscari botryoides*
Hawaiian ti *Cordyline terminalis*
Hen-and-chickens *Sempervivum tectorum*
Hibiscus *Hibiscus* spp.
Honeysuckle *Lonicera* spp.
Impatiens *Impatiens* spp.
Inch plant (Wandering Jew) *Tradescantia fluminensis*
Jade plant *Crassula argentea*
Lady's slipper *Cypripedium* spp.
Lilac *Syringa* spp.
Lipstick plant *Aeschynanthus lobbianus*
Magnolia *Magnolia* spp.
Monkey plant *Ruellia Makoyana*
Moses-in-the-cradle *Rhoeo spathacea*
Mother-in-law-tongue *Sansevieria trifasciata*
Palm *Palmaceae* spp.
Patient Lucy *Impatiens Sultanii*
Peperomia *Peperomia* spp.
Piggyback plant *Tolmiea menziesii*
Pilea *Pilea* spp.
Pink polka-dot plant *Hypoestes sanguinolenta*
Prayer plant *Maranta leuconeura kerchoviana*
Pregnant plant *Kalanchoe daigremontiana*
Rattlesnake plant *Calathea insignis*
Rose *Rosa* spp.
Rose begonia (wax begonia) *Begonia semperflorens*
Rose of Sharon *Hibiscus syriacus*
Rubber plant *Ficus elastica*
Sensitive plant (touch-me-not) *Mimosa pudica*
Snake plant *Sansevieria* spp.
Snapdragon *Antirrhinum* spp.
Spider plant *Anthericum* spp. or *Chlorophytum* spp.
Swedish ivy *Plectranthus australis*
Thanksgiving cactus *Zygocactus truncatus*
Umbrella tree *Brassaia actinophylla Schefflera*
Violet *Viola* spp.
Wandering Jew *Zebrina pendula* or *Tradescantia fluminensis*
Wax plant *Hoya carnosa*
Weeping fig *Ficus benjamina*

*List supplied by Long Island Regional Poison Control Center, Nassau County Medical Center, East Meadow, N.Y.

7. Do not store plants, particularly bulbs that could be mistaken for onions or garlic, in the same areas used for storing food.

8. Get to know the poisonous plants that exist in your area.

9. Keep ipecac syrup and activated charcoal in the medicine cabinet.

10. Learn the telephone number of your local poison control center and keep it where you can find it quickly.

Beware of these berries!*

Poisonous berries or fruits

Apple of Peru *Nicándra physalodes*
Balsam pear *Momordica charantia*
Baneberry *Actacea* spp.
Belladonna *Atropa belladonna*
Betel nut *Areca cathecu*
Bittersweet *Celastrus scandens*
Blue cohosh *Caulophyllum thalictroides***
Chinaberry *Melia azedarach*
Coontie, Florida arrowroot *Zamia* spp.
Coyotillo *Karwinskia humboldtiana*
Cycad, false sago palm *Cycas circinalis*
Daphne *Daphne mezereum*
English ivy *Hedera helix*
Jessamine *Cestrum* spp.
Lantana *Lantana* spp.
Manchineel *Hippomane mancinella*
Mistletoe *Phoradendron serotinum*
Moonseed *Menispermum canadense*
Nightshade *Solanum* spp.
Ochrosia plum *Ochrosia elliptica*
Pigeonberry *Duranta repens*
Poison ivy, oak, sumac *Toxicodendron* spp.
Poisonwood *Metopium toxiferum*
Purge nut *Jatropha*

**Berries are poisonous; roasted seeds are safe and may substitute for coffee beans.

Strawberry bush *Euonymus* spp.
Strychnine *Strychnos nux-vomica*
Tiger apple *Thevetia peruviana*
Tung nut, candlenut *Aleurites fordii*
Virginia creeper *Parthenocissus quinquefolia*
Yew—ground hemlock, seed portion of berry only *Taxus* spp.

Plants with berries that sometimes may be poisonous

Akee *Blighia sapida*
Akia *Wikstroemia* spp.
Ampelopsis, cissus *Ampelopsis* spp.
Asparagus *Asparagus officinalis*
Blackberry lily *Belamcanda chinensis*
Buckthorn, cascara *Rhamnus* spp.
Buffalo nut *Pyrularia pubera*
Cashew apple *Anacardium occidentale*—raw nut may be poisonous
Chili pepper *Capsicum frutescens*
Christmas berry *Schinus terebinthifolius*
Clintonia *Clintonia borealis*
Devilwood, osmanthus *Osmanthus* spp.
Downy myrtle, finger cherry *Rhodomyrtus* spp.
False Solomon's seal, scurvyberry *Smilacina racemosa*
Firethorn, pyracantha *Pyracantha* spp.
Fishtail palm *Caryota* spp.
Fringe tree, old man's beard *Chionanthus virginica*
Holly *Ilex* spp.
Indian cucumber *Medeola virginiana*
Lily-of-the-valley (wild) *Maianthemum canadense*
Lily turf *Liriope* spp.
Mandarin, wild cucumber, liverberry, twisted stalk, scootberry *Streptopus* spp.
Mast-wood *Calophyllum inophyllum*
Nandina *Nandina domestica*
Pawpaw, dog apple *Asimina* spp.
Pitch apple *Clusis rosea*
Privet *Ligustrum* spp.
Queen palm *Arecastrum romanzoffianum*
Rouge plant *Rivina humilis*
Sarsparilla, Hercules' club, spikenard (poisonous if raw, generally safe if cooked, used in making jelly) *Aralia* spp.
Snowberry, waxberry *Symphoricarpos* spp.
Soapberry *Sapindus*
Solomon's seal *Polygonatum* spp.
Stinking cedar *Torreya* spp.
Supplejack *Berchemia scandens*
Tallowwood plum, hogplum (considered more dangerous if eaten raw) *Ximenia americana*
Trillium, wake-robin *Trillium* spp.

*Not all fruits commonly referred to as "berries" are berries in the strict botanical sense. This list includes fleshy and nonfleshy fruits botanically classified as drupes, pomes, and other fruits, as well as "true" berries. Some are known to be poisonous, and others are suspect or are poisonous in certain circumstances.

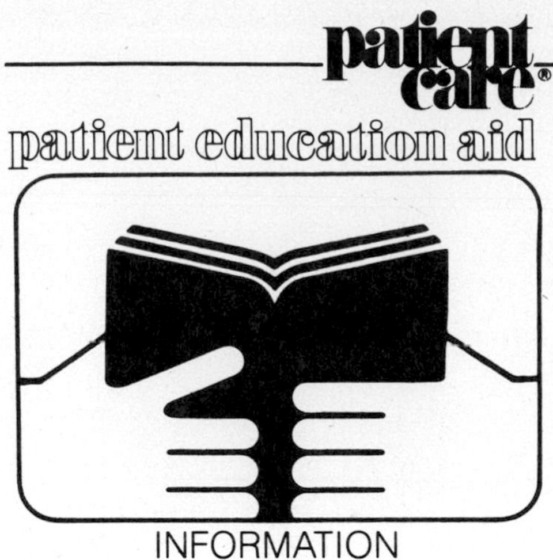

Questions and answers about carbon monoxide poisoning

What is carbon monoxide?
Carbon monoxide is a gas that is a by-product of burning fuel. It is given off from automobiles; campfires; coal, oil, and gas furnaces; and charcoal and kerosene heaters. The smoke from cigarettes also contains carbon monoxide. Carbon monoxide can be dangerous if you breathe too much of it. But because it is colorless, odorless, and tasteless, you may not be aware it is present in the air you breathe. Be extremely careful of this danger in poorly ventilated or closed spaces.

How is carbon monoxide dangerous to humans?
When you inhale air into your lungs, oxygen is transferred from the air to your blood. Oxygen attaches to a component of blood called hemoglobin; the hemoglobin carries the oxygen to the body's tissues. Carbon monoxide is also capable of attaching to the hemoglobin in the blood. If the air you breathe contains carbon monoxide (or if you inhale it in cigarette smoke), the carbon monoxide attaches to the hemoglobin in place of oxygen.

How dangerous is carbon monoxide poisoning?
Carbon monoxide poisoning can be fatal; you have probably heard of accidental or intentional deaths from exposure to carbon monoxide. In such cases, the carbon monoxide level in the blood became so high that the person could not get enough oxygen to stay alive. This may happen if an automobile is run in a closed garage or if a heater (especially charcoal) designed for outdoor use is used in a tightly closed room or house. This danger is also present if the recently developed kerosene heaters are used incorrectly.

Sometimes, people are exposed to carbon monoxide in amounts that do not threaten their lives, but do make them feel dizzy or sick. Since the symptoms are indistinguishable from those of a viral infection such as the flu (headache, nausea, chills, dizziness, tiredness), the person may not even realize what is causing the discomfort.

What would make me suspect carbon monoxide is causing me to feel sick?
Carbon monoxide may be present in your blood in high enough levels to cause a headache or other discomfort if you:

- Are in a closed but running car with a faulty exhaust system
- Live in a house with a faulty fireplace or furnace flue
- Use a kerosene heater that is not properly vented
- Use a charcoal heater in a closed space
- Work in a poorly ventilated space with gasoline- or diesel-powered vehicles

You are most likely to feel sick if two or more of these conditions are combined. Also, as suggested, smoking can be an aggravating factor.

For example, if you are a heavy smoker who drives a long distance in a closed car with a faulty exhaust system, you would have a higher carbon monoxide level in your blood than you would if you did not smoke.

What are the signs of carbon monoxide poisoning?

In low levels, carbon monoxide can cause such symptoms as headache, nausea, and tiredness. As the blood level increases, the person may complain of poor vision, may be dizzy, and may vomit. He or she may be in a stupor or experience convulsions. Eventually, he will lose consciousness and stop breathing if ventilation is not restored.

What should I do if I suspect carbon monoxide poisoning?

If you suspect carbon monoxide poisoning, remove the person from the source of the carbon monoxide, put out any fire, and ventilate the area. Then, base your actions on the patient's condition:

≫ If the person is conscious, take him to a doctor who will perform a blood test to determine the level of carbon monoxide.

≫ If the person is unconscious, place him on his side with his head resting on his arm. Loosen tight clothing and maintain body heat with a blanket. Call a doctor or an ambulance.

≫ If the person has stopped breathing, administer artificial respiration if you have been trained in cardiopulmonary resuscitation. Have someone call a doctor or an ambulance.

Even when you are certain that only mild symptoms, such as headache or nausea, are due to carbon monoxide, it may be a good idea to check with a doctor. You may be mistaken about the cause of the symptoms, and, in any event, the doctor can offer helpful advice about avoiding future exposure.

How can carbon monoxide poisoning be avoided?

You can lessen your risk of carbon monoxide poisoning by following the guidelines listed below:

1. Keep your car's exhaust system maintained by regular examination and replacement when needed.

2. Have your furnace serviced by a qualified person once a year.

3. If you are an auto mechanic or otherwise work indoors with gasoline- or diesel-powered vehicles, insist that your employer provide safe, well-ventilated working conditions.

4. If you use a kerosene heater, be sure that you follow the instructions provided by the manufacturer to the letter.

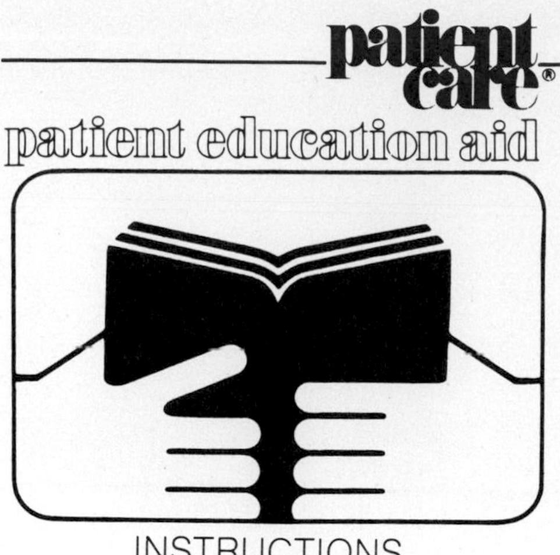

Tips for protecting yourself against sunburn

Sunbathing sensibly is an important protection against the harmful effects of the sun's rays for everyone, not only the fair skinned. You can enjoy developing a good tan this summer without sunburn disrupting your activities if you follow these simple guidelines:

1. Plan to sunbathe before 10 AM and after 2 PM. The sun rays that burn and may cause skin cancer after years of exposure are most intense two hours before and two hours after noon. Remember that during Daylight Savings Time, "noon" becomes 1 PM.

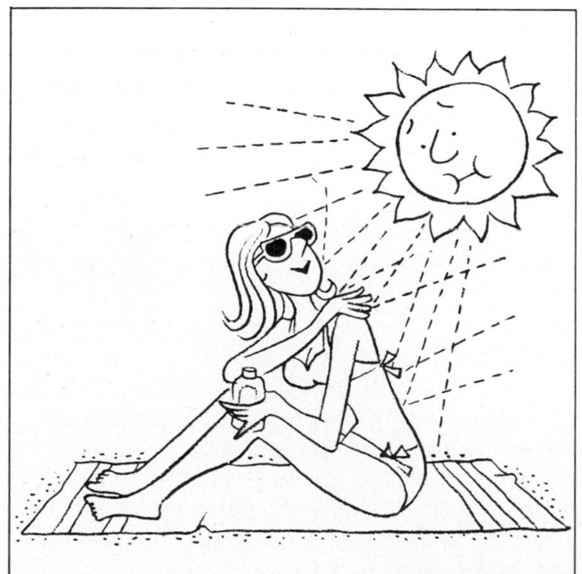

2. Use one of the many sunscreens on the market. You can select a preparation according to its sun-protection factor—2 to 15 or higher—which is printed on the label. The higher the number, the greater the protection. For instance, using a sunscreen with a protection factor of 10 generally means that you can stay in the sun without reddening 10 times longer than you could otherwise. If you are very fair skinned or have had skin cancers, use a product with a sun-protection factor of 15 or higher. If you tan easily, a preparation with a lower sun-protection factor is appropriate. Don't consider that you need little or no protection if you tan easily. Your skin will still absorb light energy and develop more wrinkling, freckling, and aging than the skin of those who protect their skin.

3. Swimming and perspiration can remove much of the sunscreen you initially apply, so be sure to reapply the preparation 1-2 times while you are in the sun.

4. Don't use preparations that dye the skin. They provide no photoprotection and merely stain the skin. Since the resultant brownish coloration is not a protective tan, you may develop a severe sunburn.

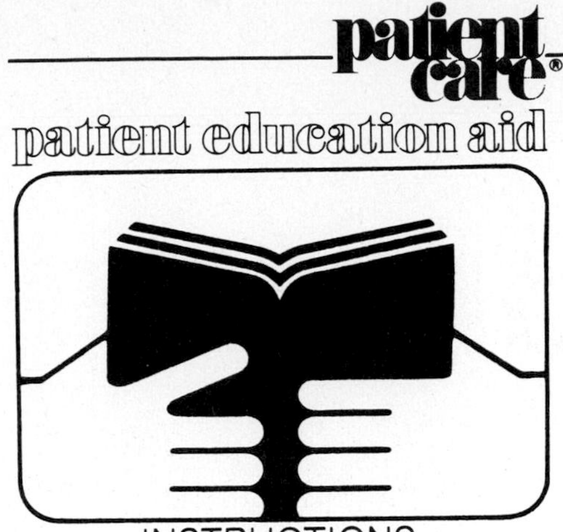

First aid for burns

Emergency Phone Numbers

Fire department ____________

Physician ____________

Emergency room ____________

Prompt first aid for a burn injury can minimize its severity and may even save a life. Become familiar with these first-aid instructions. Read them several times, then post them in a convenient spot.

Remember, the principles behind providing first aid for a burn are to relieve pain and to stop the burning process. Important basic steps are:

1. *Immediately move the victim from the source of the burn.*

2. *Place the burned area under cool, running tap water (see "How to apply cool water to the burned area"). Use cool compresses, refreshed frequently under cool water, on areas difficult to immerse in running water.*

3. *Get help quickly.*

Here are more specific first-aid steps for the four kinds of burns—those caused by flame, scalding water or other liquid, electricity, and chemicals.

Burns caused by flames

1. Move the victim away from the flames. Air feeds a fire, so do not let a person whose clothes are on fire run around.

2. Immediately spray the victim with water or wrap the burned person in a blanket, a heavy coat, or a rug.

3. If the flames were caused by a flammable liquid such as gasoline, make the burned individual avoid exposure to heat or to the fire. Either could cause clothing to reignite.

4. Spray the fire itself with water or smother it with a heavy blanket, rug, sand, or baking soda.

CAUTION: Always use baking soda to extinguish a grease fire. Water not only *does not* extinguish grease fires but can make the flaming grease splatter.

5. Remove any of the victim's clothing that is soaked by flammable substances.

6. Cool the burned area with cool, running water or cool compresses.

Burns caused by scalding

1. Remove the victim from the hot water or other liquid.

2. Remove any wet clothing.

3. Cool the burned area with cool, running water or cool compresses.

> **CAUTION:** Water does not have to be boiling to cause scalding. Water at 160°F (71.1°C) can burn through all layers of skin in one second. Even water at 125°F (51.6°C) can cause a severe burn, but it takes 2-3 minutes. *Be sure your water heater is set no higher than 124°F (51.1°C).* (In some cases the utility company must be called to reset the temperature.)

Burns caused by electricity
1. *Before touching the victim, stop the source of the current*, if possible, by unplugging the appliance or shutting off the electricity at the fuse box. This is important to avoid injury to the rescuer.

2. Use a dry towel, dry rope, or some other nonconductive means of avoiding direct contact to carefully remove the victim from the electrical current.

3. Cool the burned area with cool, running water or cool compresses.

Burns caused by chemicals
1. When a chemical such as lye or acid causes a burn, place all areas of burned skin under cool, running water. For an acid burn, irrigate the injured area for 15 minutes; for lye, irrigate for one hour.

2. Summon help after beginning the irrigation for a burn caused by lye. Do not wait until irrigation is completed.

How to apply cool water to the burned area
Hold the injured area under cool (about 55°F [12.7°C])—not cold—running water, immerse it in a sink or tub, or apply cool compresses (rewet frequently to keep cool). *Do not* apply burn creams, ointments, or other home remedies such as butter, lard, milk, or petroleum jelly.

If the person was burned by molten tar, first use very cold water or ice. Cold rapidly cools the tar and makes it brittle. Brush or flake it off the burned area, and then change to *cool* water.

For severe burns (and those caused by lye), summon help as soon as you've started the cooling process. For a small burn (less than the size of the victim's palm) that is red with no signs of blistering or loss of skin, continue cooling until the burned person reports no pain when removed from the water.

How to get help
Call your doctor, an emergency medical squad, or take the victim to the emergency room if the burn is larger than the size of the victim's palm, if blistering or loss of skin occurs, if there are other severe injuries, or if the person is unconscious. While waiting for an ambulance and en route to the hospital, keep the victim wrapped in a blanket or coat to protect him from being chilled. Do not be afraid of touching the wound with the blanket; contact is less harmful to the victim than loss of too much body heat.

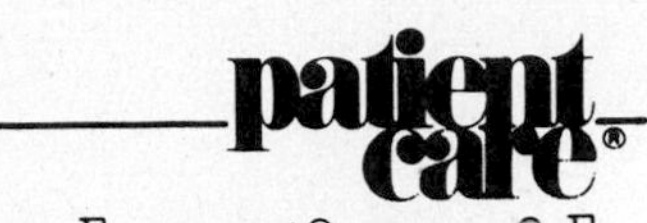

INSTRUCTIONS

Caring for a burn injury at home

Following are instructions for caring for a burn wound that your doctor says may be treated at home. Gently bathe the wounded area(s) every 24 hours, and reapply the dressings as demonstrated in the doctor's office or emergency room and as reviewed here. Especially if the person burned is a child, explain all the procedures as you change the dressing, asking for assistance and cooperation. If you have any questions, call your doctor.

Equipment you will need

A workable area with a clean, flat surface in a warm room
A bathtub, sink, or small basin
Strong abrasive cleanser
Mild detergent
A pair of bandage scissors
Aluminum foil
Clean washcloth and towel
A small, clean cup
A tongue blade
Bandages (Kerlix) and silver sulfadiazine cream (Silvadene)

Procedure

To prepare the work area and dressings:

1. Wash the tub, sink, or basin with a strong abrasive cleanser and rinse thoroughly with water.
2. Wash your hands thoroughly with soap and water.
3. Prepare the clean dressings for application:
≫ Take a 30-inch length of aluminum foil and lay it on a clean, firm, flat surface.
≫ Unroll enough bandage on the foil to cover the burn area.
≫ Using a tongue blade, spread silver sulfadiazine on the bandage. A generous tablespoonful covers 10-12 inches of gauze.
≫ Cut this portion from the roll.
≫ Cut off enough dry bandage to wrap the wound 6-7 times.
4. Fill the tub, sink, or basin with lukewarm water and ¼ cup of mild detergent.

To wash the wound and change the dressings:

1. Remove the old dressings by cutting off the outer layer and then rolling off the rest. *Do not* pull the dressing off if it is sticking to the wound; soak it off in the tub.
2. Soak the burn for 10-15 minutes in the detergent solution. Gently wash over the burned area with a soft washcloth to remove any old blood, cream, loose skin, or dry, yellow matter.
3. Using a small cup, rinse the wound with clear water. Pat the area dry with a freshly laundered soft towel. (This towel should not be used by anyone else in the family until the wound is healed.)
4. Dress the largest area first. Cover the wound with one layer of bandage treated with silver sulfadiazine, and wrap snugly with 6-7 layers of dry bandage.
5. Wash tub, sink, or basin again with a strong cleanser and rinse with water.
6. Launder towel so it will be clean and ready to use in 24 hours.

Call your doctor immediately:

☎ If the patient develops a fever of 102°F (38.9°C) or higher, and if it persists for 18-24 hours

☎ If redness or red streaking occurs around the wound

☎ If pain increases

Your next appointment is ____________.
Do not change the dressing on the day of your appointment.

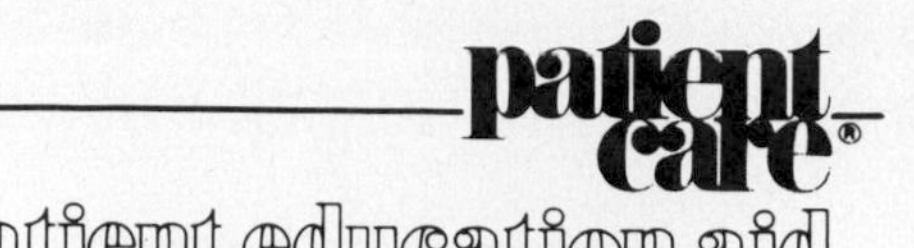

INFORMATION

How to avoid frostbite

General information

A person gets frostbite when a part of the body freezes. The areas most often affected are the hands, feet, ears, nose, and cheeks.

To avoid frostbite, protect yourself against cold and also against dampness and wind. Moisture on the skin makes the body lose heat faster. This is true whether the dampness comes from rain, snow, or perspiration. Thus, one important rule for avoiding frostbite in cold weather is: Stay dry.

Wind also steals heat from the skin. If the thermometer reads 20 °F (−6.7 °C) and the wind speed is 20 mph, exposed parts of your body lose heat as fast as they would if it were −10 °F (−23.3 °C). This is called the *windchill factor.* The harder the wind blows, the colder it feels.

You can find the windchill factor by looking up the outside temperature and wind speed on the chart below. To get an idea of how hard the wind

Windchill factors

Wind can chill exposed skin, making a cold temperature feel even colder and increasing the risk of frostbite. To find out how cold the windchill factor makes it seem outside, find today's temperature at the left and read across to the column for today's wind speed. In that box, you'll find the windchill temperature in degrees Fahrenheit (and, in parentheses, degrees Celsius).

Actual temperature	**Estimated wind speed in mph (and kph)**									**Danger of frostbite**
	calm	**5 (8)**	**10 (16)**	**15 (24)**	**20 (32)**	**25 (40)**	**30 (48)**	**35 (56)**	**40 (64)**	
50°F (10°C)	50 (10)	48 (8.9)	40 (4.4)	36 (2.2)	32 (0)	30 (−1.1)	28 (−2.2)	27 (−2.8)	26 (−3.3)	LITTLE DANGER (for properly clothed person) Maximum danger from false sense of security
40°F (4.4°C)	40 (4.4)	37 (2.8)	28 (−2.2)	22 (−5.6)	18 (−7.8)	16 (−8.9)	13 (−10.6)	11 (−11.7)	10 (−12.2)	
30°F (−1.1°C)	30 (−1.1)	27 (−2.8)	16 (−8.9)	9 (−12.8)	4 (−15.5)	0 (−17.8)	−2 (−18.9)	−4 (−20)	−6 (−21.1)	
20°F (−6.7°C)	20 (−6.7)	16 (−8.9)	4 (−15.5)	−5 (−20.5)	−10 (−23.3)	−15 (−26.1)	−18 (−27.8)	−20 (−28.9)	−21 (−29.4)	
10°F (−12.2°C)	10 (−12.2)	6 (−14.4)	−9 (−22.8)	−18 (−27.8)	−25 (−31.6)	−29 (−33.9)	−33 (−36.1)	−35 (−37.2)	−37 (−38.3)	INCREASING DANGER from freezing of exposed flesh
0°F (−17.8°C)	0 (−17.8)	−5 (−20.5)	−24 (−31.1)	−32 (−35.5)	−39 (−39.4)	−44 (−42.2)	−48 (−44.4)	−51 (−46.1)	−53 (−47.2)	
−10°F (−23.3°C)	−10 (−23.3)	−15 (−26.1)	−33 (−36.1)	−45 (−42.7)	−53 (−47.2)	−59 (−50.5)	−63 (−52.7)	−67 (−55)	−69 (−56.1)	
−20°F (−28.9°C)	−20 (−28.9)	−26 (−32.2)	−46 (−43.3)	−58 (−50)	−67 (−55)	−74 (−58.8)	−79 (−61.6)	−82 (−63.3)	−85 (−65)	GREAT DANGER
−30°F (−34.4°C)	−30 (−34.4)	−36 (−37.7)	−58 (−50)	−72 (−57.7)	−82 (−63.3)	−88 (−66.6)	−94 (−70)	−98 (−72.2)	−100 (−73.3)	

is blowing, use these rules of thumb:

≫ If you can feel the wind on your face, the speed is at least 10 mph.

≫ If the wind moves small branches or blows dust or snow around, the speed is about 20 mph.

≫ If large branches are moving, the speed is about 30 mph.

≫ If whole trees bend with the wind, the speed is at least 40 mph.

Selecting clothing for cold weather

Proper clothing for winter weather insulates you from cold, lets perspiration evaporate, and protects against wind, rain, and snow. If possible, wear several layers of light, loose clothing that will trap air yet provide adequate ventilation. Trapped air is a very effective insulator. Avoid wearing one bulky, heavy, or constricting coat. Wool fabric and polyester substitutes for down provide some protection when wet. Cotton, goose down, and duck down do not.

For ideal protection in very cold weather, wear underclothing made of wool or propylene, a substance used in making synthetic materials. Over that, wear layers of wool or synthetic down. As an outer layer, wear something that is water-repellent and windproof. Waterproof clothing that holds in perspiration is not recommended; weather-resistant fabrics like Gore-Tex keep outside water out but allow inside moisture to escape.

Protect your head and neck with a scarf and a hat or hood, and protect your face with a mask. Wear two pairs of socks. It is best to have both pairs made of wool or one of cotton and the other of wool. To protect your feet, wear well-fitted boots high enough to cover the ankles.

Mittens protect your hands better than gloves. On the other hand, mittens limit what you can do with your fingers. If you find yourself taking off your mittens often because they get in your way, consider wearing lightweight gloves under mittens. That way, you will still have protection against heat loss if you remove the mittens.

Be sure your clothing is not tight. Anything that cuts down blood flow to your arms and legs will make it harder to keep them warm and increase the risk of frostbite. For the same reason, do not remain in a sitting or kneeling position for long periods; doing so can reduce circulation of blood. Smoking can also reduce circulation, because it constricts your blood vessels. Avoid smoking if you are out in the cold for long.

If you become stranded in your car

Many people suffer frostbite when their cars break down in freezing weather. Be sure to keep protective clothing in your car if there is any risk of breakdown in an isolated area. When working on a car in the cold, avoid getting gasoline on your hands. It evaporates quickly and cools your skin. Avoid touching metal with bare skin, too. Cold metal can absorb heat quickly. Do not try to make repairs without gloves.

If you do not have boots and other appropriate protective clothing, stay in the car, with the hood up to alert passersby that the car is not deserted. As a rule, a rescue team is more likely to find you if you remain close to your vehicle. Do not walk through the snow in low shoes.

You can use the auto heater to keep warm, but *be sure to keep a window open slightly*. This will help protect against carbon monoxide poisoning. If for some reason you cannot stay in the car, build a fire if possible. Protect yourself from the wind as much as you can. You may be able to make a shelter with tree boughs, snow, or a car blanket. Insulate yourself from the ground if you can. Use tree boughs for this, too, if nothing better is at hand. Do not work so fast that you get overtired or damp from perspiration, both of which tend to make you even more susceptible to cold injury. □

Additional information: ______________________

____

____

____

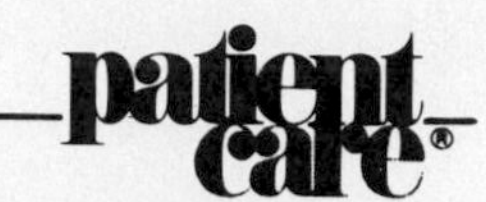

patient education aid

INFORMATION

What you should know about hypothermia

Even when you feel cold, the temperature inside your body usually stays the same—about 98.6 °F (37 °C). *Hypothermia* occurs when the internal body temperature drops several degrees. It often results from exposure to cold weather, but the weather does not have to be very cold. Even in the summer, a tired hiker exposed to wind and rain may develop hypothermia.

Prevention

The key to prevention is to be prepared for cold when you will be outdoors—whether for half a day or for weeks. Also, remember that it is best not to be alone. A person can slip into hypothermia without realizing it.

To prevent heat loss, protect yourself against cold *and* against moisture and wind. Water on the skin, whether from rain, snow, or perspiration, draws heat away from the body about 26 times as fast as air. Wind can also increase heat loss. If the thermometer reads 40 °F (4.4 °C) and the wind speed is 20 mph (32 kph), the effect on exposed skin is comparable to 18 °F (−7.8 °C). This is called the *windchill factor*.

Protective clothing

Clothing for cool or wet weather should insulate you from the cold, keep the wind out, repel water, and allow perspiration to evaporate.

Wearing several layers of light, loose clothing that will trap air is better than wearing one bulky, heavy, or tightly fitting coat. Be sure your head, neck, and legs are covered. These are areas of high heat loss. Polyester fiberfill (a substitute for down) and wool both retain some protective value when wet; cotton and goose or duck down do not. Also wear a windproof and waterproof outer garment. Weather-resistant fabrics such as Gore-Tex are recommended; they are very water resistant, but they allow moisture to escape from inside.

Other precautions for the outdoors

Here are some additional guidelines for preventing hypothermia:

- Stay in good physical condition.
- Have emergency equipment with you, even on day hikes. This can include space blankets, a knife, large plastic bags, a waterproof container of matches or a fire starter, candy, and cord. If a companion gets hurt, you will want to keep him or her covered and insulated from the ground while waiting for rescue.
- Make sure you get enough food and water while outdoors.
- Do not tire yourself.
- Take off layers of clothing before you get so warm that your clothing is soaked with perspiration. Put on layers before you get so cold you start shivering.
- On long hikes, camp early at night, while you still have enough energy to make a shelter from wind and rain. Valleys are coldest, and hilltops are windiest.

Recognizing hypothermia

Hypothermia gives little warning. Two of the body's first reactions to cold are goose pimples and shivering. If the heat produced by shivering does not keep up with heat being lost, the body's temperature will fall. If the cooling process is not stopped, mental and physical changes begin to occur. The person drops out of conversation and appears discouraged or depressed. He becomes uncoordinated; his movements become slow and labored. Simple tasks become difficult. He loses memory, and his judgment fails. He grows sleepy, lethargic, and confused. He may be combative and refuse care. He may hallucinate. If his body temperature drops below 80 °F (26.6 °C), he will probably lose consciousness and his muscles will become stiff.

Treatment in the field

The best "treatment" is to prevent hypothermia before it occurs. If a companion is shivering, remove any wet clothing and place him in a sleeping bag or blankets insulated from the ground. Get into the sleeping bag with him to share your body heat, if necessary. It is best to warm the vital organs first, so try to maintain contact only with his trunk. Avoid touching his arms and legs if possible. If the person is conscious, can talk with you, can breathe well, and generally seems to be thinking clearly, have him drink warm—or hot—fluids. Find shelter and build a fire. Keep the person warm, and move him to a hospital as soon as possible.

Someone with severe hypothermia needs different handling. If the hypothermia is severe enough that the person is very confused, uncoordinated, semiconscious, or unconscious, *do not* attempt to warm him with a fire or hot fluids. Rewarming will cause major bodily changes that need to be handled in a hospital. Protect the patient from further heat loss by wrapping him in blankets or taking him into a shelter. Do not perform cardiopulmonary resuscitation even if you are fully trained; it may trigger abnormal heartbeat. Handle the person gently, and move him to a hospital. □

Additional information: ____________________

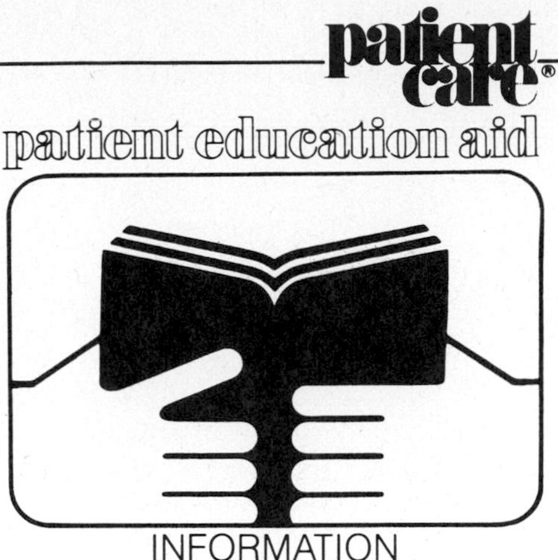

Understanding and treating heat disorders

What are heat disorders?
Anyone who works or exercises too hard in hot, muggy weather can develop a heat disorder—*heat cramps*, *heat exhaustion*, or *heatstroke*. This is especially likely to happen to joggers and other athletes who push themselves too hard when they are not fully conditioned.

≫ *Heat cramps* are muscle spasms in the stomach, arms, or legs. They occur when a person sweats a great deal and doesn't drink enough salty liquid to replace what's been lost. The cramps can be mild or very painful. They may begin either during or after heavy activity.

≫ *Heat exhaustion* usually occurs when a person exercises strenuously in hot, humid weather and doesn't replace body salt and water lost by sweating. It can also occur in an elderly or infirm person who has not been overly active but doesn't have enough body salt. The person with heat exhaustion may become extremely weak. He or she may feel nauseated and may vomit or become dizzy and faint. The person's skin turns pale, cold, and moist with sweat.

≫ *Heatstroke* is a life-threatening emergency. When exposure to heat and humidity causes the body temperature to rise to 105-110 °F (41-43 °C), the person collapses with heatstroke. He loses consciousness, and his skin becomes red, hot, and dry because the body can no longer produce sweat.

How can I help the person who has a heat disorder?
≫ *For the person with heat cramps:*
- Give him all the water he can drink. Salted water is even better: Use bouillon or add a teaspoon of salt to about a quart of water.
- Get the person out of the heat as quickly as possible.
- Don't give him salt without liquid.
- Don't try to work out the cramps by massaging the muscles. It won't help, and the cramps may even get worse.
- Have the person rest for the remainder of the day and avoid heavy activity for the next few days.

☎ Call the doctor if *any* other symptoms develop.

≫ *For the person with heat exhaustion:*
- Get him to a cool place.
- If he is conscious, give him bouillon or salted water (1 teaspoon salt in a quart of water).
- If he is unconscious, remove his clothing and sponge him down with cool or cold water.

☎ Call the doctor.

- Take his temperature periodically. If it is above 101 °F (38.5 °C) or begins to rise, get the person to a doctor as soon as possible.
- See that he rests for at least 2-3 days. This is especially important if the person is elderly or suffers from a chronic disease such as heart trouble or diabetes.

≫ *For the person with heatstroke:*

- *Act fast.* Remove the person from the source of heat.
- Cool off his body as fast as you can. Remove his clothing. If possible, put him into a tub of cold water or ice water. Otherwise, pack ice around him, rub him with ice, or run cold water from a hose over him. Get bystanders to help if you can.

☎ As soon as you've started cooling him off, call an ambulance. Tell the person you talk to that the patient has heatstroke so the ambulance attendants come prepared.

- Don't be reassured if the victim regains consciousness and says he feels all right. Anyone with heatstroke needs to be hospitalized and watched closely by medical personnel.

How can I help prevent heat disorders?

≫ Drink plenty of cold water on hot summer days, especially before and during heavy physical activity. The only way the body can lose extra heat in very hot, humid weather is by sweating. Sweat is mostly water. If you don't drink enough, your body can't make enough sweat to keep you cool. You can drink water up to an hour before you exercise, and take small amounts of water every 15-30 minutes during a workout. This is especially important if you sweat a lot. Drinking water won't give you cramps, make you bloated, or slow you down.

≫ *Don't push or overwork yourself when you're not yet used to hot, humid days.* Start with short bouts of light activity in the morning or late afternoon. Avoid heavy activity at midday.

≫ *Don't take salt in tablet or other form unless you also drink plenty of water.* If you tend to sweat a lot during heavy physical activity, your doctor may recommend drinking a mixture containing one teaspoon salt to one quart of water. This will help replenish body water and salt you lose through sweating.

≫ *Wear light-colored, porous clothing.* It can absorb sweat and help cool the body. Covering your head with a light kerchief or hat is a good idea. Never wear clothing or gear made of synthetic materials such as polyester, nylon, or plastic during heavy exertion in the summer heat. Cotton clothing is good for the heat, and khaki and tan are good colors.

≫ *Stop working or exercising and move out of the heat* if you feel even mild symptoms of a heat syndrome.

≫ *When indoors during a heat wave, be sure to keep some windows open and use fans to keep the air flowing.* If possible, keep at least one room air-conditioned so you can take a break from the heat. □

Additional information: ____________________

____

____

____

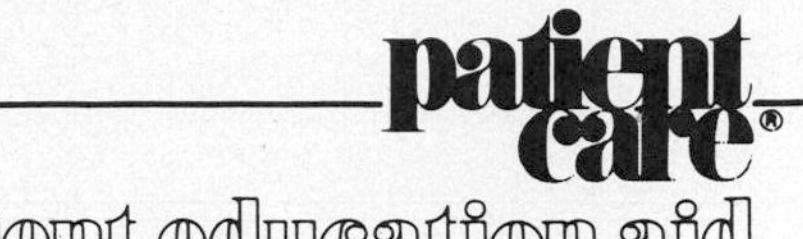

INFORMATION

Recognizing heart attack

If a person is having a heart attack, quick recognition of his or her problem and prompt medical care can mean the difference between life and death. To recognize a heart attack in its earliest stages, familiarize yourself with the following information. Then if you—or someone you are with—develops these symptoms, get medical help immediately.

Symptoms of heart attack

Most people describe the feeling of a heart attack as a discomfort in the center of the chest, unlike anything experienced before. Some further define the discomfort as a gripping or squeezing pain, while others say it is as if a great weight has been placed on the chest. Still others say they have a hot feeling—like that from a live coal—in the center of the chest.

Frequently, the chest pain or discomfort of a heart attack travels to one or both arms, the fingers, the throat, the jaw, or the upper back. It may be accompanied by shortness of breath, sweating, dizziness, and/or weakness.

Often a heart attack victim mistakenly thinks he has the type of indigestion commonly called heartburn. This doesn't mean that every time you have indigestion, you should call your doctor. But if the "indigestion" feels different from any you've had before and worsens with activity, it may signal a heart attack.

Occasionally, a heart attack causes no feeling of pain or discomfort in the chest but appears as unusual pain in the shoulder or arm alone. Such pain—unless it has an obvious cause, such as a strained or pulled muscle—is especially suggestive of heart attack if it worsens with activity and gets better with rest.

Sometimes a heart attack causes no pain at all—just numbness, severe shortness of breath, dizziness, or sweating.

Even if these problems seem to be going away, it's still important to get medical help. The pain or discomfort of a heart attack may disappear and then return.

What to do if you think you are having a heart attack

1. Call your doctor. (If you are unable to do so, have someone else call.) Your doctor will tell you whether to come to his office or go to the emergency room.

2. If you can't reach your doctor, leave a message that explains the problem and tells which hospital you are going to. Call an ambulance or have someone drive you to the emergency room, whichever is quicker.

Keep these phone numbers near your phone:

Doctor ____________________

Ambulance ____________________

Hospital ____________________

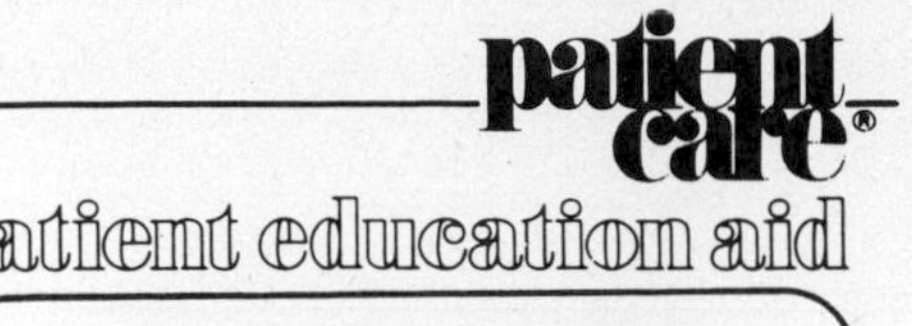

Understanding stroke

If a person in your family has had a stroke, it is natural for you to worry. Probably one of your biggest concerns is whether he or she will get better. Stroke is a serious illness that often leaves the individual partially disabled. However, many people who have had a stroke improve greatly and lead full lives again; others could recover more fully if they and their families knew more about the process of getting well and what they could do to help it along. Only a few people who have had a stroke remain completely incapacitated as a result.

This information sheet explains what stroke is, what effects it might have on the individual, and how recovery takes place. Your doctor can provide more information on how you can help your relative recover to the fullest extent possible.

What is a stroke and what effects does it have?
A stroke occurs when something suddenly interrupts the blood supply to a portion of the brain. As a result, some brain cells are damaged, and the body functions controlled by those cells are affected. A stroke may cause some degree of paralysis; it may cause the individual to lose control of his bladder or bowels; it may affect the emotions, making the individual quick to laugh or cry, easily irritated, or depressed; or it may interfere with his ability to understand or use speech.

Does stroke cause mental illness?
The brain controls our thinking and the way we feel, which is one reason why an illness that damages the brain, such as stroke, can be particularly frightening. In many cases, a stroke may make a person say meaningless words, laugh or cry for no apparent reason, or act confused or depressed. Such behavior does not mean that the individual is mentally ill. He is simply a person whose physical illness has affected his ability to control the way he behaves. The effect on an individual's behavior may be temporary or it may be long lasting.

What causes stroke?
In most cases, one of three things happens to interrupt the blood supply to a portion of the brain and cause stroke:

1. A blood clot may form in an artery leading to the brain, or in an artery in the brain, thus blocking the flow of blood. The blood clot is called a *thrombus*, and it forms because the process of arteriosclerosis has narrowed and roughened the lining of the artery (see illustration, page 299).

2. A blood clot may form somewhere else in the body and travel to the brain, interrupting the blood flow when it reaches an artery too small to pass through. A blood clot that travels in this way is called an *embolus*.

3. A *hemorrhage*—the escape of blood when an arterial wall breaks—may occur in the brain (see illustration).

Can the damaged brain cells heal?

Yes. Following stroke, small blood vessels near the damaged brain area enlarge, providing part of the circulation that was lost. Consequently, some nerve cells in the brain—those that were not permanently damaged—begin to heal and to function again. Some cells will recover completely. Brain cells unaffected by the stroke may take over the functions of those cells that do not recover.

How long does recovery take?

Most stroke patients regain some of their strength a few days after the stroke. But further recovery takes much time and work—all part of the process called *rehabilitation*, in which the individual exercises weakened muscles and relearns activities that he can no longer do. If you become discouraged because recovery is slow, it may help to remember that the majority of stroke patients who are paralyzed on the left or right side can learn to walk again. In time, the majority of patients can also relearn the daily activities an adult normally is able to do for himself, such as combing his hair, brushing his teeth, and going to the bathroom.

Thrombus

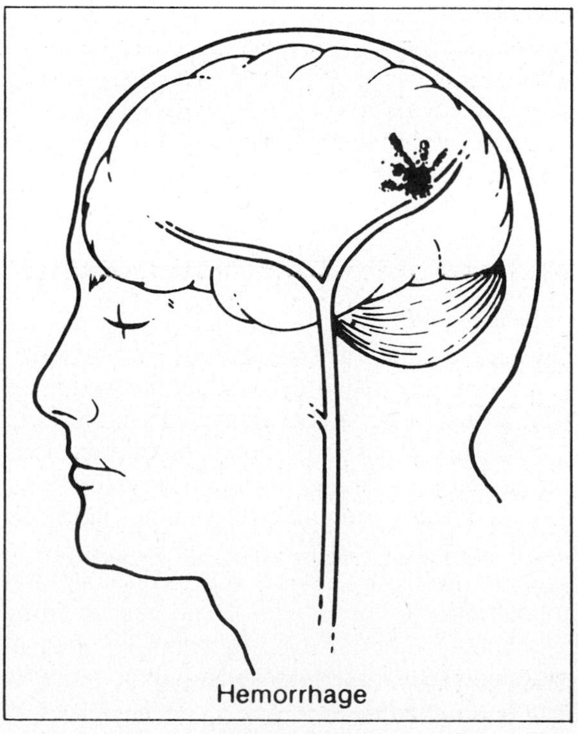

Hemorrhage

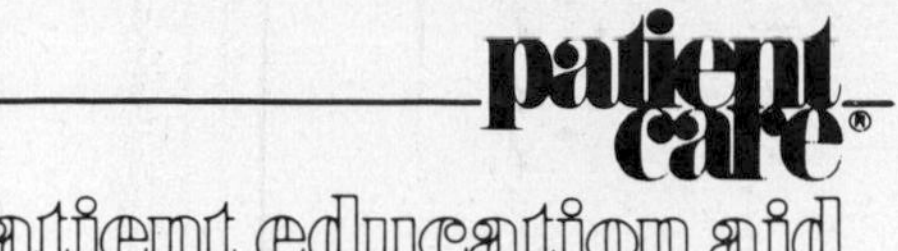

INFORMATION/INSTRUCTIONS

Understanding diabetic emergencies

People with poorly controlled diabetes are always at risk of two emergency situations. The first, *hypoglycemia*, or very low blood sugar, can occur in both type 1 (also called insulin-dependent or ketosis-prone) diabetes and type 2 (also called adult-onset, insulin-dependent, or ketosis-resistant) diabetes, but it is rare with type 2. The second, *diabetic ketoacidosis*, occurs only in type 1 diabetes. You and your family must be able to distinguish between these two emergencies. Since immediate treatment is always important and sometimes critical, protect yourself by learning to recognize early symptoms.

A summary of the following information on diabetic emergencies, for family use ("For the diabetic's family: How to recognize and treat a diabetic emergency"), is also provided.

Hypoglycemia

Causes The amount of insulin you inject each day to control your diabetes has been determined from an estimate of your usual diet and level of physical activity. If you exercise more or eat less than usual, you may be getting more insulin than you need. This excess of insulin causes the blood sugar level to drop too low for your body to function normally. If you are taking an oral antidiabetes agent for type 2 diabetes, you may get hypoglycemia by missing meals, by unusual exercise, or by inadvertently taking too much of your oral medication.

How to recognize early clues Hypoglycemic reactions come on suddenly. Early signs differ from person to person, but any of these may occur:

- ☐ Mood change
- ☐ Hunger
- ☐ Trembling
- ☐ Sweating
- ☐ Pallor
- ☐ Light-headedness
- ☐ Pounding heartbeat
- ☐ Confusion and disorientation
- ☐ Drowsiness
- ☐ Inability to concentrate
- ☐ Inability to focus your eyes while reading or watching television

If hypoglycemia is allowed to progress, you may become unconscious.

What to do at the earliest sign If you are exercising, *stop*. Immediately eat a simple, fast-acting sugar such as:

- ☐ A half cup of orange juice sweetened with 1 teaspoon of sugar, if handy

continued

What to do at the earliest sign continued

- ☐ 6-7 Life Savers or other small candies
- ☐ 2 teaspoons of sugar dissolved in a half cup of lukewarm water
- ☐ Instant glucose
- ☐ 1 tablespoon Karo or other corn syrup, honey, or maple syrup, alone or added to a half cup of orange juice
- ☐ Any other available candy or sweet such as jam or jelly

Make sure you always carry a sweet with you—hard candy, sugar cubes, or a tube of commercial cake frosting.

What to do for a severe reaction Your parents, teachers, and friends should be familiar with the symptoms of a hypoglycemic reaction and should know what to do if it becomes severe. The first step is to give sugar. In case you are unable to swallow, they should know how to give you an injection of glucagon. Instructions for your family on injecting glucagon are on the next page.

Diabetic ketoacidosis and coma

Causes Diabetic ketoacidosis may result from unusual and/or prolonged stress to your body caused by illness, an accident, surgery, or, perhaps, severe emotional stress. The immediate effect of this stress is a greatly increased blood sugar level. Also, excessive amounts of stress hormones are excreted; they further increase the blood sugar level by lowering the insulin supply. Since your insulin supply is inadequate to handle this high level of blood sugar, your body gets the heat and energy it needs by "burning" large amounts of fats in a process called fat metabolism. Products of fat metabolism—ketones—ordinarily are well utilized by the body, but under these circumstances, so many ketones are produced that they back up into the blood. Some of these ketones are acid; they acidify the blood, leading to ketoacidosis.

How to recognize early clues Ketoacidosis develops slowly over 8-24 hours. At first, there may be no symptoms. To detect it as early as possible, conscientiously test your urine as often as your doctor recommends—*at least every day without fail*. The first warning signs are tests showing large amounts of sugar—1-2 percent—in your urine, accompanied by a positive test for urinary ketones. At this point, call your doctor immediately.

During the early stages of ketoacidosis, you may also experience excessive thirst, excessive urination, and often nausea, vomiting, stomach pains, and rapid breathing. Later, you may feel drowsy, and your breath will have a fruity odor. You are sick and your body is telling you so.

Remember that an infection, fever, or intestinal upset increases your body's need for insulin and can cause ketoacidosis to develop quickly. If you become ill, be sure to continue testing your urine and increase your insulin dosage if test results are high. Your doctor has already given you instructions for adjusting your insulin dosage if you have several successive positive urine tests. Call him if you are vomiting, if signs of ketoacidosis accompany your illness, or if you have trouble adjusting your insulin dosage. If you become stuporous or unconscious, you should be taken to the hospital immediately.

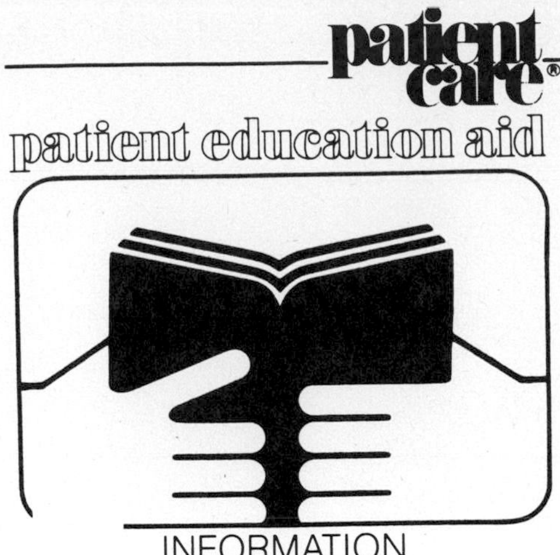

Questions and answers about epilepsy

You have recently learned that you (or someone close to you) have epilepsy. You probably have many questions about the disease. This information sheet will answer some of your questions, as well as clear up misunderstandings that some people have about epilepsy.

What is epilepsy?
Epilepsy is not a single disease; it is the name given to a group of disorders that cause a person to have *seizures* (or convulsions). To understand what happens during an epileptic seizure, it is important to recognize that the normal activities of the brain—thinking, feeling, remembering, and so on—require electrical energy. When someone has a seizure, a sudden, abnormal discharge of electrical energy occurs in the brain. This electrical "storm" causes him or her to lose control of certain bodily functions and, frequently, mental abilities for a short time—anywhere from a few seconds to several minutes.

There are several different types of seizures, each identified by what happens during the attack. For instance, the person who has a *generalized, tonic-clonic seizure* loses consciousness (blacks out) and falls to the ground. His body stiffens, and he may cry out. Then, in a second phase of the seizure, his body begins to jerk violently, and he may froth at the mouth. After the seizure, he may sleep for several hours.

Someone who has an *absence seizure*, on the other hand, seems to lose awareness of his surroundings for a few seconds during an attack. He may stare off into space, twitch, or blink several times, then suddenly become alert again, and the seizure is over. Sometimes no one notices that the absence seizure took place.

Partial seizures involve only part of the brain. The result may be the sudden jerk of an arm, leg, or other part of the body. The person having a partial seizure may appear to be in a dreamlike state. He may pick at his clothes, fidget, smack his lips, or walk around aimlessly. Sometimes a partial seizure causes the person to see or hear imaginary things.

What causes epilepsy?
Often, no definite medical explanation can be found for a person's seizures. In some individuals, epilepsy can be traced to a birth injury, a head injury, a serious infection, or a high fever affecting the brain.

Is epilepsy inherited?
The person whose mother or father (or both) has epilepsy is a little more likely than other people to have epileptic seizures. But even if both his parents have epilepsy, the chances are good that he will *not* have epilepsy.

Does epilepsy cause mental retardation or mental illness?
Epilepsy does not directly cause mental retardation or mental illness. Many children who are retarded, however, do have seizures because the injury to the brain that affects mental function also causes the seizures. Epilepsy can cause psychological stress, but this is due to the person's emotional reaction to the condition and *not* to any damage to the brain caused by the seizures.

Can a person die from having a seizure?
The seizure itself usually poses no danger to life. But sometimes people have seizures while driving or doing some other activity in which losing consciousness is dangerous. Rarely, a person

with epilepsy has a continuous series of seizures. This condition, called *status epilepticus*, requires immediate medical care. If you witness a seizure lasting longer than 10-15 minutes, take the person to an emergency room or call an ambulance.

How is epilepsy treated?
The doctor cannot *cure* epilepsy, but the drugs used to treat epilepsy—called *antiepileptics*, or *anticonvulsants*—usually prevent seizures quite well. Antiepileptics work by suppressing the abnormal electrical discharges in the brain that cause seizures. Sometimes a child outgrows the tendency to have seizures, but often a person must take antiepileptics for life.

If you are taking antiepileptics, follow the doctor's instructions carefully. It may take the doctor a while to find the best drug or drugs for you. *Never stop taking an antiepileptic drug without checking with the doctor first*, even if you have not had a seizure for a long time. Sudden stopping of an antiepileptic can cause you to have one seizure after another until medical care is obtained.

Do antiepileptic drugs have side effects?
You may have to cope with a few side effects to be free of seizures. Your doctor will help you find the right types and amounts of drugs to control your seizures with a minimum of troublesome side effects. The doctor will also provide detailed instructions for handling any side effects that cannot be avoided.

What can I do to avoid seizures in addition to taking my medication?
Try to eat nutritious, well-balanced meals at regular intervals and get enough sleep every night. Overtiring yourself and not eating properly can lower your resistance and make you more likely to have seizures.

Should I limit my activities because I have epilepsy?
Once seizures are under control with drugs, few restrictions are necessary:

≫ *Exercise* Avoid any activity where losing consciousness, even temporarily, could result in injury or death. For example, avoid scuba diving, climbing (of mountains, trees, or ropes), hang gliding, and wind surfing. Swim only with someone who can bring you safely ashore should you have a seizure. Swimming in clear water or a pool is preferable.

≫ *School* A child with epilepsy can attend regular schools and camps once his seizures are under control. The teachers or camp supervisors should be informed of the child's condition and know what to do if a seizure occurs.

≫ *Driving* Individuals with epilepsy may drive if they have been free of seizures involving loss of consciousness for a significant time. This period varies from state to state, so contact your motor vehicle department for more information.

≫ *Showers and baths* If you have epilepsy, don't take a bath or shower while in the house alone and never lock the bathroom door. Young children with epilepsy should not be left alone while bathing.

≫ *Employment* Unless seizures have been completely controlled for several years, avoid jobs where losing consciousness, even for a moment, could put you or others in danger. For example, don't drive a taxi, bus, truck, or train. Don't operate heavy machinery or work either underground or underwater.

Where can I get more information?
Your doctor will try to answer any questions not answered here. You can also call the local chapter of the Epilepsy Foundation of America (check your phone book) or write to its national headquarters (4351 Garden City Drive, Landover, MD 20785).

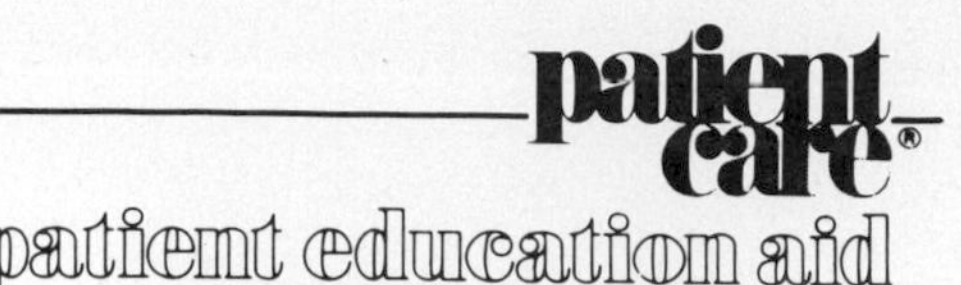

INFORMATION

First aid for epileptic seizures

A seizure can be a very frightening experience for the individual with epilepsy and for you, the family members who may witness an attack. Although your doctor has prescribed medication that should prevent further seizures almost entirely, you'll need to know what to do if another seizure occurs. First, try to remain calm and remember:

≫ Most seizures are brief.
≫ Most aren't life threatening.
≫ Most need only the simplest care.

Try to remember exactly what happens during and after the seizure so you can give your doctor the best possible description.

Care for a generalized tonic-clonic seizure

When an individual with epilepsy falls down, becomes rigid, makes jerking movements, has difficulty breathing, and becomes pale or blue complexioned, he or she is having an attack called a *generalized tonic-clonic seizure*. Emergency care consists of the following steps:

≫ Leave the person where he is unless he is endangered (for instance, if he is on a busy street).
≫ Remove eyeglasses and loosen tight clothing.
≫ Clear the area of sharp, hard, or hot objects that could injure him during his seizure.
≫ *Do not* force anything into his mouth. You can damage the individual's teeth if you try to force a stick, pencil, or other object between his teeth.
≫ *Do not* try to restrain him; you cannot stop the seizure.
≫ After the seizure, try to turn him on his side to allow any saliva, mucus, food, or vomitus that has collected to drain from his mouth.
≫ Do not offer him any food or drink until he is completely alert.
≫ Let him rest awhile if he wishes.

The person who has had a generalized tonic-clonic seizure may need to sleep for as long as several hours after the seizure. Make sure you or another adult remains with him until he is fully awake and oriented; at that time, you can accompany him to a more comfortable place.

Care for a complex partial seizure

During another kind of epileptic attack, called a *complex partial seizure*, the person may sit, stand, or walk about aimlessly, make lip-smacking or chewing movements, and fidget with his clothing. He may have a glassy stare and give either no response or an inappropriate one when you ask him a question. He may appear to be drunk, drugged, or even psychotic during the episode. When a family member with epilepsy experiences a seizure of this sort, immediate care consists of the following precautions:

≫ Remove harmful objects from his pathway, if possible, or gently coax him away from them.
≫ Avoid agitating or provoking him.
≫ Try to remain calm even if he seems angry or irrational.
≫ *Do not* restrain the person.
≫ After the seizure, remain with him until he is alert and oriented.

When to call for help

Always be alert for signs that a seizure may be unusually dangerous. Call an ambulance if *any* of the following occurs:

☎ The person having a seizure injures himself.
☎ He does not start breathing after the seizure.
☎ He seems to pass from one seizure to another without regaining consciousness.

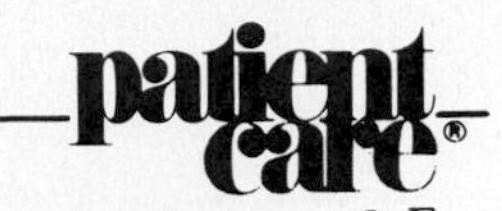

Questions and answers about asthma

This information sheet will answer many of your questions about asthma, its causes, and its treatment. Do not hesitate to ask your doctor or nurse any other questions you may have.

What is asthma?
You are already familiar with one or more of the symptoms of asthma—shortness of breath, wheezing, and coughing. These discomforts occur because asthma is a disease affecting the bronchi, tubes that carry air through the lungs. Illustration **A** shows bronchi in their normal state.

During an episode of asthma, the bronchi become obstructed, making it difficult for you—or your child, if he or she has asthma—to move air in and out of the lungs. The obstruction is caused by one or more of three conditions:

1. The muscles surrounding the bronchi contract, narrowing the passageways, or airways, through which air flows.
2. The membranes that line the bronchi swell.
3. Thick mucus fills the bronchi.

Illustration B shows the bronchi during an asthmatic attack.

How often do episodes of asthma occur?
The frequency and duration of episodes of shortness of breath, wheezing, and coughing vary from person to person. Some people with asthma experience fewer than two attacks a year; for others, difficult breathing is a daily occurrence. However, *obstruction of the bronchi is reversible*; that is, treatment is available that provides relief by opening up the airways.

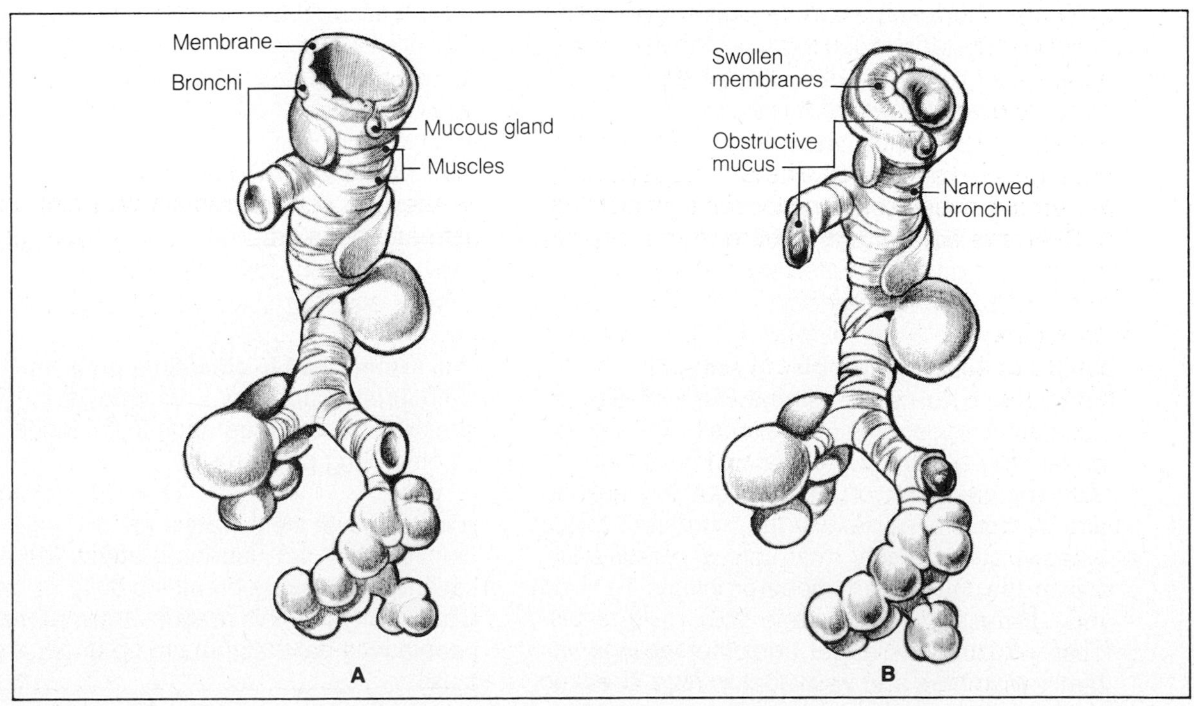

What causes asthma?
The cause of asthma is not known. For some reason, certain people develop what physicians call "reactive airways." Their airways react to such stimuli as allergy, exercise, or cigarette smoke by becoming obstructed. The list of possible stimuli is quite long, and not every item on the list affects all people with asthma. Sometimes, a specific stimulus can not be identified. It is also not known why some people are susceptible to asthma while others are not. In many cases, such susceptibility is inherited.

Is asthma an allergy?
In many people with asthma, episodes of wheezing, coughing, and shortness of breath are allergic reactions to the inhalation of certain substances, called allergens. Common allergens include mold spores, pollen from plants, animal dander, house dust, house mites, and feathers; many of these can be avoided. Allergy to foods is a rare cause of asthma and is more prevalent in children than adults. Not all people with allergies, however, develop asthma; some have hay fever or skin rashes.

Also, not all asthma is due to specific allergens. Irritating substances can trigger asthmatic attacks in people with reactive airways; for example, cigarette smoke, fumes from industrial and household chemicals, and cold or damp air are potential triggers of bronchial obstruction. Some people react to exercise or to a cold or other viral infection of the nose, throat, and/or lungs. Certain drugs, such as aspirin, also can bring on an asthmatic attack in some people.

What role does emotion play in asthma?
Emotions *do not cause* asthma. But if you already have asthma, becoming emotionally upset or experiencing a stressful situation may trigger or worsen an episode of difficult breathing. In addition, asthma, especially in the infrequent cases when it considerably interrupts a person's life, can be the cause of emotional problems. To avoid this, discuss—or encourage your child to discuss—frustrations, anger, and other feelings with family members and your doctor. Also, check to see if a support group is available in your area and, if necessary, seek professional counseling.

How is asthma treated?
Many asthmatic attacks can be prevented by avoiding the triggers that cause them. Your doctor can help you identify those substances that bother you by questioning you about the circumstances in which attacks occur and by skin testing. In a skin test, a small amount of a suspected allergen is placed on the skin, and the area is observed for a reaction.

Avoiding substances that trigger your asthmatic attacks may not be possible all the time. Fortunately, medications called *bronchodilators* are available that enlarge, or dilate, the airways. These drugs work by relaxing the muscles that surround the bronchi, by reducing swelling, and by loosening mucus. If treatment with bronchodilators is unsatisfactory, your doctor may prescribe another type of medication.

With asthma due to specific allergens, a treatment called *hyposensitization*, or *immunotherapy*, is sometimes used. In hyposensitization, small amounts of an allergen are injected into your body. These injections make you less sensitive to that allergen and, therefore, less likely to experience an asthmatic attack when you are exposed to it.

Can a child outgrow his asthma?
In many cases, as the child approaches young adulthood, the frequency of attacks lessens or they even stop completely, but a recurrence is always possible.

Will asthma lead to other lung problems?
With proper treatment, asthma is not likely to cause irreversible damage to the lungs and lead to other lung problems.

Is asthma ever life threatening?
Occasionally, an untreated attack increases in severity and severe breathing difficulty becomes a possibility. For this reason, it is important for all people who have asthma to be under a doctor's care.

Helpful hints for controlling asthma

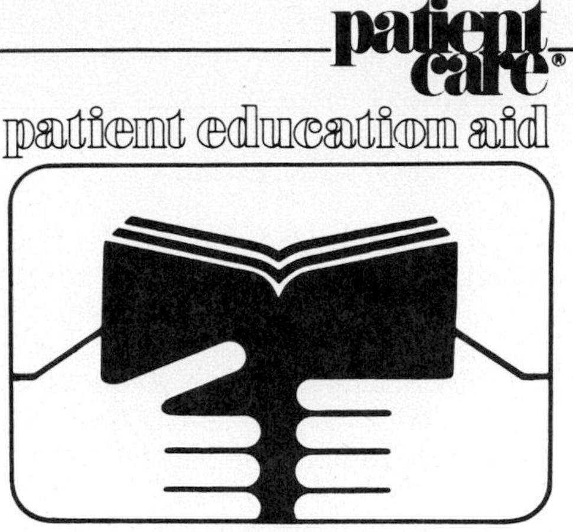

You can do several things to reduce the severity and frequency of your—or your child's—asthmatic attacks. Your doctor will work closely with you to find the appropriate treatment program that is best suited for you. The general guidelines below will help you follow your doctor's specific instructions.

1. *Avoid substances that trigger asthmatic symptoms.* Your doctor will help you determine what these are and provide suggestions for avoiding them. For many people with asthma, staying away from everything that causes wheezing would mean staying confined in a sparsely furnished, air-conditioned room. Fortunately, treatment is available to help you live with irritants and allergens that can't be avoided in your daily home or work environment.

2. *Exercise.* Do not avoid exercise. In the long run, it will improve your general well-being and your lungs' ability to function. Most people with asthma can tolerate the same level of physical activity as other people. Follow your doctor's recommendations for finding the best type of activity for you and for dealing with any discomfort it causes. For some, resting a while when difficult breathing occurs, then resuming activity, is sufficient. Or, your doctor may prescribe medication for you that you can take before you begin to exercise.

Swimming is an excellent exercise for many people with asthma. It improves lung function and conditions the body but is less likely to aggravate asthma than other strenuous activities, such as running, tennis, or football. Exercise in cold air, in particular, may cause problems.

3. *Avoid infection.* Follow a nutritious diet to keep up your resistance to infection. Any illness, but especially infections of the throat, sinuses, or lungs, can aggravate your asthma, so get prompt treatment when you are sick.

4. *Drink plenty of fluids.* Drinking lots of water or other fluids will help thin the mucus in your lungs so that it is less likely to plug the bronchial tubes and cause an asthmatic attack.

5. *Do not smoke, and avoid other air-polluted environments such as smoke-filled rooms.* Cigarette, cigar, and pipe smoke are irritants that may trigger asthmatic symptoms.

6. *Do not use any medication for asthma that is available without a prescription* unless you have discussed it with your doctor. This precaution is especially important if you are taking prescription medication, because the two drugs may have adverse effects when taken together.

7. *Carefully follow your doctor's instructions about taking medication.* No one drug or combination of drugs is ideal for all people with asthma, so you may be taking one type of medication, and a friend, another. You may need medication only when difficult breathing occurs, or you may need daily medication to prevent severe discomfort. Do not take more than the prescribed amount of medication. If you take medication every day, do not stop the drug on your own; doing so might trigger an asthmatic attack.

Finding the best medication or combination of medications for you may take several weeks. Often one drug is tried first. If the maximum dose that you can tolerate without side effects does not control your discomfort, your doctor will prescribe another drug to take in addition to the first.

Call your doctor:

- ☎ If your usual medication fails to provide relief.
- ☎ Your asthma suddenly worsens.
- ☎ You develop a fever or other sign of infection.

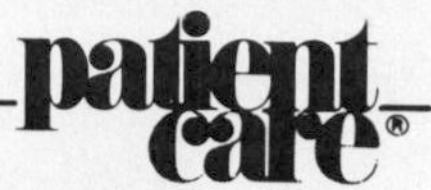

patient education aid

INSTRUCTIONS

Constipation

There is no one pattern of bowel function that is right for all people. Many people have one bowel movement a day, but some normally have 2-3 a day and others only 3-4 a week. Consider yourself constipated only if you are moving your bowels less frequently than what is normal for *you*. For example, if you usually have one movement a day, the doctor will probably consider you constipated if you report fewer than three movements a week.

Occasional constipation is common and is no cause for concern. If constipation persists or becomes a frequent problem, see your doctor.

Causes of constipation

A number of situations can cause constipation:

≫ Most often, constipation is the result of a diet low in fiber or the tendency to ignore the urge to have a bowel movement, such as while traveling.

≫ You may be constipated if you frequently use laxatives. The muscles of the bowel have become lazy—dependent on the laxative.

≫ Other medicines may contribute to constipation. These include those you buy independently, such as aspirin, and those prescribed by your doctor.

≫ If you have hemorrhoids (piles), the fear of pain may cause you to postpone trips to the bathroom and thus lead to constipation.

Often, simple changes in diet or bowel habits are all that are necessary to prevent constipation.

Tips for preventing constipation

1. *Do not ignore the urge to have a bowel movement.* While the stool remains in the bowel, water is reabsorbed by the body, making the stool hard and difficult to pass. The urge to move the bowels often follows shortly after a meal, particularly breakfast. Arrange your schedule so as to take advantage of this urge.

2. *Eat more fiber.* All fruits, vegetables, and grains have fiber. Just eating more of these foods every day may be enough prevention for you. If constipation is still a problem, however, select foods especially high in fiber from the list at right.

Bran, in particular, is an excellent source of fiber. Cooked bran may not be as effective as raw bran, but you may find it easier to tolerate. For many people, eating a bowl of bran cereal in the morning and a bran muffin and a salad during the day prevents constipation. Remember that refining processes decrease the amount of fiber in a food, which is the reason whole wheat bread is a better fiber source than white bread.

Note: To avoid indigestion and gas, gradually increase the amount of fiber you eat daily.

3. *Eat breakfast every day*, preferably one that includes a high-fiber cereal. Eating three or more small meals a day rather than one big one at night also promotes improved bowel function.

4. *Drink enough water or other fluids*—at least 2-3 8-oz glasses a day.

5. *Exercise regularly* (but remember to replace water lost through perspiration).

6. *Avoid laxatives*, unless prescribed by your doctor. A daily bowel movement is *not* essential to good health. If you follow the above recommendations, your body will eliminate waste as necessary for you (if not, see your doctor).

Taking a laxative may cause you to think mistakenly that you are constipated a day or two later. The laxative cleans you out so thoroughly that several days may pass before the bowel fills enough for you to have an urge to have a movement. Repeated use of laxatives can also alter the balance of substances in your blood called electrolytes, a balance that is essential to good health. For example, laxatives can deplete your body of one of those substances—potassium.

Foods with a high fiber content

Cereals and grains
Bran, including breads, muffins, and cereals made with bran
Whole-grain breads and muffins
Whole-grain cereals

Fruits
Bananas
Dates
Figs

Fruits continued
Prunes
Raisins

Nuts
Brazil nuts
Peanuts

Vegetables
Baked beans
Broccoli
Brussels sprouts
Peas

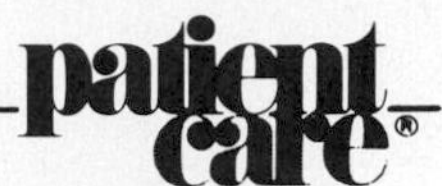

patient education aid

INSTRUCTIONS

Home care for diarrhea

Diarrhea (frequent, watery bowel movements) is commonly caused by a virus or mild food poisoning. This so-called uncomplicated diarrhea usually runs its course in 24-48 hours if you follow a few simple dietary measures. Sometimes, however, diarrhea can be a symptom of a more severe illness, or the diarrhea may become complicated due to a loss of too much fluid (dehydration). In these cases, a doctor's care is necessary. These guidelines will help you determine whether to call the doctor when you or a family member has diarrhea. They also provide information on home care of uncomplicated diarrhea.

Call your doctor:

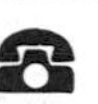 If *fever* is present.

 If there are signs of *dehydration*—decreased urination, lack of saliva, sunken eyeballs, lethargy or listlessness, or absence of tears. Dehydration can occur rapidly in infants and the elderly, especially when vomiting accompanies the diarrhea. Call the doctor if an infant younger than age 6 months has one episode of vomiting and/or diarrhea soon followed by another; closely watch an older infant who has more than one attack.

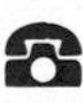 If diarrhea or abdominal pain continues *more than 24-48 hours* with little or no improvement. (If an infant or small child has diarrhea or vomiting and is under a doctor's care, be sure to check with the doctor every 48-72 hours until the diarrhea or vomiting stops.)

 If there is *blood* in the stool.

 If *abdominal pain* is severe and steady. (Milder cramping pain that comes and goes occurs frequently with diarrhea.)

Dietary measures

To promote recovery from uncomplicated diarrhea, give the irritated intestines a rest and replace lost fluids. These instructions may be helpful:

1. Stop eating solid foods and milk products until bowel movements return to normal; also drink only clear, cool, or lukewarm (not hot or ice-cold) liquids. (An infant with diarrhea may continue breast-feeding, but formula and cow's milk should be stopped.) Suggested beverages include:

≫ Water

≫ Flat, or decarbonated, cola or ginger ale (Remove carbonation by letting an opened bottle stand for several hours. Or, you can place your thumb over the mouth of an opened bottle and shake the bottle over the sink.)

≫ Liquid gelatin dessert (Jell-O or Royal desserts, for instance, made with twice the recommended amount of water and not permitted to jell)

≫ Gatorade (available in grocery stores)

≫ Pedialyte or Lytren for mild diarrhea (available in drugstores)

2. When diarrhea has stopped, begin eating small amounts of easily digested foods such as bananas, rice, baked potato (without butter), or applesauce. Continue fluids.

3. Slowly resume normal diet while avoiding milk products, alcohol, and spicy or fatty foods for several days, preferably for at least a week.

Medication

Although these dietary measures are the best treatment for uncomplicated diarrhea, a busy schedule may occasionally make it difficult to tolerate loose stools until the condition runs its course. In such cases, take Pepto-Bismol as directed on the bottle. Do not give Pepto-Bismol to children under age 3 unless your doctor recommends it. (Do not be alarmed if Pepto-Bismol darkens your stool, but call your doctor if, after you've stopped taking the medication, you continue to have dark stools.)

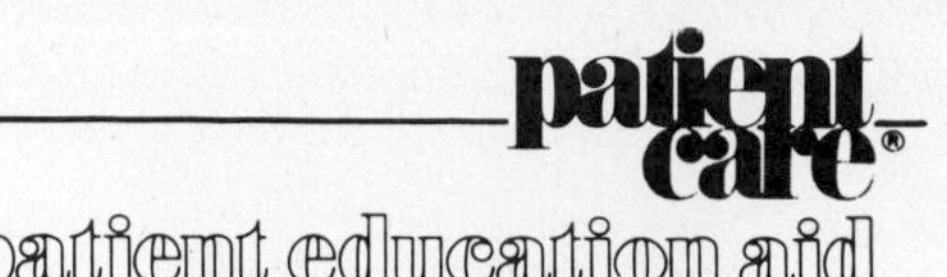

INFORMATION

Tips for managing diarrhea while traveling

Despite your best efforts to avoid contaminated food and water while traveling to help prevent diarrhea, you may experience the disorder. If so, remember that the diarrhea is ridding your body of the offending agent. Thus, the goal of treatment is *not* to stop the diarrhea suddenly but to make sure that you do not become depleted of the fluids and salts your body needs. The key to treatment is replacement of the fluid and electrolytes you lose in your stools.

As a rule, diarrhea is self-limited, and correction requires only taking readily available fluids—canned or fresh fruit juice, hot tea, or carbonated drinks. Be certain to avoid iced drinks and noncarbonated bottled fluids made from water of uncertain quality. *Do not attempt self-medication if the diarrhea is severe or does not abate within several days, if there is blood and/or mucus in the stool, if you have fever with shaking chills, or if you experience persistent diarrhea with dehydration (dry skin, dry nails, dry tongue); consult a physician immediately.*

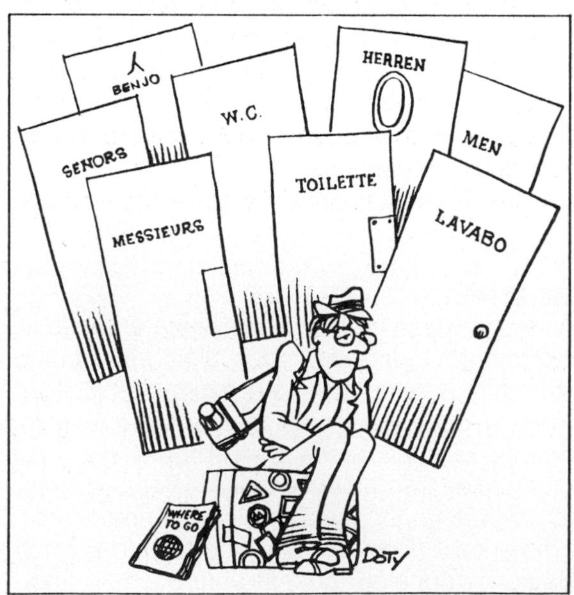

Nondrug treatment

For the usual type of self-limiting diarrhea, a good formula for treatment is:

1. Combine the following in a glass—
≫ Eight ounces of orange, apple, or other fruit juice (these are rich in potassium, one of the salts lost in diarrheal stools)
≫ One-half teaspoon honey or corn syrup (contains glucose, which is needed by the body for absorption of essential salts)
≫ One pinch table salt (contains sodium and chloride, which are lost in diarrheal stools)

2. Combine the following in a second glass—
≫ Eight ounces of water (either carbonated or boiled)
≫ One-quarter teaspoon baking soda (contains sodium bicarbonate)

3. Drink alternately from each glass, supplementing as you wish with carbonated beverages, water, or tea made with boiled or carbonated

Prepared with the assistance of the staff of the quarantine division, Center for Prevention Services, Centers for Disease Control, Public Health Service, U.S. Department of Health and Human Services, Atlanta, Ga.

water. Forgo solid foods and milk until you have recovered. (Infants with diarrhea should receive plain [boiled] water as desired while taking these salt solutions.)

Drug treatment

Antibiotics Use of an antibiotic prophylactically against diarrhea is not recommended. Not only might you experience side effects from the drug, but it may reduce the protective effect of your own bacterial flora against disease. Also, the diarrhea-causing pathogens may become resistant to the drug, rendering it valueless when pathogens do attack. In addition, an antibiotic may lessen the severity and duration of diarrhea caused by certain organisms but possibly may be useless for diarrhea that is caused by a number of other organisms.

An antibiotic that may be effective in preventing diarrhea due to enterotoxigenic *Escherichia coli* is doxycycline (Vibramycin, Vibra-Tabs). However, in some areas of the world, enterotoxigenic organisms are not sensitive to this drug. Also, use of doxycycline may result in extreme sensitivity to sunlight as well as increased risk of developing a more serious gastrointestinal infection from organisms that may not respond to it. Because complete information on the risks and benefits of doxycycline in the prevention of diarrhea in travelers is not available, the Public Health Service makes no specific recommendations about this drug. The decision whether to use doxycycline prophylactically is one that should be made only by your physician.

Antimotility agents Drugs that slow the movement of the bowels, such as diphenoxylate HCl and atropine sulfate (Lomotil) and loperamide HCl (Imodium), may relieve severe abdominal cramps associated with diarrhea. These drugs may worsen some illnesses causing diarrhea, though, and should not be taken for more than 2-3 days; they are not to be used if there is fever or blood and/or mucus in the stools.

Other agents Kaolin-pectin preparations, such as Kaopectate, do not shorten the illness, although they may alter the consistency of the stool.

Iodochlorhydroxyquin (Entero-Vioform) is ineffective in preventing or treating travelers' diarrhea, and prolonged use carries the risk of severe neurologic side effects.

Bismuth subsalicylate (Pepto-Bismol) may be helpful in preventing and treating travelers' diarrhea in adults; its use in children has not been evaluated. Two ounces, four times a day has been used successfully to prevent diarrhea in adults. For treatment, 1-2 ounces every 30 minutes for a maximum of eight doses has been found to decrease diarrhea. Definitive information on the possibility of adverse effects that may occur with such use of bismuth subsalicylate is presently unavailable.

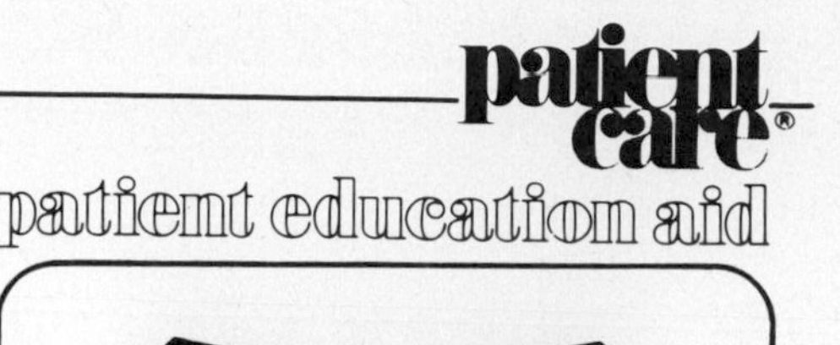

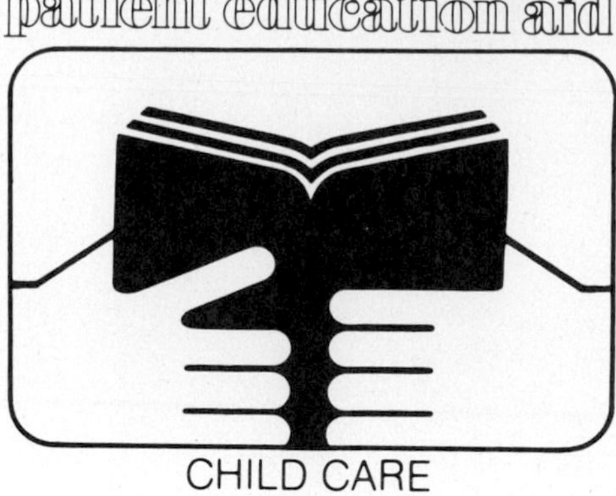

CHILD CARE

How to take your child's temperature

Doctors agree that the most reliable way to take your child's temperature is with a standard thermometer. Research suggests that a newer method—placing a commercially available plastic fever strip on the forehead—may result in readings that are too low.

Whether you take the temperature rectally, orally, or axillarily (under the arm) depends upon your child's age and upon how cooperative he is about having his temperature taken.

Reminder: Before taking a temperature, shake down the mercury to below 97°F (36.1°C) by grasping the thermometer firmly at the end opposite the bulb and, with your elbow bent, by sharply "snapping" your wrist and hand a couple of times. (Hold the thermometer over a bed or other soft surface so it won't break if it slips out of your hand.)

Axillary (under the arm)

If your child is younger than 3 months or if he protests against rectal temperature taking, use the axillary method. Axillary readings are somewhat less accurate than rectal or oral readings, but the axillary method is preferable whenever a child's age or behavior might increase the risk of breaking the thermometer.

1. Using an oral thermometer,* place the bulb end high up in the armpit, about halfway between the front and back of the arm, as shown in the illustration. Hold the arm down gently but firmly at the side of the body in order to keep the thermometer sufficiently secure.

continued

*NOTE: The oral thermometer has a longer, more slender bulb than the rectal thermometer. A rectal thermometer may be used to take temperature orally *only* if it has never been used for rectal temperature taking. Because of its long, slender bulb, an oral thermometer is *not* appropriate for taking rectal temperatures.

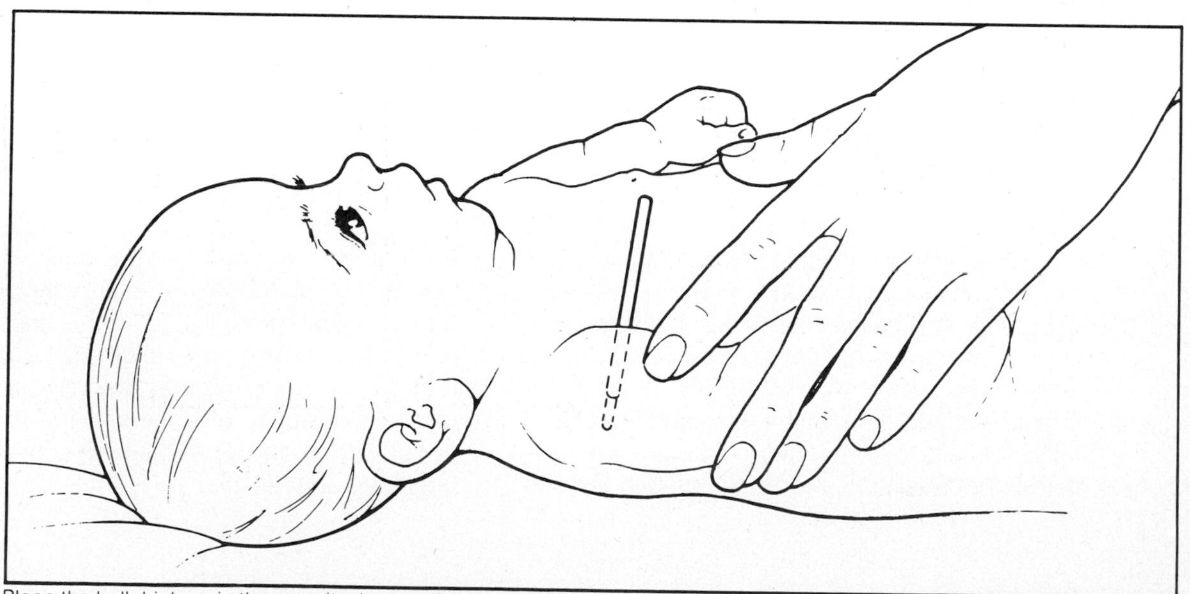

Place the bulb high up in the armpit, about halfway between the front and the back of the arm.

2. After *five minutes*, remove the thermometer and read it. (See "How to read a thermometer," next page.)

Rectal

From age 3 months until the child can understand how to keep a thermometer under the tongue without biting down on it—usually about age 6—take the temperature rectally *if he is cooperative*. If not, use the axillary method.

1. Using a rectal thermometer, lubricate the bulb end with petroleum jelly. Lay the child face down across your lap, as shown in the illustration. Then spread the buttocks and insert just the bulb end of the thermometer into the rectum. Do not push in any farther. You may prefer to place the child on a bed or other flat surface or to hold him over your shoulder with one arm, using the other hand for the thermometer.

2. Keep the thermometer in place for *three minutes*, then remove and read it. (See "How to read a thermometer," next page.)

Oral

Once your child understands how to hold a thermometer under his tongue, you may take his temperature orally, *but only if he will cooperate*. To ensure an accurate reading, wait at least 20 minutes after the child has taken food or drink.

1. Use an oral thermometer. With the child lying or sitting down, place the bulb end of the thermome-

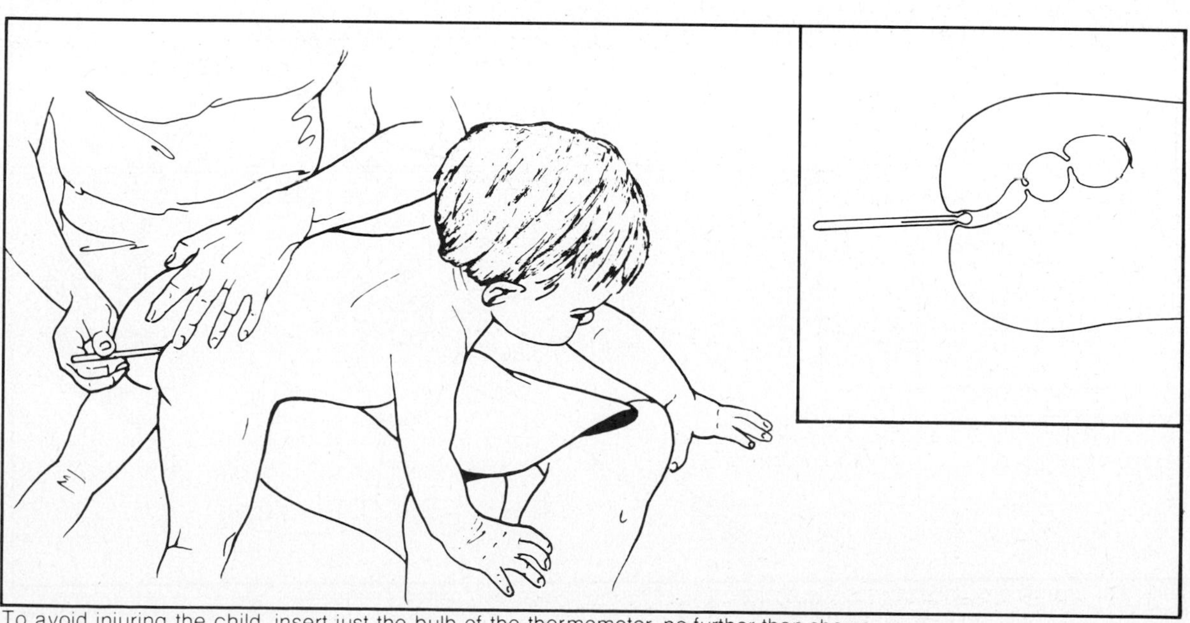

To avoid injuring the child, insert just the bulb of the thermometer, no further than shown.

ter under his tongue, at either side of the membrane connecting the tongue with the floor of the mouth. Ask him to hold the thermometer gently with his lips and to breathe through his nose. Warn against pressing too hard with the lips or teeth.

2. After *three minutes*, remove the thermometer and read it. (See "How to read a thermometer," below.)

How to read a thermometer

Practice reading a thermometer with someone who knows how. First, shake the thermometer down, run it under warm (*never hot*) water, and then read it. Repeat until you catch on.

1. Hold the end of the thermometer opposite the bulb the same way you would hold a pencil—between the thumb and index finger and resting on the third finger, as illustrated on the next page.

2. Turn the thermometer so the white or opaque surface is away from the eye.

3. Slowly rotate it back and forth until you can see the solid silver or red line of mercury. The child's temperature reading is the point where this line stops.

4. The long lines on the thermometer (running perpendicular to the line of mercury) represent degrees; the short lines represent 0.2 degrees.

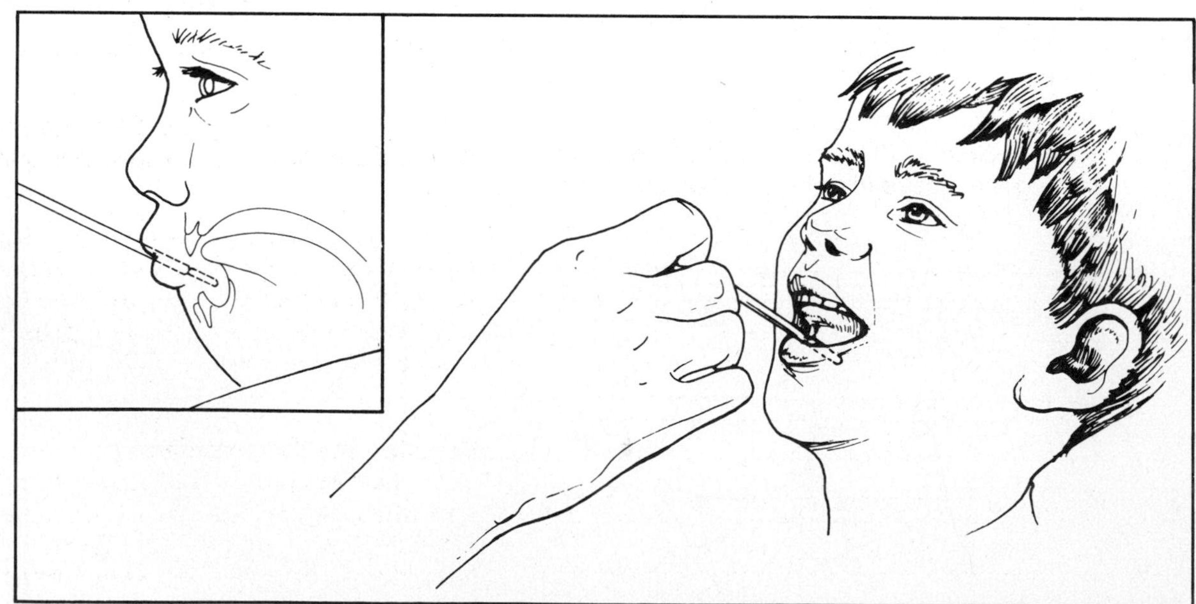

Place the thermometer under the tongue, at either side of the membrane that connects the tongue and the floor of the mouth. Tell the child to hold the thermometer in place with his lips.

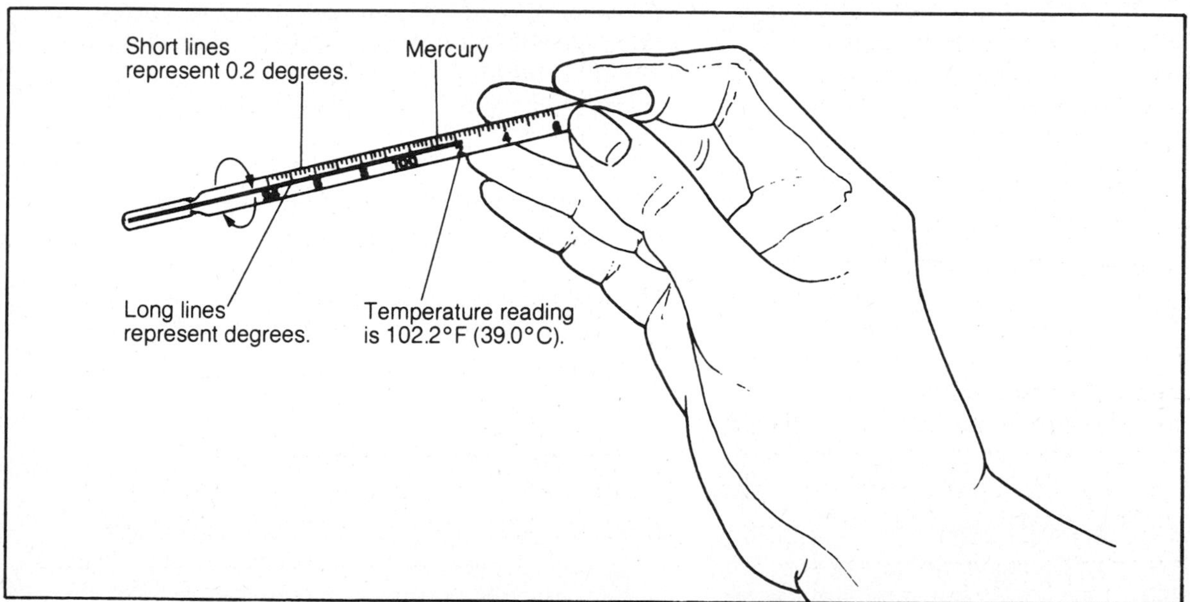

On most thermometers, the average body temperature—98.6°F (37°C)—is also represented by a long line. The reading in the drawing above is 102.2°F (39.0°C).

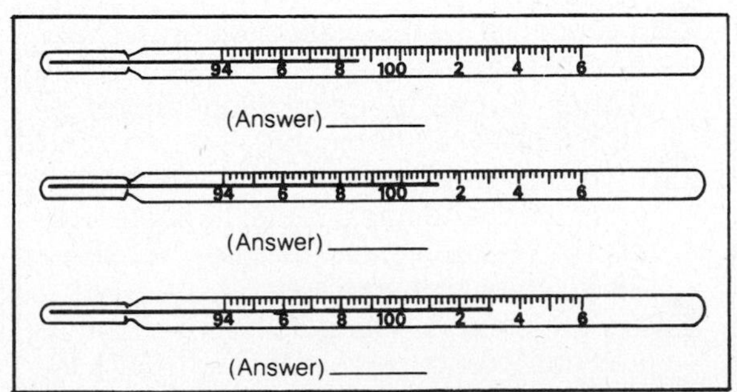

*Answers to thermometer readings: 98.6°F (37°C); 101.3°F (38.5°C); 103.1°F (39.5°C).

Practice by reading the drawings at the left; answers are shown upside down below the drawings.

5. Because the temperature under the arm or orally is lower than that taken rectally, tell your doctor which method you used when reporting your child's temperature. For example, say "Billy's temperature is 101.8°F orally."

Cleaning the thermometer

Wash the thermometer with soap and cool (*never hot)* water before replacing it in its case. The scrubbing action removes the germs. The common practice of placing the used thermometer in a glass of alcohol without washing it first is an inadequate cleaning method.

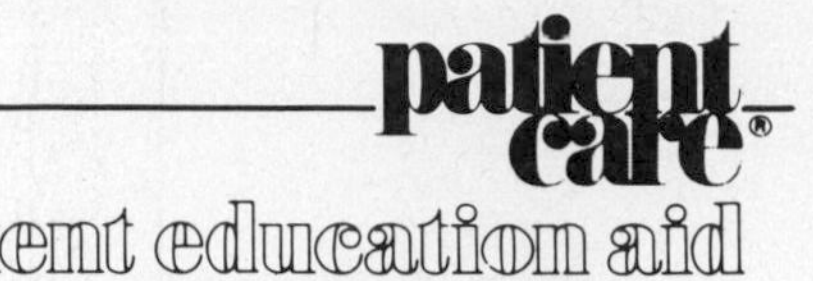

When your child has a fever

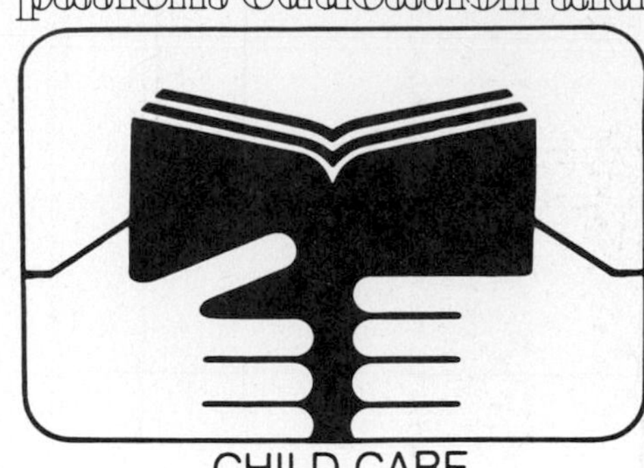

CHILD CARE

When your child's temperature is elevated, remember that fever is a symptom of an underlying illness. Determining the cause of the fever is important so that appropriate treatment can be given. In some cases, the cause will be obvious—a cold or other viral infection—and you can care for the child without your doctor's assistance.

How to lower the child's fever

Unless your child's temperature is very high, the main reason for lowering the fever is to relieve his discomfort. Here are a few suggestions for reducing your child's fever to help him feel more comfortable:

1. *Give aspirin, acetaminophen, or both.* Rather than following the instructions on the package, which base the amount you give on age, calculate the dose on the basis of your child's weight:

Weight of child	Dose of aspirin or acetaminophen
5-10 kg, or 11-22 lbs	60-120 mg
10-20 kg, or 22-44 lbs	120-240 mg
20-30 kg, or 44-66 lbs	240-360 mg
30-40 kg, or 66-88 lbs	360-480 mg
40-50 kg, or 88-110 lbs	480-650 mg

The package will tell you how many milligrams (mg) are in each tablet, teaspoonful, or milliliter. Give the appropriate dose every 4-6 hours for as long as your child is uncomfortable. If your child is still very uncomfortable after 1-2 doses of aspirin or acetaminophen alone, you may give one full dose of each every 4-6 hours.

2. *Bathe the child.* If aspirin, acetaminophen, or both together don't lower the temperature, try sponging your child with cool to lukewarm water. (Some children find a cool bath uncomfortable; do not force the child if he resists.) These instructions may be helpful:

≫ The sponge bath will be most effective if the room you use is not too warm—68°F (20°C) in winter.

≫ Prepare a surface by covering it with waterproof material, such as a plastic or rubber sheet, shower curtain, oilcloth, or large plastic bag.

≫ Place a bath towel, moistened with lukewarm water, over the waterproof material.

≫ Undress your child and place him on the towel.

≫ Sponge his entire body with water.

3. *Allow heat to escape from the child's body.* Do not overdress your child or bundle him up with several blankets. Allowing heat to escape from the body is especially important if you're giving aspirin. If the child taking aspirin is dressed too warmly, his fever may increase.

4. *Try to keep the child quiet.* Older children may prefer to stay in bed, but many children resist such confinement. Do not force the child to stay in bed when he's not sleepy. Instead, have him participate in quiet activities such as reading, watching television, or coloring.

What not to do for fever

The following procedures usually are not recommended because most children find them too uncomfortable or frightening:

1. Bathing with a solution that is half water and half alcohol.

2. Bathing with iced water or iced alcohol.

Use these only if your doctor specifically instructs you to do so to bring down a *very high* fever. A cold or iced water enema also is not recommended because it is dangerous.

Call your doctor:

- ☎ If your child seems sicker than you would expect him or her to be with a cold or other viral infection.
- ☎ If your child's fever lasts more than 2-3 days.
- ☎ If your child is unusually irritable or sleepy or if he has a stiff neck, earache, or sore throat.
- ☎ If your child is age 1 year or older and has an oral temperature of 102°F (38.9°C) or higher or has a rectal temperature of 103°F (39.4°C) or higher.
- ☎ If your child is between ages 6 months and 1 year and has a rectal temperature of 102°F or higher (axillary, 101°F—38.3°C—or higher).
- ☎ If your child is younger than 6 months and has a rectal temperature of 101°F or higher (axillary, 100°F—37.8°C—or higher).

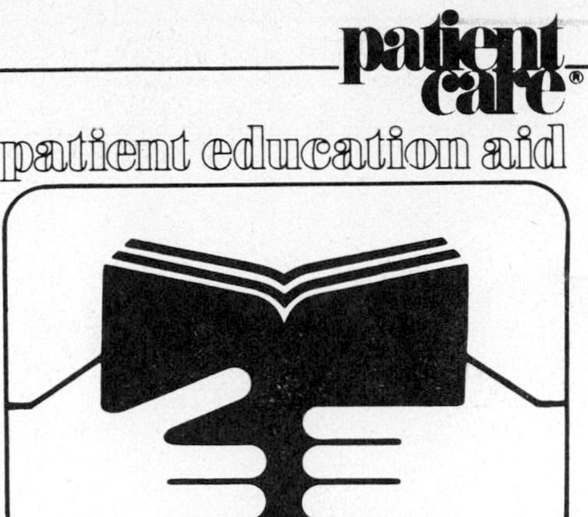

Questions and answers about sore throat

General information

The two principal causes of sore throat are irritation and infection. Painful irritation can result from one of several things—an allergy, low humidity, toxic fumes, or an unusual amount of talking, yelling, or singing. Infection of the throat may be either viral or bacterial. Sometimes both infection and irritation are to blame for a sore throat. The degree of discomfort from a sore throat ranges from a dry, scratchy feeling to severe pain interfering with swallowing. If your sore throat is due to an infection, you may have other signs of illness such as fever, chills, or a runny nose.

What is tonsillitis?

Although researchers believe that the tonsils probably help the body fight infection, the tonsils themselves sometimes become infected. When infection causes the tonsils to become inflamed, swollen, and painful, you have *tonsillitis*. The infection may be due to a virus or bacterium.

What is "strep throat"?

"Strep throat" is a common term used when the tonsils or the throat is infected by a germ called *Streptococcus*. The pain of strep throat is often severe and accompanied by fever and swollen glands. A child may also have stomach pain or vomiting. Unless strep throat is treated with antibiotics, it may develop into a more severe illness. More than one family member often has strep throat at the same time because it is passed easily from one person to another by close contact.

How do I know whether a sore throat is due to a streptococcal infection?

Your doctor can determine whether you have a streptococcal infection. However, you do not need to call the doctor every time you or a family member has a sore throat. For example, a mild sore throat lasting only 1-2 days and accompanied or followed quickly by a runny nose, aches and pains, sneezes, and other signs of a cold is most likely caused by a common cold. In general, follow the guidelines listed below when deciding whether to call the doctor.

Call your doctor if:

- ☎ The pain is so severe it interferes with swallowing.
- ☎ You notice pus on the back of the throat or tonsils.
- ☎ The sore throat is accompanied by a fever or a skin rash.
- ☎ Your child has a sore throat with any of the following: fever, headache, vomiting, stomach pain, or swollen glands.
- ☎ The sore throat, even a mild one, persists for more than two days.
- ☎ You or a family member develops a sore throat after exposure to someone with strep throat.
- ☎ You or the family member with a sore throat, even a mild one, has or has had rheumatic fever or kidney disease.

Will the doctor want to see me?

Most likely, your doctor will want to look at your throat and, perhaps, remove a small amount of mucus from the back of the throat for laboratory testing (culture). He places the mucus in a special laboratory container to "grow" bacteria in sufficient numbers for easy identification and to determine which antibiotics will kill them. Since the results of the culture will not be available for a day or two, your doctor may prescribe an antibiotic immediately if he strongly suspects you have a streptococcal or other bacterial infection. Otherwise, he may decide to wait and prescribe an antibiotic only if the culture is positive, meaning it shows that the mucus taken from your throat is infected.

A strep throat is usually treated with penicillin, unless you are allergic to it. Although you may feel better within a day or two after starting the medication, the infection will not clear up completely unless you take the drug for as long as indicated on the label of the prescription bottle. As an added precaution, your doctor may want to take another throat culture a few days after you have finished the medication to make sure the infection has cleared up.

What does a negative culture indicate?

A negative culture indicates that infective bacteria are probably not present and that your sore throat is most likely due to a virus or some type of irritation, such as smoking. In such a case, an antibiotic would not cure the sore throat or help you feel better.

What can I do to relieve sore throat pain?

Here are some suggestions for easing throat irritation or pain as well as any other discomforts that may accompany an infection:

1. *Gargle* with *salt water* (about 1/2 tsp salt per cup of warm water).

2. Let *throat lozenges* dissolve slowly in your mouth.

3. Take *aspirin* or *acetaminophen* as directed on the bottle to relieve pain and reduce fever. Ask your doctor for dosage instructions for children under age 3.

4. *Drink* plenty of fluids to help keep the throat moist and, if fever is present, to replace lost body fluid.

5. *Get plenty of rest* until your fever drops and you feel well enough to carry out your usual daily activities.

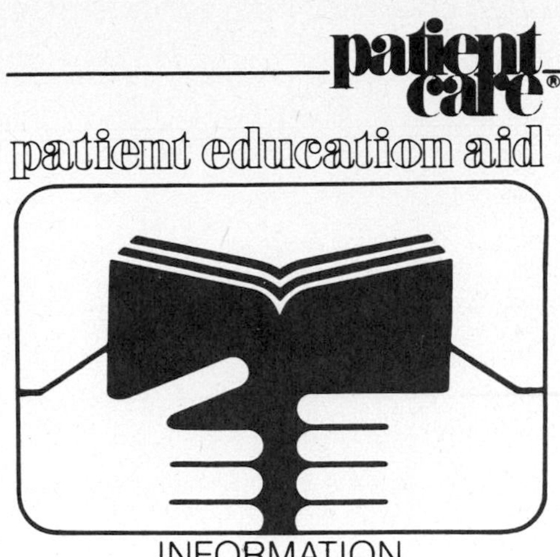

Facts about the common cold

What causes the common cold?
The common cold—runny or stuffy nose, scratchy throat, sneezing, watery eyes, dry cough—is caused by a virus. A virus is a tiny organism that can only live within the cells of larger organisms such as humans. Of the thousands of types of virus that exist, more than 300 of them are believed capable of causing the discomforts of the common cold.

How do I "catch" a cold?
Colds are *not* easy to catch. This is one of the few facts known about colds. Cold-causing viruses can only enter your body when you come into contact with the fluid from the eyes, nose, or mouth of a person who has a cold. For example, the mother who wipes her child's nose with a tissue may get some of the mucus on her fingers; if she then touches her fingers to her eyes or nose, she has a chance of coming down with the cold. Or, cold viruses may be transmitted through the air in tiny droplets when the sick person coughs or sneezes.

Most colds are acquired in the home from family members. You are also likely to come in contact with a cold virus in places where large numbers of people are confined in a small area for a long time, such as a classroom, dormitory, or barracks.

The best way to avoid a cold is to stay away from people who have one. If contact cannot be avoided, frequent handwashing and keeping fingers away from eyes and nose may help. If you do have a cold, help keep it to yourself by carefully disposing of tissues; by not sharing towels, glasses, or eating utensils; and by covering your mouth and nose when you sneeze.

Why do I seem to have so many colds when my neighbor hasn't had one for years?
During any infection, your body produces proteins called antibodies to fight the infection. The antibodies remain in your bloodstream to help prevent infection by the same virus again. Some antibodies stay in the bloodstream for a short time; others remain permanently. Your susceptibility to colds (how likely you are to get them) depends on which and how many antibodies you have.

Children are most likely to catch colds because they haven't had the opportunity to develop resistance to many types of virus. And they are apt to introduce new viruses to their families. A young child may have 10-12 colds a year, while his parents have 4-5; but the childless couple next door may have only 1-2 colds a year.

Stress, diet, and exercise appear to have little effect on susceptibility to the common cold, although research is still being done. Also, getting chilled or wet does not make you more likely to get a cold.

Will I have more colds if I smoke?
You may not have *more* colds if you smoke, but the ones you do catch are likely to be more severe than they would be if you did not smoke.

Does vitamin C prevent colds?
At present there is no conclusive evidence that taking large amounts of vitamin C can prevent a cold. Some studies have *suggested*—not proved—that taking the vitamin *may* help reduce the severity of a cold.

What should I do for a cold?
Usually, you can take care of your (or your child's) cold without your doctor's assistance. Your doctor, however, will go over the medication suggestions below with you to be sure they are suited to you. Nonetheless, keep in mind that medications for colds provide relief of symptoms, but they do not kill viruses as antibiotics do in bacterial infections. The following suggestions may help reduce your discomfort:

1. For muscle aches, headache, sore throat, or fever, take either *aspirin* or *acetaminophen* as recommended on the label. (Some doctors prefer acetaminophen for children since aspirin has been associated with a severe condition called Reye's syndrome.)

2. For nasal stuffiness, drink plenty of *fluids* to help loosen nasal secretions. You may also find an over-the-counter *decongestant drug* helpful. The sprays and drops are more effective than decongestants in pill or tablet form. *Do not use* these sprays or drops for more than three days unless your doctor advises otherwise.

3. For cough, choose a cough medicine with the cough suppressant *dextromethorphan HBr*. This medication is as effective as codeine for many people.

4. How much *rest* you need depends on how you feel. Try not to get overly tired. Staying home from either work or school for approximately 1-2 days at least will prevent further spread of the infection to others.

Shouldn't I take an over-the-counter cold medication?
Most doctors recommend treating a cold as described above. You may find, however, that a particular cold medication works for you. Remember that most cold remedies contain an antihistamine that can make you drowsy and impair judgment. Also, antihistamines may worsen a cough. Additionally, the decongestant would work better if applied directly to the nose in a spray or drop form.

When should I call the doctor?
Expect a cold to last 7-10 days (even longer in children). You may feel "under the weather" for a few days after the stuffy nose and other symptoms have gone. There is no need to call the doctor unless one of the following occurs:

☎ The cold becomes worse.

☎ The cold persists beyond 7-10 days.

☎ A fever develops.

☎ Cough or sore throat is particularly severe. (Keep in mind that mild-to-moderate sore throat can occur with a certain type of bacterial infection—streptococcal infection—which requires treatment with an antibiotic.)

☎ A severe headache develops suddenly.

☎ Ear pain develops.

☎ Difficulty in swallowing increases.

GLOSSARY

A

ABC's: Airway, Breathing and Circulation; the first three steps in the examination of any victim; basic life support.

abdomen: The large body cavity below the diaphragm and above the pelvis.

abnormal: Not normal; malformed.

abrasion: An injury consisting of the loss of a partial thickness of skin from rubbing or scraping on a hard, rough surface; also called a brush burn, friction burn.

activated charcoal: Powdered charcoal that has been treated to increase its powers of absorption; used in a slurry to absorb ingested poison.

acute: Having rapid onset, severe symptoms, and a relatively short duration.

acute abdomen: A serious intra-abdominal condition causing irritation or inflammation of the peritoneum, attended by pain, tenderness, and muscular rigidity (board-like abdomen).

acute myocardial infarction: The acute phase of a heart attack wherein a spasm or blockage of a coronary artery produces a spectrum of signs and symptoms, commonly including chest pain, nausea, diaphoresis, anxiety, pallor, and lassitude.

Adam's apple: The projection on the anterior surface of the neck, formed by the thyroid cartilage of the larynx.

afterbirth: The placenta and membranes expelled after the birth of a child.

air: The gaseous mixture which composes the Earth's atmosphere; composed of approximately 21% oxygen and 79% nitrogen, plus trace gases.

air passage: Any of several tubes that normally transmit air into the lungs.

air splint: A double-walled plastic tube that immobilizes a limb when sufficient air is blown into the space between the walls of the tube to cause it to become almost rigid.

airway: An air passage.

allergic reaction: A local or general reaction to an allergen, usually characterized by hives or tissue swelling or dyspnea.

allergy: Hypersensitivity to a substance, causing an abnormal reaction.

AMI: Abbreviation for acute myocardial infarction.

amniotic fluid: The fluid surrounding the fetus in the uterus, contained in the amniotic sac.

amniotic sac: A thick, transparent sac that holds the fetus suspended in the amniotic fluid.

amputation: Complete removal of an appendage.

analgesic: A pain-relieving drug; a class of drugs used to reduce pain.

anaphylaxis: An exaggerated allergic reaction, usually caused by foreign proteins.

anatomic position: The presumed body position when referring to anatomical landmarks; upright, facing the observer, with hands and arms at sides, thumbs pointing away from the body, legs and feet pointing straight ahead.

aneurysm: A permanent blood-filled dilation of a blood vessel resulting from disease or injury of the blood vessel wall.

angina pectoris: A spasmodic pain in the chest, characterized by a sensation of severe constriction or pressure on the anterior chest; associated with insufficient blood supply to the heart, aggravated by exercise or tension and relieved by rest or medication.

angulation: The formation of an angle; an abnormal angle in an extremity or organ.

anoxia: Without oxygen; a reduction of oxygen in body tissues below required physiology levels.

ante-: A prefix meaning before in time or place.

anterior: Situated in front of, or in the forward part of; in anatomy, used in reference to the ventral or belly surface of the body.

anti-: A prefix that shows a negative or reversal of the word root placed after it.

antidote: A substance to counteract or combat the effect of poison.

antivenin: An antiserum containing antibodies against reptile or insect venom.

arm: The upper extremity, specifically that segment between the shoulder and elbow.

arterial blood: Oxygenated blood.

artery: A blood vessel, consisting of three layers of tissue and smooth muscle, that carries blood away from the heart.

artificial ventilation: Movement of air into and out of the lungs by artificial means.

asphyxia: Suffocation.

aspirate: To inhale foreign material into the lungs; to remove fluid or foreign material from the lungs or elsewhere by mechanical suction.

asthma: A condition marked by recurrent attacks of dyspnea with wheezing due to spasmodic constriction of the bronchi, often as a response to allergens, or by mucous plugs in the bronchioles.

avulsion: An injury that leaves a piece of skin or other tissue either partially or completely torn away from the body.

axilla: The armpit.

axillary temperature: A measured body temperature obtained by placing a thermometer in the axilla while holding the arm close to the body for a period of 10 minutes.

B

Babinski reflex: A reflex response of movement of the big toe; positive reflect is determined when, on stroking the sole, the toe turns upward; negative is determined by a downward or no movement of the toe.

bag of waters: The amniotic sac and its contained amniotic fluid.

ball-and-socket joint: A joint wherein the distal bone has a rounded head (ball) that fits into the proximal bone's cup-like socket; the hip and should joints, for example.

bandage: A material used to hold a dressing in place.

basal skull fracture: A fracture involving the base of the cranium.

basic life support: Maintenance of the ABC's (airway, breathing, and circulation) without adjunctive equipment.

Battle's sign: A contusion on the mastoid process of either ear; sign of a basilar skull fracture.

biological death: A condition present when irreversible brain damage has occurred, usually from 3 to 10 minutes after cardiac arrest.

blanch: To become white or pale.

blister: A collection of fluid under or within the epidermis.

blood: The fluid that circulates through the heart, arteries, capillaries, and veins, carrying nutriment and oxygen to the body cells, and removing waste products such as carbon dioxide and various metabolic products for excretion.

blood clot: A soft, coherent, jelly-like mass resulting from the conversion of fibrinogen to fibrin, thereby entrapping the red blood cells and other formed elements within the fibrinic web.

bone: The hard form of connective tissue that constitutes most of the skeleton in a majority of vertebrates.

bowel: See intestine.

brain: A soft, large mass of nerve tissue that is contained within the cranium.

brain contusion: See cerebral contusion.

breech birth (breech delivery): The delivery during which the presenting part of the fetus is the buttocks or foot instead of the head.

bronchial asthma: The common form of asthma.

bruise: An injury that does not break the skin but causes rupture of small underlying blood vessels with resulting tissue discoloration; a contusion.

burn: An injury caused by heat, electrical current, or chemical of extreme acidity or alkalinity.

> **first-degree burn:** A burn causing only reddening of the outer layer of skin; sunburn usually is a first-degree burn.
>
> **second-degree burn:** A burn extending through the outer layer of skin, causing blisters and edema; a scald is usually a second-degree burn.
>
> **third-degree burn:** A burn extending through all layers of skin, at times through muscle or connective tissue, having a white leathery look and is insensitive; grafting is more often necessary with a third-degree burn; a flame burn is usually third degree.

burn center: A medical facility especially designed, equipped, and staffed to treat severely burned patients.

C

capillary: Any one of the small blood vessels that connect arteriole and venule, and through whose walls various substances pass into and out of the interstitial tissues, and thence on to the cells.

carbon monoxide: CO; a colorless, odorless, and dangerous gas formed by the incomplete combustion of carbon; it combines four times as quickly with hemoglobin than oxygen; when in the presence of heme, replaces oxygen and reduces oxygen uptake in the lungs.

cardiac arrest: The sudden cessation of cardiac function with no pulse, no blood pressure, unresponsiveness.

cardiopulmonary arrest: The cessation of cardiac and respiratory activity.

cardiopulmonary resuscitation (CPR): The application of artificial ventilation and external cardiac compression in victims with cardiac arrest to provide an adequate circulation to support life.

carotid artery: The principal artery of the neck, palpated easily on either side of the thyroid cartilage.

carpals: The eight small bones of the wrist.

cartilage: A tough, elastic, connective tissue that covers opposite surfaces of movable joints and also forms parts of the skeleton, such as ear and nose.

caustic: Corrosive, destructive to living tissue.

centigrade scale: The temperature scale in which the freezing point of water is 0° and the boiling point at sea level is 100°; Celsius scale.

cerebral contusion: A bruise of the brain, causing a characteristic symptomatic response.

cerebral hemorrhage: Bleeding into the cerebrum; one form of stroke or cerebrovascular accident.

cerebrospinal fluid: The fluid contained in the four ventricles of the brain and the subarachnoid space around the brain and spinal cord.

cerebrovascular accident (CVA): The sudden cessation of circulation to a region of the brain due to thrombus, embolism, or hemorrhage; also, a stroke or apoplexy.

cervical: Pertaining to the neck.

cervical collar: A device used to immobilize and support the neck.

chief complaint: The problem for which a person seeks help, stated in a word or short phrase.

chills: A sensation of cold, with convulsive shaking of the body.

circulatory system: The body system consisting of the heart and blood vessels.

clammy: Damp and usually cool.

clavicle: The collarbone; attached to the uppermost part of the sternum at a right angle, and joined to the scapular spine to form the point of the shoulder.

clinical death: A term that refers to the lack of signs of life, when there is no pulse and no blood pressure; occurs immediately after the onset of cardiac arrest.

clot: A semisolid mass of fibrin and cells.

coffee grounds vomitus: A vomitus having the appearance and consistency of coffee grounds; indicates slow bleeding in the stomach and represents the vomiting of partially digested blood.

coma: A state of unconsciousness from which the victim cannot be aroused even by powerful stimulation.

comminuted fracture: A fracture in which the bone ends are broken into many fragments.

communicable disease: A disease that is transmissible from one person to another.

compound fracture: An open fracture; a fracture in which there is an open wound of the skin and soft tissues leading down to the location of the fracture.

compress: A folded cloth or pad used for applying pressure to stop hemorrhage or as a wet dressing.

concussion: A violent jar or shock; the central nervous system injury results from the impact.

conscious: Capable of responding to sensory stimuli and having subjective experiences.

consent: An agreement by patients to accept treatment offered as explained by medical personnel.

> **implied consent:** An assumed consent given by an unconscious adult when emergency lifesaving treatment is required.
>
> **informed consent:** A consent given by a mentally competent adult who understands what the treatment will involve; can also be given by parent or guardian of a child, as defined by the State, or for a mentally incompetent adult.

constrict: To be made smaller by drawing together or squeezing.

constricting band: A band used to restrict the lymphatic flow of blood back to the heart.

contagious: A term that refers to a disease that is readily transmitted from one person to another.

contagious disease: An infectious disease transmissible by direct or indirect contact; now synonymous with communicable disease.

contaminated: A term used in reference to a wound or other surface that has been infected with bacteria; may also refer to polluted water, food, or drugs.

contusion: A bruise; an injury that causes a hemorrhage in or beneath the skin but does not break the skin.

convulsion: A violent involuntary contraction or series of contractions of the voluntary muscles; a fit or seizure.

core temperature: A body temperature measured centrally, from within the esophagus or rectum.

coronary: A term applied to the cardiac blood vessels that supply blood to the walls of the heart.

coronary artery: One of the two arteries arising from the aortic sinus to supply the heart muscle with blood.

CPR: Abbreviation for cardiopulmonary resuscitation.

cramp: A painful spasm, usually of a muscle; a gripping pain in the abdominal area; colic.

cravat: A type of bandage made from a large triangular piece of cloth and folded to form a band; used as a temporary dressing for a fracture or wound.

crepitus: A grating sound heard and the sensation felt when the fractured ends of a bone rub together.

crowning: The stage of birth when the presenting part of the baby is visible at the vaginal orifice.

CVA: Abbreviation for cerebrovascular accident.

cyanosis: A blueness of the skin due to insufficient oxygen in the blood.

D

dehydration: Loss of water and electrolytes; excessive loss of body water.

depressed fracture: A skull fracture with impaction, depression, or a sinking in of the fragments.

diabetes: A general term referring to disorders characterized by excessive urine excretion, excessive thirst, and excessive hunger.

diabetes mellitus: A systemic disease marked by lack of production of insulin, which causes an inability to metabolize carbohydrates, resulting in an increase in blood sugar.

diabetic coma: Loss of consciousness due to severe diabetes mellitus that has not been treated or to treatment that has not been adequately regulated.

diarrhea: The passage of frequent watery or loose stools.

digestive tract: The passages of tubes leading from the mouth and pharynx to the anus; the alimentary tract; mouth, pharynx, esophagus, stomach, small intestine, large intestine, rectum, and anus.

dilated pupil: An ocular pupil enlarged beyond its normal size.

dilation: The process of expanding or enlarging.

drag: A general term referring to methods of moving victims without a stretcher or litter, usually employed by a single rescuer.

> **blanket drag:** A method by which one rescuer encloses a victim in a blanket and then drags the victim to safety.
>
> **clothes drag:** A method by which one rescuer can drag a victim to safety by grasping the victim's clothes and pulling him away from danger.
>
> **fireman's drag:** A method by which one rescuer crawls with a victim, looping the victim's tied wrists over the rescuer's neck to support the victim's weight.

dressing: A protective covering for a wound; used to stop bleeding and to prevent contamination of the wound.

E

-ectomy: Suffix meaning surgical removal, as in appendectomy.

edema: A condition in which fluid escapes into the body tissues from the vascular or lymphatic spaces and causes local or generalized swelling.

electrocution: Death caused by passage of electrical current through the body.

embolism: The sudden blocking of an artery or vein by a clot or foreign material that has been brought to the site of lodgement by the blood current.

EMS: Emergency Medical Services.

EMT: Emergency Medical Technician.

epidermis: The outermost and nonvascular layer of the skin.

epiglottis: The lid-like cartilaginous structure overhanging the superior entrance to the larynx and serving to prevent food from entering the larynx and trachea while swallowing.

epilepsy: A chronic brain disorder marked by paroxysmal attacks of brain dysfunction, usually associated with some alteration of consciousness, abnormal motor behavior, or psychic or sensory disturbances; may be preceded by aura.

epistaxis: Nosebleed.

esophagus: The portion of the digestive tract that lies between the pharynx and the stomach.

exhalation: The act of breathing out; expiration.

extremity: A limb, an arm, or a leg.

extrication: Disentanglement; freeing from entrapment.

F

Fahrenheit scale: The temperature scale in which the freezing point is 32° and the boiling point at sea level is 212°.

fainting: A momentary loss of consciousness caused by insufficient blood supply to the brain; syncope.

feces: The product expelled by the bowels; semisoft waste products of digestion.

femur: The bone that extends from the pelvis to the knee; the longest and largest bone of the body; the thigh bone.

fever: An elevation of body temperature beyond normal.

fibula: The smaller of the two bones of the lower leg; the most lateral bone of the lower leg.

first-degree burn: A burn causing only reddening of the outer layer of skin; sunburn usually is a first-degree burn.

first responder: A person who arrives first at the scene of a medical emergency, usually police or fire fighters.

flail chest: A condition in which several ribs are broken, each in at least two places or a sternal fracture or separation of the ribs from the sternum producing a free-floating segment of the chest wall that moves paradoxically on respiration.

forearm: The part of the upper extremity between the elbow and the wrist.

fracture: A break or rupture in a bone.

- **closed fracture:** A simple fracture, one that does not cause a break in the skin.
- **comminuted fracture:** A fracture in which the bone is shattered, broken into small pieces.
- **compound fracture:** An open fracture, one in which the bone ends pierce the skin.
- **greenstick fracture:** An incomplete fracture, the bone is not broken all the way through, seen most often in children.
- **impacted fracture:** A fracture in which the ends of the bones are jammed together.
- **oblique fracture:** A fracture in which the break crosses the bone at an angle.
- **open fracture:** A compound fracture, one in which the skin is open.
- **simple fracture:** A closed fracture, one in which the skin is not broken.
- **spiral fracture:** A fracture in which the break line twists around and through the bone.
- **transverse fracture:** A fracture in which the break line extends across the bone at right angle to the long axis.

fracture of the hip: A fracture that occurs at the upper end of the femur, most often at the neck of the femur.

frost nip: The superficial local tissue destruction caused by freezing; limited in scope and does not destroy the full thickness of skin.

frostbite: The damage to tissues as a result of prolonged exposure to extreme cold.

G

gangrene: Local tissue death as the result of an injury or inadequate blood supply.

gastrointestinal tract: The digestive tract, including stomach, small intestine, large intestine, rectum, and anus.

grand mal: A type of epileptic attack; characterized by a short-term, generalized, convulsive seizure.

gullet: Esophagus; the passage from the pharynx to the stomach.

H

half-ring splint: A traction splint with a hinged half-ring at the upper end that allows the splint to be used on either right or left leg.

heart: A hollow muscular organ that receives the blood from the veins, sends it through the lungs to be oxygenated, then pumps it to the arteries.

heart attack: A layman's term for a condition resulting from blockage of a coronary artery and subsequent death of part of the heart muscle; an acute myocardial infarction; a coronary.

heat cramps: A painful muscle cramp resulting from excessive loss of salt and water through sweating.

heat exhaustion: A prostration caused by excessive loss of water and salt through sweating; characterized by clammy skin and a weak, rapid pulse.

hematoma: A localized collection of blood in an organ, tissue, or space as a result of injury or a broken blood vessel.

hemiplegia: Paralysis of one side of the body.

hemorrhage: Abnormally large amount of bleeding.

hemorrhagic shock: A state of inadequate tissue perfusion due to blood loss.

hemothorax: Bleeding into the thoracic cavity.

hives: Red or white raised patches on the skin, often attended by severe itching; a characteristic reaction in allergic responses.

humerus: The bone of the upper arm.

hyper-: Prefix meaning excessive, or increased.

hypertension: High blood pressure, usually in reference to a diastolic pressure greater than 90-95 mm Hg.

hyperventilation: An increased rate and depth of breathing resulting in an abnormal lowering of arterial carbon dioxide, causing alkalosis.

hyphema: Hemorrhage within the anterior chamber of the eye.

hypo-: A prefix meaning less than, lack of, a deficiency.

hypothermia: Decreased body temperature.

hypovolemic shock: Shock caused by a reduction in blood volume, such as caused by hemorrhage.

hypoxia: A low oxygen content in the blood; lack of oxygen in inspired air.

I

immobilization: To hold a part firmly in place, as with a splint.

impaled object: An object that has caused a puncture wound and remains embedded in the wound.

incision: A wound usually made deliberately in connection with surgery; a clean cut as opposed to a laceration.

infarction: The death (necrosis) of a localized area of tissue by cutting off its blood supply.

infection: An invasion of a body by disease-producing organisms.

inflammation: A tissue reaction to disease, irritation, or infection, characterized by pain, heat, redness, and swelling.

ingestion: Intaking of food or other substances through the mouth.

inhalation: The drawing of air or other substances into the lungs.

insulin: A hormone secreted by the islets of Langerhans in the pancreas; essential for the proper metabolism of blood sugar.

insulin shock: Not a true form of shock; hypoglycemia caused by excessive insulin dosage, characterized by sweating, tremor, anxiety, unusual behavior, vertigo, and diplopia,; may cause death of brain cells.

intestine: The portion of the alimentary canal extending from the pylorus to the anus.

intoxicate: To poison; commonly, to cause diminished mental control by means of drugs or alcohol.

ipecac syrup: A medication used to induce vomiting.

-itis: A suffix meaning inflammation.

J

jaw thrust maneuver: A procedure for opening the airway, wherein the jaw is lifted and pulled forward to keep the tongue from falling back into the airway.

joint: The point at which two or more bones articulate, commonly, portion of marijuana.

jugular: Pertaining to the neck; large vein on either side of the neck, draining the head via its portion named external jugular, or draining the brain via the internal jugular.

K

kidneys: The paired organs located in the retroperitoneal cavities that filter blood and produce urine; also act as adjuncts to keep a proper acid-base balance.

knee: A hinge joint between the femur and the tibia.

L

labor: The muscular contractions of the uterus designed to expel the fetus from the mother.

laceration: A wound made by tearing or cutting of body tissues.

ladder splint: A flexible splint consisting of two stout parallel wires and finer crosswires; resembles a ladder.

laryngospasm: A severe constriction of the vocal cords, often in response to allergy or noxious stimuli.

larynx: The organ of voice production.

leg: The lower limb generally, specifically, that part of the lower limb extending from the knee to the ankle.

lesion: A distinct area of pathologically altered tissue; an injury or wound.

lethal: Fatal.

lethargy: A lack of activity; drowsiness; indifference.

ligament: A tough band of fibrous tissue that connects bone to bone or that supports any organ.

limb presentation: A delivery in which the presenting part of a fetus is an arm or a leg.

linear fracture: A fracture running parallel to the long axis of the bone.

linear skull fracture: A skull fracture that runs in a straight line.

litter: Stretcher.

liver: The large organ in the right upper quadrant of the abdomen that secretes bile, produces many essential proteins, detoxifies many substances, and stores glycogen.

log roll: A method for placing a person on a carrying device, usually a long spineboard or a flat litter; the person is rolled on his side, then back on the litter.

lungs: The paired organs in the thorax that effect ventilation and oxygenation.

lymph: A straw-colored fluid that circulates in the lymphatic vessels and interstitial space.

M

metacarpal bones: The five cylindrical bones of the hand extending from the wrist to the fingers.

metatarsal bones: The five cylindrical bones of the foot extending from the ankles to the toes.

morbidity: A synonym for illness; generally used to refer to an untoward effect of an illness or injury.

mortality: Refers to death from a given disease or injury; generally thought of as a statistic to state the ratio of death to recovery.

motion sickness: A sensation induced by repetitive motion, characterized by nausea and lightheadedness.

mottled: Characterized by a patchy, discolored appearance.

mouth-to-mouth ventilation: The preferred emergency method of artificial ventilation when adjuncts are not available.

mouth-to-nose ventilation: An emergency method of artificial ventilation when mouth-to-mouth cannot be used.

mucus: A viscid, slippery secretion that lubricates and protects various body structures.

muscle: A tissue composed of elongated cells that have the ability to contract when stimulated, thus causing bone and joints to move, or other anatomical structures to be drawn together.

myocardial infarction: The damaging or death of an area of heart muscle resulting from a lack of blood supplying the area.

N

nausea: An unpleasant sensation, vaguely referred to the epigastrium and abdomen, often culminating in vomiting.

necrosis: A death of an area of tissue, usually caused by the cessation of blood supply.

nerve: A cord-like structure composed by a collection of fibers that convey impulses between a part of the central nervous system and some other region.

nervous system: The brain, spinal cord, and nerve branches from the central, peripheral, and autonomic systems.

noxious: Injurious.

O

oblique fracture: A fracture that runs diagonally to the long axis of the bone.

occipital: Pertaining to the back of the head.

ointment: A semisolid preparation for external application to the body usually containing a medicinal substance.

open fracture or dislocation: A fracture or dislocation exposed to the exterior; an open wound lies over the fracture or dislocation.

open wound: A wound in which the affected tissues are exposed by an external opening.

oral: Pertaining to the mouth.

-otomy: A suffix meaning surgical incision into an organ, as in tracheotomy.

oxygen: A colorless, odorless, tasteless gas essential to life and comprising 21% of the atmosphere; chemical formula: O_2.

P

pallor: A paleness of the skin.

palpation: The act of palpating; the act of feeling with the hands for the purpose of determining the consistency of the part beneath.

palpitation: A sensation felt under the left breast when the heart "skips a beat" caused by premature ventricular contractions.

paralysis: Loss or impairment of motor function of a part due to a lesion of the neural or muscular mechanism.

paraplegia: The loss of both sensation and motion in the legs and lower parts of the body; most commonly due to damage to the spinal cord.

patella: A small, flat bone that protects the knee joint; the kneecap.

pediatrics: The medical specialty devoted to the diagnosis and treatment of diseases of children.

penetrate: To pierce; the pass into the deeper tissues or into a cavity.

perfusion: The act of pouring through or into; the blood getting to the cells in order to exchange gases, nutrients, etc., with the cells.

petit mal seizure: A type of epileptic attack, characterized by a momentary loss of awareness but not accompanied by loss of motor tone.

pharynx: The portion of the airway between the nasal cavity and the larynx.

placenta: A vascular organ attached to the uterine wall that supplies oxygen and nutrients to the fetus; also called the afterbirth.

pneumothorax: An accumulation of air in the pleural cavity, usually entering after a wound or injury that causes a penetration of the chest wall or laceration of the lung.

point tenderness: An area of tenderness limited to 2 or 3 centimeters in diameter; point tenderness can be located in any area of the body; usually associated with acute inflammation, as in peritonitis (abdominal point tenderness.)

posterior: Situated in the back of or behind a surface.

precordial thump: A sharp blow delivered to the mid-sternum for the purpose of terminating ventricular tachycardia or stimulating the heart to beat in systole. No longer recognized by the American Heat Association as an effective maneuver.

presenting part: The part of the baby that emerges first during delivery.

pressure dressing: A dressing with which enough pressure is applied over a wound site to stop bleeding.

pressure point: One of several places on the body where the blood flow of a given artery can be restricted by pressing the artery against an underlying bone.

pressure splints: An inflatable plastic circumferential splint that can be applied to an extremity and inflated to achieve stability after a fracture.

prognosis: A probable outcome of a disease based on assumptive knowledge.

prolapsed cord: A delivery in which the umbilical cord appears at the vaginal opening before the head of the infant.

prone: A position of lying face down.

psychogenic shock: A fainting spell as a result of transient generalized cerebral ischemia; not a true shock condition.

psychosomatic: An indication of an illness in which some part of the cause is related to emotional factors.

pulse rate: The heart rate determined by counting the number of pulsations occurring in any superficial artery.

pupil: The small opening in the center of the iris.

Q

quadrant: One of the four quarters of the abdomen.

quadriplegia: A paralysis of both arms and legs.

R

radial artery: One of the major arteries of the forearm; the pulse is palpable at the base of the thumb.

radiation sickness: The condition that follows excessive irradiation from any source.

radius: The bone on the thumb side of the forearm.

rape: Sexual intercourse by force.

rash: An eruption of the skin, either localized or generalized.

rectal temperature: The core body temperature obtained by insertion of a thermometer into the rectum and retaining it for a minute; normally 1°F higher than oral temperature.

regurgitation: A backward flowing, as the casting up of undigested food from the stomach to the mouth.

rescue: The freeing of persons from threatening or dangerous situations by prompt and vigorous action.

respiration: The act of breathing; the exchange of oxygen and carbon dioxide in the tissues, lungs.

respiratory system: A system of organs that controls the inspiration of oxygen and the expiration of carbon dioxide.

resuscitation: The act of reviving an unconscious victim.

rib: One of the 24 bones forming the thoracic cavity wall.

rigid splint: A splint made of a firm material that can be applied to an injured extremity to prevent motion at the site of a fracture or dislocation.

roller dressing: A strip of rolled-up material used for dressings.

S

saliva: The clear, alkaline fluid secreted by the salivary glands.

scab: A crust formed by the coagulation of blood, pus, serum, or any combination of these on the surface of an ulcer, erosion, abrasion, or any other type of wound.

scapula: The shoulder blade.

sclera: The white, opaque, outer layer of the eyeball.

second degree burn: A burn penetrating beneath the superficial skin layers producing edema and blisters.

seizure: A sudden attack or recurrence of a disease; a convulsion; an attack of epilepsy.

semiconscious: Stuporous; partially conscious.

shell temperature: The temperature of the extremities and surface of the body.

shivering: A trembling from cold or fear; produces heat by muscular contractions.

shock: A state of inadequate tissue perfusion that may be a result of pump failure (cariogenic shock), volume loss or sequestration (hypovolemic shock), vasodilation (neurogenic shock), or any combination of these.

> **anaphylactic shock:** A rapidly occurring state of collapse caused by hypersensitivity to drugs or other foreign materials (insect venom, certain foods, inhaled allergenic); symptoms may include hives, wheezing, tissue edema, bronchospasm, and vascular collapse.
>
> **septic shock:** A shock developing in the presence of, and as a result of, severe infection.

sign: Any objective evidence of physical manifestation of a disease.

simple fracture: A fracture that is not compound; the skin is not broken over the break in the bone.

skeleton: The hard, bony structure that forms the main support of the body.

skin: The outer integument or covering of the body, consisting of the dermis and the epidermis; the largest organ of the body; contains various sensory and regulatory mechanisms.

skull: The bony structure surrounding the brain; consists of the cranial bones, the facial bones, and the teeth.

sling: A triangular bandage applied around the neck to support an injured upper extremity; any wide or narrow material long enough to suspend an upper extremity by passing the material around the neck; used to support and protect an injury or the arm, shoulder, or clavicle.

sling and swathe: A bandage in which the arm is placed in a sling and is bound to the body by another bandage placed around the chest and arm to hold the arm close to the body.

small intestine: The portion of the intestine between the stomach and colon.

snowblindness: Obscured vision caused by sunlight reflected off snow.

spasm: A sudden, violent, involuntary contraction of a muscle, or group of muscles, attended by pain and interference with function; a sudden but transitory constriction of a passage, canal, or orifice.

spineboard: A wooden or metal device primarily used for extrication and transportation of victims with actual or suspected spinal injuries.

spiral fracture: A fracture in which the line of break runs diagonally around the long axis of the bone.

spleen: The largest lymphatic organ of the body; located in the left upper quadrant of the abdomen.

splint: Any support used to immobilize a fracture or to restrict movement of a part.

sprain: A trauma to a joint causing injury to the ligaments.

sputum: Expectorated matter, especially mucus or matter resulting from diseases of the air passages.

status asthmaticus: A severe, prolonged asthmatic attack that cannot be broken with epinephrine.

status epilepticus: The occurrence of two or more seizures with a period of complete consciousness between them.

sterile: Free from living organisms, such as bacteria.

sterilize: To render sterile or free from bacterial contamination; to make an organism unable to reproduce.

sternum: The long, flat bone located in the midline in the anterior part of the thoracic cage; articulates above with the clavicles and along the sides with the cartilages of the first seven ribs.

stoma: A small opening, especially one artificially created.

stomach: A hollow digestive organ in the epigastrium that receives food from the esophagus.

stool: Feces; the matter discharged at defecation.

stove-in chest: See flail chest.

strain: An injury to a muscle caused by a violent contraction or an excessive forcible stretching.

stretcher: A carrying device that enables two or more persons to lift and carry a patient who is lying down.

stroke: A cerebrovascular accident of sudden onset.

sublingual: Under the tongue.

sucking chest wound: An open pneumothorax.

suffocate: To impede respiration, to asphyxiate.

suicide: The act of deliberately taking one's own life.

sunstroke: A form of heatstroke due to prolonged sun exposure.

supine: Lying horizonal in a face-upward position.

suture: The material used in closing a surgical wound or in repairing a gaping wound.

swathe: A cravat tied around the body to decrease movement of a part.

swimmer's ear: A condition that results from an inflammation of the external ear canal caused by growth of bacteria and fungi in the warm, wet orifice; causes exquisite pain with edema.

symptom: A subjective sensation or awareness of disturbance of bodily function.

syncope: Fainting; a brief period of unconsciousness.

syndrome: A complex of symptoms and signs characteristic of condition.

synovial fluid: A clear, viscid fluid that lubricates joints; secreted by the synovial membrane.

T

tablet: A small disc that has been molded or compressed from a powdered drug.

tachycardia: Abnormally rapid heart rate, over 100 beats per minute.

tarsal: Pertaining to the tarsus, the ankle.

temperature: The degree of heat of a living body; varies in cold-blooded animals with environmental temperature and is constant, within a narrow range, for warm-blooded animals; 98.6°F oral temperature and 99.6°F rectal are considered normal for humans.

tendon: a tough band of dense, fibrous, connective tissue that attaches muscles to bone and other parts.

tetanus: An infectious disease caused by an exotoxin of a bacteria, *Clostridium tetani*, that is usually introduced through a wound, characterized by extreme body rigidity and spasms, trismus, or opisthotonos, of voluntary body muscles.

thermal: Pertaining to heat.

thigh: The portion of the lower extremity between the hip and knee.

third degree burn: A full-thickness burn destroying all skin layers and underlying tissue; has a charred or white, leathery appearance; insensitive.

Thomas splint: A rigid metal or plastic splint that provides support for and a steady longitudinal pull on the lower extremity.

thoracic: Pertaining to the chest.

three-man lift: A method by which a number of persons may lift and move a victim smoothly.

thrombosis: Formation of a blood clot or thrombus.

tibia: The larger of the two bones in the leg; the shin bone.

tissue: An aggregation of similarly specialized cells and their intercellular substance united in the performance of a particular function.

tourniquet: A constrictive device used on the extremities to impede venous blood return to the heart or obstruct arterial blood flow to the extremities.

toxin: Any poison manufactured by plant or animal life.

trachea: The cartilaginous tube extending from the larynx to its division into the primary bronchi; windpipe.

traction: The act of exerting a pulling force.

triage: A system used for sorting victims to determine the order in which they will receive medical attention.

triangular bandage: A piece of cloth cut in the shape of a right-angled triangle; used as a sling, or folded for a cravat bandage.

trunk: The body, excluding the head and limbs; torso.

U

ulcer: An open lesion of the skin or mucous membrane.

ulna: The larger bone of the forearm, on the side opposite that of the thumb.

umbilical cord: A flexible structure connecting the fetus to the placenta.

umbilicus: The navel.

unconscious: Without awareness, the state of being comatose.

universal access number: A telephone number that can be called in emergency situations of all kinds and will tie in with the police, fire, and emergency medical services; in most areas the number is 911.

universal dressing: A large (9 by 36 inches) dressing of multilayered material that can be used open, folded, or rolled to cover most wounds, to pad splints, or to form a cervical collar.

uterus: The muscular organ that holds and nourishes the fetus, opening into the vagina through the cervix; the womb.

V

vagina: The canal in the female extending from the uterus to the vulva; the birth canal.

vasoconstriction: The narrowing of the diameter of a blood vessel.

vein: Any blood vessel that carries blood from the tissues to the heart.

venom: A poison, usually derived from reptiles or insects.

venous blood: Unoxygenated blood, containing hemoglobin in the carboxyhemoglobin state.

ventilation: Breathing; supplying fresh air to the lungs.

ventricular fibrillation: A rapid, tremulous, and ineffectual contraction of the cardia myofibrils, producing no cardiac output; cardiac arrest.

vertebra: Any one of the 33 bones of the spinal column.

vertigo: A dizziness; an hallucination of movement; a sensation as if the external world is spinning; may be right or left, upward or downward.

vital signs: The indication of life through values that reflect mental status, blood pressure, pulse rate, and respiration rate.

vitreous fluid: A jelly-like, transparent substance filling the inside of the eyeball.

voice box: The larynx.

vomiting: A forceful, active expulsion of stomach contents through the mouth, as opposed to regurgitation, which is passive.

vomitus: The matter ejected from the stomach by vomiting.

W

wheal: A swelling on the skin, produced by a sting, an injection, external force, or internal reaction.

wheeze: A high-pitched, whistling sound characterizing an obstruction or spasm of the lower airways.

wheezing: Breathing noisily and with difficulty.

wind-chill factor: The relationship of wind velocity and temperature in determining the effect of the factor on a living organism.

windpipe: The trachea.

womb: The uterus.

wrist: The joint or the region of the joint between the forearm and the hand.

X

xiphoid process: A sword-shaped cartilaginous process at the lowest portion of the sternum that ossifies in the aged and has no ribs attached to it.

Source: Adapted from National Highway Traffic Safety Administration *Emergency Medical Care* (Washington, D.C., U.S. Government Printing Office).

Notes

Notes

Notes

Notes